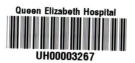

This book is due for return on or before the last date shown below.

Clinical Perfusion MRI

Techniques and Applications

Clinical Perfusion MRI

Techniques and Applications

Edited by

Peter B. Barker DPhil
Professor of Radiology and Oncology, The Russell H. Morgan
Department of Radiology and Radiological Science, The Johns Hopkins
University School of Medicine, MD, USA

Xavier Golay PhD
Professor and Chair of MR Neurophysics and Translational Neuroscience, Department of Brain
Repair and Rehabilitation, UCL Institute of Neurology, University College London, London, UK

Greg Zaharchuk MD, PhD
Associate Professor of Radiology, Stanford University, Stanford, CA, USA

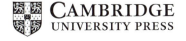
CAMBRIDGE
UNIVERSITY PRESS

CAMBRIDGE UNIVERSITY PRESS
Cambridge, New York, Melbourne, Madrid, Cape Town,
Singapore, São Paulo, Delhi, Mexico City

Cambridge University Press
The Edinburgh Building, Cambridge CB2 8RU, UK

Published in the United States of America by
Cambridge University Press, New York

www.cambridge.org
Information on this title: www.cambridge.org/9781107013391

First published 2013

Printed and bound by Grafos SA, Arte sobre papel, Barcelona,
Spain

A catalog record for this publication is available from the British Library

Library of Congress Cataloging in Publication data

Clinical Perfusion MRI: Techniques and Applications / [edited by]
    Peter B. Barker, Xavier Golay, Greg Zaharchuk.
        p. ; cm.
    Includes bibliographical references and index.
    ISBN 978-1-107-01339-1 (Hardback)
    I. Barker, Peter B., 1959–   II. Golay, Xavier.   III. Zaharchuk, Greg.
    [DNLM: 1. Magnetic Resonance Angiography–methods.
    2. Cerebrovascular Disorders–diagnosis. WN 185]
    616.1'307548–dc23

                         2012039634ISBN 978-1-107-01339-1 Hardback

Contents

Section 1:   Techniques

Section 2:   Clinical applications

Contributors

Hongyu An DSc
Biomedical Research Imaging Center and
Department of Radiology,
University of North Carolina at Chapel Hill,
Chapel Hill, NC, USA

Ramon Francisco Barajas Jr. MD
Department of Radiology and Biomedical Imaging,
University of California at San Francisco,
San Francisco, CA, USA

Peter B. Barker DPhil
Russell H. Morgan Department of Radiology and
Radiological Science, Johns Hopkins University
School of Medicine, and F. M. Kirby Research
Center for Functional Brain Imaging, Kennedy
Krieger Institute,
Baltimore, MD, USA

David A. Bluemke MD, PhD, MsB, FAHA, FACR
Radiology and Imaging Sciences,
Clinical Center, Bethesda, MD, USA

David Bonekamp PhD
Russell H. Morgan Department of Radiology
and Radiological Science, Johns Hopkins
University School of Medicine,
Baltimore, MD, USA

Jonathan Burdette MD
Wake Forest Baptist Health,
Department of Radiology,
Section of Neuroradiology,
Winston-Salem, NC, USA

Soonmee Cha MD
Departments of Radiology and
Biomedical Imaging, and Neurological Surgery,
University of California at
San Francisco,
San Francisco, CA, USA

Manus J. Donahue PhD
Departments of Radiology and Radiological Sciences,
Neurology, Psychiatry, and Physics and Astronomy,
Vanderbilt University School of Medicine,
Nashville, TN, USA

Robert R. Edelman MD
Department of Radiology,
NorthShore University HealthSystem,
Evanston, IL, USA

Riham H. El Khouli MD, PhD
Suez Canal University School of Medicine,
Ismailia, Egypt, and Russell H. Morgan
Department of Radiology and Radiological Science,
Johns Hopkins University,
Baltimore, MD, USA

James R. Ewing PhD
Department of Neurology,
Henry Ford Hospital, Detroit, MI, USA

Andria D. Ford MD
Department of Neurology,
Washington University School of Medicine,
Washington University, St. Louis, MO, USA

Xavier Golay PhD
Department of Brain and Rehabilitation,
UCL Institute of Neurology, University College
London, London, UK

Isky Gordon
ICH – Imaging and Biophysics Unit,
Department of Neurosciences & Mental Health,
University College London, London, UK

P. Ellen Grant MD
Center for Fetal Neonatal Neuroimaging and
Developmental Science, and Departments of
Medicine and Radiology, Children's Hospital Boston,
Harvard Medical School, Boston, MA, USA

Peter Jezzard PhD
FMRIB Centre, Nuffield Department of Clinical
Neurosciences, Oxford University, Oxford, UK

Jin-Moo Lee MD PhD
Departments of Neurology and Radiology,
Washington University School of Medicine,
Washington University,
St. Louis, MO, USA

Weili Lin PhD
Biomedical Research Imaging Center and
Department of Radiology,
University of North Carolina at Chapel Hill,
Chapel Hill, NC, USA

Hanzhang Lu PhD
Advanced Imaging Research Center,
University of Texas Southwestern Medical Center,
Dallas, TX, USA

Katarzyna J. Macura MD, PhD
Russell H. Morgan Department of Radiology and
Radiological Science,
Johns Hopkins University,
Baltimore, MD, USA

Neel Madan MD
Department of Radiology,
Tufts Medical Center,
Tufts University School of Medicine,
Boston, MA, USA

Joseph A. Maldjian MD
Wake Forest Baptist Health,
Department of Radiology,
Section of Neuroradiology,
Winston-Salem, NC, USA

Blake E. McGehee MD
Wake Forest Baptist Health,
Department of Radiology,
Section of Neuroradiology,
Winston-Salem, NC, USA

James P. B. O'Connor
Centre for Imaging Sciences,
University of Manchester,
Manchester, UK

Geoff J. M. Parker PhD
Centre for Imaging Sciences,
Biomedical Imaging Institute,
University of Manchester, Manchester, UK

Pottumarthi V. Prasad PhD
Department of Radiology,
NorthShore University HealthSystem,
Evanston, IL, USA

Norbert Schuff PhD
Center for Imaging of Neurodegenerative Diseases,
Veterans Affairs Medical Center, and Department of
Radiology and Biomedical Imaging,
University of California at San Francisco,
San Francisco, CA, USA

Jürg Schwitter MD
University Hospital Lausanne,
Lausanne, Switzerland

Huan Tan PhD
Department of Radiology,
NorthShore University HealthSystem,
Evanston, IL, USA

Paul S. Tofts PhD
Brighton and Sussex Medical School,
Falmer, Sussex, UK

Jinsoo Uh PhD
Advanced Imaging Research Center,
University of Texas Southwestern Medical Center,
Dallas, TX, USA

Matthias J. P. van Osch PhD
C. J. Gorter Center for High Field MRI,
Department of Radiology,
Leiden University Medical Center,
Leiden, the Netherlands

Katie L. Vo MD
Department of Radiology,
Washington University School of Medicine,
Washington University, St. Louis, MO, USA

Greg Zaharchuk MD, PhD
Radiological Sciences Laboratory, Stanford
University, Stanford, CA, USA

Foreword

Diseases of the brain remain the largest single cause of human suffering worldwide [1], and an extraordinarily wide range of symptoms can be observed with brain ischemia, including both acute and chronic neurological and/or psychological deficits. These two facts have prompted a very long quest to better understand, observe, and quantify blood flow in the living human brain – more than a century-long quest, in fact [2]. The advent of in vivo advanced imaging techniques in humans has therefore perhaps naturally been put to use to study blood flow to the brain, and indeed all organs.

While routine imaging of the larger vessels has become relatively straightforward, with a variety of imaging methods ranging from ultrasound to X-rays and beyond to magnetic resonance imaging (MRI), the measurement of tissue-level blood flow has been more challenging. The ability to measure capillary-level blood flow, or tissue perfusion, is of perhaps greater medical importance since the cell is the critical functional entity of human biology. However, methods to measure the various parameters that characterize tissue perfusion have been frankly more challenging than the imaging of the larger vessels in living humans. A variety of methods were initially developed using radioactive tracers, including planar imaging as well as tomographic methods such as positron emission tomography (PET) or single-photon emission computed tomography (SPECT). The fundamental principles of these methods have since been adapted for use with the currently far more widely available modalities of X-ray computed tomography (CT) and MRI.

In 1991, Belliveau and colleagues [3] at the Massachusetts General Hospital demonstrated that brain perfusion could be measured in humans with MRI using bolus injection of MR contrast agent, a technique which has become known as dynamic susceptibility contrast (DSC) MRI. This technique is a use of contrast agents that has regulatory approval in some countries, with more countries actively considering approval at the time of this writing. Initial applications were in the brain, most notably for studying functional brain activation and the evaluation of patients with cerebrovascular disease, and this methodology is now widely used in clinical practice. The related technique of dynamic contrast-enhanced (DCE)-MRI also looks at contrast agent kinetics following bolus injection, but over a slightly slower time scale, and has found application in oncological imaging applications, perhaps most frequently in the clinical evaluation of lesions of the breast. In the early 1990s, landmark papers by Detre *et al.* and Williams *et al.* [4, 5] demonstrated the ability to image cerebral blood flow entirely non-invasively, without the injection of an exogenous tracer, a technique now known as arterial spin labeling (ASL)-MRI. Although the utilization of this method in routine clinical neuroimaging has been somewhat less compared to DSC, perhaps because of some of the technical difficulties (now mostly overcome), the method is beginning to be used with increasing frequency. For all of these methods, the greatest volume of studies to date have been performed in the brain, with applications to other organ systems mostly still at an earlier stage of development.

In 2000, when Peter Reimer and I wrote the book *Cerebral MR Perfusion Imaging: Principles and Current Applications* [6], only DSC was in routine clinical use. Since then, the use of ASL, DCE, and DSC has steadily progressed, both for neuro- and non-neuro imaging applications. The current book covers these more recent advances, and gives the reader an excellent understanding of the theoretical and experimental aspects of perfusion MRI. For the clinician or researcher, in addition to a knowledge of data acquisition methods, it is of particular importance to understand the algorithms and analysis methods used to generate perfusion maps from the raw MR image data. Careful consideration of many factors is required in order to generate reproducible, quantitative perfusion images. This book not only describes recommended acquisition and analysis procedures, but also discusses limitations and potential pitfalls that may be encountered. While not every clinical case may require quantitative measurement, without a firm grasp of the techniques and their associated strengths and weaknesses, the interpreter will ultimately be limited in their ability to draw conclusions, and hence the need for this book. Case reports at the end of the clinical chapters describe how such methods can be applied in real-life situations.

With the popularity of perfusion MRI and its ability to aid in sorting through clinical questions has come greater support from equipment manufacturers. All major equipment vendors now provide substantial support for clinical perfusion MRI, and the role of microvascular flow continues to be of critical importance, indeed increasingly appreciated importance, in many diseases. One recent example is the advent of anti-angiogenic therapy, where the need to understand tumor- and organ-level microvascular flow has taken on tremendous importance. I expect that many additional areas will emerge as we gain greater insight into human physiology, and I also expect perfusion MRI to continue to develop and mature technically. This book, therefore, is timely and needed, as it provides both clinicians and researchers with a comprehensive and state-of-the-art evaluation of perfusion MRI.

Gregory Sorensen
Chief Executive Officer Siemens Healthcare North America
Boston, Massachusetts
2012

References

1. World Health Organization. *The Global Burden of Disease: 2004 Update*. Geneva: WHO, 2008.

2. Roy CS, Sherrington CS. On the regulation of the blood-supply of the brain. *J Physiol* 1890;**11**:85–108.

3. Belliveau JW, Kennedy DN Jr., McKinstry RC, *et al.* Functional mapping of the human visual cortex by magnetic resonance imaging. *Science* 1991;**254**:716–19.

4. Detre JA, Leigh JS, Williams DS, Koretsky AP. Perfusion imaging. *Magn Reson Med* 1992;**23**:37–45.

5. Williams DS, Detre JA, Leigh JS, Koretsky AP. Magnetic resonance imaging of perfusion using spin inversion of arterial water. *Proc Natl Acad Sci U S A* 1992;**89**:212–16.

6. Sorensen AG, Reimer P. *Cerebral MR Perfusion Imaging: Principles and Current Applications*. New York, NY: Thieme, 2000.

Preface

Blood flow is one of the most fundamental physiological parameters. Maintenance of adequate blood flow is vital for the health of biological tissue. The growth and function of many organ systems are linked tightly to their blood supply. In addition, many disease processes are associated with either increases or decreases in flow compared with normal values. The development and validation of non-invasive tools for the measurement of flow have been longstanding goals, both in biomedical research and in clinical practice.

Traditionally, the imaging of flow, or perfusion, has been accomplished using either nuclear medicine-based techniques involving radioactive isotopes, or X-ray computed tomography (CT) methods using radio-opaque contrast agents. However, soon after the introduction of magnetic resonance imaging (MRI) for anatomical imaging, research began on techniques for depicting flow. Since then, progress has been rapid, not least because MR methods have the advantage of not involving radiation, and in the case of arterial spin labeling-based techniques, are completely non-invasive. This makes them particularly appealing for use in a wide range of populations, including children and normal subjects. In addition, MR perfusion can be combined with the armamentarium of other structural, vascular, physiological, metabolic, and functional techniques available with MR to provide a comprehensive, "one-stop" examination for the patient.

Perfusion MRI is now a part of clinical practice, most notably for evaluating neurological disease. In particular, these techniques have been most developed for studying cerebrovascular disease and tumors of the central nervous system (CNS). However, perfusion MRI also has had a major impact in certain organ systems outside the CNS, including the breast, heart, and prostate. Techniques and applications continue to be developed, and over time perfusion MRI is likely to become widely used in organ systems throughout the body.

This book is divided into two major parts, the first section covering the theoretical background of the measurement of perfusion, technical aspects of dynamic susceptibility contrast (DSC) and dynamic contrast enhancement (DCE), and arterial spin labeling (ASL). Chapters are also included on its use in neuroscience (including functional MRI), and MRI methods for measuring blood volume and oxygenation. The second section contains a comprehensive review of clinical applications of perfusion MRI, in neurological diseases including stroke and brain tumors, neurodegeneration, as well as applications throughout the body (breast, heart, prostate, and other organ systems). Finally, there is a chapter dedicated to perfusion MRI in pediatrics.

This book is mainly focused on perfusion MRI in humans; however, on occasion, reference is made to preclinical studies when appropriate. However, it is not intended to be a reference work for researchers using preclinical MRI in animal models, even if many of the principles and techniques for clinical and preclinical perfusion MRI are similar. Other areas that this book does not specifically cover include vascular imaging (i.e., MR, CT, or X-ray angiography), MR perfusion using unconventional or unapproved tracers, or other non-MR methods of measuring perfusion, such as X-ray CT perfusion (CTP) or positron emission tomography (PET). These topics are beyond the scope of the current volume.

Despite the popularity of perfusion MRI in clinical use, there is currently a need for a book that covers this topic in detail. *Clinical Perfusion MRI: Techniques and Applications* aims to fill this gap, and to provide the reader with a comprehensive, yet readable, treatment of this topic. In a single volume, it provides clinicians with the basic knowledge needed to use this technique in their clinical practice. The widespread adoption of high-quality, clinical perfusion MRI will result in improved diagnoses and management decisions, resulting in better clinical outcomes in individual patients worldwide.

Abbreviations

AAT	arterial arrival time		DWI	diffusion-weighted imaging
aBV	arterial blood volume		EBCT	electron beam CT
ACA	anterior cerebral artery		EBRT	external beam radiation therapy
ACE-I	angiotensin-converting enzyme inhibitor		ECG	electrocardiogram
ACS	acute coronary syndrome		EES	extravascular extracellular space
ACZ	acetazolamide		EPI	echo-planar imaging
AD	Alzheimer's disease		EPISTAR	EPI-based signal targeting by alternating radiofrequency pulses, an early pulsed ASL sequence
ADC	apparent diffusion coefficient			
AIF	arterial input function			
AMI	acute myocardial infarction		FA	flip angle
ASE	asymmetric spin echo		FAIR	flow alternating inversion recovery, one of the early pulsed ASL sequences
ASL	arterial spin labeling			
ASPECTS	Alberta Stroke Program Early CT Score		fMRI	functional MRI
ATA	arterial transit artifact		FSE	fast spin echo
ATT	arterial transit time (ms)		FSL	Functional magnetic resonance imaging of the brain Software Library, a freeware post-processing imaging toolkit from the Univeristy of Oxford
AUC	area under the curve (for ROC analysis)			
AV	atrioventricular			
BAT	bolus arrival time (ms)			
BOLD	blood oxygenation level-dependent contrast		FTD	frontotemporal dementia
BV	blood volume		FTLD	Frontotemporal lobar degeneration
CA	Contrast agent		GABA	gamma-aminobutyric acid, an inhibitory neurotransmitter
CAD	computer-assisted diagnosis; or coronary artery disease			
			GE	gradient echo
CAS	carotid artery stenting		GESSE	gradient echo sampling under the spin echo
CBF	cerebral blood flow (ml/100 g/min)		GFR	glomerular filtration rate
CBV	cerebral blood volume (ml/100 g)		GM	gray matter
cCBV	corrected cerebral blood volume (usually corrected for leakage of contrast)		GRASE	gradient and spin echo
			GRE	gradient echo
CFR	cardiac flow reserve		HbO$_2$	oxyhemoglobin
CHD	congenital heart disease		Hct	hematocrit
CMRO$_2$	Cerebral metabolic rate of oxygen consumption (mmol O$_2$/100 g/min)		HHT	hereditary hemorrhagic telangiectasia
			HII	hypoxic-ischemic insult
CNR	contrast-to-noise ratio		ICA	internal carotid artery
CNS	central nervous system		ICDs	implanted cardioverter-defibrillators
COMI	cerebral oxygen metabolic index		ICV	intracranial volume (cm^3)
CPP	cerebral perfusion pressure (mmHg)		IVD	ischemic vascular dementia
CS	coronary sinus		JPA	juvenile pilocytic astrocytoma
CT	computed tomography		K^{trans}	Forward rate constant for transfer of a contrast agent between the vascular and extravascular space
CTA	CT angiography			
CTA	Computed tomography angiography			
CTC	contrast concentration versus time curve		LGE	late gadolinium enhancement, a marker of dead tissue on cardiac MR
CTP	CT perfusion			
CXA	coronary X-ray angiography		LV	left ventricular
DCE	dynamic contrast enhancement		MACE	major adverse cardiac events
dHb	deoxyhemoglobin		MAGIC	multiple acquisitions with global inversion cycling
DMN	Default mode network			
DNP	Dynamic nuclear polarization		MCA	middle cerebral artery
DSA	digital subtraction angiography		MCI	mild cognitive impairment
DSC	dynamic susceptibility contrast		MDCT	multi-detector CT

MEG	magnetoencephalography
MEGESE	multi-echo gradient echo/spin echo
MION	monocrystalline iron oxide nanoparticles, a type of USPIO
MITR	maximum intensity change per unit time interval ratio
MRA	magnetic resonance angiogram
mRS	modified Rankin score
MRS	magnetic resonance spectroscopy
MRV	magnetic resonance venography
MT	magnetization transfer
MTT	mean transit time (in seconds)
NAC	neo adjuvant chemotherapy
NASCET	North American Symptomatic Carotid Endarterectomy Trial, from which a standard grading system for arterial stenosis has been derived
NPV	negative predictive value
NSF	nephrogenic systemic fibrosis
PASL	pulsed arterial spin labeling
PC	phase contrast
PCA	posterior cerebral artery
pCASL	pseudo-continuous ASL, sometimes also called pulsed-continuous ASL
PCI	percutaneous coronary intervention (angioplasty and stent placement)
pCT	perfusion CT
PE	pulmonary embolism
PET	positron emission tomography
PFS	progression-free survival
PH	peak height
PICORE	Proximal inversion with a control for off-resonance effect
PK	pharmacokinetic
PLD	post-label delay (in seconds), used primarily for continuous or pseudo-continuous ASL sequences
PNET	primitive neuroectodermal tumor
PPV	positive predictive value
PS	permeability surface area product
PSR	percentage of signal recovery (in bolus DSC)
PVL	periventricular leukomalacia
PWI	perfusion-weighted imaging
Q2TIPS	Second version of quantitative imaging of perfusion by using single subtraction with addition of thin-section periodic saturation after inversion and time delay
qBOLD	quantitative blood oxygenation level-dependent contrast
QSM	quantitative susceptibility mapping
QUASAR	Quantitative signal targeting by alternating radiofrequency labeling of arterial regions, a multi-delay ASL sequence
QUIPSS I	Quantitative Imaging of Perfusion using a Single Subtraction method I
QUIPSS II	Quantitative Imaging of Perfusion using a Single Subtraction method II
QUIXOTIC	QUantitative Imaging of Extraction of Oxygen and Tissue Consumption

$R(t)$	Residue function, or fraction of tracer remaining in the voxel following an infinitely sharp bolus
R_2	$=1/T_2$, Relaxivity rate for spin echo experiments
$R_2^*=1/T_2^*$	R_2^*, Relaxivity rate for gradient echo experiments
RAS	renal artery stenosis
RCC	renal cell carcinoma
RECIST	Response Evaluation Criteria in Solid Tumors
ROC	receiver operator characteristic
ROI	region of interest
rs-fMRI	resting state functional MRI
RVD	renovascular disease
SAGE	Spin and gradient echo
SAR	specific absorption rate
SE	spin echo
SI	signal intensity
SNR	signal-to-noise ratio
SPECT	single photon emission computed tomography
SPM	Statistical Parameter Mapping, a freeware software program that runs within Matlab, from the University College of London
SSFP	steady-state free precession, a method of image readout
STEMI	ST-segment elevation myocardial infarction
SVD	singular value decomposition, a popular method of performing deconvolution
SWI	susceptibility-weighted imaging
TDL	tumefactive demyelinating lesion
TE	echo time
TEE	transesophageal echocardiogram
THM	tissue homogeneity model
TI	inversion time or delay (in pulsed ASL)
T_{max}	normalized bolus delay (in seconds)
TR	repetition time
TRUST	T_2 relaxation under spin tagging
TTE	transthoracic echocardiogram
USPIO	ultrasmall superparamagnetic iron oxide
V/Q scan	ventilation perfusion scan, used in the lung to diagnose pulmonary emboli
VASO	vascular space occupancy
vCBV	venous CBV
VEGF	vascular endothelial growth factor
Venc	velocity-encoding level, used for phase contrast angiography
VOF	venous output function
VS-ASL	velocity-selective ASL
WHO	World Health Organization, a grading system for brain tumors
WM	White matter
WML	White matter lesions
Xe-CT	Xenon-enhanced CT
Y_v	tissue oxygen saturation (%)

1

Imaging of flow: basic principles

James R. Ewing, David Bonekamp, and Peter B. Barker

Key points

- Indicator dilution techniques for measuring blood flow have existed for more than 100 years.
- Indicators may be either intravascular, or freely diffusible.
- Early techniques establishing the mathematical framework for flow (the Fick principle, Kety–Schmidt method, and central volume principle) were mainly based on arterial and venous blood sampling.
- Tissue perfusion measured by MR techniques may be either based on bolus contrast agent injection, or non-invasive, endogenous "magnetic" labeling of inflowing blood.
- MR perfusion is one of a variety of techniques now available for tomographic imaging of flow; competing techniques such as SPECT, PET, and CT are also able to produce perfusion images.

Introduction

The flow of blood to an organ is a fundamental physiological factor affecting tissue health, growth, and repair. Blood flow and volume are perturbed in many disease conditions, most notably in vascular disease and in tumors. The ability to determine non-invasively blood flow and blood volume using imaging methods therefore has important diagnostic and therapeutic implications. Since the early days of radiological imaging, scientists and physicians have been searching for methods that can accurately and non-invasively depict the major blood vessels of the body, and measure blood flow in tissue. For instance, X-ray projection imaging of blood vessels

(angiography) was first demonstrated in 1927 by Moniz [1], using iodinated contrast agents injected intravascularly, while early measurements of tissue blood flow were based on the inhalation of freely diffusible tracers (e.g., nitrous oxide [N_2O] [2], or radioactive xenon or krypton [3]). Subsequently, stable (i.e., non-radioactive) xenon was used in conjunction with X-ray computed tomography (CT) to image cerebral blood flow (CBF) [4], while other methods such as single-photon emission CT (SPECT) [5, 6] and positron emission tomography (PET) [7, 8] imaging using a variety of radiotracers also became available. More recently, dynamic CT perfusion imaging using bolus injection of iodinated contrast agents has been growing in popularity [9], particularly as fast multi-slice CT scanners have become widely available.

With the emergence of magnetic resonance imaging (MRI) as a clinical imaging modality in the 1980s and 1990s, MRI methods were developed for both angiography and perfusion. Perfusion imaging methods based on exogenous contrast media [10, 11] as well as completely non-invasive methods based on "magnetic labeling" of inflowing blood [12, 13] were developed. Compared to radioactivity- or X-ray-based perfusion methods, MR perfusion offers the advantage of the absence of radiation (particularly important for patients sensitive to radiation, such as children) as well as a synergistic combination with other MRI techniques that offer exquisite soft tissue contrast and spatial resolution. Today, MR perfusion imaging is increasingly being used in clinical practice. However, accurate quantitative perfusion imaging using MRI also involves many technical challenges.

This chapter describes methods for measuring blood flow, looks back at the history of such

Clinical Perfusion MRI: Techniques and Applications, ed. Peter B. Barker, Xavier Golay, and Greg Zaharchuk. Published by Cambridge University Press. © Peter B. Barker, Xavier Golay, and Greg Zaharchuk 2013.

measurements, and presents the central concepts for flow measurements with their corresponding mathematical expressions. Indicator dilution techniques are the main focus, and will be discussed mainly in the context of perfusion in the brain, but with the understanding that such techniques can often be applied to other organ systems. While this chapter will briefly consider measures of bulk flow in large vessels, it will principally focus on measures of perfusion, i.e., measures of flow that estimate the delivery of blood to the microvessels of an organ.

The Fick principle

Modern measurements of vascular physiology began with Adolf E. Fick's description of a method based on the conservation of mass [14]. The heart-lung system has a single flow input, the vena cava, and a single output, the aorta. The difference in oxygen concentration in arterial and venous blood, $c_a - c_v$, is the change of oxygen concentration in the blood as a result of oxygen consumption by the body's metabolism. If we assume that the rates of cardiac flow (F_c – the cardiac output or "minute volume") and oxygen consumption are constant, then $F_c(c_a - c_v)$ is the amount of oxygen per unit time consumed by the body. Mass balance requires that the quantity per unit time of oxygen exiting the heart-lung system via the aorta equals the amount that came in *via* venous blood, plus the amount of oxygen added during blood passage through the lungs:

$$F_c c_a = F_c c_v + VO_2 \qquad (1.1)$$

where VO_2 is the rate of oxygen extraction from the lungs. Thus, cardiac output can be calculated as:

$$F_c = \frac{VO_2}{c_a - c_v} \qquad (1.2)$$

The Fick principle, relying as it does on mass balance in flow, provides a robust and remarkably simple basis for an important physiological measurement, cardiac output. However, it is invasive in that it requires arterial and venous blood sampling, and the measurement of VO_2 requires that a closed-circuit breathing apparatus be constructed, with provision for in-line carbon dioxide capture, and a means of replacing the oxygen consumed by the patient. While the Fick principle's clinical significance as a means of measuring cardiac output has declined, its underlying principle – mass balance

in flow – remains the theoretical basis for nearly every method of flow measurement.

The central volume principle

The central volume principle was first stated by Stewart [15] as a corollary of the Fick principle, and reiterated by Hamilton *et al.* [16]. Using a linear systems approach, Meier and Zierler [17] generated a closely reasoned presentation of this principle. That paper and subsequent elaborations [18, 19] remain the most elegant and easily understood presentations of indicator dilution theory.

Figure 1.1, similar to that in Meier and Zierler's article [17], represents all the paths that a particle of indicator might take in a vascular system (with volume V) from point A to B. It is assumed that the system is stationary or time-invariant, i.e., that flow rates and paths do not change with time, and that the system has a single input and output. The separate pathways show additive behavior in this linear system, and the system can be decomposed into a sum of smaller and smaller components with single inputs and outputs, until only single capillaries remain. In linear systems terminology, the microvasculature is a "passive reciprocal linear two-port network" [20]. It is reciprocal because the same behavior of the system would be observed if the input and output (points A and B in Figure 1.1) were reversed. It is also assumed that all possible pathways are in-line with the supplying and draining vessels. The indicator injected at point A can be freely diffusible, entirely intravascular, or confined to the vasculature plus specific tissue compartments. The only restriction is that the indicator not be trapped in the system, which is equivalent to the absence of pools in the system (which would equal unaccounted losses of mass flow). Note, however, that the nature of the indicator does affect the inference drawn about the volume of the system.

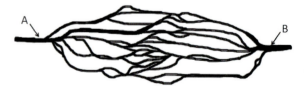

Figure 1.1 A schematic illustration of the paths of the particles of a flow indicator in a vascular system with a single input (A) and output (B). For a freely diffusible indicator, these paths do not necessarily correspond to the paths taken by blood.

mgm/l

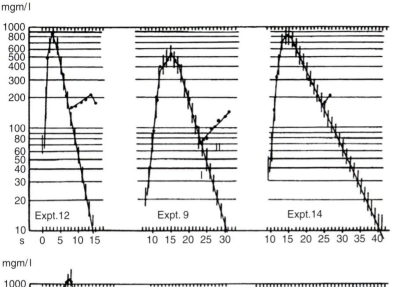

Figure 1.2 Concentration of phenolphthalein dye sampled at various points in the arterial tree of a dog after a bolus venous injection (left ventricle, expts 9, 10, 11, 13; right ventricle, expt. 12; and femoral artery, expt. 14). The log-linearity of a portion of each of the clearance curves is evident. There was very good agreement between estimates of cardiac blood flow made by this method and estimates made by the Fick procedure [21].

mgm/l

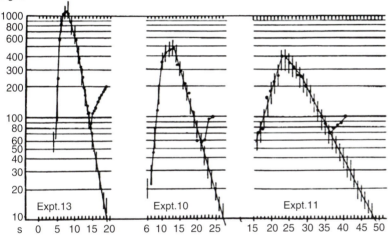

If a quantity Q of indicator is injected at point A as an ideal bolus (i.e., a Dirac "delta function") at time $t = 0$, there will be a time lag before the first appearance of the indicator at the exit of the flow system (point B), followed by a rapid rise to a peak concentration, and a more gradual clearance. Figure 1.2, taken from experiments conducted in dogs by Moore *et al.* [21], shows examples of such data, with the concentration of an easily detectable dye (phenolphthalein) sampled at various points in an arterial tree. Note the semi-logarithmic scale of the ordinate in those plots, and the log-linearity of the terminal portion of each clearance curve, indicating that the tracer concentration is decreasing exponentially with time, a sign of a "well-mixed" flow system. The logarithmic slope of the clearance in a well-mixed system should be proportional to the system's flow divided by its volume. The early use of dyes such as phenolphthalein in flow experiments generated the label of "dye dilution," or "indicator dilution" for experiments that utilized a substance that could be assumed not to be metabolized or otherwise trapped in the system.

To derive the central volume principle, consider $Q(t)$, the quantity of tracer that has left the system at point B at time t. The instantaneous quantity of the tracer ($dQ(t)/dt$) leaving the system at point B during the time interval dt equals the (assumed constant) flow F times the instantaneous concentration $c_B(t)$ at point B times dt: $dQ(t) = F \times c_B(t) \times dt$. Thus, if Q is the total amount of tracer injected,

$$\int_0^\infty \frac{d}{dt} Q(t)dt = Q \tag{1.3}$$

and thus

$$Q = F\int_0^\infty c_B(t)dt \tag{1.4}$$

If tracer quantities and concentrations can be measured directly, this leads to the calculation of the flow according to

$$F = \frac{Q}{\int_0^\infty c_B(t)dt} \tag{1.5}$$

The *transport function*, or the frequency function of transit times, $h(t)$, is defined as follows

$$h(t) = \frac{Fc_B(t)}{Q} \tag{1.6}$$

This quantity has units of inverse time (e.g., 1/min or 1/s). These units result because the product $h(t)dt$ – a unitless quantity – represents an infinitesimal (or instantaneous) probability that a particle of indicator injected at point A at time $t = 0$ will appear at point B at time t. The product $h(t)dt$ therefore is the probability density function (i.e., normalized distribution) of transit times. The ratio on the right-hand side of Eq. (1.6) expresses the amount of tracer passing through point B at the instant t as a fraction of the total injected amount Q. Therefore $\int_0^\infty h(t)dt = 1$.

To continue with the analogy to probability theory, the cumulative density function (or cumulative distribution function, $H(t)$) and the residue function $R(t)$ are defined:

$$H(t) = \int_0^t h(\tau)d\tau \tag{1.7}$$

$$R(t) = 1 - H(t) \tag{1.8}$$

$H(t)$ is the proportion of indicator particles that have traversed the system from A to B from time 0 to time t, and $R(t)$ is the proportion that remain in the system. Clearly, since all the fluid that enters the system must eventually leave, $H(t) \to 1.0$ as $t \to \infty$.

Note that the major difference between classical indicator dilution experiments and modern imaging-based perfusion techniques is the sampling location

(see below, External monitoring of indicator concentration). After a bolus input in classical indicator dilution experiments, with sampling performed at point B, the common output vessel of the system, the recorded concentration over the time course of the experiment is a scaled version of the transport function $h(t)$. In imaging experiments, the concentration of indicator in the tissue under observation (voxel) measured over time is a scaled version of the tissue residue function $R(t)$.

The flow rate at which the subset of fluid with transit time t leaves the system is $Fh(t)dt$, where F is the flow in unit volume per unit time. The volume of fluid contained in all microvascular pathways with common transit time τ therefore is $\tau Fh(\tau)d\tau$. To calculate the total volume occupied by tracer (i.e., the distribution volume) between points A and B, we can sum all these separate microvascular pathways, by integrating over all possible values of τ, assuming constant flow (F):

$$V = F\int_0^\infty \tau h(\tau)d\tau \tag{1.9}$$

Remembering that $\int_0^\infty h(t)dt = 1$, it follows from the second mean value theorem for integration that the mean transit time for all indicator (and therefore fluid) particles in the system is expressed as the $h(t)$-weighted average of transit times:

$$\bar{t} = \int_0^\infty th(t)dt \tag{1.10}$$

The combination of Eqs. (1.9) and (1.10), then, yields the *central volume theorem*:

$$V = F\bar{t} \tag{1.11}$$

where $\bar{t}$ is the mean transit time between point A and point B for an indicator particle, and V is the volume of the system accessible to the indicator between point A and point B.

Note that the residue function $R(t)$ has a special relation to the mean transit time since $R(t) = 1 - H(t)$. We can integrate by parts to demonstrate that:

$$\int_0^\infty R(t)dt = \int_0^\infty [1 - H(t)]dt = \{[1 - H(t)]t\}_0^\infty$$

$$+ \int_0^\infty th(t)dt = \int_0^\infty th(t)dt = \bar{t} \tag{1.12}$$

The relationship $\bar{t} = \int_0^\infty R(t)dt$ is intuitively clear in that a longer mean transit time results in a larger residual at each point of time.

The central volume theorem, freely diffusible indicators, and intravascular agents

It is useful to distinguish two model systems in which the indicator is either an entirely intravascular agent (never leaving the vasculature), or a freely diffusible indicator, where it is assumed that indicator concentration in tissue is in equilibrium with that in the venous drainage. While the underlying central volume theory remains the same, quite different systematic errors may occur due to the differences in clearance times of the two systems, and different experimental requirements.

In current MR practice, the labeled water of the arterial spin labeling (ASL) experiment [12, 13, 22–26] is usually considered to be a freely diffusible indicator. However, this is an approximation, since the single-pass extraction fraction of water in gray matter [27] is about 0.8. For the central volume theorem, one immediate question arises as to what volume should be considered – the whole tissue, the blood and tissue separately, or some weighted average of the blood and tissue. The tissue homogeneity model (THM) [28, 29] approach, based on the early work of Johnson and Wilson [30], can address this problem, estimating not only flow, but also vascular volume and extraction fraction. However, the signal-to-noise ratio (SNR) of ASL usually limits the practical application of THM. For CBF in small animals, careful comparison between ASL and autoradiography measurements indicates that ASL slightly overestimates CBF [31]. In humans, where the transit time from the labeling slab to the imaging plane can be comparable to the blood T_1 relaxation time (or even longer than T_1 in the presence of cerebrovascular disease), the major systematic error may be to tend to underestimate flow.

The question of extraction also applies to MR perfusion studies that use intravascular injection of contrast agents, since the central volume theory assumes that no leakage of indicator occurs, but in various organ systems (and in pathology) extravasation of contrast into tissue frequently occurs. Again, with sufficiently high-quality data (e.g., high SNR), flow, extraction fraction, vascular volume, and possibly interstitial volume can be estimated [32–34], but the technical requirements for the MR sequence are formidable, as are the post-processing procedures. Even if no leakage occurs, problems in the application of the central volume theorem to imaging data can persist. Note that the volume of the system is defined by the two sampling points (Figure 1.1). If A is placed in the middle cerebral artery (MCA), and B is placed at a collecting venule, then the volume of the system is the entire path volume taken by indicator particles that eventually exit at the collecting venule. If indicator particles are freely diffusible, then the volume V is the entire tissue volume plus vascular volume, while if indicator particles are confined to the vasculature, the volume of the system is restricted to the vascular volume. Note also that classical tracer dilution experiments measure vascular tracer concentration in the input and output vessels by direct blood sampling, while MRI experiments usually estimate arterial and tissue tracer concentrations from MR signal changes. In addition, the apparent vascular and tissue concentrations estimated from MR are affected by partial volume considerations because of the finite spatial resolution of MRI. Even when not contaminated by a major vessel, the "tissue" concentration determined by MR will be a combination of tissue and capillary concentrations. For an intravascular tracer, the microvascular concentration can be estimated by knowledge of the blood volume (fractional volume of vessels in the tissue), which is important for consideration of transport gradients between microvessels and interstitium in models of leaky vessels.

The effect of input functions: convolution

So far, only the case of the response of the vascular system to an impulse (i.e., the Dirac delta function) has been considered. In practice, contrast agents are administered over a period of time, and are further mixed by their passage through the heart-lung system, thus resulting in an input function to the organ system under study that has significant duration and also non-uniform amplitude with time. However, in linear systems, if the response to a delta function is known, the response to any other physically realizable input function can be constructed via convolution.

The input concentration of the indicator in the blood, $c_A(t)$, is known as the arterial input function (AIF), and generally will be a smoothly varying function of time, with a finite integral. At each time t, the venous output $c_B(t)$ will no longer just reflect pathways of transit time t, as in the case of an ideal impulse input function. Instead, $c_B(t)$ represents a weighted sum of pathways with different transit times. A typical arterial

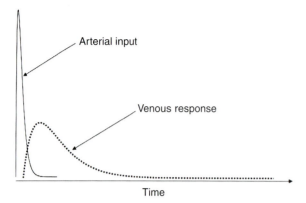

Figure 1.3 The arterial input and the venous response are related by the tissue residue function; due to dispersion in the tissue, the venous response has lower amplitude and delayed clearance compared to the arterial input.

input is illustrated in Figure 1.3, as well as a corresponding venous response. If the first small time interval (dt) of the input is represented as a delta function (with an appropriate weighting), then the response of the system to this input is well understood – it is the transport function, $h(t)$. Likewise, the next small interval of the AIF can be represented as a delta function with appropriate weighting, and so on until the entire AIF up to a time t is covered. Then the portion of the venous response from $\tau = 0$ to $\tau = t$, $c_A(0)$ to $c_A(t)$, can be expressed as the sum of responses to the weighted inputs, or in the limit as the AIF intervals are brought to zero, as an integral. Mathematically, this is expressed as a convolution:

$$c_B(t) = \int_0^t c_A(\tau)h(t - \tau)d\tau = (c_A \otimes h)(t) \qquad (1.13)$$

where the symbol $\otimes$ denotes convolution, as defined in the integral expression. Equation (1.13) describes the response of most flow systems to an arbitrary, physically realizable, input. Since it is so general, it is the basic equation of nearly every measure of flow.

Applications of the central volume principle

The heart-lung and brain vascular systems are two critically important systems. For an entirely intravascular indicator, assuming a total heart volume of about 350 ml, a lung vascular volume of about 2.2 ml/kg body weight, a cardiac output of 5 l/min (83.3 ml/s), and a 70 kg body weight [35], one arrives

at a heart-lung vascular volume of about 500 ml and a mean transit time (MTT = $\bar{t}$) of about 6 s.

In the brain, the mean vascular volume and flow are about 3.5 ml/100 g, and 50 ml/100 g/min [36], respectively. This yields a mean transit time (and dominant time constant) of about $(3.5 \times 60)/50$ s, or 4.2 s for an entirely intravascular indicator such as gadopentetate dimeglumine (Gd-DTPA) in normal cerebral microvasculature. If the indicator used is freely diffusible (e.g., one of the noble gases or water, here assumed to be freely diffusible), the working volume becomes about 1 ml/g (here assuming idealized values of a density of 1.0 for tissue and a blood–brain partition coefficient, λ, of 1.0), and the mean transit time becomes about 7 min. As noted above, λ is actually slightly less than 1.0 for water (commonly estimated at 0.9 ml/g as a whole brain average [37]), which should be applied as a small correction factor in ASL experiments.

These order-of-magnitude calculation for two systems in series should serve both as an illustration of the use of the central volume principle, and a caution as to the difficulties of using a purely intravascular indicator for estimating CBF. As we have shown, the time constant of the heart-lung system at rest is about 6 s, which is the dominant time constant. Although this shortens under exercise, it also lengthens with age and pathology. In a clinical setting, then, 6 s is probably a lower limit for the time constant of the heart-lung system. A bolus venous injection will then have a major concentration–time output behavior that is shaped by the heart-lung vascular system. This output is then directed to the input of the brain vascular system, with its 4.2 s time constant. The difficulty then becomes apparent when CBF is to be estimated from the relationship $\bar{t} = \frac{V}{F}$, i.e., from an estimate of the time constant of the brain vascular system. The problem is that if the input to a downstream system has slower time constants than the characteristic times of the downstream system, the major response of the downstream system is simply to follow, with a small time lag, the shape of the input. This makes the inference of the time constants of the downstream system difficult and inherently unstable.

The Kety–Schmidt technique

We return to the Fick principle, but now applied to flow in the brain, and specifically using a freely diffusible gaseous indicator. In the initial studies by Kety and Schmidt, the indicator was N_2O which was measured via in vitro analysis in arterial and venous samples [2, 38, 39], while in later studies the use of the inert radiogases ^{85}Kr and ^{133}Xe, detected by external scintillation detectors, became more common. N_2O studies continued for many years, and were even still in use for comparison in early MRI-based CBF studies which used fluorinated hydrocarbons as the MRI indicator [40].

In the Kety–Schmidt N_2O clearance technique, the indicator N_2O is administered in non-anesthetic concentrations *via* inhalation for a period of time that is long compared to the longest expected time constant of clearance. Conversely, an uptake experiment can be performed, in which the concentration of N_2O starts at zero and approaches saturation. In either case, the Fick principle can be applied to the system as depicted in Figure 1.1, so that the differential change in the quantity of indicator in the system during any differential period of time is equal to the amount of indicator carried in minus the amount carried out:

$$dQ_{tis}(t) = (Q_{in} - Q_{out})dt \qquad (1.14)$$

where $Q_{tis}(t)$ is the quantity of indicator in the tissue, Q_{in} and Q_{out} are the quantities of indicator carried in and out of the tissue, respectively, and t is time. If both sides of the equation are divided by the mass of the tissue compartment, M, and it is noted that $Q_{in} = FC_p(t)$, and $Q_{out} = FC_v(t)$, where F is the total flow to the tissue compartment, $c_p(t)$ is concentration of indicator in the arterial plasma as a function of time, and $c_v(t)$ is the venous concentration, then

$$dc(t) = f(c_p(t) - c_v(t))dt \qquad (1.15)$$

where $c(t)$ is the concentration of the indicator in the tissue compartment, and f is the *specific* flow, *i.e.*, the flow per unit mass of the tissue compartment. If a freely diffusible indicator is in use, then the tissue concentration is in equilibrium with the effluent venous concentration, with a proportion described by the blood–brain partition coefficient, λ.

If direct measurements of both arterial and venous concentrations are available, as in the Kety–Schmidt technique, the analysis stops at this point. With the substitution $c(t) = \lambda\, c_v(t)$, Eq. (1.15) can be directly integrated to yield an expression for flow. For a clearance experiment where indicator concentration approaches a constant value with increasing time, specific flow, with units of ml/100 g/min, is determined as:

$$f = \frac{100\,\lambda\,c_{sat}}{\int_0^\infty [c_p(t) - c_v(t)]\,dt} \qquad (1.16)$$

where c_{sat} is the equilibrium concentration of freely diffusible indicator in cerebral venous blood. Examples of the type of data typically produced by a Kety–Schmidt experiment are shown in Figure 1.4.

The Kety–Schmidt technique has the unique advantage that it is an essentially model-independent estimate of total CBF. Among its results that should be taken as "benchmarks" are that average CBF (remembering that this is a specific measure of perfusion, i.e., perfusion per

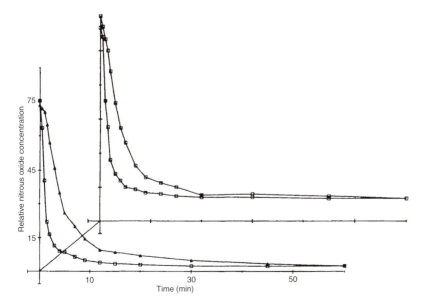

Figure 1.4 Typical data (N_2O concentration vs. time) from a washout Kety–Schmidt experiment in a cat under control conditions (foreground) and after administration of freon-22 (background). First, a steady-state concentration is achieved in which the arterial and venous N_2O concentrations are the same, at which point, the N_2O is switched out of the breathing circuit. In both studies, the lower curve is arterial concentration and the upper curve is venous concentration of N_2O. CBF is proportional to the saturation concentration of indicator divided by integrated arteriovenous difference. In this instance, application of freon-22 increased CBF, as evidenced by the smaller arteriovenous difference during the washout period.

Relative nitrous oxide concentration

75

45

15

10   30   50
Time (min)

unit mass of tissue) in the general population decreases from the age of 20 onward by about 3% per decade [41], and that average CBF in a healthy young population is about 60 ml/100 g/min [42]. Interestingly, if the aging population is selected such that conditions which in younger subjects would be judged pathological (e.g., white matter hyperintensities on MRI, or atrophy) are absent in the aged population, CBF is not significantly different from that of a young and healthy population.

The central volume and the Kety–Schmidt principles [Eq. (1.16)] are related. Clearly, the quantity $[c_p(t) - c_v(t)]$ must be related to the residue function, $R(t)$, since the instantaneous arteriovenous difference is a measure of the instantaneous difference between indicator delivered and indicator leaving the system. Thus, an integral of the arteriovenous difference over time must yield a quantity related to the mean transit time of the indicator.

As a simple example, suppose that $c_p(t)$ is a step function (Heaviside function) ($c_p(t) = c_0$ for $t < 0$, $c_p(t) = 0$ for $t \geq 0$), and that the tissue compartment has a uniform specific flow of $f = \frac{F}{V} = k$ (units ml/100 g/min). The specific flow f equals CBF. Per the central volume theorem: $k = f = \text{CBF} = \text{CBV}/\text{MTT}$, where CBV is cerebral blood volume. In a well-mixed situation, the log linear tail of a concentration–time curve in a Kety–Schmidt experiment has a negative slope of F/V: $c(t) = \exp(-kt)$. Then the integral in the denominator of Eq. (1.16), $\int_0^\infty [c_p(t) - c_v(t)]dt$, becomes $-\lambda c_{sat} \int_0^\infty e^{-kt}dt$, or $\frac{\lambda c_{sat}}{k}$, as due to the step function input, the venous concentration equals the equilibrium (saturation) concentration c_{sat} at $t = 0$. For $t \geq 0$, the operand of the integral reduces to $c_v(t)$, as $c_p(t) = 0$. Thus, the venous output can be modeled with a single exponential decay $c_v(t) = \exp(-kt)$. Considering the scaling factor of 100, one sees that this calculation produces an identity in Eq. (1.16), thus demonstrating the quantity $\int_0^\infty [c_p(t) - c_v(t)]dt$ to be equal to the mean transit time $\bar{t}$, scaled by $\frac{\lambda c_{sat}}{\text{CBV}}$.

External monitoring of indicator concentration

Up to this point, all discussion of tissue flow estimation has been based on measurements of input and output concentrations of an indicator. Since in practice this would usually require invasive arterial and venous sampling for each organ system, it is seldom used. Rather, imaging-based CBF techniques will usually measure indicator concentrations in tissue. Various "indicator-detection pairs" that have been used are: inert xenon gas with CT detection of xenon's X-ray absorption [4, 43–47] (Figure 1.5), iodinated contrast agent with X-ray absorption [48–54] (Figure 1.6), gamma-emitting radiotracers with detection by SPECT [6, 55], positron-emitting radiotracers with detection by PET [8, 36, 56–58] (Figure 1.7), paramagnetic contrast agents with MRI detection that utilizes either T_2^* [59–64] (Figure 1.8) or T_1 [32–34] contrast as a measure of tissue concentration, and spin-labeled endogenous blood with MRI detection [12, 13, 65–67].

If we begin with the ideal situation of a Dirac delta function input of a quantity q_0 of indicator into the system at time t = 0, then at any time after the introduction of the indicator, an external detector will sense the amount of indicator *remaining* in the system, $Q_T(t)$:

$$Q_T(t) = q_0[1 - H(t)] = q_0 R(t) \tag{1.17}$$

The quantity of tracer in the tissue $Q_T(t)$ at each point in time t is $Q_T(t) = V c_t(t)$, where V is the tissue volume under observation and $c_t(t)$ is the tissue concentration. Consequently, the integral of the detected tissue concentration over time curve multiplied by the tissue volume will be the mean transit time scaled by the introduced tracer amount q_0:

$$\int_0^\infty V c_t(t)dt = V \int_0^\infty c_t(t)dt = \int_0^\infty Q_T(t)dt$$

$$= \int_0^\infty q_0[1 - H(t)]dt = q_0\bar{t} \tag{1.18}$$

While the total quantity of tracer entering the system is $q_0 = F \int_0^\infty c_a(t)dt$ under all circumstances, Eqs. (1.17) and (1.18) are no longer accurate representations of the tissue tracer quantity over time if the AIF is not instantaneous. Here, the key to the mathematical examination of the processes governing the relationship between the AIF and the tissue concentration lies in the decomposition of the problem into the components of tracer quantities entering and leaving the tissue at each point in time.

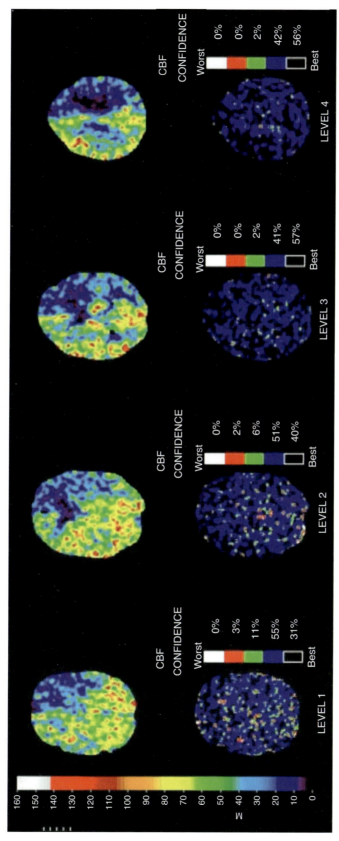

Figure 1.5 Xe–CT CBF maps from four slices (levels) in a patient with a right MCA occlusion and corresponding flow deficit. Note that the right side of the image corresponds to the patient's right-hand side. CBF was measured using the freely diffusible indicator, inert xenon, and CT Hounsfield units to estimate the indicator concentration–time curve in each pixel. Accompanying maps of goodness-of-fit for each slice are provided. Figure courtesy of Dr. Howard Yonas, University of New Mexico, Albuquerque, NM, USA.

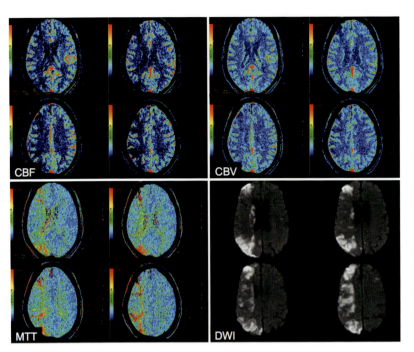

Figure 1.6 CT perfusion images from four slices calculated using bolus injection of non-ionic iodine-based contrast agent (iopamidol) in a 60-year-old male with an embolic right MCA stroke. CBF, CBV, and MTT maps showing reduced blood flow and blood volume and increased mean transit time respectively in the ischemic right hemisphere, corresponding areas of restricted water diffusion suggesting acute ischemic infarction seen on diffusion-weighted MRI scan (DWI). Figure courtesy of Dr. Rajan Jain, Henry Ford Hospital, Detroit, MI, USA.

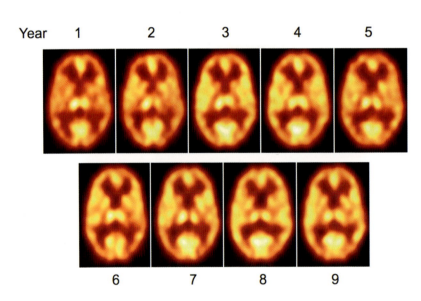

Figure 1.7 $H_2{}^{15}O$-PET CBF images in a normal elderly subject scanned every year over a 9-year period. Pixel resolution is 6.5 mm with data collection of 1 minute following intravenous injection of ^{15}O-labeled water. Excellent reproducibility and relatively stable flow from year to year is observed. Figure courtesy of Dr. Susan Resnick, National Institute on Aging, Baltimore, MD, USA.

The quantity $Q_I(t)$ of indicator entering the tissue at time t is

$$Q_I(t) = FC_a(t)dt \qquad (1.19)$$

where $C_a(t)$ is the arterial concentration of the tracer. The quantity of tracer $Q_o(t)$ leaving the tissue at time t is, following from Eq. (1.18) and the definition of:

$$Q_o(t) = Fc_V(t)dt = F . \int_0^\infty c_a(t-\tau)h(\tau)d\tau dt$$

$$= F . \int_0^\infty c_a(\tau)h(t-\tau)d\tau dt \qquad (1.20)$$

where $c_v(t)$ is the venous concentration of the tracer. The quantity remaining $Q_T(t)$ in the tissue at time t is

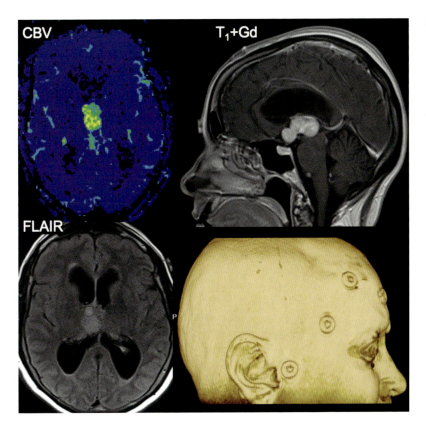

Figure 1.8 1.5 Tesla MR perfusion images (CBV) recorded using bolus-injection of a gadolinium-based contrast agent (gadobenate dimeglumine) in a 58-year-old female with a third ventricular meningioma, showing high blood volume and avid contrast enhancement on post-Gd T_1-weighted images. The lesion is also causing mild enlargement of the lateral ventricles, as seen on FLAIR MRI.

then the difference of all tracer introduced into the tissue since $t = 0$ and all tracer removed in the same interval, $Q_T(t) = \int(Q_I(t) - Q_o(t))dt$

$$Q_T(t) = Vc_t(t) = F.\int_0^t c_a(\tau)d\tau - F.\int_0^t c_v(\tau)d\tau$$

$$= F.\int_0^t c_a(\tau)\left[1 - \int_0^t h(\tau-u)du\right]d\tau \qquad (1.21)$$

$$= F.\int_0^t c_a(\tau)R(t-\tau)d\tau$$

Division by the tissue volume yields an expression which both introduces specific flow f and represents the most commonly used form in MRI perfusion experiments:

$$c_t(t) = f.\int_0^t c_a(\tau)R(t-\tau)d\tau \qquad (1.22)$$

The specific flow f is flow per unit volume of the tissue, in units of, e.g., ml/100 ml/min = %/min. In typical brain perfusion MRI exams, the specific flow

f is reported as CBF (units 1/time, e.g., 1/min); the fractional CBV (unit-less) represents the fraction of volume in the tissue voxel accessible to tracer; and the MTT with units of time, e.g., seconds. In the interpretation of all perfusion experiments one should carefully distinguish between specific flow and vascular volume fraction and absolute flow and direct volume measurement, as the choice of names for the parameters CBF and CBV does not intuitively make this distinction apparent.

Another common representation of the important formula (1.22) is:

$$f = \frac{c_t(t)}{\int_0^t c_a(\tau)R(t-\tau)d\tau} \qquad (1.23)$$

Equation (1.23) matches equation 6 of the 1996 paper by Ostergaard *et al.*, one of the two simultaneously published papers [63, 64] describing the theory of dynamic susceptibility contrast (DSC)-MRI estimates of CBF. Essentially, Eq. (1.23) states that the tissue-specific flow in an image volume is equal to the initial height $c_t(t = 0)$ of the deconvolved tissue concentration curve, relative to the arterial concentration. This is a "common sense" result: if it were possible to introduce indicator to the vasculature of the brain as a unit impulse function, the amount of indicator that would arrive in an individual voxel, and be present at time $t = 0$ would be proportional to the flow to that voxel.

Equation (1.23) is also commonly used for freely diffusible indicators. In these cases, a multi-compartmental analysis (using N compartments) is commonly used. In the brain, N is usually assumed to be 2, with the faster rate constant associated with gray matter, and the slower rate constant associated with white matter, although other tissue types may be included in the model. For instance, in the xenon inhalation technique [68], and also MRI studies performed using fluorocarbon indicators ("freons," with a single surface coil placed over the head of an experimental animal [40, 69]), the tissue concentration of indicator as a function of time, measured by the external detector, can be expressed as:

$$c(t) - \sum_{t-1}^{N} W_t C_t(t) - \sum_{t-1}^{N} P_t \int_0^i C_a(\tau) e^{-k(t-r)} d\tau$$

$$(1.24)$$

where $C(t)$ is a signal proportional to the tissue concentration of the indicator, W_i is a proportionality constant that includes the relative contribution (weight) of the ith tissue compartment to the signal; P_i is a proportionality constant equal to W_i times scaling differences between the amplitude of the arterial signal and the tissue signal; $c_i(t)$ is the tissue concentration of indicator in the ith tissue compartment as a function of time; k_i, is the clearance constant of the ith tissue compartment; $c_a(t)$ is the arterial concentration of the indicator. Equation [1.24] assumes a well-mixed compartment model. Blood flow in the ith compartment can be calculated as $f_i = k_i \lambda_i$, where f_i is the specific flow in milliliters per ml per unit time and λ_i is the blood–brain partition coefficient for the ith tissue compartment.

It should be noted that a multi-compartmental analysis of indicator dilution data demands very high primary data. This is a well-known characteristic of transfer functions with exponential kernels. Therefore, for fitting of MR perfusion data to produce reliable values, excellent signal-to-noise ratios (SNR) and temporal resolution is required both for the AIF and tissue response, and in general it is inadvisable to try to over-fit too many parameters (or too complicated a model) to data that are often quite limited in this regard.

Practical considerations for MR perfusion imaging

This introductory chapter has covered the fundamental aspects of measuring blood flow using the indicator dilution technique, with some examples given from a historical perspective, and also with some examples from other (mainly nuclear medicine, or X-ray-based) flow imaging methods for comparison. It has mainly focused on ideal models, and has not considered many of the practical issues which occur when performing MR perfusion imaging. These will be covered in later chapters of the book, and will include the relationship between tracer concentration and MR signal intensity (here assumed to be linear, but in practice may often be a complicated relationship), or the choice of contrast agent and technique used (for instance, comparison of contrast agent-based methods versus non-invasive ASL). Later chapters will also discuss how to measure tissue permeability with MRI (i.e., the rate at which a tracer moves from the intravascular space to the extravascular tissue space), and how flow and permeability measurements relate to each other. This book focuses exclusively on MR perfusion techniques, and will not cover topics such as MR angiography or alternative perfusion imaging techniques (e.g., currently competing techniques such as CT perfusion [70]). While the greatest number of perfusion studies performed to date have been in the brain, particularly for the evaluation of cerebrovascular disease and tumors, perfusion MRI is finding increasing use in other organ systems for a variety of applications. Subsequent chapters will also include discussion of extra-cerebral applications.

References

1. Moniz E. Arterial encephalography: importance in the localization of cerebral tumors. *Rev Neurol (Paris)* 1927;2:72–90.

2. Kety S, Schmidt C. The nitrous oxide method for the quantitative determination of

cerebral blood flow in man: theory, procedure, and normal values. *J Clin Invest* 1948;**27**:476–83.

3. Lassen NA, Ingvar DH. The blood flow of the cerebral cortex determined by radioactive krypton. *Experientia* 1961; **17**:42–3.

4. Yonas H, Gur D, Latchaw R, Wolfson SK, Jr. Stable xenon CT/CBF imaging: laboratory and clinical experience. *Adv Tech Stand Neurosurg* 1987;**15**:3–37.

5. Holman BL, Hill TC, Magistretti PL. Brain imaging with emission computed tomography and radiolabeled amines. *Invest Radiol* 1982;**17**(3):206–15.

6. Neirinckx RD, Canning LR, Piper IM, *et al.* Technetium-99m d, l-HM-PAO: a new radiopharmaceutical for SPECT imaging of regional cerebral blood perfusion. *J Nucl Med* 1987;**28**(2):191–202.

7. Herscovitch P, Markham J, Raichle ME. Brain blood flow measured with intravenous $H_2^{15}O$. I. Theory and error analysis. *J Nucl Med* 1983; **24**(9):782–9.

8. Raichle ME, Martin WR, Herscovitch P, Mintun MA, Markham J. Brain blood flow measured with intravenous $H_2^{15}O$. II. Implementation and validation. *J Nucl Med* 1983; **24**(9):790–8.

9. Axel L. Cerebral blood flow determination by rapid-sequence computed tomography: theoretical analysis. *Radiology* 1980;**137**(3):679–86.

10. Belliveau JW, Kennedy DN, Jr., McKinstry RC, *et al.* Functional mapping of the human visual cortex by magnetic resonance imaging. *Science* 1991;**254** (5032):716–19.

11. Villringer A, Rosen BR, Belliveau JW, *et al.* Dynamic imaging with lanthanide chelates in normal brain: contrast due to magnetic

susceptibility effects. *Magn Reson Med* 1988;**6**(2):164–74.

12. Williams DS, Detre JA, Leigh JS, Koretsky AP. Magnetic resonance imaging of perfusion using spin inversion of arterial water. *Proc Natl Acad Sci U S A* 1992;**89**(1):212–16.

13. Detre JA, Leigh JS, Williams DS, Koretsky AP. Perfusion imaging. *Magn Reson Med* 1992;**23**(1):37–45.

14. Fick A. Uber die Messung des Blutquantums in der Herzventrikeln. *Sitz der Physik-Med Ges Wurzburg* 1870;**2**:16–28.

15. Stewart G. Researches on the circulation time and on the influences which affect it. The output of the heart. *J Physiol* 1897; **XXII**:159–83.

16. Hamilton WF, Moore JW, Kinsman JM, Spurling RG. Studies on the circulation. IV. Further analysis of the injection method, and of changes in hemodynamics under physiological and pathological conditions. *Am J Physiol* 1932;**99**(3):534–51.

17. Meier P, Zierler KL. On the theory of the indicator dilution method for measurement of blood flow and volume. *J Appl Physiol* 1954;**6**:731–43.

18. Zierler K. Equations for measuring blood flow by external monitoring of radioisotopes. *Circ Res* 1965;**16**:309–21.

19. Zierler K. Theory of the use of arteriovenous concentration differences for measuring metabolism in steady and non-steady states. *Circ Res* 1961;**40**:2111–25.

20. Skilling HH. *Electrical Engineering Circuits.* New York: John Wiley and Sons, Inc., 1961.

21. Moore J, Kinsman J, Hamilton W, Spurling R. Studies on the circulation. *Am J Physiol* 1929; **89**(2):331–9.

22. Wong EC, Buxton RB, Frank LR. Implementation of quantitative perfusion imaging techniques for

functional brain mapping using pulsed arterial spin labeling. *NMR Biomed* 1997;**10**(4–5):237–49.

23. Buxton RB, Frank LR, Wong EC, *et al.* A general kinetic model for quantitative perfusion imaging with arterial spin labeling. *Magn Reson Med* 1998;**40**(3):383–96.

24. Wong EC, Luh WM, Liu TT. Turbo ASL: arterial spin labeling with higher SNR and temporal resolution. *Magn Reson Med* 2000;**44**(4):511–15.

25. Wong EC, Buxton RB, Frank LR. Quantitative imaging of perfusion using a single subtraction (QUIPSS and QUIPSS II). *Magn Reson Med* 1998;**39**(5):702–8.

26. Ewing JR, Cao Y, Fenstermacher J. Single-coil arterial spin-tagging for estimating cerebral blood flow as viewed from the capillary: relative contributions of intra- and extravascular signal. *Magn Reson Med* 2001;**46**(3):465–75.

27. Raichle M, Eichling J, Straatmann M, *et al.* Blood-brain barrier permeability of ^{11}C-labeled alcohols and ^{15}O-labeled water. *Am J Physiol* 1976;**230**:543–52.

28. St Lawrence KS, Lee TY. An adiabatic approximation to the tissue homogeneity model for water exchange in the brain: I. Theoretical derivation. *J Cereb Blood Flow Metab* 1998;**18** (12):1365–77.

29. Wang J, Fernandez-Seara MA, Wang S, St Lawrence KS. When perfusion meets diffusion: in vivo measurement of water permeability in human brain. *J Cereb Blood Flow Metab* 2007; **27**(4):839–49.

30. Johnson JA, Wilson T. A model for capillary exchange. *Am J Physiol* 1966;**210**(6):1299–303.

31. Ewing JR, Wei L, Knight RA, *et al.* Direct comparison of local cerebral blood flow rates measured by MRI arterial

spin-tagging and quantitative autoradiography in a rat model of experimental cerebral ischemia. *J Cereb Blood Flow Metab* 2003; **23**(2):198–209.

32. Sourbron S. Technical aspects of MR perfusion. *Eur J Radiol* 2010;**76**(3):304–13.

33. Sourbron S, Heilmann M, Biffar A, *et al.* Bolus-tracking MRI with a simultaneous T1- and T2*-measurement. *Magn Reson Med* 2009;**62**(3):672–81.

34. Sourbron S, Ingrisch M, Siefert A, Reiser M, Herrmann K. Quantification of cerebral blood flow, cerebral blood volume, and blood-brain-barrier leakage with DCE-MRI. *Magn Reson Med* 2009;**62**(1):205–17.

35. Guyton AC, Hall JE. *Textbook of Medical Physiology*, 11th edn. Philadelphia: Elsevier Inc., 2006.

36. Grubb R, Raichle M, Eichling J, Ter-Pogossian M. The effects of changes in $PaCO_2$ on cerebral blood volume, blood flow, and vascular mean transit time. *Stroke* 1974;**5**:630–9.

37. Petersen ET, Zimine I, Ho YC, Golay X. Non-invasive measurement of perfusion: a critical review of arterial labeling techniques. *Br J Radiol* 2006;**79**:688–701.

38. Kety S, Schmidt C. The effects of altered arterial tension of carbon dioxide and oxygen on cerebral blood flow and cerebral oxygen consumption of normal young men. *J Clin Invest* 1948;**27**:484–92.

39. Kety S, Schmidt C. The determination of cerebral blood flow in man by the use of nitrous oxide in low concentrations. *Am J Physiol* 1945;**143**:53–66.

40. Ewing JR, Branch CA, Helpern JA, *et al.* Cerebral blood flow measured by NMR indicator dilution in cats. *Stroke* 1989; **20**(2):259–67.

41. Kety SS. Human cerebral blood flow and oxygen consumption as related to aging. *J Chron Dis* 1956;**3**:478–86.

42. Sokoloff L. Cerebral circulatory and metabolic changes associated with aging. *Res Publ Assoc Res Nerv Ment Dis* 1966;**41**:237–54.

43. Carlson AP, Brown AM, Zager E, *et al.* Xenon-enhanced cerebral blood flow at 28% xenon provides uniquely safe access to quantitative, clinically useful cerebral blood flow information: a multicenter study. *AJNR Am J Neuroradiol* 2011;**32**(7):1315–20.

44. Gupta R, Jovin TG, Yonas H. Xenon CT cerebral blood flow in acute stroke. *Neuroimaging Clin N Am* 2005;**15**(3):531–42, x.

45. Yonas H, Pindzola RR. Clinical application of cerebrovascular reserve assessment as a strategy for stroke prevention. *Keio J Med* 2000;**49 Suppl** 1:A4–10.

46. Yonas H, Pindzola RP, Johnson DW. Xenon/computed tomography cerebral blood flow and its use in clinical management. *Neurosurg Clin N Am* 1996;**7**(4):605–16.

47. Yonas H, Gur D, Claassen D, Wolfson SK, Jr., Moossy J. Stable xenon-enhanced CT measurement of cerebral blood flow in reversible focal ischemia in baboons. *J Neurosurg* 1990; **73**(2):266–73.

48. Nabavi DG, Cenic A, Henderson S, Gelb AW, Lee TY. Perfusion mapping using computed tomography allows accurate prediction of cerebral infarction in experimental brain ischemia. *Stroke* 2001;**32**(1):175–83.

49. Cenic A, Nabavi DG, Craen RA, Gelb AW, Lee TY. A CT method to measure hemodynamics in brain tumors: validation and application of cerebral blood flow maps. *AJNR Am J Neuroradiol* 2000;**21**(3):462–70.

50. Nabavi DG, Cenic A, Craen RA, *et al.* CT assessment of cerebral perfusion: experimental validation and initial clinical experience. *Radiology* 1999;**213**(1):141–9.

51. Cenic A, Nabavi DG, Craen RA, Gelb AW, Lee TY. Dynamic CT measurement of cerebral blood flow: a validation study. *AJNR Am J Neuroradiol* 1999;**20**(1):63–73.

52. Jain R, Ellika SK, Scarpace L, *et al.* Quantitative estimation of permeability surface-area product in astroglial brain tumors using perfusion CT and correlation with histopathologic grade. *AJNR Am J Neuroradiol* 2008; **29**(4):694–700.

53. Jain R, Scarpace L, Ellika S, *et al.* First-pass perfusion computed tomography: initial experience in differentiating recurrent brain tumors from radiation effects and radiation necrosis. *Neurosurgery* 2007;**61**(4):778–86; discussion 786–7.

54. Ellika SK, Jain R, Patel SC, *et al.* Role of perfusion CT in glioma grading and comparison with conventional MR imaging features. *AJNR Am J Neuroradiol* 2007;**28**(10):1981–7.

55. Royal HD, Hill TC, Holman BL. Clinical brain imaging with isopropyl-iodoamphetamine and SPECT. *Semin Nucl Med* 1985; **15**(4):357–76.

56. Fox PT, Burton H, Raichle ME. Mapping human somatosensory cortex with positron emission tomography. *J Neurosurg* 1987;**67**:34–43.

57. Fox P, Mintun M, Raichle M, Herscovitch P. A noninvasive approach to quantitative functional brain mapping with $H_2^{15}O$ and positron emission tomography. *J Cereb Blood Flow Metab* 1984;**4**:329–33.

58. Herscovitch P, Raichle M, Kilbourn M, Welch M. Positron emission tomographic measurement of cerebral blood flow and permeability – surface area product of water using [^{15}O]water and [^{11}C]butanol. *J Cereb Blood Flow Metab* 1987;**7**:527–42.

59. Guckel F, Brix G, Schmiedek P, *et al.* Noninvasive quantification of cerebral blood volume and blood flow with dynamic MR tomography. Studies of probands and patients with cerebrovascular insufficiency. *Radiologe* 1995;**35**(11):791–800.

60. Guckel F, Brix G, Rempp K, *et al.* Assessment of cerebral blood volume with dynamic susceptibility contrast enhanced gradient-echo imaging. *J Comput Assist Tomogr* 1994;**18**(3):344–51.

61. Rempp KA, Brix G, Wenz F, *et al.* Quantification of regional cerebral blood flow and volume with dynamic susceptibility contrast-enhanced MR imaging. *Radiology* 1994;**193**:637–41.

62. Ostergaard L, Johannsen P, Host-Poulsen P, *et al.* Cerebral blood flow measurements by magnetic resonance imaging bolus tracking: comparison with [^{15}O]H$_2$O positron emission tomography in humans. *J Cereb Blood Flow Metab* 1998;**18**:935–40.

63. Ostergaard L, Weisskoff RM, Chesler DA, Gyldensted C, Rosen BR. High resolution measurement of cerebral blood flow using intravascular tracer bolus passages. Part I: Mathematical approach and statistical analysis. *Magn Reson Med* 1996;**36**(5):715–25.

64. Ostergaard L, Weisskoff RM, Chesler DA, Gyldensted C, Rosen BR. High resolution measurement of cerebral blood flow using intravascular tracer bolus passages. Part II: Experimental comparison and preliminary results. *Magn Reson Med* 1996;**36**(5):726–36.

65. Silva AC, Zhang W, Williams DS, Koretsky AP. Multi-slice brain perfusion imaging of the rat brain by arterial spin labeling using two actively decoupled RF coils. *Proc Int Soc Magn Reson Med,* New York, USA, 1993;632.

66. Zhang W, Silva AC, Williams DS, Koretsky AP. NMR measurement of perfusion using arterial spin labeling without saturation of macromolecular spins. *Magn Reson Med* 1995;**33**(3):370–6.

67. Zhang W, Williams DS, Koretsky AP. Measurement of rat brain perfusion by NMR using spin labeling of arterial water: *in vivo* determination of the degree of spin labelling. *Magn Reson Med* 1993;**29**(3):416–21.

68. Ewing JR, Keating EG, Sheehe PR, *et al.* Concordance of inhalation rCBFs with clinical evidence of cerebral ischemia. *Stroke* 1981;**12**(2):188–95.

69. Ewing JR, Branch CA, Fagan SC, *et al.* Fluorocarbon-23 measure of cat cerebral blood flow by nuclear magnetic resonance. *Stroke* 1990;**21**(1):100–6.

70. Hoeffner EG, Case I, Jain R, *et al.* Cerebral perfusion CT: technique and clinical applications. *Radiology* 2004;**231**(3):632–44.

Chapter

2

Dynamic susceptibility contrast MRI: acquisition and analysis techniques

Matthias J. P. van Osch

Key points

- Dynamic susceptibility contrast MRI is based on monitoring the first passage of a bolus of MR contrast agent through brain tissue.
- Imaging is performed with fast T_2- or T_2*-weighted imaging.
- Either amplitude or phase changes of the MR signal in or around a large artery may be used to measure the arterial input function.
- MR signal changes in brain tissue are transformed to $\Delta R_2^{(*)}$-curves, which are assumed to be linearly related to the concentration contrast agent.
- Deconvolution of the concentration–time curve in the brain tissue with the arterial input function yields the residue function from which the cerebral blood flow (maximum of the residue function), cerebral blood volume (area under the residue function), mean transit time (ratio of cerebral blood volume over cerebral blood flow), and timing parameters can be calculated.
- MR contrast agents can lead to nephrogenic systemic fibrosis in patients with renal failure, and use of MR contrast agent (especially the less stable types) should be restricted in this patient group.

Introduction

From the early start in history man employed "contrast media" to measure flow: Hero of Alexandria proposed for example in 62 AD the use of debris in combination with a sundial to calculate the velocity of the water in Egyptian rivers. Leonardo da Vinci improved this method by using a pig's bladder

attached to a stick with a stone on the other side. Early implementations to measure cerebral blood flow similarly introduced a tracer upstream from the brain, such as nitrous oxide or xenon gas. Even before these early blood flow measurements, functional brain experiments were introduced by monitoring changes in brain volume upon functional activity as an indicator and proof of vasodilatation [1]. It is therefore not surprising that when contrast agents for MRI based on gadolinium chelates were introduced, blood flow measurements were among the first applications. Interestingly, in 1990, for the first time the possibility of localization of neuronal activation was shown using repeated injections of a bolus of contrast agent [2], two years before the BOLD (blood oxygenation level-dependent) effect emerged as the prime tool for functional MRI (fMRI) [3].

Dynamic susceptibility contrast (DSC) perfusion MRI and dynamic CT perfusion (CTP) are the two most employed tracer kinetic perfusion techniques in clinical brain imaging. As discussed in Chapter 1, tracer kinetic techniques rely on the introduction of a contrast agent upstream to measure perfusion in an organ by monitoring how the injected contrast agent is diluted and dispersed while flowing through the vascular system. Both DSC and CTP monitor dynamically the first passage of intravenously injected contrast agents through the brain tissue and a brain-feeding artery: when the contrast agent passes quickly through cerebral tissue this reflects a high blood flow or perfusion, whereas a slow passage corresponds to low blood flow. Another MRI method, steady-state susceptibility contrast imaging, primarily enables the measurement of cerebral blood volume (CBV), using the stable vascular concentration of a blood pool contrast agent. This method has primarily been used in animal studies, but will become increasingly important now that US Food and Drug Administration (FDA)-approved blood pool agents (such as gadofoveset trisodium [Ablavar]) are available for use in humans.

The methodology of DSC-MRI is illustrated in Figure 2.1: dynamic T_2- or T_2^*-weighted scanning visualizes the passage of contrast agent through the brain tissue as loss of MR signal intensity. These signal changes are subsequently converted into $\Delta R_2^{(*)}$ curves ($R_2^{(*)} = 1/T_2^{(*)}(t)$ and $\Delta R_2^{(*)} = 1/T_2^{(*)}(t) - 1/T_2^{(*)}(0)$), which are usually assumed to be linearly proportional

to the concentration–time curve [CTC]). For the rest of this chapter, the notation $\Delta R_2^{(*)}$ will mean that the results are equally applicable to changes in either R_2 or R_2^*, which can be measured by spin- and gradient-echo images, respectively. By selecting voxels in or near a large artery, such as the middle cerebral artery (MCA), an arterial input function (AIF) is measured. This AIF is used to recalibrate the experiment: by measuring the actual shape of the bolus of contrast agent before it enters the cerebral vasculature, the measurements can be corrected for the injection profile and the dispersion of the bolus of contrast agent during the transport

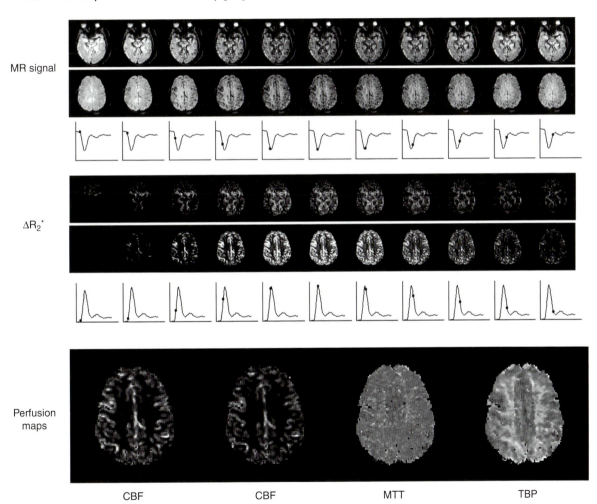

Figure 2.1 Graphical illustration of a DSC-MRI experiment. Upper two rows show dynamic T_2^*-weighted images, demonstrating signal decreases during the passage of contrast agent both near large arteries (upper) and in brain tissue. The graphs below these images indicate the timing as shown on top of the average MR signal evolution during the bolus passage. Middle panel: the MR signal changes are translated into ΔR_2^*-curves, which are proportional to concentration–time curves of the contrast agent. Lower panel: perfusion maps are obtained by deconvolution of the concentration–time curves in tissue with the arterial input function. The maximum value of the residue function equals the cerebral blood flow (CBF), the area under the residue function yields the cerebral blood volume (CBV), the mean transit time (MTT) can be calculated as the ratio of CBV over CBF, and the time-to-bolus-peak (TBP) represents the time point when the maximum concentration is reached.

from the injection site in the arm, via heart and lungs, towards the brain. Subsequently, the $\Delta R_2^{(*)}$-time curve is deconvolved with the AIF for each voxel in the brain tissue, resulting in an estimate of the residue function. As described in Chapter 1, the scaling factor for the residue function is equal to the cerebral blood flow (CBF), the area under the residue function equals the CBV, and the mean transit time (MTT) can be calculated as the ratio of CBV/CBF, assuming no leakage of the agent. Finally, timing parameters can be calculated, such as the time to peak defined as the time point of maximal signal change of the $\Delta R_2^{(*)}$-tissue passage curve. Frequently, these timing parameters are taken relative to the corresponding values of the AIF.

Theory: tracer kinetic model

To derive the theoretical framework of DSC, we start from a model of the microvasculature as a tubular network (Figure 2.2) and we assume that an instantaneous injection is performed in the main artery. The injection is defined as an instantaneous Dirac-like function of a single unit (i.e., 1 ml) produced by the bolus of contrast agent in the artery. Such an injection is of course not possible in real life, but is a mathematical tool to consider in order to derive the theoretical basis of DSC. When this spike of contrast agent arrives at the first bifurcation, the contrast agent will be split according to the ratio of the flows of the branches. In the example shown in Figure 2.2,

the flow in one artery is 60% of the flow in the main artery and therefore 60% of the contrast agent will enter this artery; likewise, the remaining 40% of the contrast agent will enter the other vessel. This process of subdividing the contrast agent will occur at each and every bifurcation and the total amount of contrast agent that arrives in a voxel will, therefore, be equal to the fraction of the flow to this voxel compared with that of the artery (F_{voxel}/F_{artery} with F the flow in ml/s).

When applying this tracer kinetic model to DSC-MRI, two adaptations must be made to this model. First, the contrast agent resides in the plasma and therefore only reflects plasma flow, whereas the aim of perfusion imaging is usually to measure the flow of whole blood (plasma, red blood cells, platelets, white blood cells, etc.). To calculate the concentration of contrast agent ($c(t)$) in whole blood from the concentration of contrast agent in the plasma, the latter has to be multiplied by the hematocrit (H) (i.e., the percentage by volume of red blood cells in whole blood). A complicating factor is that the hematocrit in large vessels is different from the hematocrit in small vessels [4]. Second, as already mentioned, it is not possible to perform an instantaneous injection into an artery. DSC relies therefore on recalibration of the experiment by measuring the arterial CTC. This is known as the AIF. After incorporating these two effects, the following formulas describe the amount of contrast agent ($n(t)$) that arrives at the first bifurcation of our simplified model of the microvasculature:

$$n_{artery}^{plasma}(t) = c_{artery}^{plasma}(t) \cdot F_{artery}^{plasma} = \frac{c_{artery}^{blood}(t)}{1 - H_{large\ vessel}} \cdot F_{artery}^{plasma}$$

$$= AIF(t) \cdot \frac{F_{artery}^{plasma}}{1 - H_{large\ vessel}} \quad (2.1)$$

Subsequently, the contrast agent will move downstream in the vascular tree, which will result in a smaller amount of contrast agent arriving in the voxel:

$$n_{input\ of\ voxel}^{plasma}(t) = AIF(t) \cdot \frac{F_{artery}^{plasma}}{1 - H_{large\ vessel}} \cdot \frac{F_{voxel}^{plasma}}{F_{artery}^{plasma}}$$

$$= AIF(t) \cdot F_{voxel}^{blood} \frac{1 - H_{small\ vessel}}{1 - H_{large\ vessel}} \quad (2.2)$$

Once the contrast agent has entered the microvasculature, it will disperse in the microvasculature bed. This dispersion is caused by the different paths that

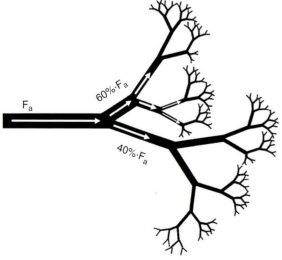

F_a

60%·F_a

40%·F_a

Figure 2.2 Schematic depiction of an arterial tree. In this example the large artery splits into two second-level arteries with 60% of the blood flowing into the upper branch and 40% in the lower artery.

the contrast agent can take through the capillary bed. Transport time differences between shorter and longer paths lead to dispersion. This dispersion is described by the residue function $R(t)$, which reflects the amount of contrast agent residing in the voxel after an instantaneous injection in the feeding artery (Figure 2.3). Since in this hypothetical experiment, the contrast agent will arrive instantaneously in the voxel, the amount of contrast agent residing in the voxel can be calculated as the difference between the total amount of contrast agent (input) and the amount of contrast agent that has left the voxel (output). The residue function can therefore be expressed as a function of distribution times, frequently depicted as $h(t)$ (= the fraction of contrast agent molecules that takes t seconds to transverse the voxel):

$$R(t) = 1 - \int_0^t h(\tau)d\tau \qquad (2.3)$$

It should be noted that $R(0) = 1$, which corresponds to the statement that all contrast agent enters the voxel instantaneously and that outflow of contrast agent only starts at that moment. In a real experiment, the input to the voxel is, however, not an instantaneous injection, but has the shape of the AIF (see Eq. (2.2) and Figure 2.3)[lower row]. This shape can be modeled as a series of instantaneous injections (Figure 2.3)[middle row] and each of these instantaneous injections will result in the retention of contrast agent in the voxel according to the residue function. The total amount of contrast agent present in the voxel is equal to the sum of all responses from the series of instantaneous injections. This procedure is mathematically known as *convolution* and depicted with the symbol $\otimes$:

$$n_{voxel}(t) = AIF(t) \cdot F_{voxel}^{blood} \cdot \frac{1 - H_{small\,vessel}}{1 - H_{large\,vessel}} \otimes R(t)$$
$$(2.4)$$

The above formula can be written as the well-known basic formula of DSC [5]:

$$c_{voxel}(t) = \frac{n_{voxel}(t)}{V_{voxel}}$$
$$= \frac{F_{voxel}^{blood}}{V_{voxel}} \cdot \frac{1 - H_{small\,vessel}}{1 - H_{large\,vessel}} \cdot AIF(t) \otimes R(t)$$
$$= CBF \cdot \frac{1 - H_{small\,vessel}}{1 - H_{large\,vessel}} \cdot AIF(t) \otimes R(t) \quad (2.5)$$

where CBF is the cerebral blood flow in ml/s/ml tissue; multiplication by 6000 yields the familiar units of ml/min/100 ml tissue.

In a DSC experiment $c_{voxel}(t)$ and AIF(t) are measured and the goal is to calculate CBF. From Eq. (2.5) it is clear that this is equivalent to asking the question: "What function can change the AIF into the measured $c_{voxel}(t)$ in tissue?". Mathematically this is equivalent to a deconvolution operation:

$$c_{voxel}(t) \otimes^{-1} AIF(t) = CBF \cdot \frac{1 - H_{small\,vessel}}{1 - H_{large\,vessel}} \cdot R(t)$$
$$(2.6)$$

After noting that $R(0) = 1$ (i.e., all of the tracer remains in the voxel at time 0) and using a literature value for the ratio of large and small vessel hematocrit, the CBF is obtained as the scaling factor of the residue function.

CBV (in ml/100 ml tissue) can be obtained in two different ways:

1. For each contrast agent that traverses a certain route through the microvasculature the volume of its path can be calculated as the product of the flow and the transit time. Taking the integral over the total transit time distribution yields the blood volume:

$$CBV = \frac{Traversed\ volume}{V_{voxel}} = \int_0^\infty \frac{F_{voxel}}{V_{voxel}} \cdot h(t) \cdot dt$$
$$= \int_0^\infty CBF \cdot h(t) \cdot dt$$
$$= -[CBF \cdot R(t) \cdot t]_0^\infty + CBF \cdot \int_0^\infty R(t)dt$$
$$= CBF \cdot \int_0^\infty R(t)dt \qquad (2.7)$$

That is, the volume can determined by calculating the area under the residue function and multiplying by the CBF.

2. From Eq. (2.1), it follows that direct integration of the CTC and AIF can also be used for calculating the CBV as long as the CTC reflects the complete response to the AIF. This is frequently achieved by limiting both the AIF and CTC to the first passage of contrast through the circulatory system.

$$CBV = \frac{\int^{first\,passage} c(t)dt}{\int^{first\,passage} AIF(t)dt} \qquad (2.8)$$

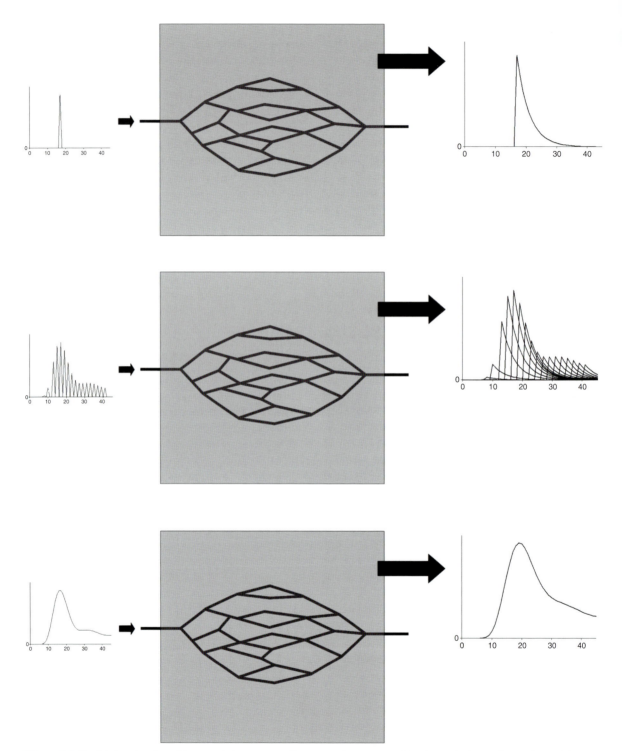

Figure 2.3 Graphical explanation of the convolution operator. First row: an instantaneous injection at the input of a voxel containing a microvascular bed (shown as gray square) results in, for example, an exponentially decaying residue function (graph on the right). Second row: if a series of instantaneous injections is performed at the input to the voxel, each instantaneous injection would result in a similar exponential-shaped response, and the total response would be equal to the sum of all individual responses. Lower row: an arbitrarily shaped AIF can be thought of as a series of instantaneous injections (comparable to the situation of the middle row) and the response is therefore equal to the sum of the response of all instantaneous injections.

Experimental methods: MR contrast agents

Gadolinium chelates were proposed in 1981 as potential MRI contrast agents. These contrast agents were based on the observation that the ion of the rare earth metal gadolinium has a strong influence on the spin-lattice (longitudinal) relaxation rate (R_1) [6]. However, because of the toxicity of the gadolinium ion, it is necessary to encapsulate it using a chelate [7]. The earliest approved contrast agent (1988), Magnevist, employs an ionic linear chelate called diethylenetriaminepentaacetic acid (DTPA) and is primarily excreted by the kidneys, leading to a half-life time in plasma of approximately 60–90 min. Gadodiamide (Gd-DTPA-BMA) is based on a non-ionic linear chelate and is known under the commercial term Omniscan. Later, cyclic ligands have been approved that bind gadolinium extremely tightly; examples are gadoteridol (Gd-HP-DO3A, ProHance) and gadoterate meglumine (Gd-DOTA, Dotarem). Another example of a cyclic molecular structure is gadobutrol (Gadovist), which is provided in a higher concentration of 1.0 mol/l compared to 0.5 mol/l for the other contrast agents. Table 2.1 is an overview of generic and trade names and some properties of both gadolinium and iron oxide agents that have been used for perfusion imaging. Of relevance to MR perfusion imaging, gadolinium-based agents also shorten transverse relaxation times, T_2 and T_2^*, which is usually the basis of most DSC studies.

Whereas gadolinium-based contrast agents were initially considered safe, they have since been linked with the syndrome of nephrogenic systemic fibrosis (NSF, previously known as nephrogenic fibrosing dermopathy) [8]. NSF is characterized by symptoms including scaling, hardening, and tightening of the skin; red or dark patches on the skin; and stiffness. NSF can also cause fibrosis of internal organs. All NSF patients were reported to have renal dysfunction, which has led to new 2010 guidelines of the FDA not to use Magnevist, Optimark (gadoversetamide) and Omniscan in patients with acute kidney injury or with chronic, severe kidney disease and to screen for patients with these conditions or chronically reduced kidney function [9]. After the initial recognition of gadolinium contrast agent involvement in NSF and the introduction of appropriate exclusion criteria, a sharp decline in the number of new cases has been reported; a recent study performed at a large, single hospital showed that when these guidelines were employed, no new cases of NSF were identified among more than 50 000 patients who underwent contrast-enhanced MRI examinations [10]. In summary, NSF is

Table 2.1. Different agents used for perfusion and hemodynamic MR imaging

Generic name	Trade name	Properties, comments
Agents for dynamic susceptibility contrast imaging		
Gadopentetate dimeglumine (Gd-DTPA)	Magnevist	0.5 M
Gadodiamide (Gd-DTPA-BMA)	Omniscan	
Gadoteridol (Gd-HP-DO3A)	ProHance	
Gadoversetamide	OptiMark	
Gadoterate meglumine (Gd-DOTA)	Dotarem	
Gadobenate dimeglumine (Gd-BOPTA)	MultiHance	Slightly higher relaxivity compared with agents listed above, due to transient protein binding
Gadubutrol	Gadovist 1.0, Gadograf	1 M Gd concentration (others are 0.5 M)
Agents for steady-state susceptibility contrast imaging		
Gadofosveset trisodium	Ablavar, Vasovist	Albumin binding leads to longer plasma half-life
Ferumoxytol	Feraheme	Ultrasmall superparamagnetic iron oxide (USPIO). Approved for iron replacement therapy, not as a contrast agent

21

a serious disease, but risk for NSF seems only to exist in patients with renal failure. The use of MR contrast agent in these patients should therefore be avoided, whereas in other patients the use can still be considered relatively safe.

Experimental methods: from MR signal to contrast agent concentration

The first step in the post-processing of DSC data is to convert the measured changes in MR signal intensity to the concentration of the contrast agent. The approach for this may differ for the AIF and the tissue passage curves, and depends on the employed sequence, i.e., spin or gradient echo sequences.

Arterial input function: spin echo sequences

When measuring the properties of contrast agents in human or bovine blood plasma with spin echo sequences, several properties emerge. First of all, the longitudinal and transverse relaxation of most contrast agents shows a linear relationship with concentration. Moreover, larger relaxivities (both R_1 and R_2) are found at lower field strengths [11]. Also, it has been observed that the AIF measurement is problematic within an artery for several reasons, most important of which are flow-related artifacts. Therefore, it is common practice to measure the AIF in a region just outside a major artery, usually the middle cerebral artery (MCA). In this approach, 5–10 voxels are selected in the neighborhood of a main artery that show typical characteristics of an AIF, as explained in Chapter 1 (early time of arrival, high amplitude, small full-width-at-half-maximum, etc.). Average ΔR_2 vs. time curves are then calculated. By calculating the signal decrease of the MR signal relative to the mean MR signal prior to the arrival of contrast agent, other determinants of the MR signal unrelated to the passage of contrast agent are corrected for:

$$\Delta R_2(t) = \frac{1}{TE} \ln \frac{\overline{S}_{pre-bolus}}{S(t)} \qquad (2.9)$$

where $\overline{S}_{pre-bolus}$ is the mean signal intensity prior to contrast agent arrival and TE is the echo time.

The main justification for the selection of the AIF outside from a main artery comes from a study in dogs that has only been published in the form of an abstract [12]. In this abstract, an average correlation between spin echo AIF measurements and blood

sampling of 0.82 was found. This is a rather low correlation and certainly justifies more research on this topic, especially because of the recent renewed interest in spin echo sequences. Moreover, the apparent contradiction between the selection of the AIF outside a major artery and the supposedly exclusive microvascular sensitivity of spin echo sequences has yet to be resolved.

Arterial input function: gradient echo sequences

In vitro experiments in whole blood have shown that for gradient echo sequences the relaxation rate depends quadratically on the concentration of contrast agent [13–15]. Furthermore, studies have also shown that the phase of the MR signal changes as a function of contrast agent concentration, in addition to the amplitude. Finally, as with spin echo sequences, partial volume effects can lead to non-linearities in the relation between the contrast agent concentration and the relaxation rate. These three effects are discussed in the next sections.

Intra-arterial measurement of the AIF: magnitude of MR signal

MR contrast agents reside within the plasma of blood and remain extracellular. This implies that red blood cells and other blood cells create contrast agent-free pockets of a different, constant susceptibility within the blood plasma that has a homogeneous, but dynamically changing concentration of contrast agent. The contrast agent in the blood plasma will lead to a shorter transverse relaxation time (T_2 effect) and the spins in the blood plasma exchange relatively quickly with the spins within the red blood cells, as the mean time for diffusive flow of water is approximately 5 ms [16]. Probably more important is the fact that the compartmentalization of contrast in blood due to the presence of red blood cells leads to field inhomogeneities that result in a fast dephasing of the transverse magnetization and therefore a much shorter T_2^*. The importance of compartmentalization due to red blood cells is evidenced by the observation that the relaxivity is dependent on the hematocrit [13, 14]. These processes therefore result in a quadratic relation between ΔR_2^* and concentration of contrast agent [13–15]. As stated above, however, this quadratic relation is dependent on the hematocrit, thereby hampering the quantification of the contrast agent concentration.

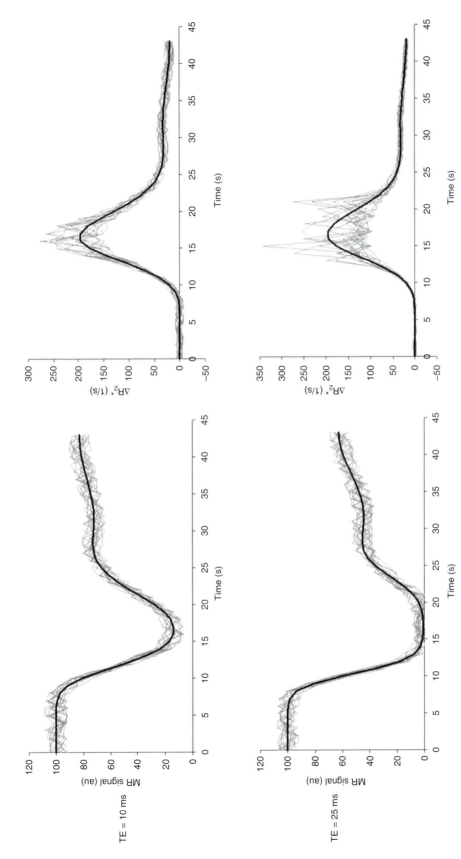

Figure 2.4 When measuring the AIF within an artery with a gradient echo sequence, signal depletion to the noise level is a major issue. When using a dual echo sequence with a short first echo time of 10 ms (see upper row), the MR signal at peak concentration is just a little bit higher than zero (black line), with noise present on the signal (gray curves), the noise amplification on the ΔR_2^*-curves is evident (see right graphs, signal-to-noise ratio (SNR) = 20 as defined as the pre-bolus signal over the standard deviation of the pre-bolus signal). When using a single echo time of 25 ms (lower row) the effects are amplified. Figure based on an AIF typical for a double dose contrast agent at 1.5 T or a single dose at 3 T and quadratic relation between ΔR_2^* and concentration of contrast agent.

When measuring the AIF based on the intravascular signal, a complication is the signal depletion during the passage of contrast agent. Figure 2.4 models a single dose injection at 3 T or a double dose injection at 1.5 T [17]. At the peak of the bolus passage, the concentration of contrast agent is so high (approximately 6.5 mM for a single dose contrast agent of 0.1 mM/kg body weight or 13 mM for a double dose) that the MR signal is almost completely gone. When noise is present, a further complicating factor is that noise is rectified, i.e., by looking at the amplitude of the MR signal, the sign of the signal is lost, leading to a "Rician" noise distribution instead of Gaussian distributed noise. This will amplify the noise during the peak of the bolus passage and lead to an underestimation of the peak concentration [18]. A possible solution for this problem is the use of dual- or multi-echo gradient echo sequences with a short echo time for the AIF measurement and a longer echo time for the measurements in brain tissue [19–21].

Intra-arterial measurement of the AIF: phase of MR signal

MR contrast agents have a significantly higher magnetic susceptibility than blood or other human tissues. This implies that during the passage of contrast agent the susceptibility of the artery will change and will differ from the surroundings. Any inhomogeneous distribution of magnetic susceptibility leads to changes of magnetic field as governed by the Maxwell equations. If the artery is modeled as an infinitely long cylinder, the magnetic field disturbances can be calculated analytically; for more arbitrary geometries or configurations, the resulting magnetic field can only

be estimated numerically. After taking the sphere of Lorentz into account, the internal and external magnetic field disturbance for an infinite cylinder can be obtained analytically from the Maxwell equations:

Inside cylinder : $\quad \Delta B = \dfrac{\Delta\chi}{6} \cdot \left(3\,cos^2\theta - 1\right) \cdot B_0$

$$(2.10)$$

Outside cylinder : $\quad \Delta B = \dfrac{\Delta\chi}{2} \cdot \dfrac{a^2}{\rho^2} \cdot sin^2\theta \cdot cos2\phi \cdot B_0$

$$(2.11)$$

where $\Delta\chi$ is the magnetic susceptibility difference between the interior and exterior of the cylinder, a the radius of the cylinder, ρ and φ the polar coordinates in the plane perpendicular to the cylinder, and θ the angle of the cylinder with respect to the main magnetic field (Figure 2.5). It is important to note that the magnetic field changes are highly dependent on the angle of the cylinder with respect to the main magnetic field. For a cylinder parallel to B_0, there are no magnetic field changes outside the vessel and there is a positive field change inside; for a cylinder at the "magic angle" (i.e., $3cos^2\theta - 1 = 0$, or $\theta = 54.7°$) the internal magnetic field change is zero and for a cylinder perpendicular to B_0 there is a negative magnetic field change inside the cylinder and the external magnetic field changes are maximized. For all other angles, there are both internal and external magnetic field changes. Finally, it should be noted that the internal magnetic field change is homogeneous over the cylinder. For DSC, the magnetic susceptibility difference is linearly related to the concentration of contrast agent and changes in the local magnetic field translate linearly into a phase change of the MR signal:

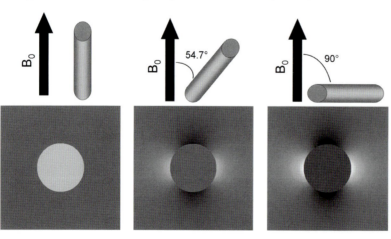

Figure 2.5 Magnetic field disturbances around a long cylinder with a different magnetic susceptibility compared to the surroundings. From left to right: a cylinder parallel to B_0 leads only to a magnetic field change within the cylinder; a cylinder at the magic angle of 54.7° does not result in magnetic field changes within the cylinder, but exhibits a multi-lobular pattern of magnetic field changes outside the cylinder; a cylinder perpendicular to B_0 experiences a magnetic field decrease internally, and a multi-lobular pattern externally.

$$\Delta\theta(t) = \theta(t) - \theta_{pre-bolus}$$

$$= \gamma \cdot TE \cdot \chi_m \cdot [Gd] \cdot \left(\frac{1}{2}\cos^2\theta - \frac{1}{6}\right) \cdot B_0 \quad (2.12)$$

where γ is the gyromagnetic constant, TE the echo time, χ_m the molar susceptibility of the contrast agent (3.4×10^{-4} for Gd-DTPA), and [Gd] the gadolinium concentration. When assuming a typical maximum concentration of gadolinium of 5 mM and an echo time of 25 ms, at 3 T, a phase change of 650° will result due to the presence of the contrast agent in an artery parallel to B_0. This implies that unwrapping of the phase signal is necessary before it can be used for concentration measurements. This can either be performed by comparing the phase of each time point with the phase of the preceding time point and keeping the phase change within $-\pi$ and $+\pi$, or by employing a multi-echo sequence with short echo time used for measuring the artery [14].

The phase of the MR signal is only seldom used, mainly because many different sources may cause phase changes, such as field inhomogeneities arising from air spaces, scanner drift, and different phase offsets for separate coil elements of multi-channel receive coils. However, using the phase for measuring the concentration of the AIF is feasible, because first of all it depends on measuring phase changes, and second because the first passage takes less than 1 min, so scanner drift should be relatively small over this time period. Recently, phase-based AIF measurements have also been adopted in DCE-MRI (dynamic contrast-enhanced MRI: a dynamic T_1-weighted technique especially used to measure the permeability of tumors, explained in Chapter 4), where the much smaller echo time results in smaller, but still detectable phase changes. The main theoretical advantages for using the phase over the amplitude of the MR signal are the higher signal-to-noise ratio (SNR) of phase images, and the fact that the phase depends on the average concentration of contrast agent within the artery, implying that the proportionality constant is independent of the hematocrit [14].

To measure the AIF by the phase of the MR signal, voxels must be selected within the artery, the angle of the artery with respect to the main magnetic field must be determined, and for each voxel the difference with the pre-bolus phase must be calculated. Subsequently, the phase–time curve needs to be unwrapped for each voxel and then all curves can be averaged. Equation (2.12) can then be used to translate the phase–time curve in a concentration–time curve.

Intra-arterial measurement of the AIF: partial volume effects

Whether you use the amplitude or the phase of the MR signal for the AIF measurement, the low spatial resolution of DSC will inevitably lead to partial volume effects. Whereas normally partial volume effects decrease the measured response proportional to the partial volume fraction, in DSC partial volume effects can lead to shape changes and can result both in an under- and overestimation of the concentration contrast agent [15]. To understand the origin of these artifacts, it is important to summarize the different factors that influence the MR signal during the passage of contrast agent: for an artery parallel to B_0, the amplitude of the intravascular signal will decrease for a higher concentration of the contrast agent, the phase of this signal will increase, and there will be no signal changes outside of the vessel; for an artery perpendicular to B_0, there will also be an amplitude decrease within the artery, but the phase of the blood signal will decrease and outside the vessel there will be regions with positive and negative phase changes (Figure 2.5). The complex MR signal of a voxel within an artery parallel to B_0 will traverse a spiral-like trajectory in the complex plane as a consequence of the decreasing amplitude and increasing phase of the MR signal during the upslope of the contrast agent passage and a reversed trajectory during the down-slope (Figure 2.6a). In a voxel composed of both tissue and artery, the total signal will be a complex sum of the blood signal and the signal from the direct surroundings. This can result in non-linear effects, because for one concentration intra- and extravascular components can add constructively, whereas for another, the signals will interact destructively (Figure 2.6b–d). When ignoring these effects and by calculating the ΔR_2^*-curves from the total voxel signal, artifacts will be apparent, including double spiking [Figure 2.6b], single spiking (Figure 2.6c), and underestimation (Figure 2.6d). Because of the unique feature that for an artery parallel to B_0 no magnetic field changes occur outside of the vessel, i.e., the MR signal from the surroundings is independent of the concentration of contrast agent within the vessel, correction for partial volume effects can be achieved. This is done by estimating the origin of the spiral in the complex plane and by shifting the spiral to the origin of the complex plane. In vivo experiments have validated this approach and did result in a more reproducible

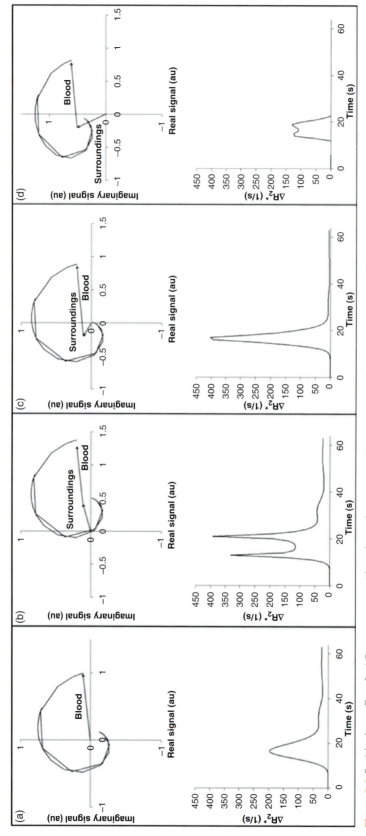

Figure 2.6 Partial volume effects for AIF measurements with gradient echo sequences. Upper row shows the theoretical evolution in the complex plane of the MR signal of intra-arterial blood and the surroundings during a bolus passage of contrast agent through an artery parallel to B_0. The lower row shows the resulting ΔR_2^*-curves calculated from the total signal of a voxel completely within the artery (left side, no partial volume) and three voxels affected by partial volume effects. The three voxels with partial volume show from left to right: shape distortion by two peaks, overestimation of the AIF, and an underestimation of the AIF. This highlights the challenge of acquiring an accurate AIF from DSC data, and is a large source of its error for quantitative hemodynamic measurements.

determination of the AIF, although the approach has only been used once in clinical studies to date [15].

Extra-arterial AIF measurement

As shown in Figure 2.5, the presence of the contrast agent within the vessel also leads to magnetic field changes outside of the vessel when the artery is not oriented parallel to the main magnetic field. This implies that both phase changes and signal loss due to dephasing will occur outside of an artery. This opens up the possibility of measuring the AIF by selecting voxels outside, but close to the artery, similar to the approach employed in spin echo DSC. Measuring the AIF outside of a vessel almost automatically implies that it is taken for granted that the height of the AIF cannot be determined and that only the correct shape can be determined. Measuring the correct amplitude of the AIF requires an accurate determination of both the radius of the vessel and the distance of the selected voxels to the vessels (see Eqs. (2.10 and 2.11.)). When aiming for the correct shape of the AIF, it is important to know where to select voxels, whether to use amplitude or phase data, whether to use a linear or a quadratic calibration curve for the amplitude data, and to study the influence of the contrast agent passage through the tissue surrounding the artery. These issues have primarily been studied by means of modeling and simulation of the physics underlying MR signal formation [22–24]. These studies show that measurements completely outside the artery provide the best option to measure the correct shape of the AIF, because partial volume effects lead to too much distortion closer to the artery. Furthermore, these studies show that when using the amplitude of the MR signal, a linear relation should be used to convert ΔR_2^* into concentration of contrast agent and that the passage of contrast agent through the tissue surrounding the artery seriously affects the shape of the measured AIF. It has been proposed to eliminate the tissue contribution from the AIF by subtracting signal from pure tissue [25]. This approach is, however, sensitive to the selection of the region of interest in the reference tissue, and more research is needed on this topic. Finally, it was shown that the phase of MR signal provides a better opportunity to measure the shape of the AIF when measuring outside an artery than the amplitude of the MR signal [23]. Therefore, it should be advised based on the current status of the literature to measure the AIF in tissue outside an artery perpendicular to B_0, such as the M1 segment of the MCA, and to use the phase of the MR signal, whenever possible.

Measuring the tissue signal

MR signal formation in heterogeneous media, such as brain tissue, is governed by processes both at the microscopic and mesoscopic scale (Figure 2.7). On the microscopic scale the MR signal behaves as it would in a tube with a homogeneous solution of contrast agent. Due to faster spin–spin interactions with increasing contrast agent concentration, the transverse relaxation time R_2 decreases. This increase is linear with the concentration of contrast agent [11, 26] and when employing gradient echo sequences, the relaxivity is higher due to dephasing near the contrast agent molecules. At the mesoscopic scale the compartmentalization of the contrast agent within the microvasculature leads to large magnetic field

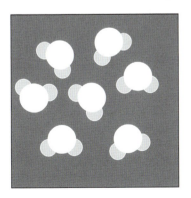 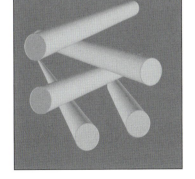 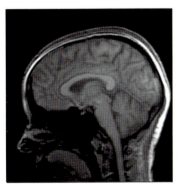

Microscopic scale   Mesoscopic scale   Macroscopic scale

Figure 2.7 The transverse relaxation rate ($\Delta R2^{(*)}$) is influenced by processes on the microscopic scale (e.g., spin–spin interactions), at the mesoscopic scale (on the scale of capillaries and other small vessels) and the macroscopic scale (e.g., air cavities that disturb the magnetic field). The micro- and mesoscopic scale are important in DSC to understand the influence of contrast agent on the MR signal in brain tissue.

inhomogeneities. This affects the MR signal in three ways: diffusion through the field inhomogeneities leads to differences in phase history between spins and thus to dephasing (both for spin and gradient echo sequences); averaging over spins precessing at different frequencies due to field inhomogeneities in tissue surrounding the vessels leads to dephasing (only in gradient echo imaging); and due to the differences in orientation of the vessels (see Eq. (2.10)) the intravascular magnetic field differs between vessels, leading as well to dephasing (only for gradient echo sequences) [27]. The relative importance of these three processes depends on the diffusion constant of tissue, the radii of the vessels, and the CBV. First, Monte Carlo simulations were performed to study the cumulative effect of all three processes [28–30]; later, analytical models were developed [29, 31–34].

In analytical models, two different regimes are recognized: the diffusion narrowing (or motionally averaged regime) and the static dephasing regime (Figure 2.8). In the diffusion narrowing regime the diffusion length (i.e., the averaged distance that a proton traverses during one echo time) is comparable to or larger than the scale of the field inhomogeneities. Or, in a more formal definition:

$$\frac{R^2}{D} \times \gamma \times B_0 \ll 1 \text{ diffusion narrowing regime} \quad (2.13)$$

where R is the radius of the vessel and D the water diffusion coefficient. In this diffusion narrowing regime, protons diffusing around the capillaries will accumulate phase dependent on the exact trajectory of the random walk. Phase history will therefore be different for each proton and dephasing will occur, which will result in an MR signal decrease. Because the path of each spin follows a random walk, the

dephasing cannot be refocused and signal loss will also occur with spin echo sequences.

In the static dephasing regime, the diffusion length is much smaller than the scale of the field inhomogeneities and the phase accumulation will be independent of the exact random walk (Figure 2.8b). The phase accumulation will therefore mainly depend on the (average) position of the proton, which can be fully refocused by spin echo sequences, but will still result in signal loss due to dephasing for gradient echo sequences. The formal definition is as follows:

$$\frac{R^2}{D} \times \gamma \times B_0 \gg 1 \text{ static dephasing regime} \quad (2.14)$$

From Eqs. (2.13 and 2.14) it is also clear that there is an intermediate regime between the diffusion narrowing and static dephasing regimes for which it has not yet been possible to develop analytical models. This regime can be approximated either by means of interpolation [31] or by Monte Carlo simulations [32].

Simulations for a realistic constellation of the vasculature consisting of a distribution of arterioles, capillaries, and venules show a linear relation between ΔR_2^* (gradient echo sequences) and concentration of contrast agent, and a non-linear relationship for ΔR_2 (i.e., spin echo), both of which also depend on CBV [31, 32]. Furthermore, it should be noted that the relaxivity in brain tissue is much higher than in blood or a homogeneous solution of contrast agent. Without correcting for these different relaxivities, CBF may be overestimated by more than a factor of 5 [31].

The most important difference between spin and gradient echo sequences was already noticed in the hallmark paper by Boxerman et al.: spin echo sequences have an exclusive microvascular sensitivity, whereas gradient echo sequences are also sensitive to

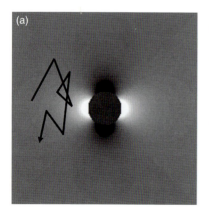
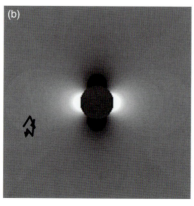

Figure 2.8 (a) In the diffusion narrowing regime, the average diffusion distance is comparable or large compared to the spatial scale of the magnetic field inhomogeneity. Dephasing due to differences in phase history cannot adequately be refocused and spin echo sequences will exhibit dephasing and more severe signal loss. (b) In the static dephasing regime (SDR), the diffusion distance of water protons is small compared to magnetic field disturbances of a vessel. This implies that spin echo sequences can adequately refocus dephasing processes, thus minimizing signal loss.

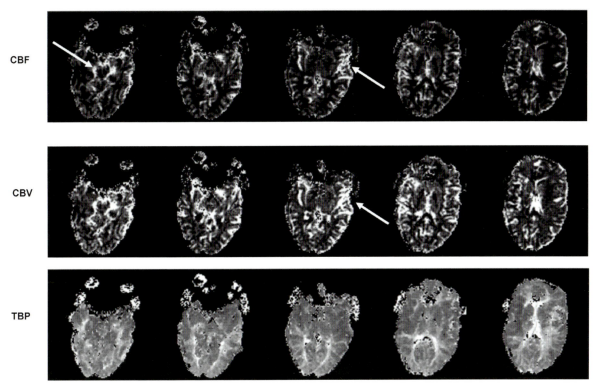

Figure 2.9 Example of large vessel artifacts in gradient echo DSC. Arrows points to large arteries showing high cerebral blood flow (CBF) and cerebral blood volume (CBV) in combination with short time-to-bolus-peak (TBP) partly obscuring the microvascular perfusion signal.

larger vessels [28]. This is caused by the fact that the diffusion length in brain tissue is small compared to the field inhomogeneities of vessels with a radius larger than 50 μm (i.e., the static dephasing regime in which spin echo sequences will refocus the dephasing). Alternatively, when the diffusion length is significant compared to the field inhomogeneities of capillaries with a radius of approximately 3–5 μm (the diffusion narrowing regime), there is signal loss on both gradient and spin echo sequences. This implies that gradient echo images will suffer from large vessel artifacts (Figure 2.9), whereas spin echo sequences will better reflect microvascular perfusion, although at a much lower SNR.

Experimental methods: acquisition optimization

For monitoring the presence of contrast agent, the sequence should be sensitive to the T_2 or $T_2^\star$ effect of the contrast agent. For an optimal sequence this implies that the echo time should be relatively large to achieve a significant reduction of the signal during the bolus passage. This results in a typical echo time of 40 ms at 1.5 T and 30 ms at 3 T for a single dose of contrast agent with gradient echo imaging and an echo time of 60–80 ms for spin echo measurements. Furthermore, it is necessary to sample the bolus passage curve at high temporal resolution to enable tracer kinetic analysis. By means of simulations it has been shown that the dynamic scan time (i.e., the time between two acquisitions of the same slice) should be 1.5 s or less [35, 36]. To enable whole brain coverage, it is clear that fast sampling schemes are necessary. Single-shot echo-planar imaging (EPI) is the most used readout acquisition, although 3D sequences that employ echo-shifting have also been used. Echo-shifting is a technique that enables the delayed readout of the echo until after the next excitation pulse: the echo time is larger than the repetition time of the sequence [37].

Analysis techniques: deconvolution

Deconvolution is the mathematical process that answers the question "How does the microvasculature change the shape of contrast agent passage from the AIF into the tissue concentration curve?" (see Eq. (2.6)). Two phenomena hamper this process: first, the

29

curves are noisy and second, the curves may be shifted in time with respect to each other, that is the tissue concentration curve can be delayed compared to the AIF, depending on where the AIF is measured and if significant vascular stenoses are present between the AIF location and tissue. Many deconvolution algorithms have been developed, but the three most important are singular value decomposition (SVD), Fourier transformation, and statistical inference approaches, such as maximum-likelihood expectation-maximization. These three methods will be briefly introduced.

Singular value decomposition (SVD)

SVD has by far been the most applied deconvolution technique due to its use in the original papers of Ostergaard *et al.* and because it has been distributed freely [38]. The basis of SVD is that the deconvolution process can be written as a matrix multiplication [38, 39]:

$$
\begin{bmatrix} c_{voxel}(0) \\ c_{voxel}(1) \\ \vdots \\ c_{voxel}(N) \end{bmatrix} = \Delta t \times \underbrace{\begin{bmatrix} AIF(0) & 0 & \cdots & 0 \\ AIF(1) & AIF(0) & \cdots & 0 \\ \vdots & \vdots & \ddots & \vdots \\ AIF(N) & AIF(N) & \cdots & AIF(0) \end{bmatrix}}_{A = U \times S \times V^T}
$$

$$
\times \underbrace{\begin{bmatrix} R(0) \\ R(1) \\ \vdots \\ R(N) \end{bmatrix}}_{b} \times F_{voxel} \qquad (2.15)
$$

The AIF data are frequently filtered to eliminate noise and to correct for discretization errors, before the AIF matrix is decomposed into three matrices with **U** and **V** orthogonal matrices and **S** a diagonal matrix. The inverse of **A** equals **V·W·U**^{T}, with **W** a diagonal matrix with values equal to 1/S along the diagonal. Noise is generally suppressed by setting values of **W** to zero when **S** is less than a certain threshold. This threshold, sometimes known as the amount of regularization, is chosen as a fixed percentage of the maximal value of **S** or can be estimated automatically depending on the SNR of the data [40]. Finally, the vector **b** can be obtained by multiplying **A**$^{-1}$ and **c(t)** and the maximum value of **b** yields the CBF.

As can be seen from Eq. (2.15), this original SVD approach assumes that the contrast agent passage through the artery always immediately precedes the tissue passage curve. However, because only a single AIF is used for all voxels in brain tissue, this assumption almost never holds. Therefore, an improved SVD implementation to correct for possible delay effects was introduced, named block-circulant SVD; other solutions for this problem have also been proposed (see [41] for an overview).

Fourier transformation

The first MRI paper to measure CBF by means of deconvolution employed the Fourier transformation, which seems a logical choice based on the well-known mathematical rule that deconvolution in the time domain is equal to division of the Fourier-transformed functions in the Fourier domain [42]:

$$
h(t) = f(t) \otimes g(t) \Leftrightarrow F(h) = F(f) \times F(g) \qquad (2.16)
$$

$$
R(t) = c(t) \otimes^{-1} AIF(t) \Leftrightarrow R(t) = F^{-1}\left(\frac{F(c(t))}{F(AIF(t))}\right)
$$

$$(2.17)$$

with **F** the Fourier operator. As with SVD-based methods, the noise should also be suppressed when using the Fourier approach. This is frequently performed by multiplying the Fourier transform of the tissue passage with a low-pass filter, like the Wiener filter, assuming that the noise has much higher frequencies than the slowly changing concentration passage through the brain tissue [38, 42]. Different timings between the AIF and the tissue passage curves (such as delay effects) affect the results of Fourier deconvolution less than SVD approaches, because the Fourier transform translates timing differences into phase differences, effectively eliminating their influence on the residue function.

Statistical inference methods

The deconvolution methods that perhaps most accurately recover the shape of residue function are based on statistical inference methods. These methods estimate the residue function by maximizing the probability of measuring the observed tissue concentration–time curve given the known AIF. The maximum-likelihood maximization-estimation method is an example of this category of deconvolution methods [43]. The residue function is estimated iteratively and noise suppression is performed by stopping the optimization process before noise amplification affects the residue function too much. Note that more sophisticated algorithms have also been proposed [44], and other related approaches such as Gaussian process deconvolution [45].

Analysis techniques: vessel-size imaging

Gradient and spin echo sequences have different sensitivities for vessels with different radii as shown in the original paper of Boxerman et al. [28]. This has led to the idea that by combining gradient and spin echo sequences, the mean radius of the vasculature can be obtained [46]. This could be of clinical importance, for instance for estimating angiogenesis in brain tumors. Vessel-size imaging is used both as a steady-state approach, especially in animals, using iron oxide particles as contrast agent, but also dynamically by interleaving gradient and spin echo acquisitions in a DSC experiment.

Analysis techniques: recalibration via other quantitative MRI techniques

Although most aspects of DSC-MRI are well understood, absolute quantification in a clinical setting is still challenging. The most quantitative techniques rely on multi-echo sequences, hampering whole brain coverage, which is preferred for clinical applications. Therefore, several methods have been proposed that combine a qualitative perfusion map with a quantitative measurement to rescale the qualitative maps to the correct units. The best-known technique that relies on this principle is the "bookend technique" that combines DSC with quantitative CBV measurements based on quantitative T_1-mapping before and after contrast agent injection [47]. However, rescaling with respect to the venous output curve [48], arterial spin labeling [49], or quantitative phase-contrast flow measurements have also been proposed [50]. All these approaches rely on the assumption that the qualitative perfusion maps provide the correct relative values, and that only a scaling factor is missing.

Analysis techniques: qualitative perfusion imaging and summary parameters

While it is clear that measurement of the AIF is necessary to calculate CBF by means of a deconvolution analysis, many clinical studies employ qualitative analysis of DSC data without any correction for the AIF. Such approaches are based on the fitting of a model function to the tissue concentration curve to limit the analysis to the first passage of the contrast agent. Subsequently, descriptive parameters of the first passage function are calculated. Frequently, a gamma variate function is used to fit the tissue signal. Often, these descriptive parameters are coined with physiological names, like MTT, CBF, and CBV [51]. However, only CBV can in fact be correctly measured in this way. To understand this, it is essential to realize that MTT could be calculated from the normalized first moment of the output of the tissue following an instantaneous injection:

$$\frac{\int_0^\infty c_{out} \cdot t \cdot dt}{\int_0^\infty c_{out} \cdot dt} = \frac{F_{tissue} \cdot \int_0^\infty h(t) \cdot t \cdot dt}{F_{tissue} \cdot \int_0^\infty h(t) dt} = \frac{CBV}{CBF} = MTT$$

(2.18)

However, first, DSC does not involve an instantaneous injection, and, second, it is not the *output* concentration that is measured, but the amount of contrast agent that still resides in the microvasculature. The first factor could ideally be corrected by dividing out the same parameters from the AIF. The second issue, however, results in a dependency on the shape of the residue function. A broad residue function would retain the contrast agent longer and therefore result in a different first moment than for a much tighter residue function [52].

Whereas qualitative analysis of DSC clearly provides useful information on the microvascular status of a patient, it is advisable to avoid the use of physiological names for the parameter maps, since this might lead to erroneous interpretations. Rather, it is better practice to use names that describe the summary parameter shown in the parameters maps (e.g., full-width-half-maximum, or first moment of the first passage).

Pitfalls: delay and dispersion

The tracer kinetic model assumes that the measured AIF reflects the shape of the input function of the microvasculature in the tissue voxel. The AIF is frequently measured in a large artery such as the MCA, and any changes in the AIF shape before entering the voxel will be included in the residue function, and will therefore be interpreted as microvascular dispersion instead of large vessel properties. AIF delay can be adequately corrected for when a proper deconvolution method is used and when the maximum value of the residue function is used as an estimate of the CBF instead of the first element of the residue function. In healthy vessels, it is also a reasonable assumption that

31

dispersion of the AIF is negligible compared with the dispersion that takes place at the capillary level. However, when pathology is present, dispersion in the large vessels can be much larger and lead to a severe underestimation of the CBF. The only way to discriminate between dispersion at the macro- and microvascular level is to measure the AIF closer to the input of the microvasculature, and this has led to the local-AIF approach. In the local-AIF approach, the measurement of an individual AIF for each voxel in brain tissue is attempted by searching for "AIF-like" voxels in the direct neighborhood, or by using the arterial signal from a principle component analysis [53, 54]. While this approach appears promising, it remains to be determined whether local AIFs are a better estimation of the actual input of the microvasculature or not. The main reservation to their use comes from the fact that as the vessels get nearer to the voxels, they are also smaller, and partial volume errors associated with tissue in the voxel increase.

Pitfalls: T$_1$ effects

Gadolinium-based MR contrast agents not only affect water transverse relaxation rates, but also increase longitudinal relaxation rates when water molecules are in close proximity to the gadolinium atom. When converting MR signal changes to concentration–time curves by calculating $\Delta R_2^{(*)}$-curves, it is implicitly assumed that the transverse effects of the contrast agent dominate. Due to the demands on a high temporal resolution, DSC relies on fast imaging. Thus, the longitudinal magnetization will not completely recover before the next excitation pulse is applied. T$_1$ effects can therefore significantly influence the MR signal. This is particularly true for the first-pass, intravascular signal where the gadolinium concentration is very high. Gadolinium does not normally enter brain tissue when the blood–brain barrier (BBB) is intact (see below), so this is less of a problem in normal brain tissue. T$_1$ effects can be minimized by using a flip angle significantly smaller than the "Ernst-angle" (which would normally be chosen to maximize SNR, but is also the flip angle that is most sensitive to T$_1$ changes). Alternatively, dual- or multi-echo sequences can be used to eliminate these T$_1$ effects by using the first echo as a reference:

$$\Delta R_2^{(*)} = \frac{1}{TE_2 - TE_1}\left(ln\frac{S_{TE_1}(t)}{S_{TE_2}(t)} - ln\frac{S_{TE_1}(0)}{S_{TE_2}(0)} \right) \quad (2.19)$$

Pitfalls: Blood–brain barrier disruption

The tight packing of endothelial cells in the brain forms the so-called "blood–brain barrier" (BBB), which protects the brain from harmful substances in the circulation, resulting in a limited passive transport from blood to the extravascular space. The BBB provides also an effective barrier for all MR contrast agents in healthy subjects, but in many diseases, including stroke, cancer, and inflammatory diseases, leakage of the contrast agent out of the vasculature is frequently observed. As described in Chapter 1, the leakage of contrast agent complicates the tracer kinetic model, and will lead to quantification errors in the measurements of the concentration of contrast agent in tissue. Both effects will lead to errors in CBF and CBV estimates, and therefore it is always important to identify BBB leakage when interpreting perfusion maps.

The leakage of contrast agent can be modeled by incorporating the leakage into the residue function. For an intact BBB, the residue function reflects the amount of contrast agent present in the (micro)vasculature of the voxel after an instantaneous injection at the input of the voxel. When the BBB is no longer intact, the contrast agent will leak out of the vasculature and the leakage will be proportional to the concentration difference between the intra- and extravascular compartments. This implies that the residue function will no longer return to zero after the contrast agent has passed through the microvascular bed, but will remain elevated. At each time point, the total amount of contrast agent that has extravasated can be calculated from the leakage during the previous time points, assuming that the back flow of contrast agent from tissue to venules is small. Because DSC is in principle restricted to the first passage of contrast agent through the brain, this is expected to be a relatively good approximation:

$$R_{total}(t) = R_{intravascular}(t) + R_{leakage}(t)$$
$$= R_{intravascular}(t) + \kappa \int_0^t R_{intravascular}(t)dt \quad (2.20)$$

where κ describes the leakage weighted by the CBV [55]. A reasonable estimate of the transfer constant can be obtained by solving this equation, but the feasibility of this approach is highly dependent on an accurate estimate of the shape of the residue function, and therefore on the SNR of the acquisition.

This approach is based on the assumption that intra- and extravascular contrast agent influences the MR signal in a similar manner. This is almost certainly an oversimplification, because the compartmentalization of intravascular contrast agent can lead to a different relaxivity compared with the more homogeneously distributed extravascular contrast agent [56].

The second problem with the leakage of contrast agent is that the T_1 shortening will lead to a higher extravascular MR signal. Indeed, since extravascular spins are in a fast exchange regime, the presence of contrast agent will quite effectively shorten the T_1 of all extravascular spins. This T_1 signal enhancement can therefore be much larger than the signal loss due to T_2 or T_2^* effects. This leads to the frequently observed post-bolus overshoot (Figure 2.10). One simple solution to mitigate T_1 effects in DSC experiments is to reduce the flip angle of the 90° radio-frequency (RF) pulse. The drawback of this approach is that this reduces the contrast-to-noise ratio of the resultant bolus passage. Also, it is important to remember that the exact behavior of the signal as a function of gadolinium concentration in tissue will depend on the sequence flip angle, repetition time, and echo time, being a balance of both T_1 and T_2^* effects. Therefore, it is also possible that the post-bolus signal shows an undershoot. Because of these two different manifestations of BBB breakdown on the ΔR_2^*-curves, the effects on CBV can also be

either an over- or an underestimation. It is advisable therefore to be cautious in the interpretation of perfusion parameters such as CBV when contrast agent leakage is present.

Finally, another approach to mitigating the adverse T_1 effects of leakage of contrast through a damaged BBB is the "pre-bolus" approach [57]. In this method, a small preload (several ml) of contrast is injected and allowed to equilibrate before the DSC experiment is performed. This preload has the effect of reducing the concentration gradients between the vessel and the tissue that drive the extravasation and lowers the T_1 of the extravascular compartment.

Steady-state susceptibility contrast

Most gadolinium contrast agents have a relatively short plasma half-life, between 60 and 90 min. The DSC approach described above relies on accurate imaging of the concentration of a rapid IV bolus of contrast during its first pass through the tissue of interest. This high-concentration contrast phase only lasts about 5–10 s in the brain due to the high CBF and low CBV. Thus, fast imaging sequences must be used, with EPI being the prototypical method. EPI has limited SNR (necessitating large voxel sizes) and usually suffers from susceptibility-induced geometric distortion, which can result in poor image quality.

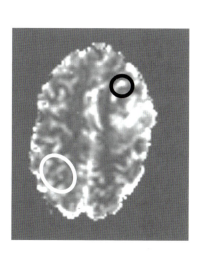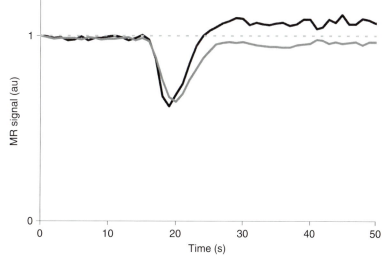

Figure 2.10 Example of a DSC study in a patient with a brain tumor. In the enhancing rim of the tumor (black curve and circle), a post-bolus overshoot can be seen, caused by T_1 enhancement due to the extravasation of contrast agent. Contralateral tissue (gray curve and white circle) depicts normal signal changes during a bolus passage. Image on the left depicts the (erroneous) CBV map.

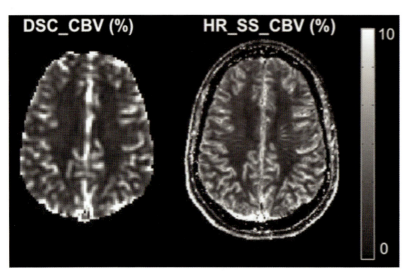

Figure 2.11 Comparison of CBV maps created using standard DSC methods (left) and steady-state susceptibility imaging (right) using the blood pool USPIO agent, ferumoxytol. Because of the stable blood concentration of ferumoxytol, one can acquire longer duration images with increased SNR and spatial resolution. Note the fine detail of the vascular structures in the white matter that can be attained using the steady-state susceptibility contrast method. It is likely such methods will provide better characterizations of small or heterogeneous lesions. Image courtesy of Dr. Thomas Christen, Stanford University, Stanford, CA, USA. HR-SS, high-resolution steady-state.

Animal studies have been performed using a different class of contrast agents known as "blood pool" agents. These agents are either large molecules or particles, such that they are retained on their passage through the kidneys, or they have high protein binding. An example of the former is ferumoxytol, an ultrasmall superparamagnetic iron oxide (USPIO), which has a mean particle diameter of about 20 nm and an intravascular half-life of about 15 hrs. It is approved in the USA not as a contrast agent, but rather as a treatment for iron-deficiency anemia. It can therefore be used "off-label." It has a very strong susceptibility effect with its greatest effect on T_2^*. Another blood pool agent that has been approved in the USA is gadofosveset trisodium (Ablavar), which is primarily a T_1 agent.

Because blood pool contrast agents have a long and stable vascular half-life, they are ideal for measuring CBV with high SNR. Instead of acquiring most of the information during the 5–10 s bolus, longer pulse sequences can be employed. The higher SNR can be traded off in a flexible fashion for higher spatial resolution, which is required to fully characterize small or heterogeneous lesions (Figure 2.11). It is important to realize that these agents can be rapidly injected and imaged using standard DSC methods to measure CBF, MTT, and other transit time parameters. However, once they reach a steady state in the vasculature, only CBV may be measured. Quantitative CBV measurements are facilitated by the lack of flow-weighting and the ability to more easily identify voxels composed of 100% blood (e.g., the superior sagittal sinus). For the T_1 gadolinium agent gadofosveset trisodium, high-resolution T_1-weighted images can be acquired pre- and post-contrast to measure CBV. Alternatively, a susceptibility agent such as ferumoxytol, which has a strong effect on T_2^*/T_2, can be used in conjunction with gradient and spin echo imaging pre- and post-contrast to measure total and microvascular CBV, respectively. Such applications may allow the calculation of mean vessel size, which is affected by angiogenesis and has found use in tumor studies [46].

Because multiple boluses do not need to be used, steady-state susceptibility contrast approaches are ideal for CBV challenge paradigms to assess vascular reactivity or functional activation. Because the contrast is in a steady state, regions of the brain experiencing increased CBV will change in signal intensity. Challenge paradigms are discussed in more detail in Chapters 7 and 8, but one example is task-based functional MRI (fMRI) for brain activation. USPIO contrast agents like ferumoxytol have been shown to confer a 2- to 3-fold increased SNR for fMRI in prior animal studies [58]. A similar SNR increase has been observed in human contrast-enhanced fMRI studies [59]. An example of USPIO-enhanced fMRI in a subject performing a simple finger-tapping paradigm is shown in Figure 2.12.

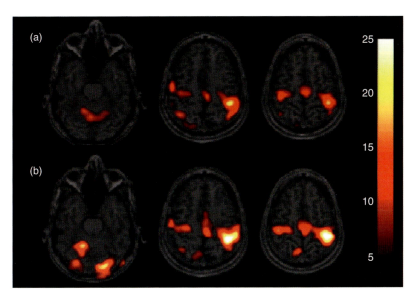

Figure 2.12 Example of task-based brain activation fMRI studies acquired (a) before and (b) after the administration of a blood pool USPIO agent, ferumoxytol. The paradigm used was right finger-tapping. Note the improved t-statistics and the increased number of activated voxels in the contrast-enhanced study, which is particularly evident in the cerebellum. Such contrast-to-noise ratio (CNR) gains in fMRI with blood pool contrast agents have been previously demonstrated in animals, but are only now beginning to be used in humans. Image courtesy of Dr. Deqiang Qiu and Dr. Michael Moseley, Stanford University, Stanford, CA, USA.

Conclusions

Both dynamic and steady-state susceptibility contrast have been used to glean hemodynamic information from brain MRI studies. DSC monitors the first passage of contrast agent through tissue and a large artery, and by deconvolution of these two curves, the residue function may be obtained, from which the hemodynamic properties of the microvasculature, including CBF, CBV, and MTT, can be derived. However, converting MR signal changes into concentration of contrast agent is challenging. Since many patients already receive gadolinium contrast agent for the detection of leakage by means of the post-gadolinium T_1-weighted imaging, DSC is readily integrated into clinical protocols. Probably for this reason, as well as the fact it can be done quickly and usually produces robust hemodynamic maps, DSC is the most often used MR perfusion technique in clinical practice. However, a remaining challenge is to transfer the accurate quantification techniques from the research community into clinical products, enabling more physiologically accurate perfusion maps to be acquired and used in clinical decision-making. Steady-state susceptibility contrast, which relies on the use of long blood half-life contrast agents, allows the potential for higher resolution and more accurate CBV maps. This previously was only possible in animal studies, but agents approved for humans are beginning to be used, and will likely improve a wide range of hemodynamic measurements, including fMRI for brain activation.

References

1. Sherrington C, Roy C. On the regulation of the blood-supply of the brain. *J Physiol* 1890;**11**(1–2): 85–108.

2. Belliveau J, Rosen B, Kantor H, *et al.* Functional cerebral imaging by susceptibility contrast NMR. *Magn Reson Med* 1990;**14**:538–46.

3. Ogawa S, Tank DW, Menon R, *et al.* Intrinsic signal changes accompanying sensory stimulation: functional brain mapping with magnetic resonance imaging. *Proc Natl Acad Sci U S A* 1992;**89**: 5951–5.

4. Fahraeus R, Lindquist T. The viscosity of the blood in narrow capillary tubes. *Am J Physiol* 1931;**96**:562–8.

5. Zierler K. Theoretical basis of indicator-dilution methods for measuring flow and volume. *Circ Res.* 1962;**10**:393–407.

6. Weinmann HJ, Brasch RC, Press WR, Wesbey GE. Characteristics of gadolinium-DTPA complex: a potential NMR contrast agent. *AJR Am J Roentgenol* 1984;**142**:619–24.

7. Runge VM. Safety of approved MR contrast media for intravenous injection. *J Magn Reson Imaging* 2000;**12**(2):205–13.

8. Grobner T. Gadolinium–a specific trigger for the development of nephrogenic fibrosing dermopathy and nephrogenic systemic fibrosis? *Nephrol Dial Transplant* 2006; **21**(4):1104–8.

9. Administration USFaD. *New Warnings for Using*

Gadolinium-based Contrast Agents in Patients with Kidney Dysfunction. 2010; Available from: http://www.fda.gov/Drugs/DrugSafety/ucm223966.htm.

10. Wang Y, Alkasab TK, Narin O, *et al.* Incidence of nephrogenic systemic fibrosis after adoption of restrictive gadolinium-based contrast agent guidelines. *Radiology* 2011;**260**(1): 105–11.

11. Pintaske J, Martirosian P, Graf H, *et al.* Relaxivity of Gadopentetate Dimeglumine (Magnevist), Gadobutrol (Gadovist), and Gadobenate Dimeglumine (MultiHance) in human blood plasma at 0.2, 1.5, and 3 Tesla. *Invest Radiol* 2006;**41**(3): 213–21.

12. Porkka I, Neuder M, Hunter G, *et al.*, editors. Arterial input function measurement with MRI. *Proc Intl Soc Magn Reson Med* San Francisco, USA, 1991;120.

13. Akbudak E, Hsu R, Li Y, Conturo T, editors. Delta R2* or delta phase contrast effects in blood. *Proc Intl Soc Magn Reson Med*, Sydney, Australia, 1998; 1197.

14. Conturo TE, Akbudak E, Kotys MS, *et al.* Arterial input functions for dynamic susceptibility contrast MRI: requirements and signal options. *J Magn Reson Imaging* 2005;**22**(6): 697–703.

15. van Osch MJ, Vonken EJ, Viergever MA, van der Grond J, Bakker CJ. Measuring the arterial input function with gradient echo sequences. *Magn Reson Med* 2003; **49**(6):1067–76.

16. Paganelli CV, Solomon AK. The rate of exchange of tritiated water across the human red cell membrane. *J Gen Physiol* 1957; **41**(2):259–77.

17. Manka C, Traber F, Gieseke J, Schild HH, Kuhl CK. Three-dimensional dynamic susceptibility-weighted perfusion MR imaging at 3.0 T: feasibility

and contrast agent dose. *Radiology* 2005;**234**(3):869–77.

18. Ellinger R, Kremser C, Schocke MF, *et al.* The impact of peak saturation of the arterial input function on quantitative evaluation of dynamic susceptibility contrast-enhanced MR studies. *J Comput Assist Tomogr* 2000;**24**(6):942–8.

19. Perman W, Gado M, Larson K, Perlmutter J. Simultaneous MR acquisition of arterial and brain signal-time curves. *Magn Reson Med* 1992;**28**:74–83.

20. Vonken EJ, van Osch MJ, Bakker CJ, Viergever MA. Measurement of cerebral perfusion with dual-echo multi-slice quantitative dynamic susceptibility contrast MRI. *J Magn Reson Imaging* 1999; **10**(2):109–17.

21. Newbould RD, Skare ST, Jochimsen TH, *et al.* Perfusion mapping with multiecho multishot parallel imaging EPI. *Magn Reson Med* 2007; **58**(1):70–81.

22. Bleeker EJ, van Buchem MA, van Osch MJ. Optimal location for arterial input function measurements near the middle cerebral artery in first-pass perfusion MRI. *J Cereb Blood Flow Metab* 2009; **29**(4):840–52.

23. Bleeker EJ, van Buchem MA, Webb AG, van Osch MJ. Phase-based arterial input function measurements for dynamic susceptibility contrast MRI. *Magn Reson Med* 2010;**64**(2):358–68.

24. Kjolby BF, Mikkelsen IK, Pedersen M, Ostergaard L, Kiselev VG. Analysis of partial volume effects on arterial input functions using gradient echo: a simulation study. *Magn Reson Med* 2009; **61**(6):1300–9.

25. Thornton RJ, Jones JY, Wang ZJ. Correcting the effects of background microcirculation in the measurement of arterial input functions using dynamic susceptibility contrast MRI of the brain. *Magn Reson Imaging* 2006; **24**(5):619–23.

26. Reichenbach JR, Hacklander T, Harth T, *et al.* 1H T_1 and T2 measurements of the MR imaging contrast agents Gd-DTPA and Gd-DTPA BMA at 1.5T. *Eur Radiol* 1997;**7**(2):264–74.

27. Albert M, Huang WE, Lee J, Patlak C, Springer C. Susceptibility changes following bolus injections. *Magn Reson Med* 1993;**29**:700–8.

28. Boxerman J, Hamberg L, Rosen B, Weisskoff R. MR contrast due to intravascular magnetic susceptibility perturbations. *Magn Reson Med* 1995;**34**:555–66.

29. Kennan R, Zhong J, Gore J. Intravascular susceptibility contrast mechanisms in tissues. *Mag Reson Med* 1994;**31**(1):9–21.

30. Buxton RB. *Introduction to Functional Magnetic Resonance Imaging.* New York: Cambridge University Press, 2002.

31. Kiselev VG. On the theoretical basis of perfusion measurements by dynamic susceptibility contrast MRI. *Magn Reson Med* 2001; **46**(6):1113–22.

32. Kjølby BF, Østergaard L, Kiselev VG. Theoretical model of intravascular paramagnetic tracers effect on tissue relaxation. *Magn Reson Med* 2006;**56**(1):187–97.

33. Yablonskiy D, Haacke E. Theory of NMR signal behavior in magnetically inhomogeneous tissues: the static dephasing regime. *Magn Reson Med* 1994;**32**:749–63.

34. Jensen JH, Chandra R. NMR relaxation in tissues with weak magnetic inhomogeneities. *Magn Reson Med* 2000;**44**(1):144–56.

35. van Osch MJ, Vonken EJ, Wu O, *et al.* Model of the human vasculature for studying the influence of contrast injection speed on cerebral perfusion MRI. *Magn Reson Med* 2003; **50**(3): 614–22.

36. Knutsson L, Stahlberg F, Wirestam R. Aspects on the accuracy of cerebral perfusion

parameters obtained by dynamic susceptibility contrast MRI: a simulation study. *Magn Reson Imaging* 2004; **22**(6):789–98.

37. Klarhofer M, Dilharreguy B, van Gelderen P, Moonen CT. A PRESTO-SENSE sequence with alternating partial-Fourier encoding for rapid susceptibility-weighted 3D MRI time series. *Magn Reson Med* 2003;**50**(4):830–8.

38. Ostergaard L, Weisskoff RM, Chesler DA, Glydensted C, Rosen BR. High resolution measurement of cerebral blood flow using intravascular tracer passages. Part I: Mathematical approach and statistical analysis. *Magn Reson Med* 1996;**36**:715–25.

39. Wu O, Ostergaard L, Weisskoff RM, *et al*. Tracer arrival timing-insensitive technique for estimating flow in MR perfusion-weighted imaging using singular value decomposition with a block-circulant deconvolution matrix. *Magn Reson Med* 2003;**50**(1): 164–74.

40. Murase K, Shinohara M, Yamazaki Y. Accuracy of deconvolution analysis based on singular value decomposition for quantification of cerebral blood flow using dynamic susceptibility contrast-enhanced magnetic resonance imaging. *Phys Med Biol* 2001;**46**(12):3147–59.

41. Knutsson L, Stahlberg F, Wirestam R. Absolute quantification of perfusion using dynamic susceptibility contrast MRI: pitfalls and possibilities. *MAGMA* 2010;**23**(1):1–21.

42. Rempp KA, Brix G, Wenz F, *et al*. Quantitation of cerebral blood flow and volume with dynamic susceptibility contrast-enhanced MR imaging. *Radiology* 1994;**193**:637–41.

43. Vonken EP, Beekman FJ, Bakker CJ, Viergever MA. Maximum likelihood estimation of cerebral blood flow in dynamic susceptibility contrast MRI. *Magn Reson Med* 1999; **41**(2):343–50.

44. Willats L, Connelly A, Calamante F. Improved deconvolution of perfusion MRI data in the presence of bolus delay and dispersion. *Magn Reson Med* 2006;**56**(1):146–56.

45. Andersen IK, Szymkowiak A, Rasmussen CE, *et al*. Perfusion quantification using Gaussian process deconvolution. *Magn Reson Med* 2002;**48**(2): 351–61.

46. Dennie J, Mandeville JB, Boxerman JL, *et al*. NMR imaging of changes in vascular morphology due to tumor angiogenesis. *Magn Reson Med* 1998;**40**:793–9.

47. Sakaie KE, Shin W, Curtin KR, *et al*. Method for improving the accuracy of quantitative cerebral perfusion imaging. *J Magn Reson Imaging* 2005;**21**(5):512–19.

48. Lin W, Celik A, Derdeyn C, *et al*. Quantitative measurements of cerebral blood flow in patients with unilateral carotid artery occlusion: a PET and MR study. *J Magn Reson Imaging* 2001; **14**(6):659–67.

49. Zaharchuk G, Straka M, Marks MP *et al*. Combined arterial spin label and dynamic susceptibility contrast measurement of cerebral blood flow. *Magn Reson Med* 2010;**63**(6):1548–56.

50. Bonekamp D, Degaonkar M, Barker PB. Quantitative cerebral blood flow in dynamic susceptibility contrast MRI using total cerebral flow from phase contrast magnetic resonance angiography. *Magn Reson Med* 2011; **66**(1):57–66.

51. Weisskoff RM, Chesler D, Boxerman JL, Rosen BR. Pitfalls in MR measurement of tissue blood flow with intravascular tracers: which mean transit time? *Magn Reson Med* 1993;**29**(4): 553–8.

52. Perthen JE, Calamante F, Gadian DG, Connelly A. Is quantification of bolus tracking MRI reliable without deconvolution? *Magn Reson Med* 2002; **47**(1):61–7.

53. Alsop DC, Wedmid A, Schlaug G, editors. Defining a local arterial input function for perfusion quantification with bolus contrast MRI. *Proceedings of the International Society for Magnetic Resonance in Medicine* Honolulu, Hawai'i, 2002.

54. Calamante F, Morup M, Hansen LK. Defining a local arterial input function for perfusion MRI using independent component analysis. *Magn Reson Med* 2004;**52**(4): 789–97.

55. Vonken EP, van Osch MJ, Bakker CJ, Viergever MA. Simultaneous quantitative cerebral perfusion and Gd-DTPA extravasation measurement with dual-echo dynamic susceptibility contrast MRI. *Magn Reson Med* 2000; **43**(6):820–7.

56. Pannetier N, Debacker C, Mauconduit F, Christen T, Barbier E, editors. Does R2* increase or decrease when contrast agent extravasates? *Proceedings of the International Society for Magnetic Resonance in Medicine*, Montreal, Canada, 2011; 3916.

57. Sorensen AG, Reimer P. *Cerebral MR Perfusion Imaging*. Stuttgart New York: Thieme, 2000.

58. Leite FP, Tsao D, Vanduffel W, *et al*. Repeated fMRI using iron oxide contrast agent in awake, behaving macaques at 3 Tesla. *Neuroimage* 2002;**16**(2):283–94.

59. Qiu D, Zaharchuk G, Christen T, Ni WW, Moseley ME. Contrast-enhanced functional blood volume imaging (CE-fBVI): Enhanced sensitivity for brain activation in humans using the ultrasmall superparamagnetic iron oxide agent ferumoxytol. *Neuroimage* 2012;**62**(3): 1726–31.

Arterial spin labeling-MRI: acquisition and analysis techniques

Xavier Golay

Key points

- ASL is a non-invasive method to measure brain perfusion.
- It is based on the "tagging" of arterial water spins using dedicated pulse sequences.
- In general two consecutive acquisitions are performed, with and without a labeling pulse, and the difference between them provides information on CBF.
- The general pulse sequence scheme can be separated into two components: a preparation scheme followed by a readout.
- Many techniques exist for ASL, combining different preparations and readouts, and specific clinical problems might require different optimized pulse sequences.
- It is an intrinsically quantitative methodology, but requires pharmacokinetic modeling to estimate values for the perfusion.
- From modeling, one can estimate at least three parameters using ASL: the blood flow (BF), the arterial part of the blood volume (aBV) and the bolus arrival time (BAT).
- The method is signal-to-noise ratio limited and benefits from high magnetic fields.

Introduction

Among the various existing MRI methods for measuring cerebral blood flow (CBF), arterial spin labeling (ASL) occupies a special position, as much for its plethora of different techniques and MRI sequences, as for the fact that each of these methods is completely non-invasive, and therefore does not require injection of any exogenous contrast agent or

tracer. Indeed, as suggested in the name of the technique, the measurement of perfusion is obtained by non-invasive labeling of arterial blood water spins (i.e., inversion or saturation) proximal to the tissue of interest. These labeled spins are then imaged at a later time point after exchange with the tissue magnetization [1]. As such, ASL can be repeated over a time period of a few seconds or minutes, and has a wide range of applications in the brain, from basic neuroscience to applied clinical neurology, as well as for the assessment of organ homeostasis anywhere in the body. A comprehensive description of the applications of ASL is given in later chapters of this book; this chapter will focus on the technique itself. While applications of ASL in the body are still an emerging topic, its application in neurology and neuroscience is now well established, and most of this introductory chapter will therefore refer to the brain, unless otherwise stated [2].

It is useful to separate the neurological applications of ASL into three main groups. The first group pertains to basic neuroscience, and refers to the applications of ASL as a means to measure CBF changes upon functional activation or pharmacological challenge [3, 4]. The second large group of applications of ASL is in neurovascular diseases, in which CBF is assessed as a surrogate marker of tissue viability [5, 6]. It should be noted that in addition to CBF, other vascular parameters, such as the bolus arrival time (BAT) or arterial blood volume (aBV) may play an important role in these diseases [7, 8]. The last group of applications refers to the use of ASL in non-neurovascular diseases, in which the distribution of flow to the tissue is not compromised, but the measurement of CBF might provide some insight into the physiology of the brain, and how it is affected by

Clinical Perfusion MRI: Techniques and Applications, ed. Peter B. Barker, Xavier Golay, and Greg Zaharchuk. Published by Cambridge University Press. © Peter B. Barker, Xavier Golay, and Greg Zaharchuk 2013.

diseases, including neurodegeneration and lesions [9–11]. As we will see later in this chapter (as well as throughout this book), the particular application will dictate the best ASL methods to be used. Note that similar comments could be made as well for non-neuro perfusion measurements, where in general, one needs to know a priori if the delivery route of the label will be affected or not, depending on the disease considered [12, 13].

In this introductory chapter, the basic principles of ASL will be described, and the important parameters defining the different sequences will be explained, so as to allow the reader to understand how they can be used in the chapters that follow. The main MRI acquisition strategies, together with their method of quantification will also be described, and finally, the potential problems and artifacts will be addressed.

Theory
Physiological parameters measured by ASL

As eluded to in the previous chapters, discussions of perfusion can be misleading without proper definition of the terms. In fact, the perfusion of an organ can be defined as the steady-state delivery rate of nutrients to this organ, as explained in detail in Chapter 1. Several parameters can define perfusion, the two most important being the quantity of blood reaching the tissue per unit of time and volume or specific blood flow (f – in the brain, the cerebral blood flow or CBF), and the amount of blood present in the tissue or blood volume (V – in the brain, the cerebral blood volume or CBV). Note that both blood flow and perfusion are sometimes used synonymously in the literature. It is important here to reiterate that the specific blood flow f considered here is really a rate and should be expressed in units of $[1/t]$ with $t =$ time, and not a flux, which would be expressed in $[D^3/t]$ with $D =$ distance. For historical reasons, f is usually given in [ml/100 g/min] or milliliters per 100 g of tissue per minute. Note that these units are not very appropriate as generally, no information can be obtained about the tissue mass of the individual voxels within an image and, in practice, a mean brain density of 1 g/ml is generally assigned to all voxels. The blood volume V is easier to understand, and is usually expressed either as a percentage of the volume (in [%]), or in [ml/100 g] or milliliters per 100 g of tissue. Note that the two units for measuring V are only identical in the case of the blood density being equal to 1 g/ml.

It is very important to note that, unlike other perfusion measurements which make use of an exogenous intravascular contrast agent, ASL is in principle unable to directly assess the entire blood volume, because it is extracted almost completely from the capillaries during the first pass through the vasculature [14–16]. Indeed, for a measurement of V to be possible, one must be able to discriminate the tracer present in the blood from that in the extravascular tissue. As such, a few studies have looked into the possibility of measuring the extraction rate of labeled water spins into the tissue to get indirect access to V [17, 18], but it is generally accepted that such ASL measurements lack the signal-to-noise ratio (SNR) to provide accurate estimates of this parameter [19].

ASL was developed mainly to measure f. However, recent improvements in the methodology enabled the estimation of other important physiological parameters. One very important parameter for neurovascular diseases is related to the time of arrival of the blood to the tissue, named in the literature as bolus arrival time (BAT), or arterial transit time (ATT) [7, 8, 20]. By measuring the signal at different time points after the labeling of the blood, it is possible to detect the first arrival of the blood in the tissue, defined as the BAT. It is interesting to note that this time is usually short because effort is made to label the blood as closely to the tissue of interest as possible. This time is generally much shorter than the one measured using exogenous contrast agents, which are injected through the antecubital vein in the arm of the patient. In addition, note that the BAT is also directly dependent on the technique used to label the blood, and it is therefore not generally comparable across studies.

In addition, it is also possible to measure the aBV, or blood present in the arteries before it exchanges with the tissue. Here as well, as long as the tracer stays within a certain compartment, it is possible to assign the signal measured to that particular compartment, and several methods have been proposed for measuring aBV, either by continuous nulling of the exchanged signal [20] or by subtraction of the ASL signal present with and without crusher gradients to selectively destroy the arterial blood signal [8].

Quantification and modeling

The theoretical basis for quantifying the ASL signal comes from indicator dilution theory [21]. As this theory has been explained in detail in the two previous chapters, only a short summary is presented here, by means of introduction to kinetic modeling for ASL. This theory describes the kinetics of an injected tracer of a known concentration into a system. For the case of an open system, corresponding to the medical use of a freely diffusible tracer such as a gas, the changes in the concentration of the tracer over time in the system will be equal to the flow multiplied by the difference in concentration between the input and output of the system, as seen in Chapter 1:

$$\frac{dc_t(t)}{dt} = f \cdot (c_a(t) - c_v(t)) \tag{3.1}$$

Where $c_t(t)$ is the measured concentration of the agent in the tissue, f is the blood flow, $c_a(t)$ is the arterial blood concentration of the tracer and $c_v(t)$ the venous blood concentration. If the tracer becomes well mixed within the organ, the measured tissue concentration is the same as the outflowing blood or venous blood concentration, corrected for the difference in densities of the agent in the organ vs. the blood. In the brain, this correction factor is called the blood–brain partition coefficient, and is written as λ: $c_t(t) = \lambda c_v(t)$. With this assumption, it is possible to find a simple solution to Eq. [3.1], which becomes:

$$\lambda c_v(t) = c_t(t) = f \cdot \int_0^t (c_a(\tau) - c_v(\tau)) d\tau \tag{3.2}$$

or

$$f(t) = \frac{\lambda c_v(t)}{\int_0^t (c_a(\tau) - c_v(\tau)) d\tau} \tag{3.3}$$

This equation is sometimes referred to as the single compartment Kety equation, as it was proposed originally by Kety and Schmidt to measure perfusion of the whole brain using nitrous oxide (N$_2$O) [22, 23]. Looking at Eq. (3.2), one can directly see that the estimated flow will vary over time and will only reach a steady-state value once the concentration in the tissue reaches a steady-state concentration. For a typical flow value of 60 ml/min/100 g, such a steady state is reached after about 12 min, as shown in Figure 3.1.

This method can easily be used in ASL, where labeled water can be assumed to act as a freely diffusible tracer. Note that this assumption is not fully correct, and measurements performed on rhesus monkeys have shown that at normal flow values only

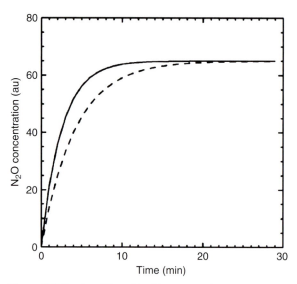

Figure 3.1 Simulated Kety–Schmidt concentration curves of N$_2$O over time. Note the delay in reaching steady state between the arterial (plain line) and venous (dotted line) tracer concentrations, directly related to the blood flow delivered to the organ.

about 80–90% of water can be considered as freely diffusible [24]. However, using ASL, it has been shown that deviations from this assumption can only be detected at high magnetic fields in small animals, where CBF can be as high as 3–5 times larger than in humans [15], while it has a very limited effect in humans, where the transit times are much larger and of the same order of magnitude as the longitudinal relaxation rate of the blood T_{1a}.

However, in order to be able to use this theory for quantification of perfusion in practice, the basic equation needs to be slightly modified to account for the fact that a short-lived pulsed input function and not a continuous infusion is being used [21]. Equation 3.2 becomes then:

$$c_t(t) = f \cdot \int_0^t c_a(\tau)(R(t - \tau)) d\tau = f \cdot c_a(\tau) \otimes R(t) \tag{3.4}$$

With $\otimes$ representing the convolution symbol. As such, the measured tissue concentration $c_t(t)$ of tracer is equal to the flow f multiplied by the convolution of the arterial input function $c_a(t)$ by the tissue response function, also known as residue function, $R(t)$.

Based on this theory, Buxton et al. [25] proposed a simple model to estimate tissue perfusion, by rewriting Eq. (3.4) in MRI terms. This is known as the general kinetic model:

$$\Delta M = 2 \cdot \alpha \cdot M_{a,0} \cdot f \cdot \int_0^t c(t) \cdot r(t - \tau) \cdot m(t - \tau) d\tau$$

$$(3.5)$$

where $M_{a,0}$ is the equilibrium magnetization of blood, $c(t)$ is the delivery function, and the arterial input function (AIF) is equal to $c_a(t) = 2 \cdot \alpha \cdot M_{a,0} \cdot c(t)$. The residue function $r(t - \tau)$ describes the washout of labeled spins from a voxel, and $m(t - \tau)$ includes the longitudinal magnetization relaxation effects, not present in Kety's original theory. To solve this equation, Buxton *et al.* originally made the general assumption of a "plug flow" or rectangular AIF [25]. In addition, they discard any effect of dispersion and dilution of the bolus, and arrive at the following equations, known as the "standard kinetic model," which gives, for the case of pulsed ASL (see below, Experimental methods):

$$c(t) = \begin{cases} 0, & t < \tau_a \\ e^{-tR_{1a}} & \tau_a \le t < \tau_d \\ 0, & t \ge \tau_d \end{cases} \quad (3.6)$$

$$r(t) = e^{\frac{-ft}{\lambda}} \quad (3.7)$$

$$m(t) = e^{-tR_{1t}} \quad (3.8)$$

Solving Eq. (3.5) using Eqs. (3.6–3.8) gives a step wise defined equation:

$$\Delta M(t) = \begin{cases} 0, & t < \tau_a \\ \dfrac{-2 \cdot \alpha \cdot M_{a,0} \cdot f}{\delta R} e^{-R_{1a} \cdot t} (1 - e^{-\delta R \cdot (t - \tau_a)}), & \tau_a \le t < \tau_d \\ \dfrac{-2 \cdot \alpha \cdot M_{a,0} \cdot f}{\delta R} e^{-R_{1a} \cdot \tau_d} (1 - e^{-\delta R \cdot (t - \tau_a)}) e^{-R_{1app} \cdot (t - \tau_d)}, & t \ge \tau_d \end{cases} \quad (3.9)$$

where, $\delta R = R_{1a} - R_{1app}$ and $R_{1app} = R_{1t} + \frac{f}{\lambda}$, also called the apparent tissue relaxation rate. A similar set of equations can be obtained for continuous ASL experiments (see below, Experimental methods), with the only difference that $c(t)$ in Eq. (3.6) will then be constant for continuous ASL (CASL), whereas it is subject to T_{1a} decay for pulsed ASL (PASL). As can be seen, various parameters such as the transit time τ_a, blood–tissue partition coefficient λ, $M_{a,0}$, R_{1a}, and R_{1t} need to be estimated or measured in order to obtain quantitative CBF values. The difference between the models used to quantify most ASL sequences lies in the number of estimated vs. measured parameters.

Experimental methods

The basic scheme used by ASL is the following (see Figure 3.2). At the most general level, ASL is based on the consecutive (interleaved) acquisition of two MRI experiments [1]. In the first experiment arterial water spins are labeled upstream from the tissue of interest by the combined application of field gradients and radiofrequency (RF) pulses. This labeling usually consists of an inversion of the arterial water magnetization. An image is then acquired after a suitable delay time, during which the RF-labeled arterial water spins have the time to travel to the tissue of interest, and to exchange there with the stationary spins located in the extravascular compartment. In the second experiment, a sham labeling is performed, to set the system in the same conditions as the first experiment, and a second image of the tissue of interest is acquired. Ideally, the only difference between the labeled acquisition and this "control" acquisition is that the latter has no manipulation of the arterial spins. Both labeling and control acquisitions are acquired after a time TI ("inversion time"). The difference between both images will provide a signal proportional to the exchanged water magnetization and therefore water delivered to the tissue at the time TI. Note that the labeling of the water spins will decrease due to longitudinal decay (T_{1blood}) during its transit to the tissue and through the capillary bed. This, combined with the fact that the blood volume in most organs is usually small – typically about 2–4% in the brain for example – makes ASL an SNR-limited technique, in particular in the white matter [26]. As such, numerous ways of improving the SNR have been introduced, from new ways to label the water spins, to advanced readout techniques providing the best possible SNR per unit time.

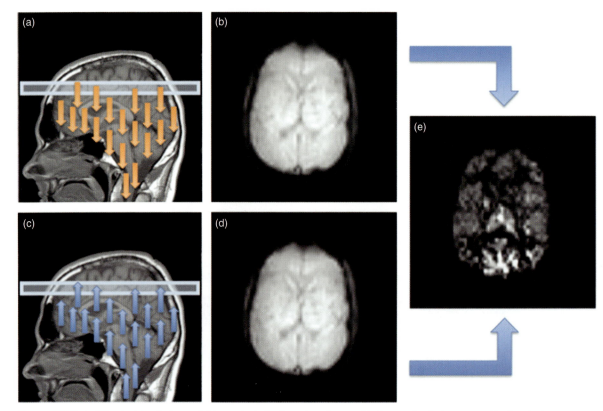

Figure 3.2 Basic ASL principles. An image (b) is acquired after inversion of magnetization proximally (represented by inverted arrows in a), followed by a second image (d) acquired after a control experiment, in which the magnetization has been left unchanged (c). The subtraction of d – b gives the perfusion-weighted image (e).

Labeling schemes

Several labeling schemes have been proposed to either invert or saturate the arterial water magnetization. The main ones are summarized on Figure 3.3. The first one is also the simplest, and consists of the simultaneous application of a long low-power RF pulse together with a gradient, usually applied along the z-axis of the scanner, to selectively invert the magnetization by flow-driven adiabatic inversion [1, 27]. In short, while the static spins only see a saturation pulse, the arterial spins will experience a large moving excitation field, of amplitude $\overline{B_{eff}} = \frac{\Delta\omega(t)}{\gamma}\,\hat{z} + A\hat{x}$, and $\Delta\omega(t) = \gamma G(r(t) - r_0)$, with $r(t) =$ position of the water spin along the z axis, $r_0 =$ labeling plane position, $\gamma =$ gyromagnetic ratio, $G =$ amplitude of the labeling gradient, and $A =$ amplitude of the applied RF field [28–30]. As such, it is really the motion of the spins along the arteries (in, e.g., the carotids or aorta) that produces the changing field applied along the z axis and therefore inverts the magnetization [29]. The main problem with this

method is the strong magnetization transfer (MT) effect produced by such long off-resonance RF pulses [1, 31]. This MT effect will affect the static tissue with almost the same amplitude as the perfusion effect, by transferring the macromolecular magnetization labeled by the long RF pulse to the free water through direct spin (chemical) exchange and spin–spin interactions [32]. For this reason, a control experiment is performed, by reversing the polarity of the gradient to produce an identical amount of MT without labeling of the arterial water spins. This control will, however, only balance out the MT effects in a single plane equidistant from each labeling plane, and precludes this method being used for multiple slices. To control for MT in more than one slice, one can either use a separate coil for labeling [33], thereby avoiding any direct saturation of macromolecules in the tissue of interest, or use more advanced control experiments, such as, e.g., using a sinusoidal modulation of the RF pulse leading to a double labeling plane inducing identical MT effects, and effectively

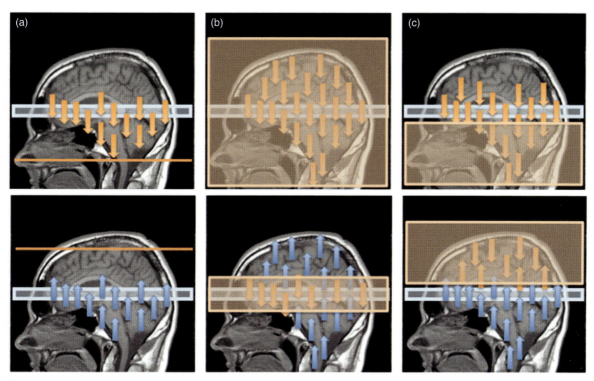

Figure 3.3 Basic ASL schemes. (a) Original continuous ASL sequence, where the spins are inverted using a combination of gradient and RF pulse over a long period of time, resulting in a very well-defined narrow inversion region, usually placed at the cervico-medullar junction for labeling, and at equidistance on the other side for control. (b) The symmetrical pulsed ASL scheme (also known as FAIR sequence, see text) in which labeling is achieved by the alternating application of a slice-selective and non-selective inversion-recovery sequence. (c) Asymmetrical pulsed ASL scheme, as originally presented in the EPISTAR sequence (see text). The labeling is achieved by a slab-selective inversion pulse, placed proximally for labeling and distally for the control acquisition.

producing a null labeling pulse by double inversion of the arterial water spins [34].

In an attempt to make continuous labeling possible on clinical scanners, on which RF duty cycle is limited, Dai and colleagues [35] have recently proposed an alternative implementation of this method, dubbed pulsed-continuous ASL or pseudo-continuous ASL (pCASL) [35, 36]. In pCASL both continuous gradient and RF pulses are replaced by a series of short RF pulses combined with strong slice-selection gradients, for the selection of a thin slab through which the arterial water spins flow. The refocusing part of this slice-selection gradient is then chosen such that it produces an additional phase for flowing spins, which will then be flipped slightly at each application of every RF pulse (see Figure 3.4 for a demonstration of this effect) [35, 36]. Briefly, the frequency difference between two consecutive pulses is given by $\Delta\omega = \gamma G \Delta r$, and is given by the difference in the slice-selection gradient G multiplied by the displacement of the arterial water spins Δr during a

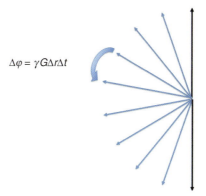

$$\Delta\varphi = \gamma G \Delta r \Delta t$$

Figure 3.4 Demonstration of the pCASL scheme, in which the magnetization is inverted after each RF pulse. The phase difference between two pulses is given by the equation; briefly, it can be calculated by the multiplication of the apparent frequency sweep $\Delta\omega = \gamma G \Delta r$ by the time during which this frequency sweep is applied Δt.

small time Δt. The phase difference is then simply given by the multiplication of $\Delta\omega$ by the time during which this frequency sweep is applied Δt.

43

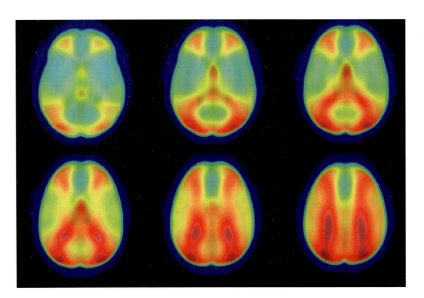

Figure 3.5 Average arrival time maps from the QUASAR study [44], averaged over >1000 scans, clearly demonstrating the difference in arrival times between main perfusion territories (blue-green) and borderzone areas (orange-red). The scale is between 0 and 1 s. Adapted from Hendrikse *et al.* [44].

Another group of labeling schemes, originally developed at around the same time as the continuous labeling approach, are the so-called pulsed labeling techniques. There are numerous variants of pulsed ASL (PASL) developed over the years, which can be split into two main categories, based on whether the labeling is symmetrical with respect to the measured plane or not. The simplest PASL sequence is based on the repeated acquisitions of an inversion recovery sequence, with and without slice-selection gradient to exclude or include the blood outside of the volume of interest (see Figure 3.3b) [37–39], and has been dubbed flow alternating inversion recovery (FAIR) [37]. Here as well, the perfusion signal comes from the difference between inverted and non-inverted blood entering the tissue of interest, leading to a difference in the apparent relaxation time between both measurements.

The original asymmetrical PASL method is called echo-planar imaging (EPI)-based signal targeting by alternating radiofrequency pulses (EPISTAR) [40]. In EPISTAR, the blood is labeled proximally to the area of interest through the application of a slab-selective inversion pulse, followed by a control pulse on the opposite side of the area of interest (see Figure 3.3c). In successive implementations, the control acquisition was replaced by two inversion slabs performed with half the power of the original inversion pulse [41, 42], in a way similar to the double inversion used in CASL [34]. Multiple other schemes have been implemented, all based on the previous two methods,

in an attempt to optimize the control acquisition. Lists of all these sequences and their abbreviations can be found elsewhere [2, 43].

One of the inherent problems of PASL techniques is that they label the whole arterial blood as a bolus and let it flow through the volume of interest. As such, one of the major sources of error is the transit time τ_a which, even in healthy subjects, varies across the brain, being longest in the territories perfused by the most distal branches, such as in the regions between main perfusion territories also known as border-zone areas [44, 45] (Figure 3.5). In the original PASL implementations, information on perfusion was assessed at a single inversion time point (Figure 3.6a), and therefore without information about the transit time. Quantification was then based on the second step in Eq. (3.9), and τ_a was assumed equal for all pixels or simply set to zero. Making this assumption leads to invalid CBF quantification in both absolute and relative terms, and therefore to incorrect estimates of perfusion values between areas [25, 46]. But τ_a is not the only parameter potentially leading to errors in the estimate of perfusion. The end of the bolus τ_d is also particularly problematic, as it cannot be estimated easily in a PASL experiment, since the bolus is essentially defined by the dimension of the labeling slab, which will take more or less time to flow through the organ (typically the brain), depending on the arterial size, stiffness, and the cardiac output fraction of the patient, among others.

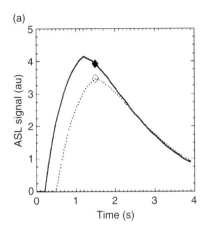
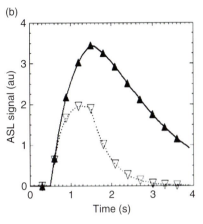

Figure 3.6 Typical arrival time curve from a PASL experiment. A single time point (a) cannot differentiate between delayed and reduced perfusion, while an acquisition of the whole curve (b) allows the clear separation of the various influences from arrival time, blood flow, and dispersion of the bolus. Adapted from Golay *et al.* [42].

In an attempt to improve the definition of the bolus and therefore simplify perfusion quantification [47], Wong and colleagues developed a simple modification of PASL sequences that circumvent the problem of variable τ_d by the introduction of additional saturation pulses. Their methods, dubbed QUIPSS (I and II) for "Quantitative Imaging of Perfusion using a Single Subtraction" are based on the application of a slab-selective 90° saturation pulse to properly define the edges of the bolus. In the QUIPSS I sequence, this saturation pulse is applied to the volume of interest, thereby defining the start of the bolus, and in the QUIPSS II method, it is applied at the level of the labeling volume to define its length. Note that in that case, the bolus width and transit time can be regulated in a way similar to CASL, using the saturation pulse to limit and define the length of the tag. It is, however, important to ensure that the application of this saturation pulse catches the end of the labeled bolus, as otherwise, it will have no effect and will lead to erroneous estimates of τ_d. As such, if TI_1 is the time at which the QUIPSS II pulse is applied and TI_2 is the inversion time post labeling, we have, if $TI_1 < (\tau_d - \tau_a)$ and $TI_2 > (TI_1 + \tau_a)$, and by rearranging Eq. (3.9):

$$\Delta M(t = TI_2) = 2 \cdot \alpha \cdot M_{a,0} \cdot f \cdot TI_1 \cdot e^{-\frac{TI_2}{T_{1b}}} \cdot q_{PASL}(t = TI_2)$$
$$(3.10)$$

where q_{PASL} is a constant term with a numerical value close to 1. Note that in this case, the magnetization difference coming from the ASL experiment depends only on the chosen sequence parameters TI_1, TI_2, and the relaxation times, in addition to flow [47, 48].

Similarly to QUIPSS II, a series of saturation pulses can be applied instead of a large volume excitation to better define the end of the bolus using sharper excitation profiles, and has been dubbed Q2TIPS for "QUIPSS II with Thin-slice TI_1 Periodic Saturation" by Luh and colleagues [48].

Note that the conditions $TI_1 < (\tau_d - \tau_a)$ and $TI_2 > (TI_1 + \tau_a)$ can generally be satisfied in volunteers and patients without vascular diseases where the difference in transit time is small (< 1.5 s) [49]. However, these methods may fail in patients with moderate to severe atherosclerosis, where the transit time can be long in affected areas (> 2.0 s) due to low perfusion velocity and, in some cases, extensive collateral perfusion. In these cases, the problem may be solved by acquiring images at multiple inversion times, and therefore measuring the entire ΔM curve (Figure 3.6b). Of course, it is important to remember that these methods will also fail if the arterial arrival times are markedly increased (> 4–6 s), since the label is almost completely gone at these time points due to T_1 decay.

Multi-delay ASL experiments can be performed using a succession of ASL experiments at various inversion times, normally at a lower resolution than the main perfusion measurement [7], and sometimes using an optimized temporal sampling strategy [50]. Alternatively, Günther *et al.* [51] introduced an elegant solution to this problem using a Look-Locker readout to measure the ASL signal at multiple inversion times in a single scan. Because of multiple low flip angle readouts, the general model needs to be modified by substituting R_{1app} in Eq. (3.9) with

$$R_{1app,eff} = R_1 + \frac{f}{\lambda} - \frac{ln(cos(\varphi))}{\Delta TI}, \quad \text{where} \quad \varphi \quad \text{is the}$$

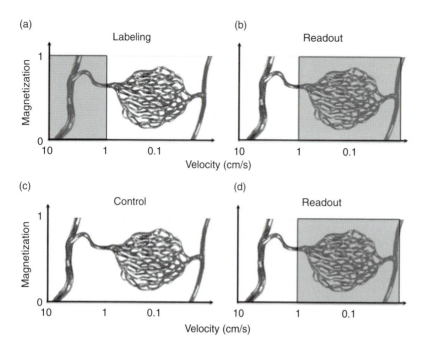

(a) Labeling

(b) Readout

(c) Control

(d) Readout

Figure 3.7 Principles of velocity-selective ASL. The signal is labeled in the large vessels (a), and only the spins that have reduced their velocity below the cut-off will be measured during the readout (b). In the control case, the labeling pulse is not applied (c), and the same readout is performed (d).

excitation flip angle and ΔTI is the interval between successive excitation pulses. Other implementations of the same readout method have been published, based either on a transfer-insensitive labeling (TILT) pulse [52, 53] or on a STAR labeling pulse [8].

Note that CASL is also sensitive to the transit time, but because the measurement is performed once the system has reached its steady state, the effects are reduced with respect to PASL. In addition, transit time insensitivity can be reached for CASL using a post-label delay (PLD) of typically 1.5–3.0 s between continuous labeling and readout [54], according to the subject's condition.

Apart from these "classical" ASL schemes, certain researchers have opted to use a different type of labeling, based on the decreasing velocity of the blood as it moves from the arteries into the microvasculature. In short, in this so-called velocity-selective ASL (VS-ASL), the blood is labeled using a global preparation scheme, not based on a specific position upstream from the tissue of interest, but everywhere in the organ. This is achieved by selectively saturating the spins flowing at a velocity larger than a chosen cut-off velocity v_c (i.e., typically larger than 1 cm/s), and then, by only imaging the spins that have decelerated to a velocity below v_c [55, 56]. The specific velocity labeling may be obtained using a pair of gradients in all ways similar to phase-contrast angiography or to the so-called crusher gradients used to remove the signal from large arteries (see below [8, 57]). Another set of crusher gradients is used during image acquisition to avoid having any signal above the cut-off frequency imaged. The control experiment is performed in the same way, except that no labeling (i.e., crushing in this case) is applied. Figure 3.7 shows the principles of this labeling technique. The main advantage of this technique is that it should be much less sensitive to long transit delay times, and may therefore be the method of choice for neurovascular diseases (see Chapter 8).

Recently, most of these labeling schemes (apart from VS-ASL) have been used to label selectively one or another artery. Such methods have been published under different names, such as perfusion territory imaging [58], regional perfusion imaging (RPI, [59]), selective [60] or territorial ASL [6], or even vessel-selective ASL [61], but are all based on the principles described in Figure 3.8. The simplest approach is to selectively label an individual artery using a separate small labeling coil [58, 62], though this requires extra hardware and limits the acquisition to arteries easily accessible in the neck. A more convenient approach is to angulate the labeling slab (for PASL) so as to include only a single artery at the time.

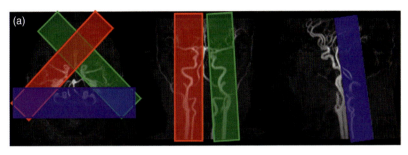

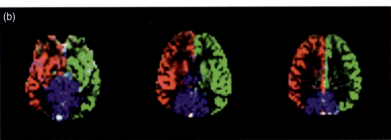

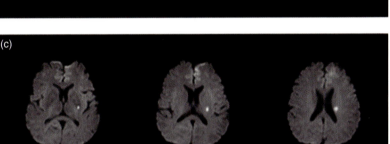

Figure 3.8 Principles of territorial ASL. Generally, each major vessel is labeled independently (a), allowing the reconstruction of an image of territorial perfusion, such as the one presented in (b). (b) Depiction of the perfusion territory in a patient with a small diffusion-weighted imaging-positive lesion in the basal ganglia (c). In this case, territorial ASL did not provide any additional information, apart from confirming that the lesion is fully in the left ICA territory, which is not always the case, as perfusion territories in this area have been shown to show a large variability [97].

The labeling pulse will then in most cases intersect with the tissue of interest, and strong pre-saturation pulses need to be applied in the brain to avoid its direct labeling, particularly difficult to achieve at 3 T [42, 59]. Thus, a careful planning of the labeling pulse needs to be performed, based on multiple maximum-intensity projections (MIPs) of a time-of-flight (TOF) MRA scan, as originally explained in [59]. Basically, the size of the oblique labeling slab can be adjusted in one direction and is infinite in the other two directions. Labeling slabs covering the internal carotid arteries (ICAs) need to be planned on the basis of both axial and coronal MIPs and aligned such that each ICA is labeled independently. Signal contribution from the contralateral ICA, as well as the basilar and vertebral arteries, needs to be avoided by appropriate angulations. The posterior circulation is planned using both axial and sagittal MIPs of the circle of Willis, using identical precautions to avoid mislabeling from other territories. The planning for all territories needs in general to be verified on the native TOF images to minimize the amount of contamination due to mislabeling of adjacent vessels, although it is not always completely avoidable, depending on the tortuosity of the vessels.

In addition, both a CASL and pCASL version of this method have been published [61, 63], the later being much easier to implement as it can be done blindly, without the careful planning needed for the PASL-based techniques. Indeed, in the pCASL-based method, the labeling efficiency is modulated in the labeling plane by additional gradients added to the labeling scheme, allowing calculation of the perfusion territories from an algebraic combination of several scans, labeling two or more vessels at the time with different efficiencies [61, 64, 65].

Finally, additional MRI tricks have been developed to limit the artifacts due to misregistration between labeling and control acquisitions and improve the SNR of ASL. One of the most widely

47

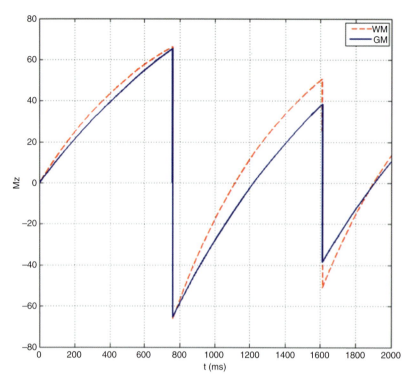

Figure 3.9 Simulations of the evolution of gray matter (blue) and white matter (dotted red) magnetization, after a saturation pulse, followed by two inversion pulses at 760 ms and 1612 ms, respectively, both optimized to null white matter (TI = 700 ms) and gray matter (TI = 1400 ms) signals 100 ms before the TI = 2000 ms (as in [7]). These simulations are made for two voxels in the frontal gray matter (M_0 = 140; TI = 1209 ms) and white matter (M_0 = 100; TI = 699 ms) as per [98]. The final fraction of magnetization for each of the tissues is 13.5% for white matter and 7.55% for gray matter respectively.

used consists of using a combination of RF pulses to selectively suppress the background tissue signal in the area of interest, without influencing the labeling scheme (see e.g. Figure 3.9) [66]. This background-suppression method can be used both with pulsed [66] or continuous ASL [67].

Readout methods

As the ASL signal is based on the difference between two images, it is very important for the acquisition techniques to be very fast. Indeed, any slight difference between labeling and control may lead to an artifactual signal of the same order of magnitude as the ASL signal itself [68]. Therefore, from the early days of ASL, snapshot imaging techniques have been used, such as multi-slice spin-echo or gradient-echo EPI [38, 40] or spiral readouts [69] (Figure 3.10). The problem with these rapid imaging techniques is that they are very sensitive to magnetic susceptibility artifacts, which lead to image distortions and signal voids [70, 71]. In addition, gradient-echo EPI produces images with a strong T_2^*-weighting, especially at high field strengths (≥ 3 T), which can produce spurious activation-related CBF changes when used in functional MRI (fMRI) [72].

Another problem with multi-slice acquisition techniques for ASL is that the time between labeling and acquisition will vary from slice to slice, leading to complications when fitting the data to obtain quantitative CBF values. The acquisition order is therefore very important for multi-slice acquisitions, and care should be taken to use an ascending acquisition order to provide a natural bolus-following acquisition scheme, as it is expected that the labeled bolus will reach the slices located more cranially at a later time point than the caudal ones [45].

As an alternative, other rapid readout techniques have recently been introduced, such as steady-state free precession (SSFP) [73] or 3D gradient and spin echo (3D-GRASE) [7, 67]. SSFP is a good technique to use, especially in the body, where fast EPI readouts lead to severe distortions of the images [74]. The drawback with SSFP however is that the technique can be quite sensitive to B_0 field variations and shimming conditions, and does show characteristic bands of signal void in areas with large off-resonance effects [75]. As such, this readout technique might be better reserved for lower field strengths (< 3.0 T). The 3D-GRASE readout is essentially a fast spin echo technique combined with a single-shot EPI readout acquisition per z phase encoding plane

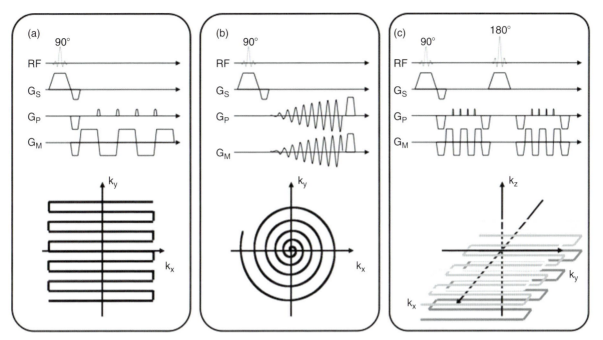

Figure 3.10 Main readouts used in ASL. The upper panels show the basic pulse sequences while the lower ones describe the k-space trajectories. (a) Single-shot EPI sequence; (b) single-shot spiral; (c) single-shot 3D-GRASE readout [7]. In the 3D-GRASE sequence, a single-shot EPI readout is applied in-between every 180° refocusing RF pulse. Note that a second version of this sequence has been published, using a stack of spiral rather than EPI readouts [34].

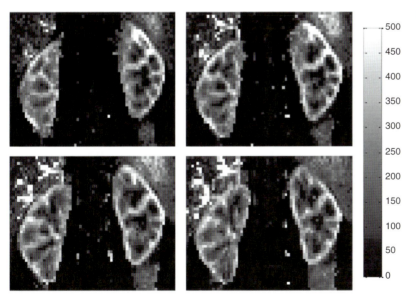

Figure 3.11 Four central slices of calculated kidney perfusion measured using a PASL sequence with a 3D-GRASE sequence at 1.5 T. Images adapted from [75].

[76] (Figure 3.10c). When combined with partial k-space coverage or parallel imaging, this readout method allows for very fast whole brain imaging acquisition of ASL data [7, 67]. Note that it has also been applied outside of the brain, albeit at 1.5 T, for measurement of kidney perfusion [77] (Figure 3.11). Its main advantages are its speed and very high SNR, due to the multiple fast spin echo readouts used [7]. In addition, it allows all slices within the perfusion volume to be sampled at the

49

same time, thereby making the analysis of the data more straightforward.

An additional variation of this method has been implemented as the product sequence on the General Electric platform, and consists of a fast spin-echo train like in the 3D-GRASE case, albeit replacing the stack of EPI readouts by spiral readouts [35], making it less susceptible to air–tissue interface artifacts, due to the shorter achievable gradient echo time of the spiral readouts (see Figure 3.10).

Analysis techniques

Even with the very best acquisition techniques, including optimized sequences, high magnet field strengths, and sensitive receiver coils, the ASL technique today is still largely SNR-limited. As such, methods for the analysis of the raw data play a very important role. Unfortunately, the data analysis techniques are often the least well documented in many publications, with a few exceptions (as e.g. [68]), leaving the reader to wonder exactly how the perfusion images presented were calculated. In the following section, two major steps are presented, the first one concerning data preparation, including correction for motion artifacts, rejection of poor-quality data, filtering, and signal enhancement techniques, recently developed in the context of ASL. In the second section, the major fitting procedures used for producing quantitative ASL data are presented.

Data processing and filtering

As a subtraction technique relying heavily on signal averaging, ASL is by definition very sensitive to motion artifacts. This problem can become particularly acute in certain patient populations, such as children, [78, 79] or patients suffering from dementia [9, 80]. To tackle this issue, two main approaches have been proposed. The first one, and also probably the simplest, is to automatically discard any pair of subtracted (control-label) images that show clear motion-related artifacts [78, 81]. This can be done simply based on the mean signal intensity of the subtracted images over time, as motion-corrupted images will show a much larger average signal than the one only related to perfusion [81]. As 30–50 averages are usually acquired, a reduction of the number of averages (by ±10–20% max) will still usually provide a meaningful perfusion-weighted image. The disadvantage of this technique is that if used in a clinical trial, it might

induce a bias as the SNR might be related to the type or severity of the disease. The other possibility is to co-register the dynamic images in a way similar to what is used in fMRI [82]. Such algorithms might, however, be difficult to use, as usually, ASL is acquired using a very anisotropic acquisition scheme (see next section), and therefore, attempted interpolation might in fact produce a more, rather than less, spurious signal. A final approach is the use of prospective motion correction (available on every clinical platform), in which low-resolution projection images are used to determine motion in run time and then a translational and rotational matrix is applied to keep the imaged volume in a single position [62]. The ideal method might be therefore to combine some elements of all of these techniques, to ensure as much as possible artifact-free perfusion weighting in the raw ASL data.

Once motion artifacts have been taken care of, de-noising and filtering techniques can be applied to enhance the SNR in ASL. There has not been much work done on this topic, but recently, a thorough study was published [83] comparing several de-noising and filtering techniques. The results suggest that temporal ICA might be the most useful technique for enhancing the SNR in ASL by discarding noise-related temporal components.

In addition to noise levels, another problem of ASL is related to its sensitivity to partial volume effects. Here as well, very little has been published so far on the topic, but one study [84] recently proposed an interesting simple method to tackle this issue, by assuming a slow-changing average CBF in gray and white matter in the brain. Figure 3.12 shows the effects of that method on CBF values in a healthy volunteer (courtesy of Ms. R. Oliver, UCL, London). By adapting this algorithm to the noise level [85] both de-noising and partial volume correction may be applied at the same time.

Fitting procedures

Once all pre-processing steps have been performed, and the quality of the "raw" ASL data is considered acceptable, several steps still remain to be performed to produce CBF maps. There are generally two ways of getting CBF images. In the first one, using a single TI, usually acquired using a QUIPSS II or Q2TIPS method [47, 48], difference images are simply transformed into CBF maps using Eq. (3.10). No fitting

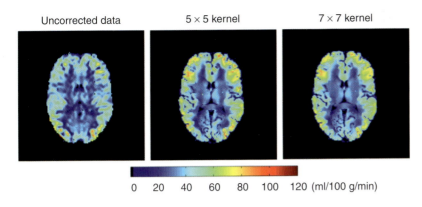

Uncorrected data 5 × 5 kernel 7 × 7 kernel

0 20 40 60 80 100 120 (ml/100 g/min)

Figure 3.12 Effect of correction for partial volume effect using the algorithm from Asllani *et al.* [82] using different kernels. Generally, gray matter values for CBF increase after partial volume correction, but a smoothing effect starts to appear when using large kernels.

is required, and the only differences between different studies are usually different assumed values for the relaxation times and blood–brain partition coefficients. The most precise estimate of CBF will be produced using T_1 and possibly λ maps; however, most commercial implementations so far simply use single T_1 and λ values, which may result in up to 20–50% error in blood flow estimates, depending on the disease. It is therefore advised for clinical applications to acquire at least a T_1 map. As for the blood T_1 values to be used, they can either be measured for each patient [86, 87], which would only be indicated in patient populations known to be prone to a large and sudden change in haematocrit, such as neonates (see Chapter 16), or taken from published literature values [88, 89]. Note that here as well, not all authors use the same value for blood T_1 and as such, a consensus should be achieved if one aims to achieve quantitative estimates of CBF that are reproducible between different users and studies.

In addition, for example in neurovascular disease, the simple timing assumptions on which the QUIPSS II and Q2TIPS methods are based will no longer be fulfilled. As such, it becomes necessary to acquire the ASL data at multiple inversion times, and then use typically Eq. (3.9) to obtain separate maps of both arrival times and CBF values [7, 8, 51]. Note that a few alternatives have been published, including using a Fourier transform to get access to timing and blood flow information [90] or a simple deconvolution of Eq. (3.5) using measured AIF [8]. Note that the latter, based on the QUASAR sequence, will also provide measurements of aBV.

Finally, a simpler solution is provided for pCASL and CASL techniques, for which it is generally assumed that the system has reached the steady state.

In such a case, an equation similar to Eq. (3.9) can be used, with the same caveats as in the PASL case concerning the use of single T_1 and λ values [43].

Recommended protocols, artifacts, pitfalls, and limitations
Problems and limitations

As mentioned earlier, ASL's major problem is its intrinsic low SNR. In fact, the measured ΔM is often in the order of 1% or less, and subtraction errors are frequent, often caused by motion artifacts, especially in clinical studies of difficult patient populations (see the previous section, Analysis techniques). In lieu of advanced image processing schemes, other acquisition tricks can be used, such as background-suppression techniques. Such methods have been developed to cancel the background (static) signal not related to perfusion. They usually achieve complete annihilation of the static signal over a wide range of T_1 values (particularly necessary for brain perfusion) using multiple inversion pulses [66]. These background-suppression methods have been used for multi-shot and single-shot 3D PASL, CASL, and pCASL, among others (Figure 3.9).

Another problem in ASL is the remaining labeled signal in the vasculature, which is an especially important potential source of error at short TIs, and when using multiple TIs to fit the labeled bolus in PASL [91]. One of the first solutions implemented was the use of small diffusion gradients (diffusion b-value = 1–10 s/mm^2) to eliminate the remaining arterial signal [92]. Note that a comparison of the signal obtained with and without crusher gradients has been used to estimate ATT in CASL [93], or both ATT and aBV in the QUASAR sequence [8]. Also, for non-vessel suppressed ASL images, the vascular signal is known as arterial transit artifact (ATA) and is indicative of slow flow in patients with cerebrovascular disease (see Chapter 8 for more detail).

Another potential source of problems for PASL techniques are the inversion pulses used, as poorly defined slice profiles will result in reduced labeling efficiency, as well as possible contamination of the volume of interest by the labeling pulse. For this reason, very sharp labeling pulses are needed, and most modern implementations use adiabatic RF pulses of one sort or another [94, 95].

Existing sequences and preferred protocols

Each major manufacturer nowadays provides a basic set of ASL pulse sequences in their neurological package. However, each chose to adopt a different basic set of technologies, which may leave the user slightly unsure as to what protocol to use. Here, we propose a series of very general guidelines to be used with each of the vendors, whenever possible. Of course, such guidelines need to be adapted to each clinical situation, and more thorough reviews and white papers are being prepared by the international community to provide more exhaustive guidelines for separate diseases [96]. But in general, such sequences are best performed at high field strength (≥ 3.0T), and the three main manufacturers of MR systems at this field strength are General Electric, Siemens Medical Solutions, and Philips Healthcare. The following discussion will therefore be limited to these manufacturers.

So far, only General Electric provides pCASL as a standard labeling sequence, while the other two major manufacturers of high field systems deliver methods based on PASL sequences. As such, the preferred protocols are different for each manufacturer. But there are main rules to follow, and they are valid on each implementation. First, the resolution needs to be chosen with care. Because of its low SNR, ASL images by definition need to be acquired at a low resolution. Typical 64×64 or up to 80×80 matrices are usually chosen (3–4 mm in-plane resolution), with a maximum in-plane resolution of 1.8 mm (matrix of 128×128, field of view of 230 mm). Such high in-plane resolution might necessitate an increase in slice thickness (up from a typical 4–6 mm), or

number of averages, though. A typical single time point acquisition with a reasonable SNR will take about 3–5 min, with a number of averages ranging from 30 to 50 at 3.0 T.

On a modern GE scanner (MR750 and later), a pCASL sequence can be used with the above-mentioned resolution. The proposed readout is a stack of spiral based on a fast spin echo sequence, and the number of interleaves as well as the number of averages can be adjusted. A pCASL labeling pulse of 1.5 s is provided by default, consisting in a series of 0.5-ms Hanning-shaped RF pulses played out every 1.0–1.2 ms [35]. An adjustable post-labeling delay can be used, and it is recommended to use at least 1.5 s to avoid intravascular artifacts in most patients [54]. The sequence contains background suppression pulses by default.

Siemens has currently two different ASL sequences, an asymmetric PASL sequence based on the PICORE scheme [97], with an EPI readout, and, on its most modern version of its software, a FAIR-based sequence [37] combined with a 3D-GRASE readout [7]. Both sequences are provided with a Q2-TIPS bolus saturation scheme [48]. The recommended protocol to use in this case for single-TI acquisitions would be a TI of at least 1.8 s (corresponding to TI2 for Q2-TIPS). The TI1 is a bit more tricky to set, but should not exceed 0.6 s for a PICORE labeling slab of 10 cm, and can be slightly longer, typically up to 1 s for a global FAIR labeling. Resolution and averages are the same as before. Certain authors have proposed the use of a quick, low-resolution (i.e., $4.5 \times 4.5 \times 4.5$ mm^3) acquisition of a multi-TI ASL sequence to map out the BAT [7], and this will be available in the upcoming version of the software on Siemens scanners.

Finally, Philips implemented a different ASL technique, based on the QUASAR sequence [8, 45]. The current product does not provide a sequence capable of measuring the AIF in every pixel as in the original paper, but just a PASL method, based on an EPISTAR scheme [42], followed by a Look-Locker acquisition combined with an EPI readout. The sequence uses an advanced pre-saturation scheme based on a spectroscopic water suppression method [42], and therefore automatically fits for both T_1 and the ASL bolus using slightly modified equations [51]. The main disadvantage of this method is that it does not permit whole brain scanning, due to the restricted time available in-between the multiple time points in the Look-Locker acquisition. Since the Look-Locker scheme necessitates the use of flip angles lower than 90°, the resolution to be chosen would typically be relatively low ($3.75 \times 3.75 \times 6\ mm^3$). The next version of the software should, however, provide the full QUASAR sequence with the interleaved acquisition of data with and without vascular crushers to estimate the AIF and therefore enable a model-free estimation of perfusion [45]. Finally, please note that Philips also provides a simple single-TI EPISTAR sequence, combinable with a QUIPSS II technique, and a choice of multiple readouts; the recommended readout is multi-slice single-shot EPI.

Conclusions

As shown in the previous section, ASL is far from being harmonized among vendors, and probably presents so far the widest variety among all modern MR pulse sequences. For this reason, it is just beginning to enter clinical use, and a considerable amount of work remains to be done to ensure that users will employ the right sequence for the right disease [96]. In addition, very simplistic post-processing procedures are available so far for analyzing ASL data on the main manufacturers' platforms, and a limited number of products are available from research groups. The Oxford-based FSL package has a toolbox (http://www.fmrib.ox.ac.uk/), and other tools exist as well [68], but this scarcity, together with the variety of existing pulse sequences and models, has led most groups working on the subject to develop their own in-house software, which complicates the comparison of results from different groups in different diseases. As such, the multiple chapters of this book in which ASL is used really represent the state of the art of the applications of this method, showing more its possibilities in diseases rather than a well-established clinical tool at present, although there are some exceptions (e.g., Chapter 10). However, because of its non-invasive nature, increasing commercial availability, and hopefully upcoming standardization, over time ASL promises to become used both in large-scale clinical trials as well as in daily clinical practice.

Acknowledgments

The author would like to thank Dr. David Thomas for his help with the editing of this chapter, Ms. Ruth Oliver for providing Figure 3.7 and Dr. Enrico De Vita for providing Figure 3.9.

References

1. Williams DS, Detre JA, Leigh JS, Koretsky AP. Magnetic resonance imaging of perfusion using spin inversion of arterial water. *Proc Natl Acad Sci U S A* 1992;**89**(1):212–16.

2. Golay X, Hendrikse J, Lim TC. Perfusion imaging using arterial spin labeling. *Top Magn Reson Imaging* 2004;**15**(1):10–27.

3. Kim SG, Tsekos NV. Perfusion imaging by a flow-sensitive alternating inversion recovery (FAIR) technique: application to functional brain imaging. *Magn Reson Med* 1997;**37**(3):425–35.

4. Hoge RD, Atkinson J, Gill B, *et al.* Linear coupling between cerebral blood flow and oxygen consumption in activated human cortex. *Proc Natl Acad Sci U S A* 1999;**96**(16):9403–8.

5. Chalela JA, Alsop DC, Gonzalez-Atavales JB, *et al.* Magnetic resonance perfusion imaging in acute ischemic stroke using continuous arterial spin labeling. *Stroke* 2000;**31**(3):680–7.

6. Chng SM, Petersen ET, Zimine I, *et al.* Territorial arterial spin labeling in the assessment of collateral circulation: comparison with digital subtraction angiography. *Stroke* 2008;**39**(12):3248–54.

7. Gunther M, Oshio K, Feinberg DA. Single-shot 3D imaging techniques improve arterial spin labeling perfusion measurements. *Magn Reson Med* 2005;**54**(2):491–8.

8. Petersen ET, Lim T, Golay X. Model-free arterial spin labeling quantification approach for perfusion MRI. *Magn Reson Med* 2006;**55**(2):219–32.

9. Alsop DC, Detre JA, Grossman M. Assessment of cerebral blood flow in Alzheimer's disease by spin-labeled magnetic resonance imaging. *Ann Neurol* 2000;**47**(1):93–100.

10. Johnson NA, Jahng GH, Weiner MW, *et al.* Pattern of cerebral hypoperfusion in Alzheimer disease and mild cognitive impairment measured with arterial spin-labeling MR imaging: initial experience. *Radiology* 2005;**234**(3):851–9.

11. Schuff N, Matsumoto S, Kmiecik J, *et al.* Cerebral blood flow in ischemic vascular dementia and Alzheimer's disease, measured by arterial spin-labeling magnetic resonance imaging. *Alzheimers Dement* 2009;**5**(6):454–62.

12. Roberts DA, Detre JA, Bolinger L, *et al.* Renal perfusion in humans: MR imaging with spin tagging of arterial water. *Radiology* 1995;**196**(1):281–6.

13. Hirshberg B, Qiu M, Cali AM, *et al.* Pancreatic perfusion of healthy individuals and type 1 diabetic patients as assessed by magnetic resonance perfusion imaging. *Diabetologia* 2009;**52**(8):1561–5.

14. St Lawrence KS, Frank JA, McLaughlin AC. Effect of restricted water exchange on cerebral blood flow values calculated with arterial spin tagging: a theoretical investigation. *Magn Reson Med* 2000;**44**(3):440–9.

15. Zhou J, Wilson DA, Ulatowski JA, Traystman RJ, van Zijl PC. Two-compartment exchange model for perfusion quantification using arterial spin tagging. *J Cereb Blood Flow Metab* 2001;**21**(4):440–55.

16. Parkes LM. Quantification of cerebral perfusion using arterial spin labeling: two-compartment models. *J Magn Reson Imaging* 2005;**22**(6):732–6.

17. Wells JA, Lythgoe MF, Choy M, *et al.* Characterizing the origin of the arterial spin labelling signal in MRI using a multiecho acquisition approach. *J Cereb Blood Flow Metab* 2009; **29**(11):1836–45.

18. Zaharchuk G, Bogdanov AA, Jr., Marota JJ, *et al.* Continuous assessment of perfusion by tagging including volume and water extraction (CAPTIVE): a steady-state contrast agent technique for measuring blood flow, relative blood volume fraction, and the water extraction fraction. *Magn Reson Med* 1998;**40**(5):666–78.

19. Carr JP, Buckley DL, Tessier J, Parker GJ. What levels of precision are achievable for quantification of perfusion and capillary permeability surface area

product using ASL? *Magn Reson Med* 2007;**58**(2):281–9.

20. Brookes MJ, Morris PG, Gowland PA, Francis ST. Noninvasive measurement of arterial cerebral blood volume using Look-Locker EPI and arterial spin labeling. *Magn Reson Med* 2007; **58**(1):41–54.

21. Meier P, Zierler KL. On the theory of the indicator-dilution method for measurement of blood flow and volume. *J Appl Physiol* 1954;**6**(12):731–44.

22. Kety SS, Schmidt CF. The determination of cerebral blood flow in man by use of nitrous oxide in low concentrations. *Am J Physiol* 1945;**143**:53–66.

23. Kety SS, Schmidt CF. The nitrous oxide method for the determination of cerebral blood flow in man: theory, procedure and normal values. *J Clin Invest* 1948;**27**:467–83.

24. Eichling JO, Raichle ME, Grubb RL, Jr., Ter-Pogossian MM. Evidence of the limitations of water as a freely diffusible tracer in brain of the rhesus monkey. *Circ Res* 1974;**35**(3):358–64.

25. Buxton RB, Frank LR, Wong EC, *et al.* A general kinetic model for quantitative perfusion imaging with arterial spin labeling. *Magn Reson Med* 1998;**40**(3): 383–96.

26. van Gelderen P, de Zwart JA, Duyn JH. Pitfalls of MRI measurement of white matter perfusion based on arterial spin labeling. *Magn Reson Med* 2008;**59**(4):788–95.

27. Dixon WT, Du LN, Faul DD, Gado M, Rossnick S. Projection angiograms of blood labeled by adiabatic fast passage. *Magn Reson Med* 1986;**3**(3):454–62.

28. Maccotta L, Detre JA, Alsop DC. The efficiency of adiabatic inversion for perfusion imaging by arterial spin labeling. *NMR Biomed* 1997;**10**(4–5): 216–21.

29. Trampel R, Jochimsen TH, Mildner T, Norris DG, Moller HE. Efficiency of flow-driven adiabatic spin inversion under realistic experimental conditions: a computer simulation. *Magn Reson Med* 2004;**51**(6):1187–93.

30. O'Gorman RL, Summers PE, Zelaya FO, *et al.* In vivo estimation of the flow-driven adiabatic inversion efficiency for continuous arterial spin labeling: a method using phase contrast magnetic resonance angiography. *Magn Reson Med* 2006; **55**(6):1291–7.

31. McLaughlin AC, Ye FQ, Pekar JJ, Santha AK, Frank JA. Effect of magnetization transfer on the measurement of cerebral blood flow using steady-state arterial spin tagging approaches: a theoretical investigation. *Magn Reson Med* 1997;**37**(4):501–10.

32. Wolff SD, Balaban RS. Magnetization transfer contrast (MTC) and tissue water proton relaxation in vivo. *Magn Reson Med* 1989;**10**(1):135–44.

33. Zhang W, Silva AC, Williams DS, Koretsky AP. NMR measurement of perfusion using arterial spin labeling without saturation of macromolecular spins. *Magn Reson Med* 1995;**33**(3):370–6.

34. Alsop DC, Detre JA. Multisection cerebral blood flow MR imaging with continuous arterial spin labeling. *Radiology* 1998; **208**(2):410–16.

35. Dai W, Garcia D, de Bazelaire C, Alsop DC. Continuous flow-driven inversion for arterial spin labeling using pulsed radio frequency and gradient fields. *Magn Reson Med* 2008;**60**(6): 1488–97.

36. Wu WC, Fernandez-Seara M, Detre JA, Wehrli FW, Wang J. A theoretical and experimental investigation of the tagging efficiency of pseudocontinuous arterial spin labeling. *Magn Reson Med* 2007;**58**(5):1020–7.

37. Kim SG. Quantification of relative cerebral blood flow change by flow-sensitive alternating inversion recovery (FAIR) technique: application to functional mapping. *Magn Reson Med* 1995;**34**(3):293–301.

38. Kwong KK, Chesler DA, Weisskoff RM, *et al.* MR perfusion studies with T1-weighted echo planar imaging. *Magn Reson Med* 1995;**34**(6):878–87.

39. Schwarzbauer C, Morrissey SP, Haase A. Quantitative magnetic resonance imaging of perfusion using magnetic labeling of water proton spins within the detection slice. *Magn Reson Med* 1996; **35**(4):540–6.

40. Edelman RR, Siewert B, Darby DG, *et al.* Qualitative mapping of cerebral blood flow and functional localization with echo-planar MR imaging and signal targeting with alternating radio frequency. *Radiology* 1994; **192**(2):513–20.

41. Edelman RR, Chen Q. EPISTAR MRI: multislice mapping of cerebral blood flow. *Magn Reson Med* 1998;**40**(6):800–5.

42. Golay X, Petersen ET, Hui F. Pulsed star labeling of arterial regions (PULSAR): a robust regional perfusion technique for high field imaging. *Magn Reson Med* 2005;**53**(1):15–21.

43. Petersen ET, Zimine I, Ho YC, Golay X. Non-invasive measurement of perfusion: a critical review of arterial spin labelling techniques. *Br J Radiol* 2006;**79**(944):688–701.

44. Hendrikse J, Petersen ET, van Laar PJ, Golay X. Cerebral border zones between distal end branches of intracranial arteries: *MR imaging. Radiology* 2008;**246**(2):572–80.

45. Petersen ET, Mouridsen K, Golay X. The QUASAR reproducibility study, Part II: Results from a multi-center arterial spin labeling test-retest study. *Neuroimage* 2010;**49**(1):104–13.

46. Wong EC, Buxton RB, Frank LR. A theoretical and experimental comparison of continuous and pulsed arterial spin labeling techniques for quantitative perfusion imaging. *Magn Reson Med* 1998;**40**(3): 348–55.

47. Wong EC, Buxton RB, Frank LR. Quantitative imaging of perfusion using a single subtraction (QUIPSS and QUIPSS II). *Magn Reson Med* 1998; **39**(5):702–8.

48. Luh WM, Wong EC, Bandettini PA, Hyde JS. QUIPSS II with thin-slice TI1 periodic saturation: a method for improving accuracy of quantitative perfusion imaging using pulsed arterial spin labeling. *Magn Reson Med* 1999; **41**(6):1246–54.

49. Wintermark M, Sesay M, Barbier E, *et al.* Comparative overview of brain perfusion imaging techniques. *Stroke* 2005;**36**(9):2032–3.

50. Xie J, Gallichan D, Gunn RN, Jezzard P. Optimal design of pulsed arterial spin labeling MRI experiments. *Magn Reson Med* 2008;**59**(4):826–34.

51. Günther M, Bock M, Schad LR. Arterial spin labeling in combination with a look-locker sampling strategy: inflow turbo-sampling EPI-FAIR (ITS-FAIR). *Magn Reson Med* 2001;**46**(5):974–84.

52. Golay X, Stuber M, Pruessmann KP, Meier D, Boesiger P. Transfer insensitive labeling technique (TILT): application to multislice functional perfusion imaging. *J Magn Reson Imaging* 1999;**9**(3):454–61.

53. Hendrikse J, Lu H, van der Grond J, Van Zijl PC, Golay X. Measurements of cerebral perfusion and arterial hemodynamics during visual stimulation using TURBO-TILT.

Magn Reson Med 2003; **50**(2):429–33.

54. Alsop DC, Detre JA. Reduced transit-time sensitivity in noninvasive magnetic resonance imaging of human cerebral blood flow. *J Cereb Blood Flow Metab* 1996;**16**(6):1236–49.

55. Duhamel G, de Bazelaire C, Alsop DC. Evaluation of systematic quantification errors in velocity-selective arterial spin labeling of the brain. *Magn Reson Med* 2003;**50**(1): 145–53.

56. Wong EC, Cronin M, Wu WC, *et al.* Velocity-selective arterial spin labeling. *Magn Reson Med* 2006;**55**(6):1334–41.

57. Schepers J, Van Osch MJ, Nicolay K. Effect of vascular crushing on FAIR perfusion kinetics, using a BIR-4 pulse in a magnetization prepared FLASH sequence. *Magn Reson Med* 2003;**50**(3): 608–13.

58. Zaharchuk G, Ledden PJ, Kwong KK, *et al.* Multislice perfusion and perfusion teritory imaging in humans with separate label and image coils. *Magn Reson Med* 1999;**41**(6):1093–8.

59. Hendrikse J, van der Grond J, Lu H, van Zijl PC, Golay X. Flow territory mapping of the cerebral arteries with regional perfusion MRI. *Stroke* 2004;**35**(4):882–7.

60. Davies NP, Jezzard P. Selective arterial spin labeling (SASL): perfusion territory mapping of selected feeding arteries tagged using two-dimensional radiofrequency pulses. *Magn Reson Med* 2003; **49**(6):1133–42.

61. Wong EC. Vessel-encoded arterial spin-labeling using pseudocontinuous tagging. *Magn Reson Med* 2007; **58**(6):1086–91.

62. Talagala SL, Ye FQ, Ledden PJ, Chesnick S. Whole-brain 3D perfusion MRI at 3.OT using CASL with a separate labeling coil.

55

Magn Reson Med 2004;**52**(1): 131–40.

63. Werner R, Norris DG, Alfke K, Mehdorn HM, Jansen O. Continuous artery-selective spin labeling (CASSL). *Magn Reson Med* 2005;**53**(5):1006–12.

64. Günther M. Efficient visualization of vascular territories in the human brain by cycled arterial spin labeling MRI. *Magn Reson Med* 2006;**56**(3):671–5.

65. Zimine I, Petersen ET, Golay X. Dual vessel arterial spin labeling scheme for regional perfusion imaging. *Magn Reson Med* 2006;**56**(5):1140–4.

66. Ye FQ, Frank JA, Weinberger DR, McLaughlin AC. Noise reduction in 3D perfusion imaging by attenuating the static signal in arterial spin tagging (ASSIST). *Magn Reson Med* 2000; **44**(1):92–100.

67. Fernandez-Seara MA, Wang Z, Wang J, *et al.* Continuous arterial spin labeling perfusion measurements using single shot 3D GRASE at 3 T. *Magn Reson Med* 2005; **54**(5):1241–7.

68. Wang Z, Aguirre GK, Rao H, *et al.* Empirical optimization of ASL data analysis using an ASL data processing toolbox: ASLtbx. *Magn Reson Imaging* 2008;**26**(2):261–9.

69. Yang Y, Frank JA, Hou L, *et al.* Multislice imaging of quantitative cerebral perfusion with pulsed arterial spin labeling. *Magn Reson Med* 1998;**39**(5): 825–32.

70. Chen Q, Siewert B, Bly BM, Warach S, Edelman RR. STAR-HASTE: perfusion imaging without magnetic susceptibility artifact. *Magn Reson Med* 1997;**38**(3):404–8.

71. Crelier GR, Hoge RD, Munger P, Pike GB. Perfusion-based functional magnetic resonance imaging with single-shot RARE and GRASE acquisitions. *Magn Reson Med* 1999;**41**(1):132–6.

72. Lu H, Donahue MJ, van Zijl PC. Detrimental effects of BOLD signal in arterial spin labeling fMRI at high field strength. *Magn Reson Med* 2006;**56**(3):546–52.

73. Boss A, Martirosian P, Klose U, *et al.* FAIR-TrueFISP imaging of cerebral perfusion in areas of high magnetic susceptibility differences at 1.5 and 3 Tesla. *J Magn Reson Imaging* 2007;**25**(5):924–31.

74. Boss A, Martirosian P, Claussen CD, Schick F. Quantitative ASL muscle perfusion imaging using a FAIR-TrueFISP technique at 3.0 T. *NMR Biomed* 2006;**19**(1):125–32.

75. Scheffler K, Lehnhardt S. Principles and applications of balanced SSFP techniques. *Eur Radiol* 2003;**13**(11):2409–18.

76. Oshio K, Feinberg DA. GRASE (Gradient- and spin-echo) imaging: a novel fast MRI technique. *Magn Reson Med* 1991;**20**(2):344–9.

77. Cutajar M, Thomas DL, Banks T, *et al.* Repeatability of renal arterial spin labelling MRI in healthy subjects. *MAGMA* 2012; **25**(2):145–53.

78. Oguz KK, Golay X, Pizzini FB, *et al.* Sickle cell disease: continuous arterial spin-labeling perfusion MR imaging in children. *Radiology* 2003; **227**(2):567–74.

79. Taki Y, Hashizume H, Sassa Y, *et al.* Correlation between gray matter density-adjusted brain perfusion and age using brain MR images of 202 healthy children. *Hum Brain Mapp* 2011; **32**(11):1973–85.

80. Schuff N, Zhu XP. Imaging of mild cognitive impairment and early dementia. *Br J Radiol* 2007;**80** Spec No 2:S109–14.

81. Tan H, Maldjian JA, Pollock JM, *et al.* A fast, effective filtering method for improving clinical pulsed arterial spin labeling

MRI. *J Magn Reson Imaging* 2009;**29**(5):1134–9.

82. Zhilkin P, Alexander ME. Affine registration: a comparison of several programs. *Magn Reson Imaging* 2004;**22**(1):55–66.

83. Wells JA, Thomas DL, King MD, *et al.* Reduction of errors in ASL cerebral perfusion and arterial transit time maps using image de-noising. *Magn Reson Med* 2010;**64**(3):715–24.

84. Asllani I, Borogovac A, Brown TR. Regression algorithm correcting for partial volume effects in arterial spin labeling MRI. *Magn Reson Med* 2008;**60**(6):1362–71.

85. Petr J, Ferre JC, Gauvrit JY, Barillot C. Denoising arterial spin labeling MRI using tissue partial volume. In: Dawant BM, Haynor DR, editors, *Proceedings of SPIE Medical Imaging 2010: Imaging Processing*, San Diego, USA, 2010;**7623**:76230L–76230L-9.

86. Qin Q, Strouse JJ, van Zijl PC. Fast measurement of blood T1 in the human jugular vein at 3 Tesla. *Magn Reson Med* 2011;**65**(5):1297–304.

87. Varela M, Hajnal JV, Petersen ET, *et al.* A method for rapid in vivo measurement of blood T1. *NMR Biomed* 2011;**24**(1):80–8.

88. Lu H, Clingman C, Golay X, van Zijl PC. Determining the longitudinal relaxation time (T1) of blood at 3.0 Tesla. *Magn Reson Med* 2004;**52**(3): 679–82.

89. Stanisz GJ, Odrobina EE, Pun J, *et al.* T1, T2 relaxation and magnetization transfer in tissue at 3T. *Magn Reson Med* 2005; **54**(3):507–12.

90. Guenther M, editor. Analytical parameter estimation in arterial spin labeling time series by fourier transformation. *Proc Intl Soc Magn Reson Med*, Miami, USA, 2005;1136.

91. Chappell MA, MacIntosh BJ, Donahue MJ, *et al.* Separation of macrovascular signal in multi-inversion time arterial spin labelling MRI. *Magn Reson Med* 2010;**63**(5):1357–65.

92. Ye FQ, Mattay VS, Jezzard P, *et al.* Correction for vascular artifacts in cerebral blood flow values measured by using arterial spin tagging techniques. *Magn Reson Med* 1997; **37**(2):226–35.

93. Wang J, Alsop DC, Song HK, *et al.* Arterial transit time imaging with flow encoding arterial spin tagging (FEAST). *Magn Reson Med* 2003;**50**(3):599–607.

94. Yongbi MN, Branch CA, Helpern JA. Perfusion imaging using FOCI RF pulses. *Magn Reson Med* 1998;**40**(6):938–43.

95. Warnking JM, Pike GB. Reducing contamination while closing the gap: BASSI RF pulses in PASL. *Magn Reson Med* 2006; **55**(4):865–73.

96. Golay X, Guenther M. Arterial spin labelling: final steps to make it a clinical reality. *MAGMA* 2012;**25**(2):79–82.

97. Wong EC, Buxton RB, Frank LR. Implementation of quantitative perfusion imaging techniques for functional brain mapping using pulsed arterial spin labeling. *NMR Biomed* 1997; **10**(4–5):237–49.

98. Lu H, Nagae-Poetscher LM, Golay X, *et al.* Routine clinical brain MRI sequences for use at 3.0 Tesla. *J Magn Reson Imaging* 2005; **22**(1):13–22.

DCE-MRI: acquisition and analysis techniques

Paul S. Tofts and Geoff J. M. Parker

Key points

- DCE-MRI uses dynamic T_1-weighted imaging after bolus administration of Gd-based contrast agent to estimate parameters which depends on blood perfusion and tissue permeability.
- Accurate measurements require an arterial input function (AIF) to be sampled, pre-contrast tissue T_1 (T_{10}) to be measured, and the flip angle of the imaging sequence to be precisely set.
- Modeling of DCE-MRI data usually yields the transfer constant (K^{trans}), volume of the extravascular extracellular space (v_e), and the rate constant k_{ep} ($k_{ep} = K^{\text{trans}}/v_e$).
- More sophisticated models also estimate other parameters such as the vascular plasma volume (v_p) and blood perfusion (F).
- Measurements may either be "flow-limited" ($K^{\text{trans}} = F(1 - Hct)$, where Hct is the blood hematocrit), or "permeability-limited" ($K^{\text{trans}} = PS$, the permeability surface area product), depending on the relative magnitudes of F and PS.
- When flow (F) and permeability (PS) are comparable, more sophisticated modeling can be used; however, care should be taken not to over-interpret the data (i.e., not to fit too many model parameters if data are limited or noisy).
- The MRI protocol to be used, and the optimal temporal resolution and duration of data acquisition, depend on the organ system to be studied; for tumors, scan time should be at least 5–10 min; if the "plateau" phase of enhancement is not reached, v_e may not be accurately estimated.
- In evaluating anti-angiogenic cancer therapies, the consensus is that K^{trans} should be the primary outcome variable from DCE-MRI measurements.

Introduction

There are increasing opportunities to use dynamic contrast-enhanced (DCE) T_1-weighted imaging to characterize tumor and other pathological biology and treatment response, using modern fast sequences that can provide good temporal and spatial resolution combined with good organ coverage [1]. Quantification in MRI is recognized as an important approach to characterize tissue biology. This chapter provides an introduction to the physical concepts of mathematical modeling, image acquisition, and image analysis needed to measure aspects of tissue biology using DCE imaging, in a way that should be accessible for a research-minded clinician.

Quantification in MRI represents a paradigm shift, a new way of thinking about imaging [2]. In qualitative studies, the scanner is a highly sophisticated camera, collecting images that are viewed by an experienced radiologist. In quantitative studies, the scanner is used as a sophisticated measuring device, a scientific instrument able to measure many properties of each tissue voxel (e.g., T_1, T_2, diffusion tensor, magnetization transfer, metabolite concentration, K^{trans}). An everyday example of quantification would be the bathroom scales, used to measure our weight. We expect that the machine output shown on the dial, in kg, will be accurate (i.e., close to the true value), reproducible (i.e., if we make repeated measurements over a short time they will not vary), reliable (the scales always work), and biologically relevant (the quantity of weight does indeed relate

Clinical Perfusion MRI: Techniques and Applications, ed. Peter B. Barker, Xavier Golay, and Greg Zaharchuk. Published by Cambridge University Press. © Peter B. Barker, Xavier Golay, and Greg Zaharchuk 2013.

to our health). An example of a clinical measurement would be a blood test; we expect it to work reliably every time. This is the aspiration for quantitative MRI: that it should deliver a high-quality measurement that relates only to the patient biology (and not the state of the scanner at the time of measurement).

A popular measurement derived from DCE-MRI is the transfer constant, K^{trans} (see below, or refer to Chapter 1), which characterizes the diffusive transport of low-molecular weight gadolinium (Gd) chelates across the capillary endothelium [3]. K^{trans} has been widely used in imaging studies to characterize tumor biology and treatment response. The fractional volume v_e of the extravascular extracellular space (EES; i.e., the interstitial space), can also be measured. A consensus recommendation [4] proposed that in assessing anti-angiogenic and anti-vascular therapies in cancer, K^{trans} should be a primary readout (endpoint). Secondary endpoints should include v_e, the rate constant k_{ep} $\left(k_{ep} = K^{\text{trans}}/v_e\right)$, and the plasma volume v_p (if available from the modeling process). The traditional clinical evaluation of tumor treatment uses the RECIST criteria, based on tumor diameter; however, effective non-cytotoxic therapies do not necessarily induce rapid tumor shrinkage, and markers such as K^{trans} and v_e may often be more sensitive markers of the effect a drug has on a tumor. There are also applications of DCE-MRI in tissues other than tumors, e.g., renal and myocardial function, and assessment of inflammation in the lung and joints; this chapter focuses on DCE-MRI methods and is illustrated with applications in tumors and other pathologies, with one example of normal renal function.

Although K^{trans} is not a direct measurement of perfusion, it is often sensitive to perfusion (see below, Eqs (4.7), and (4.8). Explicit estimation of perfusion (F) is also possible with appropriate modeling techniques (see below), although often their use demands advanced rapid imaging methods, which are not currently widely available.

Modeling

The signal data modeling process for DCE-MRI can be considered as having two components [5]. First, the Gd contrast agent concentration has to be found from the MRI signal enhancement. Second, given the Gd concentration as a function of time, pharmacokinetic analysis can then be undertaken to model how the contrast agent distributes in the body, and how this depends on physiological parameters. This is independent of the

imaging conditions (MRI field strength, etc.), and in principle also independent of imaging modality (for example whether X-ray computed tomography (CT) or MRI [6, 7]). Given the characteristics of the modeling, this then guides the choice of imaging sequence (see the section on image acquisition).

MRI modeling: finding Gd concentration from MRI signal

The MRI Gd concentration model has in turn two components. First, T_1 is reduced from its native value T_{10} by the presence of a concentration c of Gd:

$$\frac{1}{T_1} = \frac{1}{T_{10}} + r_1 c \tag{4.1}$$

Often it is more convenient to use the relaxation rate $R_1 = 1/T_1$:

$$R_1 = R_{10} + r_1 c \tag{4.2}$$

The longitudinal relaxivity r_1, (i.e., the constant of proportionality between Gd concentration and increase in relaxation rate $R_1 = 1/T_1$) is specific to a contrast agent and varies with field strength. For example, the relaxivity of Gd-DTPA (Magnevist) is usually assumed to be equal to the in vitro value of $4.5\,\text{s}^{-1}\text{mM}^{-1}$ (measured in aqueous phantoms at 1.5 T [8]), although it may be different in vivo [9, 10]. Note that in order to calculate c, the native tissue (or lesion) T_1 (i.e., the value before injection of contrast agent, T_{10}) must also be known. Note that to apply Eqs. (4.1) and (4.2) to total tissue Gd concentration one has to implicitly assume fast water exchange between tissue compartments, i.e., that all the Gd in a voxel is available to relax all of the water, whether it is residing in the blood pool, the extravascular extracellular (interstitial) space or the intracellular space.

Second, the way in which the T_1 reduction increases the signal is modeled; this is specific to each sequence type. The most common sequence used for this purpose is the simple spoiled gradient echo ("FLASH" or "GRE"), on account of its ability to combine good volume coverage, acceptable spatial resolution, acceptable precision and accuracy, and acceptable acquisition speed. The signal S from a spoiled gradient echo sequence is:

$$S = S_0 \frac{\left(1 - e^{-TR/T_1}\right)\sin\,\theta}{1 - e^{-TR/T_1}\cos\,\theta} \tag{4.3}$$

where S_0 is the relaxed signal (i.e., equal to S when $TR \gg T_1$, $\theta = 90°$), and θ is the flip angle (FA). Note that this equation assumes echo time (TE) $<<$ T_2^*. S_0

can be found from the measured pre-Gd signal (before injection of contrast agent).

The sequence must be truly "spoiled" (i.e., there is no build up of steady-state transverse magnetization) and the FA used must be known (if necessary by employing a B_1 mapping method). Provided that the three parameters (r_1, T_{10}, and FA) are known, then there is a clear relationship between signal and the change in T_1 (i.e., the Gd concentration) (Eq. (4.3)).

To find the arterial plasma concentration, which will be required if pharmacokinetic modeling is to be performed, one needs first to find the blood concentration $c_b(t)$ from the blood signal, using Eqs. (4.1) and (4.3). Blood T_{10} is about 1.4 s at 1.5 T [11]. Since the contrast agent is only present in the extracellular space, the plasma concentration $c_p(t)$ is higher, by a factor related to the hematocrit Hct, e.g., a factor of 1.7 for $Hct = 41\%$[12]. Note that Hct can vary considerably between patients and over time in patients undergoing treatment [13]:

$$c_p = \frac{c_b}{1 - Hct} \tag{4.4}$$

Some studies attempt to find Gd concentration from signal by using a phantom calibration curve; however, these approaches are usually flawed, since the signal is also proportional to proton density (which is greater in an aqueous solution than in tissue), and the FA may be different when imaging the phantom (caused for example by different coil loading and/or B_1 inhomogeneity).

Pharmacokinetic modeling: from Gd concentration to physiology

"Tofts model": K^{trans} v_e and k_{ep}

Most modeling uses the concept of a compartment; this is like a bucket: the Gd tracer inside is dissolved in water and at the same concentration everywhere, and the flow into or out of the bucket is small enough to allow the contents to remain well mixed.

The simplest compartmental model has one tissue compartment in addition to a vascular compartment. This is known as the "Tofts model" [5] (mathematically equivalent to that proposed by Teorell [14] and Kety [15] in a non-MRI context), and may be used to measure K^{trans} and v_e (see Figure 4.1). The bolus injection of Gd gives a time-varying blood plasma concentration $c_p(t)$, which can be measured in each subject, or if not available estimated from a population average [16–18]. Since the commonly used contrast agents are small ($< \approx 1000$ daltons) then the leakage across the endothelium from the capillaries into the EES is generally accepted to be diffusive, passive, and hence reversible; it is therefore proportional to the difference between the concentrations in the plasma and in the EES (c_p and c_e respectively).

$$v_e \frac{dc_e(t)}{dt} = K^{trans}\left(c_p(t) - c_e(t)\right) \tag{4.5}$$

K^{trans} is the constant of proportionality, and $v_e c_e$ is the amount of Gd in the EES. Formally, K^{trans} is the volume transfer constant between the blood plasma and the EES [3]. Clearance from the blood is usually renal, although biliary clearance is also possible, depending on the contrast agent.

The solution to this equation is a convolution of c_p with the impulse response function K^{trans} $\exp(-k_{ep}t)$ [19]; when the intravascular Gd is taken into account, the total tissue concentration is:

$$c_t(t) = v_p c_p(t) + K^{trans} \int_0^t c_p(\tau)e^{-k_{ep}(t-\tau)}d\tau \tag{4.6}$$

Thus the total Gd concentration in a voxel or region of interest (ROI) (Eq. 4.6) is the sum of the EES contribution (which usually dominates, since $v_e \approx 10$–60%) and the intravascular contribution (the "v_p term"), which is often small and in some cases ignored

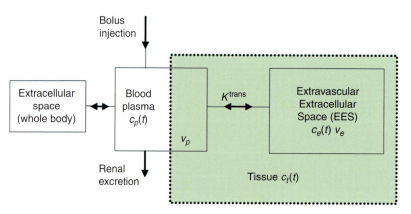

Figure 4.1 A simple compartmental model used for DCE-MRI data analysis. The Tofts model [5].

$(v_p \approx 1\text{–}10\%)$ [19]. The original "Tofts model" [5] had no v_p term. The "extended Tofts model" [19] refers to Eq. (4.6), with the v_p term present.

This model was able to explain signal enhancement in multiple sclerosis lesions [5] (Figure 4.2), and gave values of K^{trans} and v_e consistent with the known biology of acute and chronic lesions.

The differences in enhancement curve shape, and the time of peak enhancement, both apparent in Figure 4.2, are important. A model simulation [5] using typical K^{trans} values for tumors and neglecting the influence of any intravascular Gd (i.e., $v_p = 0$), shows that the initial slope depends on K^{trans} (Figure 4.3a), and is independent of v_e (Figure 4.3b). The final peak value depends on v_e, and larger v_e tumors take longer to reach their peak (Figure 4.3b). The shape of the curve is determined by k_{ep}, and if K^{trans} is increased whilst keeping k_{ep} fixed, the curve increases in amplitude but retains the same shape (Figure 4.3c) as is expected from Eq. (4.6).

In the original formulation of the model (applied to multiple sclerosis), trans-endothelial leakage was low enough that there would not be significant local depletion of Gd concentration in the capillary. Perfusion F was sufficient to maintain the capillary concentration at the arterial value. In this case, K^{trans} is just the permeability surface area product (PS), and DCE could reasonably be called "permeability imaging." This "permeability-limited" case is defined by $F \gg PS$:

$$K^{trans} = PS \qquad (F \gg PS) \qquad (4.7)$$

In tumors, the endothelium can be much more leaky, there may be local depletion from the vasculature, and K^{trans} will represent a combination of permeability and perfusion [3]. In the limiting case of very high

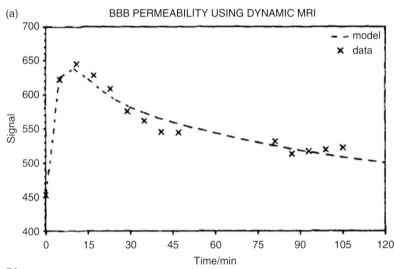

(a)

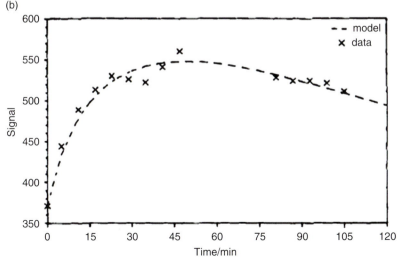

(b)

Figure 4.2 Use of DCE-MRI to measure capillary leakage in a patient with multiple sclerosis [5]. The upper plot shows enhancement in an acute multiple sclerosis lesion. The signal peaks at about 12 min, model fitting gave $K^{trans} = 0.050\ \mathrm{min}^{-1}$, $v_e = 21\%$. The lower plot shows a lesion with a less permeable blood–brain barrier ($K^{trans} = 0.013\ \mathrm{min}^{-1}$), and an enlarged EES ($v_e = 49\%$), with signal peaking later (at about 50 min). These data were collected in 1989 using a multi-slice spin echo sequence; note the poor temporal resolution by modern standards, and the missing data when the patients took a break. BBB, blood–brain barrier.

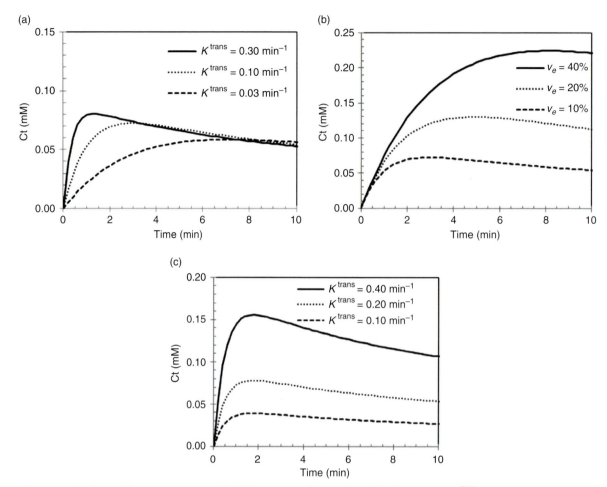

Figure 4.3 Simulations of tissue concentration after bolus injection of 0.1 mmol/kg of Gd, for a range of K^{trans} and v_e values, ignoring any intravascular contribution. (a) increasing K^{trans}, with fixed $v_e = 10\%$ (b) increasing v_e, with fixed $K^{trans} = 0.1$ min^{-1} (c) constant $k_{ep} = 2$ min^{-1}, increasing K^{trans} [5].

permeability, then K^{trans} will equal the plasma perfusion $(F_p = F(1 - Hct))$, and DCE could reasonably be called "perfusion imaging." This is the "flow-limited case", defined by $F \ll PS$.

$$K^{trans} = F(1 - Hct) \qquad (F \ll PS) \qquad (4.8)$$

The significance of K^{trans} under various values of F, PS, and v_p is explored in the reviews by Sourbron and Buckley [20, 21].

Perfusion is here used to mean the supply of blood to tissue (units: ml blood/min/100 ml tissue), and we have assumed that all blood passing into a volume of tissue is available for capillary exchange. Perfusion is the preferred term here [4]. It is sometimes called "blood flow," as used in some other chapters throughout this book. Note that in that case, the term may be ambiguous, as "flow" may also mean blood flow velocity (in m/s).

Blood perfusion F can be estimated from K^{trans} (Eq. 4.7) in the PS-limited case, provided Hct is known. However small-vessel hematocrit Hct^{small} can be considerably lower than in large vessels (where the AIF is measured). This is related to the Fahraeus effect; in small vessels the red blood cells are comparable in size to the vessel diameter, and travel faster than plasma [22]. Values for Hct^{small} are hard to measure; values of 24% (dog heart) [23], 31% (human brain) [24], 25% [25], and 8–20% [22] have been reported. The renal vasa recta (10–20 μm in diameter) have a reduced hematocrit of 40–50% compared with a large vessel [26]. Thus estimates of F are vulnerable to large uncertainties in Hct [27, 28].

Since the contrast agent is transported in the plasma, plasma perfusion F_p is more reliably measured than blood perfusion F. Thus there is a move to using F_p rather than F as the relevant biomarker in DCE-MRI [21, 27, 28].

The modeling of the capillary vasculature shown in Figure 4.1 is naive, and not surprisingly at high temporal resolution it fails. Modern sequences can sometimes provide a temporal resolution of ~1 s (depending on the organ, resolution, and coverage required), and in these cases the initial rise in signal gives information about perfusion, as Gd arrives in the capillary bed over a few seconds. More sophisticated models are then able to extract pure perfusion information [29, 30], and potentially pure permeability information as well. In DCE kidney imaging, the perfusion peak in tissue is clearly delayed (by about 4 s) with respect to the arterial peak (see Figure 4.4).

Other pharmacokinetic models

Other models have been proposed that aim to extract estimates of perfusion F from the DCE-MRI time series. These fall into three broad categories:

Bolus passage perfusion estimates

In some organs, notably the lung [31, 32] and the heart [33], T_1-weighted DCE-MRI measurements have been modeled in a similar fashion to bolus passage dynamic susceptibility contrast (DSC) measurements that historically have found application in the brain. The reason for this is partly physiological – these organs have a large blood volume – and partly pragmatic – the DCE-MRI measurements typically require breath-hold in both the lung and heart and therefore it is convenient to measure only the first passage. By restricting analysis to this early phase of the contrast agent delivery to the tissue it is often possible to ignore the effects of contrast agent leakage or to assume that any leakage that does occur is unidirectional (i.e., from the blood to the EES only, as there is not time for measureable leakage in the opposite direction). This allows methods such as the indicator dilution theorem to be applied [32], whilst not precluding full compartmental analysis if deemed necessary [33, 34]

Two-compartment exchange model (2CXM)

As discussed above, the model described in Eq. 4.6 allows the parameter K^{trans} to be interpreted either as the permeability surface area product (PS) or as perfusion (F), depending on the relative magnitudes of PS and F. The 2CXM addresses this ambiguity by explicitly modeling a perfusion component influencing the signal in the blood pool [30, 35, 36]

$$v_p \frac{dc_p(t)}{dt} = F(c_a - c_p) - K_{PS}(c_p - c_e) \qquad (4.10)$$

and

$$v_e \frac{dc_e(t)}{dt} = K_{PS}(c_p - c_e) \qquad (4.11)$$

where c_a is the AIF (i.e., the Gd concentration in a supplying artery), c_p is the tissue blood plasma concentration, and K_{PS} is the equivalent of K^{trans} (a transfer constant between the blood plasma space and the EES) but now the F versus PS ambiguity has been removed. While this is clearly an attractive benefit of this approach, the fact that an additional model parameter is extracted from the data imposes additional

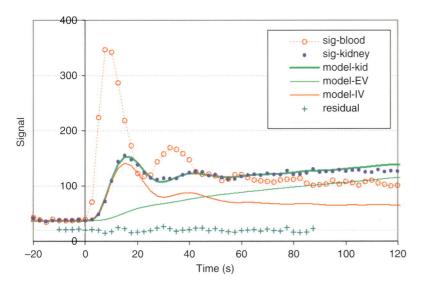

Figure 4.4 Model analysis of renal enhancement. The kidney signal (sig-kidney) is clearly delayed (by about two time points) from the blood signal (sig-blood). The model fit (model-kid) shows separately the extravascular filtered Gd (model-EV, from which glomerular filtration rate [GFR] is found) and the intravascular Gd (model-IV, from which blood volume and perfusion are estimated).

data quality requirements, and a careful statistical assessment should be performed to ensure that use of the more complex model is justified [34, 37].

Tissue homogeneity model

The tissue homogeneity model explicitly models the gradient in contrast agent concentration along a capillary induced due to the progressive leakage of contrast agent from the start to the end of the capillary bed [29, 38, 39]. It no longer conforms to the concept of a compartmental model with well-mixed compartments and is therefore sometimes referred to as a distributed parameter model. The modeling of the gradient in concentration along the capillary necessitates the incorporation of a transit time along the capillary, which in turn provides information on blood flow. The model has been simplified as the *adiabatic approximation to the tissue homogeneity model* (*AATH*) and applied to extract blood flow information using DCE-MRI in a range of tissues [29, 34]. As with the 2CXM, fitting of the AATH model requires additional parameter definition, with the subsequent need for careful assessment of the quality of the support for the model provided by the DCE-MRI data.

Heuristic methods

Other, simpler, methods are also used in DCE analysis. These include extraction of parameters such as inital slope, time to peak, and maximum enhancement. If the data acquisition is correctly configured, then these do not require knowledge of parameters that characterize the imaging sequence (e.g., FA) and the tissue (e.g., T_{10}) and are very simple to implement (there is no fitting process). However, errors in FA and variations in tissue native T_1 can have a substantial impact on image contrast and this can also affect heuristic parameterizations (an extreme example is if the FA is so small as to remove all useful T_1 contrast and no enhancement is observed). These parameterizations also usually have increased variability within and between subjects and between MR scanners, are dose-dependent, and the calculated tissue parameters may have no clear relationship to the underlying biological tissue characteristics.

Image acquisition

Imaging protocol

In DCE imaging, repeated T_1-weighted images are collected for several frames before Gd is injected, and then for several minutes afterwards. This is often preceded by a T_1 measurement. A good bolus injection can be achieved by using a power injector, with a saline flush after the Gd. The receiver and transmitter gains must be controlled for the whole series of DCE images.

Quality assurance [2, 40] can be used to ensure the scanner is stable for the DCE acquisition period. A phantom at constant temperature can be repeatedly imaged (this can also be used to check T_1 accuracy), or else one or more healthy volunteers can be repeatedly scanned (without Gd).

The sequence parameters will involve compromise between coverage, temporal resolution, and spatial resolution. Newer scanners have faster gradients (allowing shorter repetition times [TRs]), and multi-array receive coils give higher signal-to-noise ratio at short TRs. The optimal sequence will depend on the organ being measured; often frame times of 2–20 s can be achieved when using spoiled gradient echo methods. Three-dimensional (volume) sequences are preferred, since they have better FA accuracy than 2D (slice-selective) sequences and provide good volume coverage. Body coil transmission gives better FA accuracy than combined transmit/receive coils, but B_1 mapping may still be desirable, particularly in abdominal studies and at higher field strengths (3 T and above). In the abdomen, a coronal-sagittal oblique slice orientation (instead of transverse) can have two advantages: the aorta can be sampled along its length, reducing wash-in effects, and breathing movement is mostly in-plane and therefore more easily corrected. However, coronal-sagittal oblique methods are not always able to sample simultaneously the aorta and the organ or tumor of interest, so transverse acquisitions are more generally applicable, particularly if an effective motion correction strategy is employed [41].

The blood signal curve may be measured, in order to provide an AIF for the modeling. In this case a temporal resolution of ~3 s or less is desirable [42]. When examining abdominal organs or tumors the aorta is usually imaged, for thoracic imaging the ventricles of the heart or the pulmonary artery may be used, and for pelvic regions the iliac arteries may be employed; these vessels have cross-sectional areas that are large enough to allow AIFs to be extracted with minimal partial volume contamination. However, for other organs it can be a challenge to identify an adequate arterial supply and alternatives must be employed. For example, in the assessment of perfusion in breast lesions sometimes the left ventricle of the heart may be used, and in the brain the carotid may be employed, but both can suffer from problems with wash-in effects and coil sensitivity fall-off and, in the case of the carotid, substantial partial volume corruption. In such cases it may be necessary to

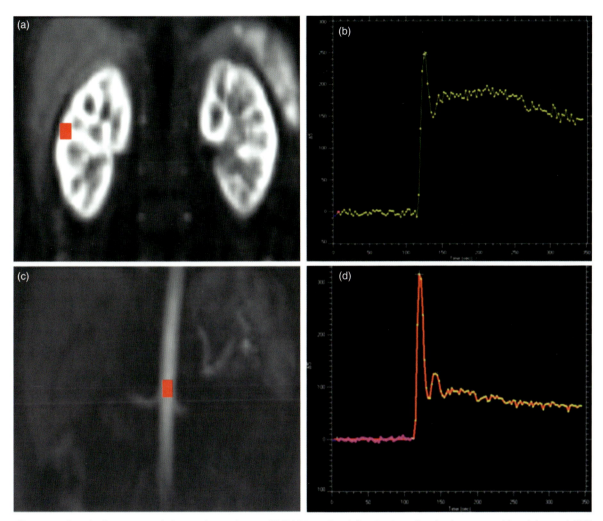

Figure 4.5 Signal enhancement in kidney and aorta. A cortical ROI (a) is used to define the time of peak enhancement (b), and the arterial ROI (c) gives the blood curve (d).

use a surrogate for the AIF, such as the concentration time course in a draining vein (such as the sagittal sinus) or a population AIF. Alternatively, it may be possible to account for partial volume effects by using alternative AIF measurement strategies, such as dual bolus methods [43, 44], phase-based correction methods [45], or reference tissue methods [46]. Wash-in effects are reduced by ensuring that the blood is fully saturated (i.e., has experienced several radiofrequency [RF] pulses) by the time it reaches the location of the ROI [47].

The DCE sequence should ideally be run long enough to sample the enhancement plateau. If not, then v_e cannot be reliably measured, given that it only affects the plateau value, but not the rising portion of the curve (see Figure 4.3b). In tumors, this means that one must often scan for quite a long duration (up to 5–10 min).

An example of rapid DCE is shown in Figure 4.5. Imaging of the kidney and aorta at a temporal resolution of 2.5 s, using half the standard dose of Gd, allows the perfusion phase of the tissue signal to be seen, and it has a clear delay with respect to the aortic peak. In this organ the blood volume is large (about 30%), and can be estimated because the perfusion peak is so distinct. A modified Tofts model fits the data well (Figure 4.4); in this model of the uptake phase (up to 90 s), the vascular delay and dispersion are accounted for, and there is no efflux from the parenchymal ROI. Renal filtration occurs mostly after bolus passage, and can be well estimated. Using this technique, GFR estimates in controls were in good agreement with normal literature values [27, 28, 48].

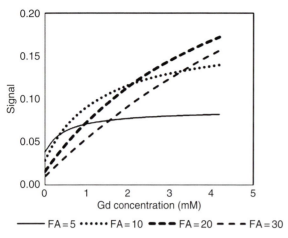

Figure 4.6 Signal intensity for a gradient echo sequence with various FA values. Eqs. (4.2) and (4.3) were used, with TR = 3 ms and $T_1 = 1$ s.

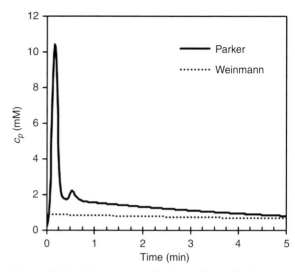

Figure 4.7 Population average AIFs (dose = 0.1 mmol/kg).

There is scope to optimize the FA when using spoiled gradient echo acquisitions. A small FA gives more signal at low concentration, but has limited dynamic range (see Figure 4.6 FA = 5°); increasing the FA gives increased sensitivity to Gd (Figure 4.6 FA = 10°); further increases (Figure 4.6 FA = 20° or 30°) give a wider dynamic range (at the expense of reduced sensitivity) and are needed if measuring the AIF (peak blood concentration 6 mM [17], see Figure 4.7) together with tissue enhancement. Non-linear dependence of signal on Gd concentration is not a concern as it is properly dealt with in the MRI model. However, large changes in T_2^* during the initial stages after contrast agent administration may affect the measurement when using spoiled gradient echo methods. This can be minimized by using the shortest possible TE.

Motion artifacts

Breathing can cause serious artifacts in body imaging, particularly in locations close to the diaphragm. Some data suggest this may only be a small effect and may not contribute significantly to overall measurement reproducibility [41]. However, we suggest some potential approaches to minimizing its effect:

1. Allow free breathing. Some centers minimize diaphragm movement by having one or both hands above the head. Any residual motion can be compensated for using image registration in post-processing, although the changing contrast observed during the DCE-MRI time course means that specially tailored registration methods may be required [41].

2. Breath-hold for first pass (~20 s) then allow breathing (although this can result in a large movement as breathing resumes). Also the position of the abdominal tissues during breath-hold may be different to all the other points in the time series, necessitating image registration. Some patients may also find it difficult to maintain a good breath-hold for 20 s.

3. Free breathe and discard data at the extremes of position (using the images, navigator gating or respiratory monitoring to detect the extrema) or apply image registration. However, discarding images can lead to important time points during the DCE-MRI and AIF series being missed, which is particularly critical during the first pass of contrast agent.

4. Guided free breathing (instructions from the imaging technologist).

Whether breathing should be controlled or not is currently unclear (this may depend on the kind of patient, and the availability of registration – see below), and is the subject of ongoing research.

Flip angle accuracy

FA accuracy is often poor, but is crucial if tissue parameters such as K^{trans} are to be determined accurately. It affects the calculation of concentration from enhancement (Eq. (4.3)), the estimation of the AIF, and the measurement of T_{10}. B_1 non-uniformity (heterogeneity), if present, means that the FA distribution is also non-uniform. There are two primary causes of such non-uniformity. First, dielectric resonance produces

Table 4.1. Sensitivity of tissue parameters to assumed T_{10} value taken from the literature. One signal dataset was analyzed using four values of T_{10}; parameters from the resulting fits are shown

Tissue	T_{10} (s)	K^{trans} (min^{-1})	v_e (%)	Residual in fit	k_{ep} (min^{-1})	$K^{trans} T_{10}$
Normal low-risk fatty portion	0.46	0.88	143	0.091	0.62	0.41
Tumor – low T_{10}	0.60	0.63	96	0.092	0.65	0.38
Normal high-risk diffuse density portion	0.71	0.51	76	0.093	0.67	0.36
Tumor – high T_{10}	1.3	0.26	36	0.095	0.72	0.34

Adapted from Tofts et al. [53]

standing waves in the subject, which are more pronounced at higher fields (e.g., 3 T) and in larger objects (the effect is greater in the body than in the head and can be significant even at 1.5 T [49]). Second, smaller transmit coils are less uniform, and therefore the body transmit coil is to be preferred (not a smaller combined transmit/receive coil). During the FA setup procedure, a good technique, if available, will optimize the FA over just the volume to be imaged (not the whole slice), and an accurate FA may then be obtained in spite of more global FA non-uniformity. An additional source of FA error is in 2D multi-slice imaging, where the slice profile is often poor, leading to varying FA across the slice [50, 51]. Therefore 3D (volume) acquisitions are preferred.

B_1 maps can be measured quite quickly [52] (< 2 min) and these may enable corrections to be made in the presence of FA inaccuracy and inhomogeneity. Transmit phased array technology is in development, which provides the ability to produce more homogeneous B_1 fields over the ROI within the subject, and these so-called "RF shimming" methods may enable acquisitions with more uniform and accurate FA values. Note that all manufacturers are developing dual- or multiple-transmitter systems for their 3 T systems, and some of these systems are already available today.

Tissue T_1

The tissue T_1 value (T_{10}) can be measured, or else a standard value from the literature used. An accurate measurement is preferred for each individual subject, since in disease this can alter; this can often be carried out in $\ll 5$ min. The most common method is the variable FA method, where gradient echo sequences with several FA values are used. These include a mostly proton density-weighted sequence (low FA) and one or more T_1-weighted sequence (higher FA). Clearly the T_{10} accuracy is crucially dependent on the FA accuracy.

Inversion recovery methods (with variable inversion time [TI], fixed FA) are more robust, but usually slower.

An error in the T_{10} value will in turn usually give an incorrect value for the tissue concentration (Eq. (4.1)). Thus if T_{10} has been measured badly, or if an incorrect standard value from the literature has been used, then gross errors in tissue parameters such as K^{trans} can ensue, particularly if literature values are used for a tissue which has a wide range of possible T_{10} values. An example from breast cancer shows that for a range of feasible T_{10} literature values used in the fitting process, the fits to a given image intensity dataset are equally good, K^{trans} can vary by at least a factor of 2, and v_e can reach impossible values ($v_e > 100\%$) [53]; see Table 4.1. k_{ep} is relatively robust (as long as the vascular volume [v_p] is negligible). An increase of 1% in T_{10} gives a resulting decrease of 1% in K^{trans}, such that the product remains approximately constant.

Choice of contrast agent

Any contrast agent can in principle be used for DCE methodology, provided it is stable and transport is passive (i.e., there is no active transport mechanism which would be concentration-dependent or favor transport in one direction over the other – see Eq. (4.5)). The initial work [5] was carried out with Gd-DTPA (Magnevist, size 938 Da). Clearly larger molecules will have lower permeability and hence possibly lower K^{trans} values (Eqs. (4.7) and (4.8)). The AIF may alter a little with viscosity (increased viscosity could slow down the mixing of the bolus into the blood pool). Contrast agents with larger molecular weight potentially can separate out the effects of permeability and perfusion on uptake, although the compound must be stable, with a single form in the bloodstream, and imaging times become longer. In view of the concerns about nephrogenic systemic fibrosis (NSF), there will be value in gaining experience using the newer cyclic compounds. In addition to Magnevist, potentially suitable candidate compounds (not all cyclic) are: Dotarem (754 Da), Eovist (725 Da), Gadovist (605 Da), Omniscan (574 Da), Optimark (662 Da), and ProHance (559 Da) (see http://www.rxlist.com). Different contrast media have different blood pool clearance rates, which may affect the AIF for DCE-MRI when long time series are being acquired. In particular, those agents that demonstrate clearance via the liver as well as the kidney (e.g., MultiHance [gadobentate dimeglumine] or Primovist/Eovist [gadoxetic acid disodium]) may demonstrate different blood kinetics to those that are cleared only via the kidneys. However, little research has been performed to date into the differences in AIFs that are likely to be observed when using different contrast media.

Image analysis

Analysis can be carried out on individual ROIs, or on a pixel-by-pixel basis to produce a map for the whole organ. The reduction of motion artifact using spatial registration, if available, is likely to improve the quality of the fit (depending on the tissue location). In-plane movement is relatively easy to remove, but because motion in the body is non-rigid, effective removal is much harder than in the brain, and a topic of ongoing research. Evidence suggests that while it is possible to correct for motion in DCE-MRI time series, the process of model fitting is relatively robust to periodic motion, meaning that quiet steady breathing may not introduce as many confounds as might be feared [41]. However, non-periodic motion (such as a bulk shift of the body) and very large breathing-related motion are likely to cause problems in the modeling output and should ideally be corrected.

The pharmacokinetic models described above require knowledge of the arterial plasma concentration $c_p(t)$; this is the arterial input function (AIF) calculated from the whole blood signal (which confusingly is sometimes called the "AIF," even though it contains both plasma and erythrocytes). It can be measured for each subject, and thus within- and between-subject variation can be taken into account, although if the technique is not implemented well, it can introduce extra variation which contaminates the final measurements of tissue physiology.

Alternatively, a population average AIF can be used. Some of these are described analytically (i.e., using mathematical equations, rather than just a list of numbers), which makes them more convenient to use. In particular they are available at any temporal resolution. The most popular are the original biexponential Weinmann plasma curve [16], derived from low temporal resolution arterial blood samples, and the more complex Parker blood function [17], derived from high temporal resolution MRI data. Horsfield's functional form [18] for the AIF needs a single measurement of absolute concentration. In the Parker function, bolus first pass and recirculation are represented. After bolus passage and recirculation, the MRI measurement for a standard dose of 0.1 mmol/kg (Parker $c_p[1 \text{ min}] = 1.53 \text{ mM}$ assuming $Hct = 42\%$) is considerably higher than the direct measurement (Weinmann $c_p[1 \text{ min}] = 0.82 \text{ mM}$); however, the estimates are within the error bars of the two experimental results used to derive the functions, indicating that they are likely to be compatible. Possible reasons for residual discrepancy include a population difference (the Parker AIFs were drawn from a population of cancer patients and the Weinmann AIFs from healthy volunteers; in neither case was a measured Hct used) and wash-in effects in the MRI method. Although the Weinmann input function was derived from blood samples with a temporal sampling too slow to capture the detail clearly present up to about 40 s (see Figure 4.7), by 1 min we expect the Weinmann values to be unaffected by this bolus mixing effect. The numerical AIFs of Fritz-Hansen et al. [54] showed excellent agreement between an inversion recovery MRI method and rapid direct blood measurements; their values (approximate mean over six subjects $c_p(1 \text{ min}) = 1.09 \text{ mM}$; range 0.86–1.64 mM; assumed $Hct = 0.42$) are closer to the Weinmann value but overlap with the Parker value (mean over 67 DCE-MRI measurements $c_p(1 \text{ min}) = 1.8 \pm 0.5 \text{ mM [SD]}$; assumed $Hct = 0.42$). The choice of AIF will depend on the tissue being studied and the sequences available.

When it comes to the modeling of the tissue signal, several versions can be considered. For "Tofts, modeling" the primary free parameters are K^{trans} and either k_{ep} or v_e (since k_{ep} and v_e are related). It is worth including v_p to see if the fit improves (but without inducing overfitting), and whether there is a systematic effect on the fitted K^{trans} and v_e values.

The onset time of the bolus t_onset should be included in the fitting process as there will be a variable delay between the location of AIF measurement and the tissue of interest. Similarly, onset time estimation will be needed if a population average AIF

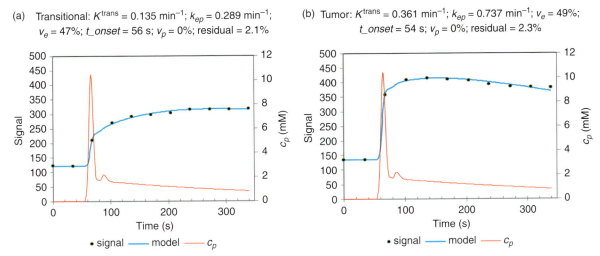

(a) Transitional: K^{trans} = 0.135 min^{-1}; k_{ep} = 0.289 min^{-1}; v_e = 47%; t_onset = 56 s; v_p = 0%; residual = 2.1%

(b) Tumor: K^{trans} = 0.361 min^{-1}; k_{ep} = 0.737 min^{-1}; v_e = 49%; t_onset = 54 s; v_p = 0%; residual = 2.3%

Figure 4.8 Modeling of prostate cancer DCE data. The Parker AIF was used (Figure 4.7), with $v_p = 0$. Although data were only acquired every 34 s, the model was calculated with a temporal resolution of 1 s. Spreadsheet output is shown for (a) transitional tissue and (b) tumor ROIs (data from University of Miami).

is used (since the timing of bolus arrival with respect to the start of tissue enhancement is unknown). The appropriate approach will again depend on the organ and the temporal resolution.

The mathematical process of fitting the model to the data works as follows. The model signal can be calculated for many combinations of the free parameters (K^{trans}, etc., Table 4.2). For each of these combinations, the differences between the model signal value (at each time point) and the measured data are found. These differences are squared and summed across each time point to provide a "total "difference." The free parameters are adjusted until this total difference is minimized. The model has then been "fitted" to the data. This is called the "least squares solution." The differences between the data and the fitted model are called "residuals" (e.g., Figure 4.5). From these can be found the "root-mean-square residual," which is a kind of average difference between the model and the data, and which gives an indication of the quality of the model and of the fit. If the residuals appear random in character then these probably derive from a random effect such as image noise or movement; if there seems to be a systematic pattern to the residuals then the model can often be improved.

For any fitting procedure, basic tests should be carried out to ensure that the procedure converges properly (i.e., that the fitted parameters are independent of the starting values), and reformulation of the free parameters to decrease their interdependence may be required. "Fit failures" can occur, particularly if the data

are noisy (e.g., deriving from single pixels instead of an ROI); no valid parameter values are produced for that dataset. In the fitting process it is important to identify and flag these failures, so that the output (i.e., invalid parameter values) does not contaminate any subsequent analysis. Values of $v_e > 100\%$ may occur if an incorrect value of T_{10} has been used (see Table 4.1), if v_p has not been incorporated in the fit when needed, or if the enhancement peak has not been reached (see Figure 4.3b). It is also helpful to test to see if any detectable enhancement has occurred prior to fitting a model in order to avoid fitting to a signal that is indistinguishable from noise, as this can lead to randomly erroneous parameters. Ithas also been shown that quantification of the amount of tumor that does not enhance is in itself a useful parameter to extract from the DCE-MRI time series [55–57]. Note that recent developments in the field allow for nested modeling of both "Tofts models", with or without v_p, with automatic selection of one model over the next one based on an F test [58].

Fitting can be implemented in three ways. The simplest and most straightforward way is to use ROI data (which are inherently low noise) and put these into a spreadsheet (e.g., Microsoft Excel running on a PC). The mathematics can be set up using inbuilt formula functions, and the "solver" function can carry out the minimization process. The more complex way is to set up pixel-by-pixel mapping, either using a standard environment (e.g., Matlab) or by obtaining this from a supplier. Pixel mapping is more likely to

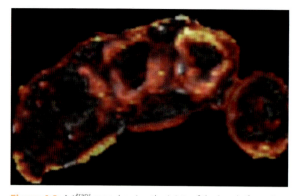

Figure 4.9 A K^{trans} map showing the joints of the hand of a patient suffering from rheumatoid arthritis. The presence of inflammation in the joints leads to additional blood vessel recruitment and leaky vasculature, making DCE-MRI a potentially useful way to monitor disease and therapeutic intervention [66].

benefit from spatial registration of the images to reduce the effect of motion; the operation is much more computer-intensive, and the single-pixel data are inherently noisy, so care must be taken to identify fit failures. The benefits of pixel mapping include the abilities to interrogate all the tissue without bias, and to generate histograms and other measures of tissue or tumor heterogeneity, which have potential utility [59, 60]. The third possibility is to use commercially available software, which is currently available from third parties and also from at least one mainstream MRI vendor.

Histograms can show the distribution of parameter values, in a region or volume of interest. By taking care of histogram generation and architecture, histograms become more useful and comparisons are more easily made [61]. The y-values can be calculated such that the area under the histogram curve is either the total volume under interrogation (in ml), or 100%

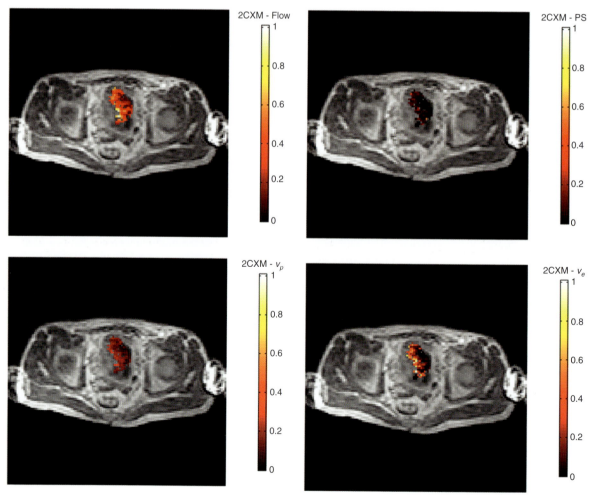

Figure 4.10 An example of the application of the 2CXM model in a patient with prostate cancer, providing measures of flow, PS, v_p, and v_e.

(i.e., the histograms are normalized). Features such as peak location and height can be extracted from histograms. Characterizing the distribution tails can have predictive value [56, 62], and principle component analysis of the histogram shape can be powerful [63].

An example of using a spreadsheet to implement modeling of ROI data is shown in Figure 4.8 [64]. The prostate data have quite low temporal resolution (34 s), T_{10} had to be assumed (1.5 s), and a Parker AIF was used. Including the v_p term did not improve the fitting (and in fact it became rather unstable), probably because prostate perfusion is low [65] and the temporal resolution coarse. In several ROIs from the same subject, fitted onset time agreed within 2 s, suggesting that it can be found quite reliably.

Examples of parametric maps based on pixel-by-pixel analysis are shown in Figures 4.9 and 4.10; Figure 4.9 shows a K^{trans} map from the hand of a patient with rheumatoid arthritis, while Figure 4.10 shows various permeability and flow parameters derived from the 2CXM model in a patient with prostate cancer.

Conclusions

The principle physiological parameters that can be measured with DCE-MRI are the transfer coefficient K^{trans} (related to capillary permeability, surface area and perfusion) and v_e, the size of the EES, although additional useful parameters are measurable given appropriate sequences and analysis methods. To do this needs good control of FA and an accurate measurement of tissue T_1 before injection of Gd. If T_1 measurement is not available, then it may be possible to use a standard value; in any case the rate constant k_{ep} can still be measured, which is probably useful. The possible and optimum acquisition protocols and models will depend on which tissue is being imaged.

Acknowledgments

David Collins and Martin Leach (both Institute of Cancer Research, UK), and David Buckley (University of Leeds, UK) contributed valuable insight into DCE imaging. Isky Gordon (University College London, UK) and Iosif Mendichovszky (University of Manchester, UK) provided data for Figure 4.5. Peter Gall (Siemens Medical) contributed the list of CAs. Radka Stoyanova (University of Miami, USA) provided data for Figure 4.9. Penny Hubbard (University of Manchester, UK) provided Figure 4.10.

References

1. Jackson A, Buckley DL, Parker GJ. *Dynamic Contrast-Enhanced Magnetic Resonance Imaging in Oncology.* Berlin: Springer, 2004.

2. Tofts PS. *Quantitative MRI of the Brain: Measuring Changes Caused by Disease.* New York: Wiley, 2003.

3. Tofts PS, Brix G, Buckley DL, *et al.* Estimating kinetic parameters from dynamic contrast-enhanced T(1)-weighted MRI of a diffusable tracer: standardized quantities and symbols. *J Magn Reson Imaging* 1999;**10**:223–32.

4. Leach MO, Brindle KM, Evelhoch JL, *et al.* The assessment of antiangiogenic and antivascular therapies in early-stage clinical trials using magnetic resonance imaging: issues and recommendations. *Br J Cancer* 2005;**92**:1599–610.

5. Tofts PS, Kermode AG. Measurement of the blood-brain barrier permeability and leakage space using dynamic MR imaging. 1. Fundamental concepts. *Magn Reson Med* 1991;**17**:357–67.

6. Naish JH, McGrath DM, Bains LJ, *et al.* Comparison of dynamic contrast-enhanced MRI and dynamic contrast-enhanced CT biomarkers in bladder cancer. *Magn Reson Med* 2011; **66**: 219–26.

7. Yang C, Stadler WM, Karczmar GS, *et al.* Comparison of quantitative parameters in cervix cancer measured by dynamic contrast-enhanced MRI and CT. *Magn Reson Med* 2010;**63**:1601–9.

8. Tofts PS, Shuter B, Pope JM. Ni-DTPA doped agarose gel–a phantom material for Gd-DTPA enhancement measurements. *Magn Reson Imaging* 1993;**11**:125–33.

9. Shuter B, Tofts PS, Wang SC, Pope JM. The relaxivity of Gd-EOB-DTPA and Gd-DTPA in liver and kidney of the Wistar rat. *Magn Reson Imaging* 1996;**14**:243–53.

10. Stanisz GJ, Henkelman RM. Gd-DTPA relaxivity depends on macromolecular content. *Magn Reson Med* 2000;**44**:665–7.

11. Spees WM, Yablonskiy DA, Oswood MC, Ackerman JJ. Water proton MR properties of human blood at 1.5 Tesla: magnetic susceptibility, T(1), T(2), T*(2), and non-Lorentzian signal behavior. *Magn Reson Med* 2001;**45**:533–42.

12. Boron WF, Boulpaep EL. *Medical Physiology.* Philadelphia: Saunders, 2008.

13. Roberts C, Hughes S, Naish JH, *et al.* Individually Measured Hematocrit in DCE-MRI studies. *Proc Intl Soc Magn Reson Med*, Montreal, Canada, 2011; 1078.

14. Teorell T. Kinetics of distribution of substances admitted to the body. I. The extravascular modes of administration. *Arch Int Pharmacodyn Ther* 1937;**57**:205–25.

15. Kety SS. The theory and applications of the exchange of inert gas at the lungs and tissues. *Pharmacol Rev* 1951;**3**:1–41.

16. Weinmann HJ, Laniado M, Mutzel W. Pharmacokinetics of GdDTPA/dimeglumine after intravenous injection into healthy volunteers. *Physiol Chem Phys Med NMR* 1984;**16**:167–72.

17. Parker GJ, Roberts C, Macdonald A, *et al.* Experimentally-derived functional form for a population-averaged high-temporal-resolution arterial input function for dynamic contrast-enhanced MRI. *Magn Reson Med* 2006;**56**:993–1000.

18. Horsfield MA, Thornton JS, Gill A, *et al.* A functional form for injected MRI Gd-chelate contrast agent concentration incorporating recirculation, extravasation and excretion. *Phys Med Biol* 2009;**54**:2933–49.

19. Tofts PS. Modeling tracer kinetics in dynamic Gd-DTPA MR imaging. *J Magn Reson Imaging* 1997;**7**:91–101.

20. Sourbron SP, Buckley DL. On the scope and interpretation of the Tofts models for DCE-MRI. *Magn Reson Med* 2011;**66**:735–45.

21. Sourbron SP, Buckley DL. Tracer kinetic modelling in MRI: estimating perfusion and capillary permeability. *Phys Med Biol* 2012;**57**:R1–33.

22. Pries AR, Ley K, Gaehtgens P. Generalization of the Fahraeus principle for microvessel networks. *Am J Physiol* 1986;**251**:H1324–32.

23. Crystal GJ, Downey HF, Bashour FA. Small vessel and total coronary blood volume during intracoronary adenosine. *Am J Physiol* 1981;**241**:H194–201.

24. Sakai F, Nakazawa K, Tazaki Y, *et al.* Regional cerebral blood volume and hematocrit measured in normal human volunteers by single-photon emission computed tomography. *J Cereb Blood Flow Metab* 1985;**5**:207–13.

25. Rempp KA, Brix G, Wenz F, *et al.* Quantification of regional cerebral blood flow and volume with dynamic susceptibility contrast-enhanced MR imaging. *Radiology* 1994;**193**:637–41.

26. Gaehtgens P. Flow of blood through narrow capillaries: rheological mechanisms determining capillary hematocrit and apparent viscosity. *Biorheology* 1980;**17**:183–9.

27. Tofts PS, Cutajar M, Mendichovszky IA, Gordon I. Accurate and precise measurement of renal filtration and vascular parameters using DCE-MRI and a 3-compartment model. *Proc Intl Soc Magn Reson Med*, Stockholm, Sweden, 2010; 326.

28. Tofts PS, Cutajar M, Mendichovszky IA, Peters AM, Gordon I. Precise measurement of renal filtration and vascular parameters using a two-compartment model for dynamic contrast-enhanced MRI of the kidney gives realistic normal values. *Eur Radiol* 2012;**22**:1320–30.

29. St Lawrence KS, Lee TY. An adiabatic approximation to the tissue homogeneity model for water exchange in the brain: I. Theoretical derivation. *J Cereb Blood Flow Metab* 1998;**18**:1365–77.

30. Donaldson SB, West CM, Davidson SE, *et al.* A comparison of tracer kinetic models for T1-weighted dynamic contrast-enhanced MRI: application in carcinoma of the cervix. *Magn Reson Med* 2010;**63**:691–700.

31. Hatabu H, Tadamura E, Levin DL, *et al.* Quantitative assessment of pulmonary perfusion with dynamic contrast-enhanced MRI. *Magn Reson Med* 1999;**42**:1033–8.

32. Ohno Y, Hatabu H, Murase K, *et al.* Quantitative assessment of regional pulmonary perfusion in the entire lung using three-dimensional ultrafast dynamic contrast-enhanced magnetic resonance imaging: preliminary experience in 40 subjects. *J Magn Reson Imaging* 2004;**20**:353–65.

33. Jerosch-Herold M. Quantification of myocardial perfusion by cardiovascular magnetic resonance. *J Cardiovasc Magn Reson* 2010;**12**:57.

34. Naish JH, Kershaw LE, Buckley DL, *et al.* Modeling of contrast agent kinetics in the lung using T1-weighted dynamic contrast-enhanced MRI. *Magn Reson Med* 2009;**61**:1507–14.

35. Brix G, Kiessling F, Lucht R, *et al.* Microcirculation and microvasculature in breast tumors: pharmacokinetic analysis of dynamic MR image series. *Magn Reson Med* 2004;**52**:420–9.

36. Sourbron S, Ingrisch M, Siefert A, Reiser M, Herrmann K. Quantification of cerebral blood flow, cerebral blood volume, and blood-brain-barrier leakage with DCE-MRI. *Magn Reson Med* 2009;**62**:205–17.

37. Brix G, Zwick S, Kiessling F, Griebel J. Pharmacokinetic analysis of tissue microcirculation using nested models: multimodel inference and parameter identifiability. *Med Phys* 2009;**36**:2923–33.

38. Johnson JA, Wilson TA. A model for capillary exchange. *Am J Physiol* 1966;**210**:1299–303.

39. Koh TS, Zeman V, Darko J, *et al.* The inclusion of capillary distribution in the adiabatic tissue homogeneity model of blood flow. *Phys Med Biol* 2001;**46**:1519–38.

40. Tofts PS. QA: quality assurance, accuracy, precision and phantoms. In: Tofts P, editor, *Quantitative MRI of the Brain: Measuring Changes Caused by Disease.* Chichester: John Wiley, 2003;55–81.

41. Buonaccorsi GA, O'Connor JP, Caunce A, *et al.* Tracer kinetic model-driven registration for dynamic contrast-enhanced MRI

time-series data. *Magn Reson Med* 2007;**58**:1010–19.

42. Henderson E, Rutt BK, Lee TY. Temporal sampling requirements for the tracer kinetics modeling of breast disease. *Magn Reson Imaging* 1998;**16**:1057–73.

43. Kostler H, Ritter C, Lipp M, *et al.* Prebolus quantitative MR heart perfusion imaging. *Magn Reson Med* 2004;**52**:296–9.

44. Risse F, Semmler W, Kauczor HU, Fink C. Dual-bolus approach to quantitative measurement of pulmonary perfusion by contrast-enhanced MRI. *J Magn Reson Imaging* 2006;**24**:1284–90.

45. Korporaal JG, van den Berg CA, van Osch MJ, *et al.* Phase-based arterial input function measurements in the femoral arteries for quantification of dynamic contrast-enhanced (DCE) MRI and comparison with DCE-CT. *Magn Reson Med* 2011; **66**:1267–74.

46. Yankeelov TE, Luci JJ, Lepage M, *et al.* Quantitative pharmacokinetic analysis of DCE-MRI data without an arterial input function: a reference region model. *Magn Reson Imaging* 2005;**23**:519–29.

47. Roberts C, Little R, Watson Y, *et al.* The effect of blood inflow and B(1)-field inhomogeneity on measurement of the arterial input function in axial 3D spoiled gradient echo dynamic contrast-enhanced MRI. *Magn Reson Med* 2011;**65**:108–19.

48. Buckley DL, Shurrab AE, Cheung CM, *et al.* Measurement of single kidney function using dynamic contrast-enhanced MRI: comparison of two models in human subjects. *J Magn Reson Imaging* 2006;**24**:1117–23.

49. Barker GJ, Simmons A, Arridge SR, Tofts PS. A simple method for investigating the effects of non-uniformity of radiofrequency transmission and radiofrequency reception in MRI. *Br J Radiol* 1998;**71**:59–67.

50. Brookes JA, Redpath TW, Gilbert FJ, Murray AD, Staff RT. Accuracy of T1 measurement in dynamic contrast-enhanced breast MRI using two- and three-dimensional variable flip angle fast low-angle shot. *J Magn Reson Imaging* 1999;**9**:163–71.

51. Parker GJ, Barker GJ, Tofts PS. Accurate multislice gradient echo T(1) measurement in the presence of non-ideal RF pulse shape and RF field nonuniformity. *Magn Reson Med* 2001;**45**:838–45.

52. Dowell NG, Tofts PS. Fast, accurate, and precise mapping of the RF field in vivo using the 180 degrees signal null. *Magn Reson Med* 2007;**58**:622–30.

53. Tofts PS, Berkowitz B, Schnall MD. Quantitative analysis of dynamic Gd-DTPA enhancement in breast tumors using a permeability model. *Magn Reson Med* 1995;**33**:564–8.

54. Fritz-Hansen T, Rostrup E, Larsson HB, Sondergaard L, Ring P, Henriksen O. Measurement of the arterial concentration of Gd-DTPA using MRI: a step toward quantitative perfusion imaging. *Magn Reson Med* 1996;**36**:225–31.

55. O'Connor JP, Jayson GC, Jackson A, *et al.* Enhancing fraction predicts clinical outcome following first-line chemotherapy in patients with epithelial ovarian carcinoma. *Clin Cancer Res* 2007;**13**:6130–5.

56. Donaldson SB, Buckley DL, O'Connor JP, *et al.* Enhancing fraction measured using dynamic contrast-enhanced MRI predicts disease-free survival in patients with carcinoma of the cervix. *Br J Cancer* 2010;**102**:23–6.

57. Mills SJ, Soh C, O'Connor JP, *et al.* Tumour enhancing fraction (EnF) in glioma: relationship to tumour grade. *Eur Radiol* 2009;**19**:1489–98.

58. Bagher-Ebadian H, Jain R, Nejad-Davarani SP, *et al.* Model selection for DCE-T1 studies in glioblastoma. *Magn Reson Med* 2011;**68**:241–51.

59. Rose CJ, Mills SJ, O'Connor JP, *et al.* Quantifying spatial heterogeneity in dynamic contrast-enhanced MRI parameter maps. *Magn Reson Med* 2009;**62**:488–99.

60. Canuto HC, McLachlan C, Kettunen MI, *et al.* Characterization of image heterogeneity using 2D Minkowski functionals increases the sensitivity of detection of a targeted MRI contrast agent. *Magn Reson Med* 2009;**61**:1218–24.

61. Tofts PS, Davies GR, Dehmeshki J. Histograms: measuring subtle diffuse disease. In: Tofts P, editor. *Quantitative MRI of the Brain: Measuring Changes Caused by Disease.* Chichester: John Wiley, 2003;581–610.

62. Tofts PS, Benton CE, Weil RS, *et al.* Quantitative analysis of whole-tumor Gd enhancement histograms predicts malignant transformation in low-grade gliomas. *J Magn Reson Imaging* 2007;**25**:208–14.

63. Dehmeshki J, Ruto AC, Arridge S, *et al.* Analysis of MTR histograms in multiple sclerosis using principal components and multiple discriminant analysis. *Magn Reson Med* 2001;**46**:600–9.

64. Tofts PS, Stoyanova R. Fast modelling of slow DCE data from prostate: rate constant (k_{ep}) and extracellular extravascular space (EES; v_e) both distinguish hypoxic regions in the tumour. European Society for Magnetic Resonance in Medicine and Biology Congress Leipzig 2011; 27.

65. Buckley DL, Roberts C, Parker GJ, Logue JP, Hutchinson CE. Prostate cancer: evaluation of vascular characteristics with dynamic contrast-enhanced T1-weighted MR imaging–initial experience. *Radiology* 2004;**233**:709–15.

66. Hodgson RJ, Barnes T, Connolly S, *et al.* Changes underlying the dynamic contrast-enhanced MRI response to treatment in rheumatoid arthritis. *Skeletal Radiol* 2008;**37**:201–7.

73

Appendix 4.1: Model parameters

There are several kinds of parameters used in the model. *Fixed* parameters (FA, TR, Hct, T_{10}, T_{10}^{blood}, r_1) have preset values which are required before fitting can start. *Free* parameters (K^{trans}, v_e, k_{ep}, and maybe v_p and t_onset) are varied and then estimated as part of the fitting process. Other parameters (c_p, etc.) are used temporarily as part of the process of modeling the signal. The fixed and free parameters are summarized in Table 4.2.

Table 4.2. Fixed and free parameters in DCE modeling

Quantity	Symbol	Units	Type
Perfusion (of blood)[a]	F	ml blood/min (100 ml tissue)$^{-1}$	Free
Flip angle[b]	FA	degrees	Fixed; may require B_1 mapping to provide accurate values
Hematocrit[c]	Hct	%	Fixed; measure independently if possible Approximate normal ranges: males 40–52%; females 36–48%. Textbook value is 41% [12]
Onset time	t_onset	s	Free
Rate constant[d]	k_{ep}	min^{-1}	Free
Transfer constant	K^{trans}	min^{-1}	Free
T_1 relaxivity	r_1	s^{-1} mM^{-1}	Fixed (4.5 s^{-1} mM^{-1}). May vary in vivo but currently not possible to measure
T_1 of blood	T_{10}^{blood}	s	Fixed (measured)
T_1 of tissue	T_{10}	s	Fixed (measured)
TR	TR	s	Fixed
Fractional volume of EES[e]	v_e	$0 < v_e < 100\%$	Free
Fractional volume of blood plasma in tissue	v_p	$0 < v_p < 100\%$	Free

[a] Plasma perfusion F_p is more reliably measured, and an unambiguous symbol for blood perfusion is F_b (see text)
[b] θ is also used to denote the flip angle (used in Eq. (4.3))
[c] Small vessel hematocrit is considerably lower (see text)
[d] $k_{ep} = K^{trans}/v_e$
[e] Extravascular extracellular space

5 Imaging of brain oxygenation

Weili Lin, Hongyu An, Andria D. Ford, Katie L. Vo, Jin-Moo Lee, and Greg Zaharchuk

Key points

- Brain oxygenation is important in many disease processes, most notably ischemic stroke and brain tumors.
- It is possible to make proton MR images sensitive to oxygenation using the blood oxygenation level-dependent (BOLD) contrast mechanism.
- Quantitative BOLD (qBOLD) approaches rely on analytical and numerical models to determine the tissue oxygenation, removing the potentially confounding effects of T_2, CBV, and magnetic field inhomogeneity.
- Quantitative susceptibility mapping (QSM) allows measurement of oxygenation in large blood vessels.
- "T_2 relaxation under spin tagging" (TRUST) methods first isolate the vascular compartment, and then measure its T_2 relaxation time, using a look-up table to convert T_2 values to oxygenation.
- By also measuring cerebral blood flow (CBF), it is possible to estimate a cerebral oxygen metabolic index (COMI), related to $CMRO_2$.
- Changes in transverse relaxation times are small over the physiological range of oxygenation, similar to background field inhomogeneities, making accurate determination difficult; MR-based methods of oxygenation imaging are therefore currently in the research realm, rather than clinical practice.

Introduction

Tissue oxygenation is a critical physiological parameter in most organ systems. In the brain, oxygenation status plays an important role in hypoxic and ischemic injuries, carotid artery disease, and tumor growth and response to therapy. Traditionally, positron emission tomography (PET) has been used to measure brain oxygen metabolism, but more recently the feasibility of measuring brain oxygenation with MRI has been explored [1–6]. This chapter discusses the theory and methodology of several approaches for measuring brain tissue oxygenation using MRI, including quantitative blood oxygenation level-dependent (qBOLD), quantitative susceptibility mapping (QSM), and T_2 relaxation under spin tagging (TRUST). Additional detail, particularly more technical aspects, can be found in a recent review article [7]. Before delving into these methods, we will present a brief review of cerebral autoregulation as it affects oxygenation measurements.

Theory

Cerebrovascular autoregulation and oxygenation measurements

When an artery becomes narrowed or completely occluded, the mean arterial pressure (MAP) in the distal circulation may fall, depending on both the degree of stenosis and the adequacy of collateral sources of blood flow [8]. If collateral flow is inadequate, MAP will fall, leading to a reduction in cerebral perfusion pressure (CPP), which is defined as the difference between MAP and venous backpressure.

When CPP falls, the cerebral vasculature can respond with two compensatory mechanisms serving to maintain the normal delivery of oxygen and nutrients. First, arterioles can dilate in order to reduce vascular resistance and maintain cerebral blood flow (CBF) at near normal levels [9]. This phenomenon, termed autoregulation, operates over a wide range of perfusion pressure reductions [10]. The second compensatory mechanism is through increases in the oxygen extraction fraction (OEF) [3, 11]. When the delivery of oxygen falls, the amount of available oxygen extracted from the blood can increase in order to maintain normal oxygen metabolism. OEF can increase from a baseline of 40% to up to 80%. This situation has been called "misery perfusion"[12]. There are slight increases in OEF through the autoregulatory range, as CBF falls at a slight, but constant rate [1, 3, 13]. OEF increases dramatically once autoregulatory capacity has been exceeded. Cerebral metabolic rate of oxygen utilization ($CMRO_2$) remains constant during both the autoregulation and misery perfusion states. However, at maximal oxygen extraction, any further reduction in CBF results in a decline of $CMRO_2$. Below a certain threshold, it has been postulated that a series of cellular and molecular death cascades are activated, leading inexorably to neural cell death. Therefore, a non-invasive means to probe alterations in cerebral oxygen metabolism may be useful in distinguishing viable tissue from tissue destined to die.

Non-quantitative and quantitative BOLD

The fundamental principle on which blood oxygenation is estimated by MRI is that hemoglobin in its oxygenated form is diamagnetic, while in its deoxygenated form is paramagnetic. Oxygen depletion resulting in increasing levels of deoxyhemoglobin therefore causes a paramagnetic shift in the resonance frequency of blood water, and due to the vascular structure, also increases signal dephasing, particularly in gradient echo images (decreased T_2^* – the "BOLD" effect). Deoxygenated blood in the microvasculature can also shorten tissue transverse relaxation times. With the advent of fast imaging techniques and the improved understanding of the biophysical basis of the BOLD effect [14–16] contrast mechanisms, MRI has the potential therefore for the estimation of brain oxygen levels. Specifically, it has been demonstrated that when the concentration of deoxyhemoglobin increases, the transverse relaxation times T_2 and T_2^* decrease, resulting in a decreased MR signal intensity on T_2- and T_2^*-weighted images, respectively. With

animal models, many studies have demonstrated that BOLD effects can be used to monitor the changes of oxygen saturation in vivo under pathophysiological conditions such as hypoxia [17–23], hyper- and hypocapnia [19, 24, 25], hemodilution [26], and ischemia [27, 28]. Figure 5.1 demonstrates how the MR signal behaves under both experimental hypercapnia and hypoxia. These images were acquired in a rat using a T_2^*-weighted sequence that is sensitive to changes of deoxyhemoglobin concentration. Figure 5.1a shows the T_2^*-weighted image acquired during the baseline condition. Under the hypercapnic condition (Figure 5.1b), an increased CBF with concurrent vasodilatation is anticipated, resulting in a reduction of OEF which in turn leads to a decrease of deoxyhemoglobin concentration and an increase in MR signal (Figure 5.1b). Notice the visibility of the venous vessels is markedly diminished. In contrast, under the hypoxic condition, the increased OEF leads to an increase of deoxyhemoglobin concentration. As a result, a reduction in MR signal is observed (Figure 5.1c). Together, these results demonstrate that the BOLD contrast approach could be used to provide insights into alterations of blood oxygenation in vivo.

In addition to the qualitative indicators of blood oxygenation, extensive effort has been devoted to developing quantitative measures of BOLD effects including experimental [29–31] and theoretical [32–35] approaches. The ability of MRI to measure blood oxygenation was demonstrated as early as 1982 by Thulborn et al. [30], who reported a linear relation between blood R_2 ($= 1/T_2$) and oxygenation ex vivo. Wright et al. [31] subsequently proposed a simplified signal model characterizing the relation between R_2 and blood oxygenation. Through imaging of blood samples with different oxygenation levels, a calibration curve was obtained, which in turn provided a means for obtaining in vivo blood oxygenation. More recently, a rapid data acquisition approach capable of obtaining in vivo blood oxygenation measures in less than a minute was proposed [36]. With this approach, in vivo experiments in human subjects for measuring blood oxygenation at both the internal carotid artery and the internal jugular vein were conducted, which in turn provided quantitative measures of global OEF. A normal global OEF of 37% was reported, which is consistent with values obtained using PET scans. However, a potential difficulty associated with the T_2-based approach is the need for a calibration curve, typically derived from ex vivo studies. Alternatively,

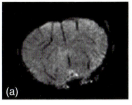 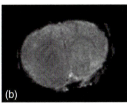 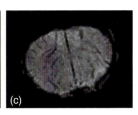

(a) (b) (c)

Figure 5.1 MR signal behaviors under baseline condition (a), hypercapnia (b), and hypoxia (c) in a rat brain using a T_2^*-weighted sequence. Notice the diminished (b) and enhanced (c) visualization of vascular structures during hypercapnia and hypoxia compared to the baseline condition, due to decreased and increased vascular deoxyhemoglobin concentrations respectively.

others [37] have modeled the blood vessels as long cylinders, for which an exact theoretical expression is available to quantify in vivo blood oxygenation, eliminating the need for an empirically derived calibration curve. While the above approaches have all been successfully applied in vivo to obtain quantitative measures of blood oxygenation, these approaches can only measure blood oxygenation in large vessels. However, in many diseases, approaches for deriving oxygenation at the tissue level are needed rather than in large vessels.

Yablonskiy and Haacke [34] have proposed a signal model focused on deoxyhemoglobin-induced signal loss outside of the intravascular space, which could potentially provide a means to quantitatively measure blood oxygenation not only in large vessels but also at the tissue level.

Assuming blood vessels form an interconnecting network of long cylinders with random orientations, a relation between R_2' ($= 1/T_2^* - 1/T_2$) and blood oxygenation can be derived as

$$R_2 = \lambda \cdot \gamma \cdot \frac{4}{3} \cdot \pi \cdot \Delta\chi_0 \cdot cHct \cdot (Y_a - Y_v) \cdot B_0 \qquad (5.1)$$

where λ is the fractional blood volume containing deoxyhemoglobin or venous cerebral blood volume (vCBV). In this discussion, λ and vCBV will be used interchangeably. γ is the gyromagnetic ratio, cHct is the fractional cerebral hematocrit, B_0 is the main magnetic field strength, Y_a and Y_v are the arterial and venous oxygen saturation, respectively, and $\Delta\chi_0$ is the susceptibility difference between the fully oxygenated and the fully deoxygenated blood, which has been measured to be 0.18 ppm/Hct in cgs units [38]. From this equation, it is evident that if R_2' and vCBV can be obtained experimentally, OEF (defined as $Y_a - Y_v$, or $1 - Y_v$ when the arterial blood is fully oxygenated) can be calculated. Below, we will discuss how these two parameters can be measured experimentally.

Experimental methods
Imaging approaches to measure CBV and R_2'

Various MR imaging methods have been developed to acquire images that can be subsequently processed using Eq. (5.1) [34] to obtain vCBV and OEF. A basic requirement is to measure R_2', the difference between the transverse relaxation rates that can be "reversed" or not by an 180° refocusing pulse. Many pulse sequences have been proposed for this purpose (e.g., [39]), and more detailed descriptions of the imaging approaches can be found elsewhere [40–44], but here we will focus on the potential applications of two approaches: multi-echo gradient echo/spin echo (MEGESE) [40, 43], also sometimes called gradient echo sampling under the spin echo (GESSE); and asymmetry spin echo (ASE) approaches [42]. In short, there are three fundamental differences between the two approaches. The MEGESE approach employs a conventional 2D spin echo sequence with additional gradient echoes centered around the spin echo. In contrast, the ASE approach employs a spin echo echo-planar imaging (EPI) sequence, where the duration between the 90° and 180° pulses is varied to acquire a series of images with different T_2^* weighting while keeping the echo time identical for all images. Second, with the differences in sequence design for the two approaches, the data analysis schemes also differ. Since the gradient echo images acquired using MEGESE are inherently weighted by T_2, it is necessary to estimate T_2 to remove effects of T_2 in different gradient echo images. Conversely, the T_2 effect is identical for all images acquired using ASE and thus the T_2 estimation step is not needed. Finally, although the ASE approach is less sensitive to motion-related artifacts, owing to the EPI acquisition scheme, the spatial resolution is limited when compared to the 2D MEGESE approach. Therefore, although both approaches are capable of providing measures of OEF and vCBV, the choice between these two

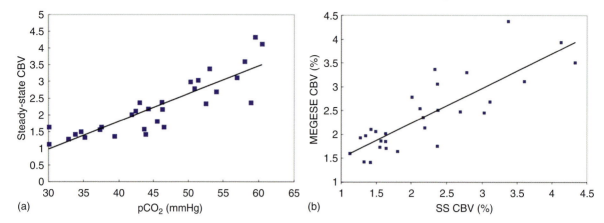

Figure 5.2 A linear relation between MR-measured CBV and PaCO$_2$ is shown in (a) consistent with the expected physiological behavior during hypercapnia. In addition, a linear relationship is found between the "MEGESE" determined CBV and the commonly used steady-state approach based on T$_1$-weighted MRI (b).

sequences needs to be considered in the context of the applications. For example, the ASE can be used for human studies, to minimize motion artifacts, while 2D MEGESE is more suitable for animal studies, to improve spatial resolution.

Venous CBV measurements

The lack of a gold standard for measuring vCBV in vivo makes it difficult to validate directly the MR MESEGE approach. Nevertheless, several experimental studies have suggested that MR is indeed capable of serving as a non-invasive means for measuring this parameter, which is necessary for the measurement of oxygenation using qBOLD.

It is well known that CBV increases in response to hypercapnia (elevated PaCO$_2$). To study how arterial and venous CBV respond individually to hypercapnia, one study acquired MEGESE images after injecting a gadolinium (Gd)-based contrast agent, OmniScan (0.05–0.1 mmol/kg) [45]. It is expected that the magnetic susceptibility effect caused by the Gd contrast agent will be much larger than that due to oxygenation changes associated with hypercapnia, and will uniformly affect both arterial and venous blood pools once a steady state of Gd concentration in the vasculature has been reached. Therefore, after Gd injection, changes in the measured R$_2'$ are expected to be dominated by changes in CBV (rather than oxygenation), and since Gd is equally distributed throughout the vasculature, this will be the total CBV, rather than venous CBV. This approach permits the direct comparison between the MEGESE-based

CBV determination, and that of more established approaches for measuring CBV, namely either steady-state and dynamic susceptibility contrast approaches (see Chapters 1, 2, and 4). A highly linear relation (r = 0.87) was observed between CBV obtained from the steady-state T$_1$-weighted MRI approach and PaCO$_2$ (Figure 5.2a), as well as a linear relation (r = 0.83) between the CBV obtained using the MEGESE approach and that from the steady-state approach (Figure 5.2b). Together, these findings suggest that the MEGESE is capable of providing measures of CBV that are consistent with the known physiological alteration during hypercapnia, and values agreed well with the established steady-state approach.

Similar studies have also been conducted in normal subjects in the absence of contrast agent. Under these circumstances, changes in vCBV in normal subjects during hypercapnia may be estimated. Figure 5.3 shows vCBV during normo- (Figure 5.3a) and hypercapnia (Figure 5.3b), demonstrating an increased vCBV during experimental hypercapnia. Estimates of vCBV in gray and white matter revealed that the mean vCBV in white matter increased from 3.3 ± 0.5% to 3.8 ± 0.8%, while in gray matter it increased from 4.2 ± 0.5% to 4.8 ± 0.6% during normocapnia and hypercapnia, respectively. These results suggest that vCBV is elevated in response to hypercapnia, similar to the total CBV (tCBV). The ratio of vCBV to tCBV in human subjects [45] was investigated by acquiring two sets of CBV images, MEGESE (Figure 5.4a) prior to the injection of a contrast agent for vCBV, and the steady-state approach for tCBV after contrast agent injection

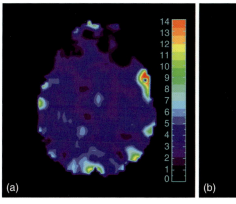 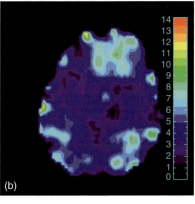

Figure 5.3 Venous CBV maps based on R_2' mapping obtained from a normal volunteer under normo- (a) and hypercapnic (b) conditions are shown, demonstrating increased vCBV during hypercapnia when compared with that during normocapnia.

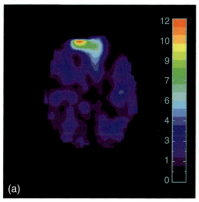 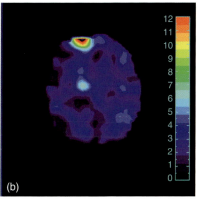

Figure 5.4 MR-measured vCBV in a normal volunteer measured (pre-contrast) from R_2' mapping (a), and tCBV estimated from steady-state T_1-weighted MRI in the presence of a contrast agent (b). Artifacts due to field inhomogeneity are seen in the frontal lobe.

(Figure 5.4b). vCBV and tCBV were found to be $2.5 \pm 0.3\%$ and $3.2 \pm 0.4\%$, respectively, which in turn provide a vCBV/tCBV ratio of 0.77 ± 0.04, in general agreement with results reported using other techniques [46, 47].

Oxygen extraction fraction

OEF is a fundamental physiological variable of importance in a number of conditions, and therefore it is critical to determine whether MR is capable of providing a measure of OEF in vivo. Ideally, a direct comparison between MR-determined OEF and that obtained using PET (which may be considered a gold standard in humans) is needed. However, a difficulty in directly comparing OEF between MR and PET is that, until very recently, it has not been possible to acquire MR and PET images simultaneously during experimental manipulation. Simultaneous acquisition

of MR and PET is of critical importance for any validation where physiological conditions are to be manipulated. For example, although an experimental manipulation (i.e., hypercapnia) can be introduced twice, one for MR and the other for PET, a major assumption is that identical physiological conditions can be maintained for both manipulations, which is clearly challenging. Hopefully, this limitation will be overcome in the near future with the availability of hybrid MR/PET scanners [48]. Alternatively, it is feasible to validate MR-measured OEF through the classical approach: namely, a direct comparison between MR measures and jugular bulb oximetry [44, 49], where blood samples are drawn from the jugular vein, reflecting the total amount of oxygen extracted by the brain, assuming that the arterial blood is fully saturated.

A study in rats with experimental manipulations including hypoxia and hypercapnia was employed to

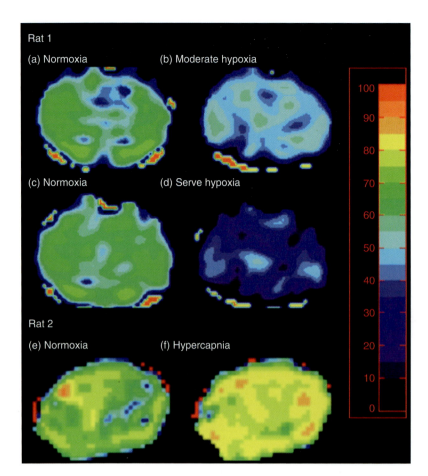

Rat 1
(a) Normoxia   (b) Moderate hypoxia
(c) Normoxia   (d) Serve hypoxia
Rat 2
(e) Normoxia   (f) Hypercapnia

Figure 5.5 MR-measured venous cerebral blood oxygenation (Y_v) in two rats under different experimental conditions, including (a, c, e) normoxia, (b, d) hypoxia, and (f) hypercapnia. Moderate and severe hypoxia cause a progressive decrease in Y_v (increase in OEF, unless Y_a is also decreased), while hypercapnia causes a mild increase in Y_v (decreased OEF).

introduce a wide range of physiologically relevant blood oxygenation conditions in order to investigate the relationship between MR OEF measurements and venous oxygenation [49]. Animals were imaged with a catheter placed in the internal jugular bulb for simultaneous blood sampling. Representative cerebral venous blood oxygenation (Y_v) maps (which can be converted to OEF maps using the relationship OEF $= Y_a - Y_v$) from one rat undergoing control, moderate hypoxia, and severe hypoxia, and another rat undergoing hypercapnia, are shown in Figure 5.5, demonstrating MRI's ability to discern expected changes of Y_v in response to experimental conditions.

To compare MR oxygenation measurements with those taken directly via blood gas measurements, ideally the samples should be withdrawn from the superior sagittal sinus where the MR measurement is made. However, the placement of a catheter in the superior sagittal sinus would induce susceptibility

effects on MR, confounding measures of blood-induced BOLD effects. Therefore, the relationship between blood oxygenation in the internal jugular vein and the superior sagittal sinus was first determined (Figure 5.6a), which was then used to derive a predicted superior sagittal sinus blood oxygenation based on a jugular blood oxygenation measurement [49]. A linear relationship was obtained between MR-measured blood oxygenation of the brain and the predicted oxygenation of the superior sagittal sinus, based on experimentally derived values from the jugular vein (Figure 5.6b).

MR estimates of OEF have also been attempted in human volunteers using measurements of R_2'. MR images acquired during both normo- (breathing of medical air) and hypercapnia (carbogen, 97% O_2 and 3% CO_2) from a representative subject are shown in Figure 5.7. The image acquired during hypercapnia shows a reduction of OEF, consistent with the

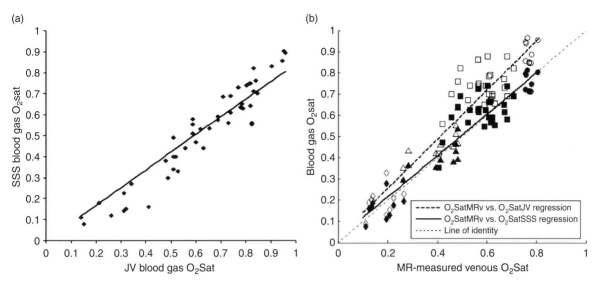

Figure 5.6 (a) A linear relation of blood oxygenation in the jugular vein (JV) and the superior sagittal sinus (SSS) is observed, although it is evident that the oxygenation of the jugular vein is higher when compared with that obtained from the superior sagittal sinus. (b) The comparison of MR-measured blood oxygenation in the brain with that obtained at the jugular vein through blood gas analysis and the converted superior sagittal sinus.

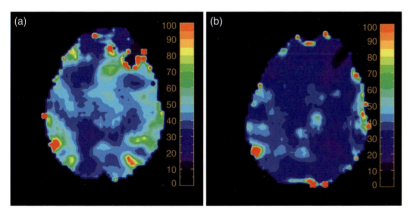

Figure 5.7 MR-derived OEF maps in a normal human volunteer during (a) normo- and (b) hypercapnia (breathing 97% O_2 3% CO_2). Quantitative estimates of OEF in gray (GM) and white matter (WM) under normo- and hypercapnia are shown in (c).

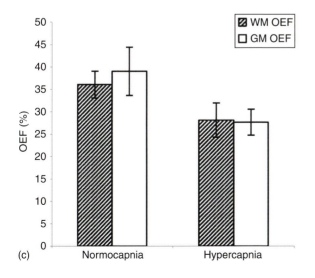

expected physiological response. Note that the images displayed in Figure 5.5 are Y_v (which is equal to $Y_a - OEF$) while OEF is provided in Figure 5.7. Quantitative OEF estimates for both gray matter and white matter during normo- and hypercapnia are shown in Figure 5.7c, demonstrating a significant OEF reduction during hypercapnia. Since BOLD effects are field strength dependent, with a higher magnetic field having a greater sensitivity to susceptibility effects, results on both OEF and vCBV from human subjects are given in Table 5.1. Both the OEF and vCBV are essentially identical between the two field strengths, with a normal OEF in the order of 45% that is consistent with that obtained using PET [40–42].

Improving oxygenation measurements using a multi-parametric approach

While the MEGESE and ASE approaches described above can measure oxygenation and CBV, it has been shown that reliable estimations are only possible in the setting of high signal-to-noise ratio (SNR) [50, 51]. In particular, if one or the other parameter is known, the other parameter may be more easily

Table 5.1. Measures of MR-based OEF and vCBV at 1.5 T and 3 T

	1.5 T (n = 12)	3 T (n = 5)
OEF	45.3% ± 5.5%	45.2% ± 5.5%
vCBV	2.68% ± 0.47%	2.89% ± 0.2%

estimated. Thus, one approach is to measure T_2 and T_2^* using separate high-resolution multi-echo gradient and spin echo sequences, and CBV using either dynamic or steady-state susceptibility contrast perfusion-weighted imaging [52, 53]. This approach can also be combined with CBF maps acquired using arterial spin labeling (ASL), enabling quantitative measurements of $CMRO_2$ (see below). An example of the increase in OEF associated with acute stroke using this approach is shown in Figure 5.8. Currently, the largest drawbacks to this method are the need for contrast administration and the need for high-resolution imaging (i.e., small voxels) for the measurement of T_2 and T_2^*, so as to minimize the effects of main magnetic field (B_0) inhomogeneity.

Measuring oxygenation using quantitative susceptibility mapping (QSM)

In addition to causing changes in the transverse relaxation rate R_2', the presence of deoxyhemoglobin also causes a change in the water resonance frequency (i.e., a bulk magnetic susceptibility effect). In gradient echo MRI, this will cause a phase shift of the MRI signal, which increases with increasing TE. This phase shift allows magnetic field differences between vessels and brain parenchyma to be detected, as well as differentiation between arteries and veins within the brain [54]. By using a mathematical model that relates magnetic field susceptibility changes to phase changes, it is possible to determine the difference in

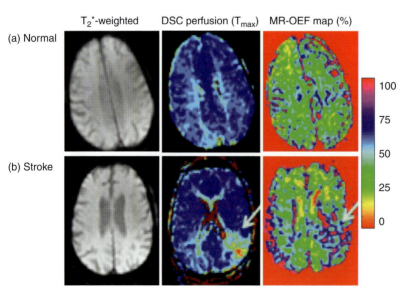

Figure 5.8 Images in a normal volunteer (a) and patient with acute stroke (b). The middle column is a map of T_{max}, the arterial input function-normalized time to the peak of the residue function, which shows a region of prolongation in the left posterior frontal lobe in the stroke patient. In this same region, there is an increased OEF (arrow), consistent with misery perfusion. OEF $(1 - Y_v)$ was measured using a multi-parametric approach in which T_2, T_2^*, and CBV were all directly measured using a multi-echo spin and gradient echo EPI sequence during bolus contrast injection.

susceptibility between veins and brain tissue [55, 56]. Since the value of magnetic susceptibility difference between tissue and fully deoxygenated blood is a known constant (0.27 ppm), this allows susceptibility maps to be scaled into maps of venous oxygenation. Using this approach, oxygenation in cerebral veins in humans was found to be Y_v of 61 ± 6% [57]. Another study used such a measurement to estimate the oxygenation of the carotid arteries and jugular veins, which, when coupled with a measurement of CBF, allowed an estimate of global Y_v (64 ± 4%) and $CMRO_2$ (127 ± 7 mol/100 g/min), both consistent with prior literature values [58]. The largest impediments towards more routine application of this methodology are the ability to assess only relatively large veins (rather than tissue) and errors due to non-vascular susceptibility sources (such as intra- and extracellular iron). Nevertheless, the field of QSM is likely to grow in importance as a tool for determining oxygenation in the human brain.

Measuring oxygenation using T_2 relaxation under spin tagging (TRUST)

It has been known for a long time that T_2 and $T_2{}^*$ of blood is dependent on its oxygenation state, first described by Thulborn *et al.* in the early days of MRI [31]. The "TRUST" method attempts to isolate the venous blood signal by suppressing the surrounding brain parenchyma signal, and then measures T_2 or $T_2{}^*$ relaxation rates free from partial volume effects. This was first demonstrated for separating large arteries and veins [32], and has been refined by subsequent investigators [39, 59, 60]. This method has been demonstrated in human brain at 3 T [61], using an ASL method to isolate arterial blood. It was found that the arterial oxygenation level decreased from 97% to 84% during a hypoxic challenge (14% O_2 inhalation). It was also found that the mean oxygenation of the superior sagittal sinus was 65 ± 8%, which also changed as expected during hypercapnia and caffeine administration [62].

Isolating venous blood in small venules is more challenging. One attempt used a velocity-selective ASL sequence with specific timing to isolate venous blood, a method called QUantitative Imaging of eXtraction of Oxygen and TIssue Consumption (QUIXOTIC) [63]. Using this approach, a venous oxygenation level of 73 ± 2% was found, slightly higher than previous methods and literature values.

The source of this difference remains a source of investigation. The limitations of QUIXOTIC include relatively low SNR, since vCBV is a small fraction of most cerebral voxels.

MR-measured cerebral oxygen metabolic index

Although there are several reported approaches capable of providing in vivo measures of $CMRO_2$, including relative and global measures [37, 38, 58, 64, 65], here we will only focus on approaches that provide both quantitative and regional measures.

Once CBF and OEF are obtained using MRI, the cerebral oxygen metabolic index (COMI) may be defined as the product of CBF and OEF. Note that there are several differences between the derivation of COMI and PET-based $CMRO_2$. First, although related, the physiological definitions of the two values are different. COMI yields the theoretical volume of blood from which 100% of oxygen can be extracted (i.e., oxygen clearance), while PET $CMRO_2$ gives an absolute value of oxygen extracted from a given volume of blood in μmol/min/g. Second, definitions of COMI and PET $CMRO_2$ are different. PET $CMRO_2$ is defined as the product of CBF, OEF, and arterial oxygen content (CaO_2), while COMI is simply the product of CBF and OEF. Finally, MR-based OEF differs from PET-based OEF. As mentioned previously, the MR-based OEF described earlier in this chapter reflects the extent to which arterial blood is desaturated as it passes through the brain. After using separate measurements of regional CBF, CBV, and arterial blood sampling to obtain arterial time activity and correcting for the signal from the un-extracted ^{15}O, quantitative OEF can be obtained. Subsequently, $CMRO_2$ can be calculated as a product of CBF, OEF, and CaO_2 [66]. Despite the aforementioned differences, the physiological implications of the two values should be similar. Figure 5.9 shows CBF, OEF, and COMI from a normal volunteer. Not unexpectedly, given its strong dependence on CBF, a clear demarcation between gray and white matter COMI is seen [67, 68]. COMI values of 29 ± 3 and 13 ± 3 ml/100 g/min for gray and white matter, respectively have been measured using this technique [65]. These results yield a gray matter to white matter COMI ratio of 2.4 ± 0.4, which is comparable to the reported range of $CMRO_2$ ratio of 1.4–2.0 in the PET literature [67, 68].

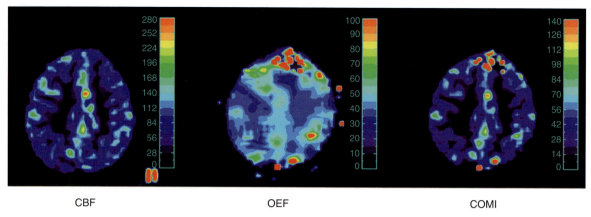

Figure 5.9 MR-measured cerebral blood flow (CBF) using DSC, OEF (using R_2' mapping), and cerebral oxygen metabolic index (COMI, the product of CBF and OEF, which is related to the $CMRO_2$) from a normal volunteer.

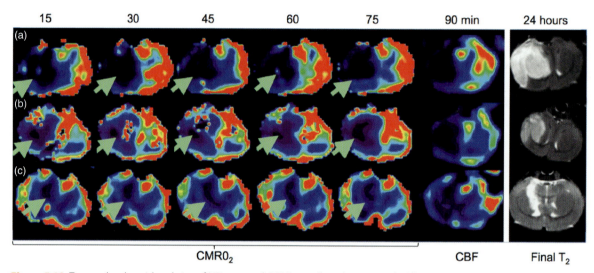

Figure 5.10 Temporal and spatial evolution of MR-measured COMI maps from three rats with different degrees of ischemic injury following permanent occlusion of the right middle cerebral artery (MCAO). In addition, the CBF and T_2-weighted images obtained at 90 min and 24 hrs after MCAO, respectively, are shown.

Applications of COMI

With the ability to provide quantitative measures of oxygen metabolism using MRI, regional measures of COMI can be obtained in a wide variety of pathological conditions. In the context of this chapter, we will focus a brief discussion specifically on its application in cerebral ischemia.

Using an intraluminal suture middle cerebral artery occlusion (MCAO) rat model, the temporal changes of COMI every 15 min during 90 min of MCAO were measured (Figure 5.10) [49]. Using the size of the T_2 lesion as a gauge for ischemic severity, the severity progressively decreases in examples from three different rats (rows a to c). In the rat shown in row a, COMI is markedly reduced immediately after occlusion and throughout the entire ischemic duration, suggesting that the brain tissue is severely injured immediately after MCAO onset. Regions with substantial COMI reduction 75 min after MCAO are similar to the final lesion seen on T_2-weighted MRI. In the second rat (row b), although a large region of mild COMI reduction is observed, only a small region with severely reduced COMI is observed immediately after MCAO, which continues to evolve as a function of time. The temporal characteristics of COMI in the third rat (row c) are similar to the second rat; the

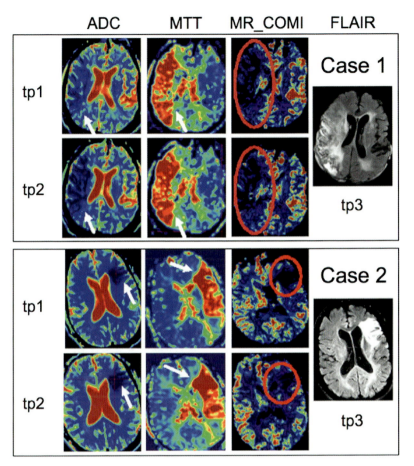

Figure 5.11 Preliminary example of MR-based COMI in two patients with acute ischemic middle cerebral artery (MCA) stroke, one with a diffusion/perfusion matched (upper panel) and one with a diffusion/perfusion mismatched lesion (lower panel). Time point 1 (tp1) is 3 hrs, tp2 6 hrs, and tp3 1 month after stroke onset. Apparent diffusion coefficient (ADC) and mean transit time (MTT) maps derived from diffusion perfusion MRI are shown at time points 1 and 2. Note that in the lower case, only the region with low COMI (similar to the ADC lesion) progresses to infarction, despite a much larger region having prolonged MTT.

region with severely diminished COMI is initially small and continues to evolve as a function of time. Nevertheless, the final T_2 lesion is much smaller than that for the first two rats, with infarction of the basal ganglia and preoptic regions only, with sparing of the cortex. Consistent with the smaller final infarct size, CBF and COMI were relatively well preserved in the cortex at earlier time points.

In addition to animal studies, human studies using MR-based COMI have been demonstrated. [5, 69] One study imaged acute ischemic stroke patients at 3 hrs, 6 hrs, and 1 month after the onset of symptoms [69]. Representative examples are provided in Figure 5.11 for two patients, one with a diffusion/perfusion matched lesion (upper panel) and the other with a mismatched lesion (lower panel). For the patient with the matched lesion, a persistently low COMI is observed for both time points, eventually evolving to infarction. In contrast, the patient with the diffusion/perfusion mismatch only shows reduced COMI in part of the region with reduced flow (similar to the region with reduced apparent diffusion coefficient [ADC]), which later evolved into final infarction. Although studies with a larger sample size will be needed to determine conclusively the utility of COMI in patients with acute stroke, these preliminary results suggest that a severely reduced COMI may be indicative of future infarction.

Conclusions

While methods to measure oxygenation and oxygen metabolism using MRI are still developmental, this remains an active area of research interest. Improved techniques will be required, which are robust enough for use in clinical studies, with suppression of artifacts from background field inhomogeneities and other experimental imperfections, and the development of appropriate post-processing tools. Studies with a larger sample size are needed to determine conclusively the potential clinical utilities of MR oxygenation imaging in this setting, and compare with existing modalities. In addition, the recent availability of hybrid MR/PET scanners may offer new means to validate MR measures of oxygenation simultaneously with the gold standard PET measurements.

References

1. Frykholm P, Andersson JL, Valtysson J, et al. A metabolic threshold of irreversible ischemia demonstrated by PET in a middle cerebral artery occlusion-reperfusion primate model. *Acta Neurol Scand* 2000;**102**:18–26.

2. Giffard C, Young AR, Kerrouche N, Derlon JM, Baron JC. Outcome of acutely ischemic brain tissue in prolonged middle cerebral artery occlusion: a serial positron emission tomography investigation in the baboon. *J Cereb Blood Flow Metab* 2004;**24**:495–508.

3. Powers WJ, Grubb RL, Darriet D, Raichle ME. Cerebral blood flow and cerebral metabolic rate of oxygen requirements for cerebral function and viability in humans. *J Cereb Blood Flow Metab* 1985;**5**:600–8.

4. Young AR, Sette G, Touzani O, et al. Relationships between high oxygen extraction fraction in the acute stage and final infarction in reversible middle cerebral artery occlusion: an investigation in anesthetized baboons with positron emission tomography. *J Cereb Blood Flow Metab* 1996;**16**:1176–88.

5. Lee JM, Vo KD, An H, et al. Magnetic resonance cerebral metabolic rate of oxygen utilization in hyperacute stroke patients. *Ann Neurol* 2003;**53**:227–32.

6. Adeoye O, Hornung R, Khatri P, Kleindorfer D. Recombinant tissue-type plasminogen activator use for ischemic stroke in the United States: a doubling of treatment rates over the course of 5 years. *Stroke* 2011;**42**:1952–5.

7. Christen T, Bolar DS, Zaharchuk G. Imaging brain oxygenation with MRI using blood oxygen approaches: methods, validation, and clinical applications. *AJNR Am J Neuroradiol.* 2012;in press.

8. Powers WJ, Press GA, Grubb RL, Gado M, Raichle ME. The effect of hemodynamically significant carotid artery disease on the hemodynamic status of the cerebral circulation. *Ann Intern Med* 1987;**106**:27–34.

9. MacKenzie ET, McGeorge AP, Graham DI, et al. Effects of increasing arterial pressure on cerebral blood flow in the baboon: influence of the sympathetic nervous system. *Pflugers Arch* 1979;**378**:189–95.

10. Rapela CE, Green HD. Autoregulation of canine cerebral blood flow. *Circ Res* 1964;**15** Suppl:205–12.

11. Powers WJ. Cerebral hemodynamics in ischemic cerebrovascular disease. *Ann Neurol* 1991;**29**:231–40.

12. Baron JC, Bousser MG, Comar D, Soussaline F, Castaigne P. Noninvasive tomographic study of cerebral blood flow and oxygen metabolism in vivo. Potentials, limitations, and clinical applications in cerebral ischemic disorders. *Eur Neurol* 1981;**20**:273–84.

13. Dirnagl U, Pulsinelli W. Autoregulation of cerebral blood flow in experimental focal brain ischemia. *J Cereb Blood Flow Metab* 1990;**10**:327–36.

14. Ogawa S, Lee TM, Nayak AS, Glynn P. Oxygenation-sensitive contrast in magnetic resonance image of rodent brain at high magnetic fields. *Magn Reson Med* 1990;**14**:68–78.

15. Ogawa S, Lee TM, Barrere B. The sensitivity of magnetic resonance image signals of a rat brain to changes in the cerebral venous blood oxygenation. *Magn Reson Med* 1993;**29**:205–10.

16. Ogawa S, Lee TM, Kay AR, Tank DW. Brain magnetic resonance imaging with contrast dependent on blood oxygenation. *Proc Natl Acad Sci USA* 1990;**87**:9868–72.

17. Rosen BR, Turner R, Hunter GJ, Fordham JA. MR depicts perfusion of brain and heart. *Diagn Imaging (San Franc).* 1991;**13**:105–10.

18. Prielmeier F, Nagatomo Y, Frahm J. Cerebral blood oxygenation in rat brain during hypoxic hypoxia. Quantitative MRI of effective transverse relaxation rates. *Magn Reson Med* 1994;**31**:678–81.

19. Jezzard P, Heineman F, Taylor J, et al. Comparison of EPI gradient-echo contrast changes in cat brain caused by respiratory challenges with direct simultaneous evaluation of cerebral oxygenation via a cranial window. *NMR Biomed* 1994;**7**:35–44.

20. Hoppel BE, Weisskoff RM, Thulborn KR, et al. Measurement of regional blood oxygenation and cerebral hemodynamics. *Magn Reson Med* 1993;**30**:715–23.

21. Rostrup E, Larsson HB, Toft PB, Garde K, Henriksen O. Signal changes in gradient echo images of human brain induced by hypo- and hyperoxia. *NMR Biomed* 1995;**8**:41–7.

22. Kennan RP, Scanley BE, Gore JC. Physiologic basis for BOLD MR signal changes due to hypoxia/hyperoxia: separation of blood volume and magnetic susceptibility effects. *Magn Reson Med* 1997;**37**:953–6.

23. Lin W, Paczynski RP, Celik A, *et al.* Experimental hypoxemic hypoxia: changes in R2* of brain parenchyma accurately reflect the combined effects of changes in arterial and cerebral venous oxygen saturation. *Magn Reson Med* 1998;**39**:474–81.

24. Davis TL, Kwong KK, Weisskoff RM, Rosen BR. Calibrated functional MRI: mapping the dynamics of oxidative metabolism. *Proc Natl Acad Sci USA* 1998;**95**:1834–9.

25. Lin W, Celik A, Paczynski RP, Hsu CY, Powers WJ. Quantitative magnetic resonance imaging in experimental hypercapnia: improvement in the relation between changes in brain R2 and the oxygen saturation of venous blood after correction for changes in cerebral blood volume. *J Cereb Blood Flow Metab* 1999;**19**:853–62.

26. Lin W, Paczynski RP, Celik A, Hsu CY, Powers WJ. Effects of acute normovolemic hemodilution on T_2*-weighted images of rat brain. *Magn Reson Med* 1998;**40**:857–64.

27. De Crespigny AJ, Wendland MF, Derugin N, Kozniewska E, Moseley ME. Real-time observation of transient focal ischemia and hyperemia in cat brain. *Magn Reson Med* 1992;**27**:391–7.

28. Ono Y, Morikawa S, Inubushi T, Shimizu H, Yoshimoto T. T_2*-weighted magnetic resonance imaging of cerebrovascular reactivity in rat reversible focal cerebral ischemia. *Brain Res* 1997;**744**:207–15.

29. Foltz WD, Merchant N, Downar E, Stainsby JA, Wright GA. Coronary venous oximetry using MRI. *Magn Reson Med* 1999;**42**:837–48.

30. Thulborn KR, Waterton JC, Matthews PM, Radda GK. Oxygenation dependence of the transverse relaxation time of water protons in whole blood at high field. *Biochim Biophys Acta* 1982;**714**:265–70.

31. Wright GA, Hu BS, Macovski A. 1991 I.I. Rabi Award. Estimating oxygen saturation of blood in vivo with MR imaging at 1.5 T. *J Magn Reson Imaging* 1991;**1**:275–83.

32. Stables LA, Kennan RP, Gore JC. Asymmetric spin-echo imaging of magnetically inhomogeneous systems: theory, experiment, and numerical studies. *Magn Reson Med* 1998;**40**:432–42.

33. Kennan RP, Zhong J, Gore JC. Intravascular susceptibility contrast mechanisms in tissues. *Magn Reson Med* 1994;**31**:9–21.

34. Yablonskiy DA, Haacke EM. Theory of NMR signal behavior in magnetically inhomogeneous tissues: the static dephasing regime. *Magn Reson Med* 1994;**32**:749–63.

35. van Zijl PC, Eleff SM, Ulatowski JA, *et al.* Quantitative assessment of blood flow, blood volume and blood oxygenation effects in functional magnetic resonance imaging. [see comments.]. *Nat Med* 1998;**4**:159–67.

36. Qin Q, Grgac K, van Zijl PC. Determination of whole-brain oxygen extraction fractions by fast measurement of blood T(2) in the jugular vein. *Magn Reson Med* 2011;**65**:471–9.

37. Fernandez-Seara MA, Techawiboonwong A, Detre JA, Wehrli FW. MR susceptometry for measuring global brain oxygen extraction. *Magn Reson Med* 2006;**55**:967–73.

38. Weisskoff RM, Kiihne S. MRI susceptometry: image-based measurement of absolute susceptibility of MR contrast agents and human blood. *Magn Reson Med* 1992;**24**:375–83.

39. Ma J, Wehrli FW. Method for image-based measurement of the reversible and irreversible contribution to the transverse-relaxation rate. *J Magn Reson B* 1996;**111**:61–9.

40. An H, Lin W. Quantitative measurements of cerebral blood oxygen saturation using magnetic resonance imaging. *J Cereb Blood Flow Metab* 2000;**20**:1225–36.

41. An H, Lin W. Cerebral oxygen extraction fraction and cerebral venous blood volume measurements using magnetic resonance imaging: effects of magnetic field variation. *Magn Reson Med* 2002;**47**:958–66.

42. An H, Lin W. Impact of intravascular signal on quantitative measures of cerebral oxygen extraction and blood volume under normo- and hypercapnic conditions using an asymmetric spin echo approach. *Magn Reson Med* 2003;**50**:708–16.

43. He X, Yablonskiy DA. Quantitative BOLD: mapping of human cerebral deoxygenated blood volume and oxygen extraction fraction: default state. *Magn Reson Med* 2007;**57**:115–26.

44. He X, Zhu M, Yablonskiy DA. Validation of oxygen extraction fraction measurement by qBOLD technique. *Magn Reson Med* 2008;**60**:882–8.

45. An H, Lin W. Cerebral venous and arterial blood volumes can be estimated separately in humans using magnetic resonance imaging. *Magn Reson Med* 2002;**48**:583–8.

46. Duong TQ, Kim SG. In vivo MR measurements of regional arterial and venous blood volume fractions in intact rat brain. *Magn Reson Med* 2000;**43**:393–402.

47. Pollard V, Prough DS, DeMelo AE, *et al.* Validation in volunteers of a near-infrared spectroscope for monitoring brain oxygenation in vivo. *Anesth Analg* 1996;**82**:269–77.

48. Schlemmer HP, Pichler BJ, Schmand M, *et al.* Simultaneous

MR/PET imaging of the human brain: feasibility study. *Radiology* 2008;**248**:1028–35.

49. An H, Liu Q, Chen Y, Lin W. Evaluation of MR-derived cerebral oxygen metabolic index in experimental hyperoxic hypercapnia, hypoxia, and ischemia. *Stroke* 2009;**40**:2165–72.

50. Sohlin MC, Schad LR. Susceptibility-related MR signal dephasing under nonstatic conditions: experimental verification and consequences for qBOLD measurements. *J Magn Reson Imaging* 2011;**33**:417–25.

51. Sedlacik J, Reichenbach JR. Validation of quantitative estimation of tissue oxygen extraction fraction and deoxygenated blood volume fraction in phantom and in vivo experiments by using MRI. *Magn Reson Med* 2010;**63**:910–21.

52. Christen T, Lemasson B, Pannetier N, *et al.* Evaluation of a quantitative blood oxygenation level-dependent (qBOLD) approach to map local blood oxygen saturation. *NMR Biomed* 2011; **24**: 393–403.

53. Christen T, Schmiedeskamp H, Straka M, Bammer R, Zaharchuk G. Measuring brain oxygenation in humans using a multiparametric quantitative blood oxygenation level dependent MRI approach. *Magn Reson Med* 2012; **68**: 905–11.

54. Reichenbach JR, Venkatesan R, Schillinger DJ, Kido DK, Haacke EM. Small vessels in the human brain: MR venography with deoxyhemoglobin as an intrinsic contrast agent. *Radiology* 1997;**204**:272–7.

55. Shmueli K, de Zwart JA, van Gelderen P, *et al.* Magnetic susceptibility mapping of brain tissue in vivo using MRI phase data. *Magn Reson Med* 2009;**62**:1510–22.

56. Wharton S, Schafer A, Bowtell R. Susceptibility mapping in the human brain using threshold-based k-space division. *Magn Reson Med* 2010;**63**: 1292–304.

57. Fan AP, Benner T, Bolar DS, Rosen BR, Adalsteinsson E. Phase-based regional oxygen metabolism (PROM) using MRI. *Magn Reson Med* 2012; **67**:669–78.

58. Jain V, Langham MC, Wehrli FW. MRI estimation of global brain oxygen consumption rate. *J Cereb Blood Flow Metab* 2010;**30**:1598–607.

59. Golay X, Silvennoinen MJ, Zhou J, *et al.* Measurement of tissue oxygen extraction ratios from venous blood T(2): increased precision and validation of principle. *Magn Reson Med* 2001;**46**:282–91.

60. Oja JM, Gillen JS, Kauppinen RA, Kraut M, van Zijl PC. Determination of oxygen extraction ratios by magnetic resonance imaging. *J Cereb Blood Flow Metab* 1999;**19**:1289–95.

61. Lu H, Xu F, Grgac K, *et al.* Calibration and validation of TRUST MRI for the estimation of cerebral blood oxygenation. *Magn Reson Med* 2012; **67**: 42–9.

62. Lu H, Ge Y. Quantitative evaluation of oxygenation in venous vessels using T2-relaxation-under-spin-tagging MRI. *Magn Reson Med* 2008;**60**:357–63.

63. Bolar DS, Rosen BR, Sorensen AG, Adalsteinsson E. QUantitative Imaging of eXtraction of oxygen and TIssue consumption (QUIXOTIC) using venular-targeted velocity-selective spin labeling. *Magn Reson Med* 2011; **66**: 1550–62.

64. Xu F, Ge Y, Lu H. Noninvasive quantification of whole-brain cerebral metabolic rate of oxygen (CMRO2) by MRI. *Magn Reson Med* 2009;**62**:141–8.

65. An H, Lin W, Celik A, Lee YZ. Quantitative measurements of cerebral metabolic rate of oxygen utilization using MRI: a volunteer study. *NMR Biomed* 2001;**14**:441–7.

66. Mintun MA, Vlassenko AG, Shulman GL, Snyder AZ. Time-related increase of oxygen utilization in continuously activated human visual cortex. *Neuroimage* 2002;**16**:531–7.

67. Law I, Iida H, Holm S, *et al.* Quantitation of regional cerebral blood flow corrected for partial volume effect using O-15 water and PET: II. Normal values and gray matter blood flow response to visual activation. *J Cereb Blood Flow Metab* 2000;**20**:1252–63.

68. Ashkanian M, Borghammer P, Gjedde A, Ostergaard L, Vafaee M. Improvement of brain tissue oxygenation by inhalation of carbogen. *Neuroscience* 2008; **156**:932–8.

69. Ford AL, An H, Vo KD, *et al.* MR-derived oxygen metabolic index (OMI) predicts gray matter infarction better than ADC during the hyper-acute phase of ischemic stroke. *J Cereb Blood Flow Metab* 2009;**29** (suppl 15):S90.

6

Vascular space occupancy (VASO) imaging of cerebral blood volume

Hanzhang Lu and Jinsoo Uh

Key points

- Vascular space occupancy (VASO) imaging is based on intrinsic T_1 differences between blood and tissue.
- The technique uses non-selective inversion recovery sequence and the inversion time is set to null the blood signal.
- This method can be used to non-invasively detect CBV changes due to brain activation or physiological challenges.
- Absolute values of CBV can be measured by performing image subtraction between post- and pre-contrast scans when Gd-based contrast agents are used.
- The post-/pre-contrast signal difference has a straightforward relationship with CBV since the pre-contrast blood magnetization is 0 and the post-contrast blood signal is at equilibrium magnetization.
- CBV quantification with VASO may be simpler than that obtained using DSC or DCE methods, and does not require the knowledge of arterial input function.

Introduction

Apart from dynamic contrast-enhanced (DCE) and dynamic susceptibility contrast (DSC) imaging, assessment of cerebral blood volume (CBV) can also be achieved by taking advantage of differences in intrinsic MR properties between blood and surrounding tissues. In this chapter, Vascular Space Occupancy (VASO) MRI, which utilizes T_1 difference between tissue and blood to separate signals from these two compartments, is described. This technique can operate in two different "modes," one intrinsic, without the use of any

exogenous contrast agent and the other following injection of a gadolinium (Gd) chelate. Since the first mode is completely based on intrinsic MR properties of the brain compartments, it can be used in subjects in whom injection of a Gd-based contrast agent might be undesirable or unsafe. For repeated measurements of CBV, the measurement can also be performed at a relatively high temporal resolution (e.g., 6 s) compared with conventional DSC or DCE methods, which require a considerable waiting time for the contrast agent to clear from the bloodstream if repetitive measurements are to be made. However, the first mode can only give relative changes in CBV but cannot be used to estimate absolute CBV. To obtain absolute CBV measurements [1], two VASO scans at pre- and post-injection of Gd-based contrast agent are needed. Compared with the other contrast agent-based methods, the VASO approach should provide higher sensitivity because it maximizes the difference in blood signal pre- and post-Gd. Also it does not require the knowledge of arterial input function, and is relatively insensitive to variations in contrast agent concentrations.

Theory

As described above, VASO MRI was first designed to non-invasively detect CBV changes following functional activation [2–9]. Later, it was combined with intravascular T_1 shortening effects of the contrast agent to measure absolute values of CBV [10–14].

Non-invasive evaluations of CBV changes using VASO MRI

The VASO sequence uses a non-slice-selective inversion recovery sequence and an optimal inversion time (TI) to null the blood signal, resulting in an

MR image that reflects the volume of extravascular tissue. Figure 6.1a shows the basic MRI pulse sequence for VASO MRI.

A radiofrequency (RF) pulse is used to invert the longitudinal magnetization of all water in the sample, after which the inverted magnetization returns exponentially to equilibrium with the longitudinal relaxation time constant T_1. Because T_1 differs between blood and tissue, the times at which their magnetizations cross zero differ. The nulling time for a spin species can be determined by solving the following equation:

$$1 - 2 \cdot e^{-TI/T_1} + e^{-TR/T_1} = 0 \qquad (6.1)$$

where TR is the repetition time, TI is the inversion time, and T_1 is the longitudinal relaxation time of the spin. Therefore, if T_1 is known, the necessary TI to null each spin species can be calculated for any TR.

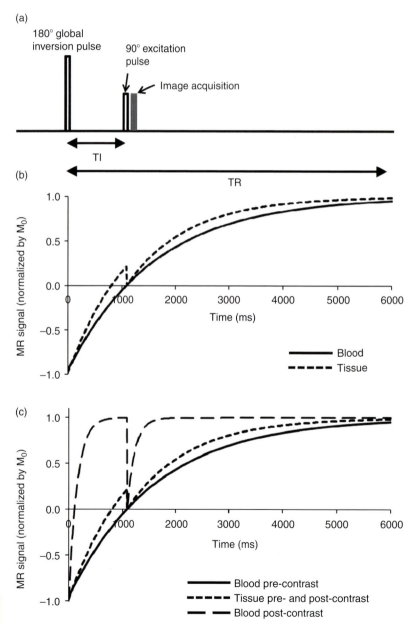

(a)

180° global inversion pulse

90° excitation pulse

Image acquisition

TI

TR

(b)

MR signal (normalized by M_0)

Time (ms)

——— Blood
- - - - Tissue

(c)

MR signal (normalized by M_0)

Time (ms)

——— Blood pre-contrast
- - - - Tissue pre- and post-contrast
— — Blood post-contrast

Figure 6.1 VASO pulse sequence. (a) Diagram of VASO MRI. The sequence consists of a non-slice-selective inversion RF pulse followed by a TI such that the blood magnetization is nulled. (b) Simulations of longitudinal magnetizations of blood and tissue as a function of time under the VASO sequence. (c) Simulations of blood and tissue magnetizations in the presence of Gd-DTPA contrast agent. TR, repetition time.

In VASO MRI [2], the TI value that nulls the blood signal is used. Since tissue T_1 is typically shorter than the blood T_1, the tissue magnetization at a blood-nulling TI is positive. Figure 6.1b shows the longitudinal magnetizations for blood (solid line) and tissue (dotted line) as a function of time during the experiment. The signal (S) depends on the longitudinal magnetization at the time of RF excitation, as given by:

$$S = S_{tissue} + S_{blood}$$
$$= M_o \cdot [C_{tissue} \cdot (1 - CBV) \cdot (1 - 2 \cdot e^{-TI/T_{1,t}} + e^{-TR/T_{1,t}}) + 0]$$
$$(6.2)$$

where the term M_0 is a constant giving the MR signal per unit volume of water protons at equilibrium; C_{tissue} is the water proton density of tissue (ml of water per ml of tissue); CBV is measured in ml of blood per ml of brain; $T_{1,t}$ is the tissue T_1 value, TI is 920 ms at 1.5 T and 1086 ms at 3 T based on whole blood T_1 values of 1350 ms and 1624 ms, respectively [2, 15], for long-enough TR ($\geq$ 6 s, see Recommended protocols). Note that the blood term, S_{blood}, is 0 due to the inversion recovery nulling of the blood magnetization. Most terms in Eq. (6.2) are constant and are not expected to vary much with the physiological variations associated with functional activation (but may not be unchanged in pathological conditions). Thus, the signal is primarily related to (1 − CBV). Note that Eq. (6.2) assumes that no exchange occurs between water in blood and in tissues, which in practice is not the case. The VASO signal change with activation can be written as:

$$\frac{S_{activated} - S_{baseline}}{S_{baseline}} = \frac{CBV_{baseline} - CBV_{activated}}{1 - CBV_{baseline}} \quad (6.3)$$

In VASO MRI, the detected MR signal is primarily related to CBV, provided that the sequence is designed to be minimally sensitive to other factors that may change during activation, such as cerebral blood flow (CBF) and blood oxygenation. To minimize the influence of blood flow on the VASO signal, the inversion pulse is chosen to be non-slice-selective and is implemented with a body transmission coil to be sure that all blood signal in the body is inverted. To reduce the effect of blood oxygenation level-dependent (BOLD) contributions to the signal, the sequence should use the shortest possible acquisition echo time (TE). Under these conditions, the measured VASO MRI signal should approximately follow the

longitudinal magnetization expression given in Eq. (6.2). Additionally, to maximize signal intensity, a 90° excitation RF pulse is often used, since TR is usually long.

When CBV increases due to functional stimulation or a physiological challenge, a larger fraction of the voxel contains the nulled blood signal (i.e., the term [1−CBV] decreases), so the observed MRI signal is reduced. With this mechanism, VASO MRI can be used as a non-invasive method for functional brain mapping based on CBV changes. This method is potentially more advantageous than BOLD functional MRI (fMRI) in detecting activated neurons because the vasodilatation during activation is restricted to microvasculature that has a diameter of less than 100 to 200 microns [16, 17], and therefore this approach might provide higher spatial specificity compared to the conventional BOLD fMRI, which is often dominated by signals from large veins which may not be especially proximal to the actual site of neuronal activity.

Quantification of absolute CBV with contrast-based VASO MRI

While the non-contrast VASO method described above is able to detect CBV changes, absolute values of CBV (in ml blood/100 ml brain) are not measured. This is primarily because the T_1 of tissue is not known; thus one cannot obtain a quantification of CBV from Eq. (6.2). Note that the T_1 of tissue cannot be obtained by simply measuring a T_1 map. The results from a T_1 map actually represent a weighted average value between tissue and blood, essentially forming a circular argument if used for VASO CBV determination. Therefore, an alternative approach based on the T_1 shortening effect of Gd-DTPA contrast agent is needed in order to estimate absolute CBV.

Intravenous injection of Gd-DTPA reduces the T_1 relaxation time [18]. When the blood–brain barrier (BBB) is intact, such changes occur only in blood and not in brain parenchyma. Therefore, when a post-contrast VASO experiment is performed with identical imaging parameters, the MR signal can be written as:

$$S_{post} = S_{tissue} + S_{blood}$$
$$= M_0 \cdot [C_{tissue} \cdot (1 - CBV) \cdot (1 - 2 \cdot e^{-TI/T_{1,t}} + e^{-TR/T_{1,t}})$$
$$+ c_b \cdot CBV \cdot (1 - 2 \cdot e^{-TI/T_{1,b,post}} + e^{-TR/T_{1,b,post}})]$$
$$(6.4)$$

where $T_{1,b,post}$ is the blood T_1 value after contrast agent injection and C_b is the water proton density of blood. Note that the first term in Eq. (6.5), the tissue signal (Figure 6.1c, dotted curve), is the same as that in Eq. (6.2) because the contrast agent is restricted to the blood, whereas the second term, the blood signal (Figure 6.1c, dashed curve), is non-zero because the contrast agent has significantly shortened the blood T_1 and the blood signal is no longer nulled at the TI used. Considering that $e^{-TI/T_{1,b,post}}$ is negligible when a long TR (> 5 sec) is used, the signal difference between post-contrast and pre-contrast images is given by:

$$S_{diff} = abs(S_{post} - S_{pre})$$

$$= M_0 \cdot CBV \cdot c_b \cdot (1 - 2 \cdot e^{-TI/T_{1,b,post}}) \qquad (6.5)$$

which is linearly related to CBV and can be used as a relative CBV map. The absolute difference is taken because the signal intensity in the post-contrast images is not always greater than that in the pre-contrast images. For example, when CSF partial volume with brain is large, the sign of the magnetization may be negative because of the long CSF T_1, in which case $S_{post} < S_{pre}$ in the modulus data.

When the $T_{1,b,post}$ is sufficiently small with respect to TI, the term $2 \times e^{-TI/T_{1,b,post}}$ vanishes and Eq. (6.5) can be simplified to:

$$S_{diff} = M_0 \cdot CBV \cdot c_b \qquad (6.6)$$

For example, when $T_{1,b,post} = 250$ ms, $2 \times e^{-TI/T_{1,b,post}} = 0.025$; when $T_{1,b,post} = 200$ ms, $2 \times e^{-TI/T_{1,b,post}} = 0.010$ (for long TR at 3 T). Note that these $T_{1,b,post}$ values are achievable with Gd-DTPA contrast agent using typical dosages [19–21]. The absolute CBV can then be calculated by:

CBV (ml blood/100 ml brain)

$$= CBV \times 100 = \frac{S_{diff}}{M_0 \cdot c_b} \times 100 \qquad (6.7)$$

where M_0 can be taken as the signal intensity in a pure CSF voxel from a scan with a long TR and a short TE, and c_b is a well-known physical parameter, 0.87 ml of water/ml of blood [22]. Alternatively, the term $M_0 \cdot c_b$ can be obtained in the post-contrast image from a voxel containing only blood, such as in regions of venous sinus or major arteries.

Experimental methods

Non-invasive evaluations of CBV changes using VASO MRI

These experiments typically contain two conditions. Depending on the goals of the particular study, these conditions can be resting state versus brain activation when performing a task, free breathing versus holdingbreath, breathing room-air versus breathing a special gas mixture containing more (or less) oxygen or carbon dioxide, normal blood pressure versus lowered blood pressure using a negative pressure device or sodium nitroprusside, or baseline condition versus condition following pharmacological intervention. For the purpose of discussion in this chapter, brain activation will be used as an example.

VASO fMRI typically uses single-shot echo-planar imaging (EPI) for image acquisition; thus it can evaluate CBV changes dynamically over short periods of time. The TR used typically ranges from 2 to 6 s, although we note that the theory presented above usually assumes a long TR. A typical experimental design is similar to BOLD fMRI. Figure 6.2a illustrates a typical VASO fMRI paradigm, in which interleaved blocks of resting state and visual stimulation are used and VASO images are acquired continuously. This particular example used flashing checkerboard with 30 s ON and 30 s OFF, and was repeated four times, resulting in a duration of 4.5 min. Other imaging parameters include field of view (FOV) 240 mm, matrix 64 × 64, one slice with thickness of 6 mm, single-shot gradient-echo EPI, parallel imaging acceleration factor 2, TE = 7.8 ms, TI = 1086 ms.

The TR value in VASO fMRI requires careful consideration. In dynamic studies, shorter TR is preferable as it provides a higher temporal resolution and also yields more images for a given scan duration, which could be used for averaging and improving statistical power. However, shorter TR in VASO may result in confounding contributions of blood inflow to the signal [3, 23]. The reason is that the RF transmission coil on a typical clinical scanner is not sufficient to homogeneously invert magnetization over the entire body and, as a result, the magnetization of the blood spins is not at a steady state. Therefore, depending on the spin history, the blood magnetization could have different values from what is predicted from the model.

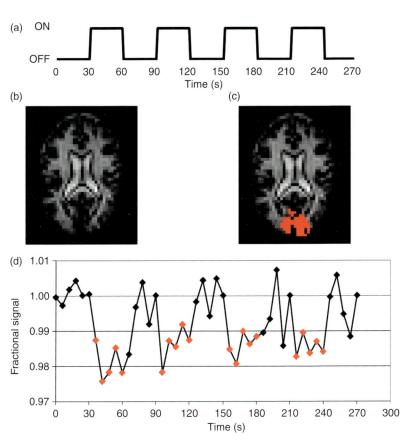

Figure 6.2 VASO fMRI as a method to non-invasively detect blood volume changes during brain activation. (a) Experiment paradigm. VASO images are acquired under interleaved blocks of resting and visual stimulation conditions. (b) An example of a VASO functional image. (c) Activation map due to visual stimulation (red voxels) overlaid on VASO image. (d) Time course of VASO signals during the experiment. Red dots indicate the activated state.

Consequently, the sequence parameters used may not be able to truly null the blood signal. When using a typical TR for fMRI (e.g., 3 s), the VASO signal will contain weightings from blood flow and, during brain activation, blood flow will increase, which results in additional signal changes observed in VASO fMRI. Due to the flow contributions and also exchange of water between blood and tissue, the amplitude of VASO fMRI signal change may be greater than that predicted by the actual change in CBV.

Figure 6.3 shows simulation results of VASO signal changes as a function of TR when the flow effect is included. These simulations were performed for a field strength of 3 T, assuming as baseline CBV of 5%, and an increase of 20% due to activation, with a delay of 1.8 s for the blood to reach the imaging slice after entering the body coil coverage. The green line indicates the expected signal change for CBV effect only. As can be seen, this should be independent of the TR value used. The signal with flow effect is shown by the blue curve, and shows a more negative signal change, attributed to flow increase associated

with activation. The effect can be reduced to some extent by adding a post-saturation RF pulse following the EPI acquisition [24]. The post-saturation pulse, however, will not completely normalize the signal. Therefore, TR of 6 s or greater is recommended for VASO fMRI studies.

Most earlier VASO studies were performed with a single slice because the inverted magnetization only crosses zero at one time point during the longitudinal recovery. Thus, after the first slice is excited at the blood-nulling point, one cannot excite any other slice, as the blood magnetization in the following slices will no longer be at zero. Therefore, the extension from single-slice VASO to multiple slice is not as trivial as that for BOLD fMRI. Two options are available to circumvent this issue. One option is to use the so-called multiple-acquisitions-with-global-inversion-cycling (MAGIC) sequence [25, 26], in which the magnetization is inverted again after crossing each zero point to make it negative and, as it recovers toward equilibrium, the blood signal will have successive nulling points. If one applied multiple

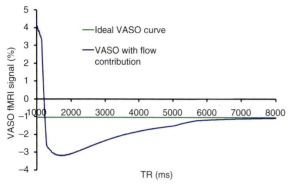

Figure 6.3 Simulation results of VASO fMRI signals as a function of TR. Under ideal conditions (green curve), the VASO signal is only determined by CBV change, and thus should not be TR dependent. However, because the transmission coil used in clinical scanners cannot cover the whole body, the VASO signal could be sensitive to flow effect when a short TR is used, resulting in an overestimation of CBV changes. Thus, a TR of 6 s is recommended for VASO experiments (see text for details about the simulation).

inversion pulses, multiple slices can be acquired with this scheme. A second option is to use single-shot 3D acquisition schemes such as the gradient-echo-and-spin-echo (GRASE) technique, in which the whole brain or a large portion of the brain is acquired following one RF excitation. This approach has been shown to have excellent spatial coverage and sensitivity [27, 28].

Quantification of absolute CBV with contrast-based VASO MRI

Absolute CBV measurement with VASO MRI consists of a pre-contrast and a post-contrast scan using identical imaging parameters. The timing of a typical experiment is shown in Figure 6.4. The pre-contrast VASO scan is performed immediately before the contrast agent injection. Gd-DTPA contrast agent (Magnevist, Berlex Laboratories, Wayne, NY) can be administered manually or using a power injector. It has been shown that a standard dosage (0.1 mmol/kg) is sufficient for the blood concentration to reach the necessary level for VASO [12]. Unlike DSC-MRI, there is no requirement for a high injection rate as the method works in the steady state. The post-contrast VASO scan can be performed at any time between 1 and 14 min after the injection. The 1 min waiting is needed to allow the contrast agent to fully mix with blood and for its concentration to reach a steady state [29]. In subjects with normal renal

function, beyond 14 min post injection the blood concentration of Gd-DTPA will probably be too low, such that the T_1 assumption described in Eq. (6.7) is no longer valid [12].

The imaging parameters for contrast-based VASO experiments are largely similar to those used for VASO fMRI, but with a number of differences. First, unlike VASO fMRI, the contrast-based VASO method does not typically use single-shot acquisition. This is because the measurement is usually focused on "baseline" values of CBV, rather than looking for changes associated with activation or physiological challenges. Thus the temporal resolution of the measurement is not a major factor. Therefore, the scans typically use segmented EPI, acquiring between three and nine gradient echoes per shot. The reduced requirement on temporal resolution allows higher spatial resolution to be attained. This is therefore an advantage over the dynamic imaging methods (such as DSC and DCE), which are usually performed at lower spatial resolutions because of time constraints. Another difference from VASO fMRI is that multiple, 2D slices can be acquired, since for segmented EPI the time interval between adjacent echo trains is relatively short. For instance, a typical acquisition might acquire 15 slices within a "readout" duration of 180 ms, and a correction factor would be applied to account for the small magnetization recovery (for the pre-contrast scan) during the 180 ms period. With these considerations, typical imaging parameters for contrast-based VASO are: FOV = 220 × 220 mm^2, matrix = 128 × 128, 11 slices acquired with descending order, slice thickness = 5 mm, TR = 6000 ms, TI = 920 ms (at 1.5 T) [2] and 1086 ms (at 3 T) [15], segmented gradient-echo EPI acquisition with seven echoes per shot or 18 shots altogether, TE = 6 ms, flip angle = 90°. The resulting scan duration for each VASO experiment is 1 min and 42 s. In order to obtain the normalizing factor "M_0," a proton-density imaging scan should be performed with identical geometric parameters (i.e., FOV, matrix, slice thickness, and slice location). Example imaging parameters are: TR = 20 s, TE = 19 ms (or shorter, if available on the scanner), flip angle = 90°, single-shot gradient-echo EPI acquisition, parallel imaging factor = 2, scan duration = 30 s. The inhomogeneity of head coil sensitivity is accounted for by referencing against the body coil signal profile, assuming the body coil has a homogeneous sensitivity within the brain and the dielectric effect is minimal.

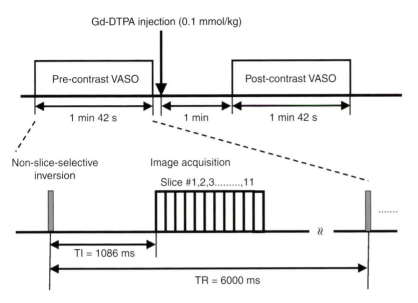

Figure 6.4 Experimental design of contrast-based VASO studies. A complete study consists of pre- and post-contrast VASO scans using identical parameters. Within each scan, multiple slices are acquired by exciting the slices sequentially around the blood-nulling time. The incomplete nulling due to imperfect TI can be corrected in the post-processing (see text for details).

Analysis techniques

Non-invasive evaluations of CBV changes using VASO MRI

Data processing procedures for VASO fMRI are largely similar to those for BOLD. Magnitude images are saved and subject motion between volumes is corrected using automated image realignment algorithms. Rigid-body method, instead of affine or elastic registration, should be used because the image volumes are of the same contrast and geometric properties. Detrending or high-pass filtering should be used to remove signal drift. The first few image volumes should be excluded to allow the subject to get used to the scanner noise and reach a hemodynamic steady state.

Detection of activated voxels is based on cross-correlation or general linear regression model between the VASO fMRI time course and the task paradigm. Care has to be taken to adapt the hemodynamic response function, as the typical VASO response is different from the BOLD one [30]. A statistical threshold can be set to detect the activated voxels. Note, however, that a negative signal change is expected when CBV increases, because VASO signal reflects $(1 - CBV)$.

Since the basic principles of VASO fMRI analysis are similar to those of BOLD, many standard fMRI software packages may be used for VASO processing, such as Statistical Parameter Mapping (SPM, University College London, UK), FSL (FMRIB Centre, University of Oxford, UK), BrainVoyager (Brain Innovation B.V., the Netherlands), and AFNI (NIMH Scientific and Statistical Computing Core, Bethesda, MD, USA).

An example of a VASO functional image is illustrated in Figure 6.2b. Note that the blood vessels are completely dark, but the tissue signals are still present. The white matter tends to be brighter compared with the gray matter because of its shorter T_1. The CSF magnetization is negative in sign because its T_1 is much longer (~4 s), but in the magnitude image the signal intensity is also relatively high. Figure 6.2c shows a VASO activation map using visual stimulation. Figure 6.2d shows the corresponding time course in the activated voxels. Note that the sign of the VASO signal change is negative as predicted from the signal mechanism.

Quantification of absolute CBV with contrast-based VASO MRI

All MR images are reconstructed on the scanner using identical scaling factors. This is important for the image subtraction and estimation of absolute CBV maps. Both magnitude and phase images should be stored on the scanner, since the phase images are required in order to determine the sign of the signal.

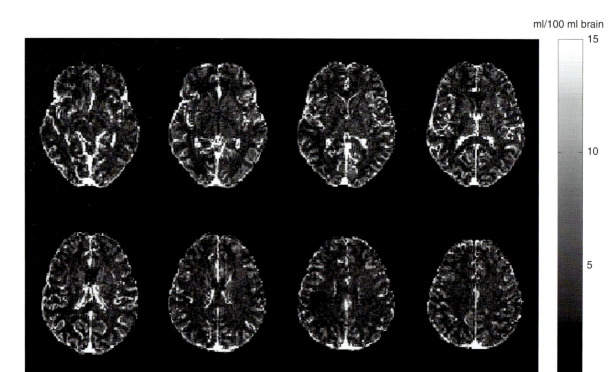

Figure 6.5 Absolute CBV maps (in ml blood/100 ml brain) obtained with VASO MRI. The scan used spatial resolution of $1.7 \times 1.7\ mm^2$ (slice thickness 5 mm). The duration of each VASO scan was 1 min 42 s.

This is important because, in an inversion recovery sequence like VASO, the magnetization may be positive or negative depending on the T_1 of the tissue type. For short T_1 tissue such as gray or white matter, the magnetization will be positive, whereas for CSF the magnetization will be negative. For mixed voxels with partial volumes, the sign of the total magnetization will depend on the volume fraction of each tissue type, and the phase of the image, Φ, can be used to determine the sign by thresholding of $-90° \leq \Phi < 90°$ as positive and $90° \leq \Phi < 270°$ as negative. The sign-corrected pre- and post-contrast VASO images can be co-registered using standard software packages such as FSL (FMRIB Centre, University of Oxford, UK). It is important to use image registration algorithms that are based on mutual information (rather than least-square differences) because the image contrast may be altered when the contrast agent is administered. CBV can then be calculated based on the algorithms described in the Theory section (Eq. (6.8)), with M_0 for each subject estimated from the ventricular voxels of the proton density images.

In multi-slice image acquisitions (see Figure 6.4), only one slice (usually slice #1) can be excited at the exact blood-nulling point. The blood signals in the later slices are not perfectly zero. Consequently, a correction factor is needed to account for such sensitivity differences. The factors can be calculated from the blood T_1 relaxation curve (Figure 6.1c solid line) and are found to be: 1.00, 0.98, 0.97, 0.95, 0.94, 0.92, 0.91, 0.89, 0.88, 0.86, and 0.85 for slice 1 through 11, respectively using the sequence timing parameters described above. Figure 6.5 shows an example of CBV maps obtained from VASO MRI.

Recommended protocols, artifacts, pitfalls, limitations, etc.

Non-invasive evaluations of CBV changes using VASO MRI

Since the VASO technique is based on blood nulling, the imaging parameters, in particular TI, are dependent on the T_1 of blood. Because T_1 of blood is field-specific, the optimal TI is different for different field strengths. Table 6.1 lists the T_1 of blood and gray and white matter, and the optimal TI for 1.5 T, 3 T and 7 T at TR = 6000 ms.

In terms of acquisition techniques, one can use single-shot gradient-echo EPI or spin-echo EPI for 2D imaging or single-shot GRASE for 3D imaging. For all schemes, the shortest possible TE should be used to minimize BOLD effects in the VASO signal. Table 6.2 lists typical acquisition parameters.

At field strengths of 3 T or lower, gradient-echo EPI is preferable due to the relatively short TE available and the small extravascular BOLD effect (note that the intravascular BOLD effect has been removed during blood signal nulling). At higher field (e.g., 7 T, 9.4 T), a spin-echo acquisition is preferred because the extravascular BOLD is the dominant form of BOLD at these field strengths [31, 32]. When 3D GRASE is used, caution should be used in selecting the number of slices and the total length of the acquisition echo train. It is recommended that the echo-train duration should be limited to 200–300 ms. Otherwise, significant image blurring will occur, in particular in the slab selective direction which is the usual fast-spin-echo turbo factor direction.

Table 6.1. T_1 of blood and brain tissues at different magnetic field strengths and the corresponding optimal TI values at a TR of 6000 ms

	T$_1$ (ms)			TI (ms)
	Blood	Gray matter	White matter	
1.5 T	1350[a]	1019[b]	586[b]	920
3 T	1624[c]	1166[b]	729[b]	1086
7 T	2212[d]	2132[e]	1220[e]	1391

[a] Lu et al. [2].
[b] Lu et al. [46].
[c] Lu et al. [15].
[d] Dobre et al. [47].
[e] Rooney et al. [48].

Compared with the BOLD method, the VASO technique has a number of advantages in studies of hemodynamic changes. First, VASO signal change can be more easily linked to physiological parameters. This is because baseline CBV is typically 0.03 to 0.06. Therefore, in Eq. (6.3), the term on the denominator can be approximated to 1. The equation thus can be simplified to:

$$\frac{S_{activated} - S_{baseline}}{S_{baseline}} = CBV_{baseline} - CBV_{activated} = -\Delta CBV$$

(6.8)

That is, the signal change in VASO MRI is directly related to ΔCBV. Second, the VASO signal is expected to originate from microvascular regions. This is because vasodilatation following brain activation primarily occurs in small resistance vessels such as small arteries and arterioles that are in the order of 100 microns [16, 33]. Therefore, if one can detect these hemodynamic changes, the location of the voxels should most closely approximate the location of activated neurons. As such, CBV-based fMRI provides a better spatial specificity compared to the BOLD fMRI method which is based on venous oxygenation changes and may be sensitive to large draining veins. A third advantage of VASO is that the signal is less sensitive to susceptibility effects related to air–brain interfaces, which may provide an advantage in areas such as the prefrontal cortex and medial temporal regions. Finally, VASO MRI can be combined with other hemodynamic methods such as BOLD and CBF-based fMRI techniques to obtain quantitative information about CBF, CBV, and oxygenation, in order to understand the physiological basis of each phase of the BOLD effect [30]. This may help to identify the BOLD component that is most related to neural activity.

Table 6.2. Typical acquisition parameters for VASO fMRI

	Gradient-echo EPI	Spin-echo EPI	GRASE
FOV	220 × 220 mm^2	220 × 220 mm^2	220 × 220 mm^2
In-plane resolution	3.4 × 3.4 mm^2	3.4 × 3.4 mm^2	3.4 × 3.4 mm^2
Slice thickness/number of slices	5 mm/1	5 mm/1	5 mm/24
TR/TE	6000 ms/7.8 ms	6000 ms/17 ms	6000 ms/14 ms
TI	1086 ms	1086 ms	1086 ms
Parallel imaging factor	2	2	4 (Y) × 2 (Z)
EPI factor	32	32	16

VASO fMRI also has some limitations. First, the signal-to-noise ratio (SNR) of VASO is lower compared to BOLD. At typical fMRI resolution, the sensitivity of VASO is about one-third of that of BOLD and is similar to that of arterial spin labeling [2]. Second, spatial coverage is still challenging in VASO. Because of the need to wait until the blood-nulling point to apply the excitation RF pulse, VASO is intrinsically less time efficient. Even with the 3D GRASE method, the typical number of slices is approximately 20, which is typically lower than the number acquired during BOLD studies. A third limitation is that the temporal resolution of VASO is in the order of 6 s which is poorer compared to BOLD. As described above, this is due to inflow confounding factor at shorter TR values.

Quantification of absolute CBV with contrast-based VASO MRI

Segmented EPI is usually used in contrast-based VASO experiments. In setting up a protocol, compromises are made between EPI factor, TE, inter-slice time interval, and the number of slices. The main considerations in deciding these parameters are that the TE should not be more than 10 ms (to minimize extravascular BOLD effect) and that the acquisition duration combining all slices should be less than 300 ms (to minimize blood signal during the pre-contrast scan). If the number of slices necessary to cover the whole brain is greater than the number allowed for the given TR, one can acquire the whole brain in multiple packages or partitions [13].

Table 6.3 shows two examples of VASO protocols. The main difference between them is that the first one is acquired at standard spatial resolution, whereas the second one uses a high resolution, allowing one to investigate subfield details in cortical regions.

Compared with the DSC-MRI method for CBV measurement (see Chapter 2), the VASO approach uses steady-state imaging rather than dynamic imaging; the temporal requirements of dynamic imaging generally result in significantly lower spatial resolution than is possible with steady-state techniques. DSC also often employs single-shot EPI acquisitions (rather than multi-shot as used in VASO), and may cause greater image distortion and susceptibility signal loss in some brain regions, in particular at the peak of the bolus when the maximum concentration of the Gd-based contrast agent leads to a strong reduction of the signal,

Table 6.3. Examples of VASO protocols for quantitative CBV measurement

	Standard resolution	High resolution
Slice orientation	Transverse	Coronal
FOV	220×220 mm^2	200×200 mm^2
In-plane resolution	1.7×1.7 mm^2	0.8×0.8 mm^2
Slice thickness/ number of slices	5 mm/11 slices	4 mm/9 slices
TR/TE	6000 ms/6 ms	6000 ms/6 ms
TI	1086 ms	1086 ms
EPI factor	7	7
Flip angle	90°	90°
Scan duration	1 min 42 s	2 min 30 s

due to a very short T_2^*. Since VASO images can be acquired with regular k-space or segmented-EPI schemes, the spatial resolution of the image is not limited by maximum echo-train length and higher-resolution CBV maps may be achieved when the SNR is sufficient. Therefore, VASO has the potential to assess blood supply in very small cortical structures such as hippocampal subfields. Furthermore, the VASO method has a relatively straightforward theory and does not require estimation of the arterial input function, which by itself is an area of intensive research [34, 35]. These features are expected to make the VASO method a useful tool for quantitatively measuring CBV in clinical applications, as well as in animal studies using long half-life contrast agents [36]. However, a disadvantage of VASO for measuring CBV compared to DSC is the significantly lower contrast-to-noise ratio, since CBV is only a small fraction of the voxel and signal changes of just a few percent are measured; in contrast, bolus DSC-MRI with gradient-echo EPI readout causes large changes in signal intensity, which are proportional to CBV.

Compared with other T_1-based methods such as DCE, the VASO technique has a number of advantages. First, the VASO sequence employs a non-slice-selective inversion pulse and the signal is not sensitive to the inflow effect of the blood. Therefore, the confounding effect from blood flow is minimized. Second, the blood signal in the pre-contrast VASO image is zero and that in the post-contrast image is 1 (equilibrium). Thus, the sensitivity to the T_1 shortening effect in blood is maximized. The maximized sensitivity makes the VASO technique more advantageous for assessing vascular health in white matter, which has been limited due to low vascularity. Third, this approach allows for simpler quantification in terms of absolute CBV, because the signal difference (between pre- and post-contrast) expected for a unit volume of blood is known. As a result, one does not necessarily need to use a voxel with pure blood for referencing and normalization, and other tissue types (e.g., CSF in ventricle) can instead be used. Fourth, blood T_1 relaxation reaches a plateau in the post-contrast image when the contrast agent concentration in the blood is above a certain level. This feature provides a relatively large acquisition window in the post-injection period as long as the concentration of the contrast agent is still above this threshold.

VASO MRI for quantitative CBV estimation shares common limitations of other T_1-based CBV methods in that a few confounding factors can cause bias in the estimated CBV values. First, the contrast agent will shorten transverse relaxation times of blood and brain, as well as T_1 relaxation, resulting in an image with undesired T_2 or T_2^* weighting. Second, extravasation of Gd-DTPA can occur in patients with a compromised BBB. This will increase the fraction of water molecules affected by the contrast agent and will cause overestimation of CBV; it may be difficult to distinguish BBB-leakage effects from CBV changes in patients with subtle leakage. Finally, water exchange between blood and tissue across the BBB may influence the quantification of CBV. However, these confounding effects can be minimized by conducting multi-echo and multi-time point acquisitions [12], although these may require trade-offs in image resolution/FOV or the total scan time.

Applications of VASO imaging

VASO in brain tumor

Gliomas are the most common type of primary brain tumor, and the prognosis for this disease remains very poor. The current gold standard for determination of glioma grade is by histopathological assessment of either surgical biopsy or resection specimens. VASO provides a potential approach to differentiate between high- and low-grade gliomas [37].

As previously described, the signal difference between pre- and post-contrast images provides a

quantitative CBV estimation when the BBB is intact and the leakage of contrast into brain parenchyma is negligible. When the BBB is significantly compromised, as in the case of many gliomas, the VASO results reflect a combined effect of CBV and vascular permeability. Previous studies have shown that the malignancy of a glioma can be characterized by rapid cellular proliferation accompanied by neovascularization [38, 39], as well as increased permeability of the vascular endothelium [40, 41]. Both effects are expected to increase the contrast-enhanced VASO signal intensity. This feature renders VASO a unique advantage in its ability to measure the combined effects of increased CBV and vascular permeability, thereby increasing the sensitivity of differentiating low-grade from high-grade tumors.

In a recent study, a total of 39 patients (9 World Health Organization [WHO] grade II, 20 grade III, and 10 grade IV as determined by histopathological assessment) were examined using VASO, with region-of-interest (ROI) analysis in tumoral regions, as well as in regions contralateral to the tumor [37].

Figure 6.6 shows examples of VASO images in different tumor grades. The ratio between tumor side and contralateral side, $VASO_{Ratio}$, showed significant differences in all three of the pairwise comparisons ($p < 0.01$) [37]. VASO values in the tumoral regions, $VASO_{Tumor}$, showed significant difference between grade II and III and between II and IV but not between III and IV. Both $VASO_{Tumor}$ and $VASO_{Ratio}$ were found to be significant predictors of tumor grade, giving diagnostic accuracies of 66.7% and 71.8%, respectively. When testing to discriminate grade II tumors from higher-grade tumors, the areas under the receiver operating characteristic curve were found to be 0.974 and 0.985 for $VASO_{Tumor}$ and $VASO_{Ratio}$, respectively [37].

VASO in Alzheimer's disease

Alzheimer's disease (AD) is a neurodegenerative disease associated with neuritic plaques composed of beta amyloid and neurofibrillary tangles made of hyperphosphorylated *tau* protein. While amyloid/tau pathology is the primary focus in the field, recent evidence indicates that vascular factors are important in the pathogenesis of AD [42–44]. In this example, the perfusion deficit in patients with AD has been assessed by CBV measured by the VASO MRI technique [13].

VASO scans were performed in patients with mild AD (n = 16, age 70.7 ± 9.3, 9 males, mini-mental state

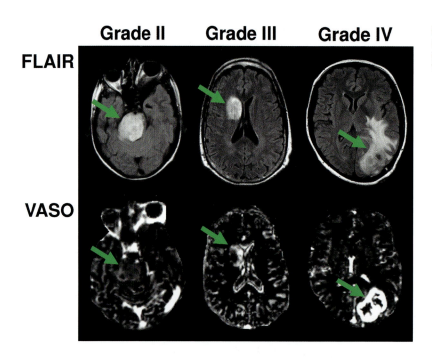

Figure 6.6 Examples of VASO images in patients with brain tumors. Generally, greater VASO signals seem to correspond to higher-grade tumors.

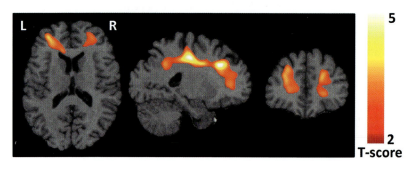

Figure 6.7 Brain regions showing lower CBV values in Alzheimer's disease (n = 16) relative to normal elderly individuals (n = 10) (two sample t-test with threshold of p < 0.005 and cluster size > 1250 mm³).

examination score = 26.6 ± 3.5) and in elderly non-demented subjects (n = 10, age 73.1 ± 4.4, 3 males). The measured CBV images were spatially normalized to a template brain space using an elastic registration algorithm [45] for voxel-wise analysis.

Figure 6.7 shows the result of the voxel-wise two sample t-test for the two groups. After applying statistical threshold (p < 0.005 for each voxel, cluster size > 1250 mm³), the regions showing CBV decline were overlaid on the T_1-weighted anatomical image. Significant CBV deficits were observed primarily in white matter, located bilaterally in frontal lobes and extending to parietal lobes [13]. No significant clusters were observed for the opposite contrast (i.e., CBV in AD group greater than CBV in controls). An ROI analysis showed consistent results: CBV in AD patients were 26.1% (p < 0.001) and 18.5%

(p = 0.015) lower than in controls in frontal and parietal white matters, respectively. This trend was also seen in occipital white matter, but the level of statistical significance was lower (p = 0.04). No significant difference was observed in temporoparietal gray matter and hippocampus.

To assess the effect of CBV deficit on neural tissue integrity, diffusion parameters in regions showing CBV deficits were calculated. A significant negative correlation (Pearson correlation p = 0.021, r = 0.41; Spearman rank correlation p = 0.027, r = 0.39) was observed between apparent diffusion coefficient (ADC) and the CBV values across subjects, suggesting that subjects with lower CBV had higher diffusion coefficients. These data suggest that the vascular contribution in AD is primarily localized to frontal/parietal white matter and is associated with brain tissue integrity.

Conclusions

VASO imaging utilizes intrinsic T_1 differences between blood and tissue to separate signal contributions from these two compartments. The imaging parameters are chosen to null blood, but maintain the tissue magnetization, making the signal reflective of $(1 - CBV)$. VASO can therefore be used to detect non-invasively CBV changes during brain activation or physiological challenges. To obtain absolute values of CBV, Gd-DTPA contrast agent can be used and, due to the blood-nulling feature of the sequence, the quantification of CBV values is simpler and does not need the knowledge of arterial input function.

References

1. Kuppusamy K, Lin W, Cizek GR, Haacke EM. In vivo regional cerebral blood volume: quantitative assessment with 3D T1-weighted pre- and post-contrast MR imaging. *Radiology* 1996;**201**:106–12.

2. Lu H, Golay X, Pekar JJ, Van Zijl PC. Functional magnetic resonance imaging based on changes in vascular space occupancy. *Magn Reson Med* 2003;**50**:263–74.

3. Donahue MJ, Lu H, Jones CK *et al.* Theoretical and experimental investigation of the VASO contrast mechanism. *Magn Reson Med* 2006;**56**: 1261–73.

4. Scouten A, Constable RT. VASO-based calculations of CBV change: accounting for the dynamic CSF volume. *Magn Reson Med* 2008;**59**:308–15.

5. Wu WC, Buxton RB, Wong EC. Vascular space occupancy weighted imaging with control of residual blood signal and higher contrast-to-noise ratio. *IEEE Trans Med Imaging* 2007;**26**:1319–27.

6. Donahue MJ, van Laar PJ, van Zijl PC, Stevens RD, Hendrikse J. Vascular space occupancy (VASO) cerebral blood volume-weighted MRI identifies hemodynamic impairment in patients with carotid artery disease. *J Magn Reson Imaging* 2009;**29**:718–24.

7. Hua J, Donahue MJ, Zhoo JM, *et al.* Magnetization transfer enhanced vascular-space-occupancy (MT-VASO) functional MRI. *Magn Reson Med* 2009;**61**:944–51.

8. Glielmi CB, Schuchard RA, Hu XP. Estimating cerebral blood volume with expanded vascular space occupancy slice coverage. *Magn Reson Med* 2009;**61**: 1193–200.

9. Wu CW, Liu HL, Chen JH, Yang Y. Effects of CBV, CBF, and blood-brain barrier permeability on accuracy of PASL and VASO measurement. *Magn Reson Med* 2010;**63**:601–8.

10. Lu H, Law M, Johnson G, *et al.* Novel approach to the measurement of absolute cerebral blood volume using vascular-space-occupancy magnetic resonance imaging. *Magn Reson Med* 2005;**54**:1403–11.

11. Lu H, Law M, Ge Y, *et al.* Quantitative measurement of spinal cord blood volume in humans using vascular-space-occupancy MRI. *NMR Biomed* 2008; **21**:226–32.

12. Uh J, Lewis-Amezcua K, Varghese R, Lu H. On the measurement of absolute cerebral blood volume (CBV) using vascular-space-occupancy (VASO) MRI. *Magn Reson Med* 2009;**61**: 659–67.

13. Uh J, Lewis-Amezcua K, Martin-Cook K *et al.* Cerebral blood volume in Alzheimer's disease and correlation with tissue structural integrity. *Neurobiol Aging* 2010;**31**:2038–46.

14. Uh J, Lin AL, Lee K *et al.* Validation of VASO cerebral blood volume measurement with positron emission tomography. *Magn Reson Med* 2011;**65**:744–9.

15. Lu H, Clingman C, Golay X, van Zijl PC. Determining the longitudinal relaxation time (T1) of blood at 3.0 Tesla. *Magn Reson Med* 2004;**52**:679–82.

16. Harrison RV, Harel N, Panesar J, Mount RJ. Blood capillary distribution correlates with hemodynamic-based functional imaging in cerebral cortex. *Cereb Cortex* 2002;**12**:225–33.

17. Kuschinsky W. Regulation of cerebral blood flow: an overview. In: Mraovitch S, Sercombe R, editors. *Neurophysiological Basis of Cerebral Blood Flow Control: An Introduction.* London: Johns Libbey & Company Ltd., 1996; 245–62.

18. Koenig SH, Brown RD, 3rd. Relaxometry of magnetic resonance imaging contrast agents. *Magn Reson Annu* 1987:263–86.

19. Donahue KM, Burstein D, Manning WJ, Gray ML. Studies of Gd-DTPA relaxivity and proton exchange rates in tissue. *Magn Reson Med* 1994;**32**:66–76.

20. Ibrahim MA, Emerson JF, Cotman CW. Magnetic resonance imaging relaxation times and gadolinium-DTPA relaxivity values in human cerebrospinal fluid. *Invest Radiol* 1998;**33**:153–62.

21. Wendland MF, Saeed M, Yu KK, *et al.* Inversion recovery EPI of bolus transit in rat myocardium using intravascular and extravascular gadolinium-based MR contrast media: dose effects on peak signal enhancement. *Magn Reson Med* 1994;**32**:319–29.

101

22. Herscovitch P, Raichle ME. What is the correct value for the brain–blood partition coefficient for water? *J Cereb Blood Flow Metab* 1985;**5**:65–9.

23. Donahue MJ, Hua J, Pekar JJ, van Zijl PC. Effect of inflow of fresh blood on vascular-space-occupancy (VASO) contrast. *Magn Reson Med* 2009;**61**:473–80.

24. Lu H. Magnetization "reset" for non-steady-state blood spins in Vascular-Space-Occupancy (VASO) fMRI. *Proc Int Soc Magn Reson Med*, Toronto, Canada, 2008;406.

25. Lu H, van Zijl PC, Hendrikse J, Golay X. Multiple acquisitions with global inversion cycling (MAGIC): a multislice technique for vascular-space-occupancy dependent fMRI. *Magn Reson Med* 2004;**51**:9–15.

26. Scouten A, Constable RT. Applications and limitations of whole-brain MAGIC VASO functional imaging. *Magn Reson Med* 2007;**58**:306–15.

27. Poser BA, Norris DG. 3D single-shot VASO using a Maxwell gradient compensated GRASE sequence. *Magn Reson Med* 2009;**62**:255–62.

28. Poser BA, Norris DG. Application of whole-brain CBV-weighted fMRI to a cognitive stimulation paradigm: robust activation detection in a stroop task experiment using 3D GRASE VASO. *Hum Brain Mapp* 2011;**32**:974–81.

29. Morris TW, Ekholm SE, Prentice LI. The effects of gadolinium-DTPA and -DOTA on neural tissue metabolism. *Invest Radiol* 1991;**26**:1087–90.

30. Lu H, Golay X, Pekkar JJ, van Zijl PC. Sustained poststimulus elevation in cerebral oxygen utilization after vascular recovery. *J Cereb Blood Flow Metab* 2004;**24**:764–70.

31. Jin T, Kim SG. Improved cortical-layer specificity of vascular space occupancy fMRI with slab inversion relative to spin-echo BOLD at 9.4 T. *Neuroimage* 2008;**40**:59–67.

32. Hua J, Jones CK, *et al.* Vascular-Space-Occupancy (VASO) MRI in human brain at 7T. *Proc Int Soc Magn Reson Med*, Montreal, Quebec, Canada, 2011; 3604.

33. Lee SP, Duong TQ, Yang G, Iadecola C, Kim SG. Relative changes of cerebral arterial and venous blood volumes during increased cerebral blood flow: implications for BOLD fMRI. *Magn Reson Med* 2001;**45**:791–800.

34. Perkio J, Aronen HJ, Kangasmäki A, *et al.* Evaluation of four postprocessing methods for determination of cerebral blood volume and mean transit time by dynamic susceptibility contrast imaging. *Magn Reson Med* 2002;**47**:973–81.

35. van Osch MJ, Vonken EJ, Viergever MA, van der Groud J, Bakker CJ. Measuring the arterial input function with gradient echo sequences. *Magn Reson Med* 2003;**49**:1067–76.

36. Mandeville JB, Marota JJ, Kosofsky BE, *et al.* Dynamic functional imaging of relative cerebral blood volume during rat forepaw stimulation. *Magn Reson Med* 1998;**39**:615–24.

37. Lu H, Pollack E, Young R, *et al.* Predicting grade of cerebral glioma using vascular-space occupancy MR imaging. *AJNR Am J Neuroradiol* 2008;**29**:373–8.

38. Aronen HJ, Gazit IE, Louis DN, *et al.* Cerebral blood volume maps of gliomas: comparison with tumor grade and histologic findings. *Radiology* 1994;**191**:41–51.

39. Law M, Yang S, Wang H, *et al.* Glioma grading: sensitivity, specificity, and predictive values of perfusion MR imaging and proton MR spectroscopic imaging compared with conventional MR imaging. *AJNR Am J Neuroradiol* 2003;**24**:1989–98.

40. Burger PC. Malignant astrocytic neoplasms: classification, pathologic anatomy, and response to treatment. *Semin Oncol* 1986;**13**:16–26.

41. Law M, Yang S, Babb JS, *et al.* Comparison of cerebral blood volume and vascular permeability from dynamic susceptibility contrast-enhanced perfusion MR imaging with glioma grade. *AJNR Am J Neuroradiol* 2004;**25**:746–55.

42. de la Torre JC. Is Alzheimer's disease a neurodegenerative or a vascular disorder? Data, dogma, and dialectics. *Lancet Neurol* 2004;**3**:184–90.

43. Iadecola C. Neurovascular regulation in the normal brain and in Alzheimer's disease. *Nat Rev Neurosci* 2004;**5**:347–60.

44. Zlokovic BV. Neurovascular mechanisms of Alzheimer's neurodegeneration. *Trends Neurosci* 2005;**28**:202–8.

45. Shen D, Davatzikos C. HAMMER: hierarchical attribute matching mechanism for elastic registration. *IEEE Trans Med Imaging* 2002;**21**:1421–39.

46. Lu H, Nagae-Poetscher LM, Golay X, *et al.* Routine clinical brain MRI sequences for use at 3.0 Tesla. *J Magn Reson Imaging* 2005;**22**:13–22.

47. Dobre MC, Ugurbil K, Marjanska M. Determination of blood longitudinal relaxation time (T1) at high magnetic field strengths. *Magn Reson Imaging* 2007;**25**:733–5.

48. Rooney WD, Johnson G, Li X, *et al.* Magnetic field and tissue dependencies of human brain longitudinal 1H2O relaxation in vivo. *Magn Reson Med* 2007;**57**:308–18.

Chapter

7

MR perfusion imaging in neuroscience

Manus J. Donahue and Peter Jezzard

Key points

- The measurement of perfusion provides an indirect access to brain metabolism through the tight coupling between oxygen consumption and delivery.
- CBF is therefore a more direct estimate of brain function than the use of the blood oxygenation level-dependent (BOLD) contrast, which arises from a complex interplay between CBF, CBV, and oxygen extraction, with influences from hematocrit and basal oxygenation levels.
- Functional perfusion imaging is more challenging to perform than BOLD fMRI, as its contrast-to-noise ratio is lower, yet provides a better localization of activation than BOLD.
- The combination of both methods provides additional insight into oxygen metabolism during functional activation.
- Oxygen metabolic responses using a combination of BOLD and ASL perfusion MRI are particularly well suited to study pharmacological responses in the brain.
- CBF has found another application when combined with resting-state fMRI to study functional connectivity in various neurodegenerative diseases.

Introduction

It is well known that elevated neuronal activity is accompanied by increased glucose and oxygen delivery to tissue. As these substrates are delivered to the tissue by the blood, changes in cerebral blood flow (CBF), or perfusion, are also closely associated with

modulations in neuronal activity. Thus, information regarding brain function can be obtained from measurements of CBF, and corresponding measurements of hemodynamic activity have emerged as the most popular approach for assessing changes in brain function [1–4]. CBF, defined in Chapters 1 and 3, is the rate at which the blood is delivered to tissue (generally reported in units of ml blood/100 g tissue/min), as opposed to the quantity or velocity of blood in vessels. It is known that functionally driven changes in hemodynamic activity are associated with complex cerebrovascular interactions between perivascular neurons, glio-vascular and intramural vascular signaling; however, the precise mechanisms by which neuronal activity elicits changes in CBF have not been fully established [5].

Until the advent of functional MRI (fMRI) in the early 1990s, the primary method for mapping brain activation in humans used positron emission tomography (PET) to provide images of perfusion change. This is achieved by counting the number of positron annihilations in the brain following injection of radioactive water ($H_2^{15}O$) during a task state versus a rest state [6, 7]. Similar tracer-based approaches have been employed using a range of imaging modalities (e.g., PET, MRI, single-photon emission computed tomography [SPECT], and computed tomography [CT]) that incorporate both metabolic (^{11}C-glucose, ^{15}O) and non-metabolic (^{133}xenon, ^{99m}Tc-ethylcysteinate dimer, nitrous oxide, gadolinium) substrates [8]. Fundamentally, these approaches record changes in image contrast following tracer injection and, by applying tracer kinetic models, attempt to quantify CBF in absolute units (e.g., ml blood/100 g tissue/min), as introduced in Chapter 1. The major disadvantage of these approaches is that they require the injection of a contrast agent,

---

Clinical Perfusion MRI: Techniques and Applications, ed. Peter B. Barker, Xavier Golay, and Greg Zaharchuk. Published by Cambridge University Press. © Peter B. Barker, Xavier Golay, and Greg Zaharchuk 2013.

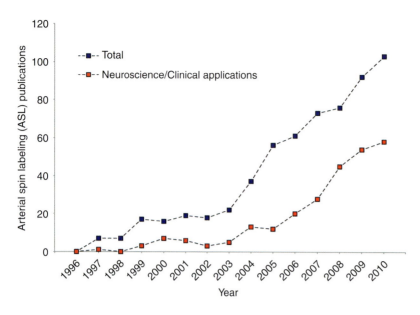

Figure 7.1 Number of total (blue) and human neuroscience (red) articles involving arterial spin labeling (ASL) appearing on PubMed.gov from 1996 to 2010. Criteria for selection of human neuroscience articles were studies that used ASL as a tool to investigate brain perfusion in a specific healthy or clinical population, in response to a pharmacological challenge, or as a physiological measure to interpret functional imaging contrast. Studies that were not included in this category pertain primarily to methodological ASL investigations, as well as applications of ASL to rodents and non-human primates, and ASL application studies outside the brain.

which limits the ability of these techniques to be applied in functional experiments where multiple, repeated measurements may be desired. Additionally, longitudinal studies aiming to track perfusion changes over time become more difficult owing to restrictions on permissible doses. Indeed, in clinical populations where contrast agents may be contraindicated [9, 10], invasive perfusion measurements are generally not performed, particularly for research purposes.

Therefore, perfusion imaging studies are increasingly utilizing new approaches that do not require contrast agent injection and can therefore be applied in a broader range of neuroscience applications. Magnetic labeling of arterial blood water using arterial spin labeling (ASL)-MRI is one especially promising approach [11] (see Chapter 3). Similar to the above invasive perfusion imaging techniques, ASL is also a tracer-based approach. However, in ASL endogenous blood water is exploited as the tracer, which can be magnetically labeled with radiofrequency (RF) pulses. This strategy creates a freely diffusible tracer (water) that can be tracked using conventional MR imaging readout schemes. Compared to $H_2{}^{15}O$-PET perfusion imaging, where the tracer decay is governed by the half-life of ^{15}O ($\sim$122 s), the blood water tracer in ASL decays with the longitudinal relaxation time (T_1) of arterial blood water ($\sim$1.7 s at 3 T) [12, 13]. Therefore, ASL perfusion measurements must be made relatively

quickly ($\sim$1.5–2 s) after labeling blood water. However, they can be repeated multiple times over several minutes, either to improve signal-to-noise ratio (SNR) or to study dynamic processes. Since the temporal resolution of CBF-weighted ASL measurements (4–6 s) is similar to that of the hemodynamic response to an infinitely short stimulus, it is possible to assess variation in cerebral perfusion approximately concurrent to flow changes associated with neuronal or vascular reactivity.

To demonstrate the gain in popularity of using ASL for neuroscience investigations, Figure 7.1 shows the total number of ASL papers published from 1996 to 2010, as well as the fraction of these studies that focus specifically on neuroscience applications in humans. Early work in ASL was largely devoted toward methodological development and animal and human validation studies; however, approximately half of all studies conducted between 2005 and 2010 were neuroscience (basic or clinical) or pharmacological studies in humans. The remaining fraction of studies over this time period focused on continued methodological development of new ASL variations, rodent and non-human primate imaging, and non-brain applications such as kidney and skeletal muscle perfusion imaging. Therefore, there is a growing interest in neuroscience studies that exploit CBF-weighted ASL contrast specifically as a tool for better understanding brain function. This chapter focuses on the use of ASL perfusion imaging in neurosciences and

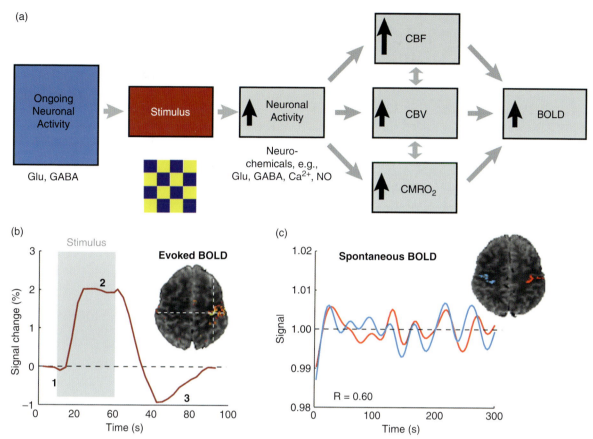

Figure 7.2 Overview of events leading to BOLD signal. (a) Ongoing neuronal activity is primarily influenced by glutamate (Glu) and γ-aminobutyric acid (GABA) signaling. In response to a stimulus, increased neuronal activity and neurochemical changes elicit a large increase in CBF, and a smaller increase in cerebral blood volume (CBV) and cerebral rate of oxygen metabolism (CMRO$_2$). (b) Evoked BOLD fMRI. A stimulus-evoked BOLD activation map (finger tapping) and response showing the (1) initial dip, (2) positive response, and (3) post-stimulus undershoot. (c) Spontaneous BOLD activation. Voxels in the motor cortex showing coherent fluctuations; the coherence of such fluctuations can be used to map regions of functional connectivity in the absence of administered tasks (so-called "resting-state fMRI"). CBF is central to eliciting BOLD responses, and therefore separate measurements of CBF can both complement and in certain applications replace BOLD fMRI. NO, nitric oxide.

specifically highlights the insights that are being gained through the use of non-invasive ASL approaches.

Theory
Functional neuroimaging with blood oxygenation level-dependent (BOLD) MRI

Currently, the most popular method for mapping brain activity utilizes the blood oxygenation level-dependent (BOLD) MRI technique [4, 14, 15]. Briefly, BOLD contrast arises from the disproportionate CBF increase relative to oxygen metabolism during increased neuronal activity, which results in an increase in the amount of oxyhemoglobin (HbO$_2$),

relative to deoxyhemoglobin (dHb), in capillaries and veins [4, 16, 17]. The MR water signal correspondingly increases in and around capillaries and veins owing to the relative reduction in paramagnetic dHb, and the consequent lengthening of the water transverse relaxation time as the microscopic field gradients surrounding the paramagnetic blood vessels are diminished in magnitude and extent. Since the BOLD fMRI signal is ultimately sensitive to the dHb content in the voxel it is only an indirect marker of neuronal activity, influenced by complex metabolic and hemodynamic modulations that occur concurrent to both ongoing and stimulus-evoked neuronal activity (Figure 7.2). Nevertheless, BOLD fMRI has become popular largely owing to its non-invasive nature, ease of implementation, ability to acquire whole brain images with relatively high SNR, and good spatial (2–4 mm) and temporal (1–3 s) resolutions. Additionally, extensive image analysis algorithms have been developed, which in most cases are made freely available, allowing for BOLD data to be processed without the need for extensive knowledge of MR physics or computing.

The ensemble stimulus-induced hemodynamic response measured with BOLD fMRI roughly corresponds to a brief reduction in signal (initial dip, though not always observed), followed by an increase in signal (stimulus-evoked signal change), followed by a signal reduction below baseline (post-stimulus undershoot) [18, 19]. However, these hemodynamic response components vary considerably between individuals and brain regions, and the precise physiological factors driving their magnitude and duration are incompletely understood. Knowledge of these factors is fundamental, as implementation of BOLD for discriminating different populations (e.g., diseased vs. healthy) and making conclusions regarding brain physiology rely on a quantitative understanding of the signal origin. While much progress has been made in understanding the hemodynamic and metabolic contributions to BOLD contrast, important gaps remain in the ability to relate BOLD signal to underlying neuronal activity and neurotransmission. These gaps significantly hinder interpretability of BOLD contrast in many applications, as substantial variability exists even between healthy individuals [20, 21], partly accounting for why BOLD data remain largely qualitative in nature. Understanding the physiological sources of this variability is crucial to using BOLD as a tool for identifying quantitative differences in brain function between individuals and conditions, and for gauging functional response to disease and treatment. Furthermore, competing functional imaging approaches, such as PET, similarly seek to infer changes in neuronal activity from surrogate hemodynamic and metabolic contrast. For this reason, understanding the relationship between neuronal, hemodynamic, and metabolic activity is of relevance beyond just BOLD fMRI.

It is difficult to quantitatively interpret BOLD signal in terms of neuronal activity for several reasons. First, the signal changes that are detected do not arise directly from neuronal activity, or even from a single hemodynamic parameter, but instead are the result of a complex set of changes in CBF, cerebral blood volume (CBV), and oxygen metabolism, and are further sensitive to differences in hematocrit and basal oxygenation levels [17, 22–24]. Furthermore, these relationships have been shown to differ in response to excitatory glutamatergic activity and inhibitory γ-aminobutyric acid (GABA)-ergic activity [20, 25, 26]. For example, ^{13}C spectroscopy data in anesthetized rats have demonstrated that both the rate of neurotransmitter cycling and glucose oxidation in GABAergic neurons is approximately 25% of corresponding levels in glutamatergic neurons [27–29]. Furthermore, mouse astrocytes exposed to glutamate (Glu) initiate uptake of glucose, whereas no uptake is observed during GABA exposure [26]. This has prompted the hypothesis that glutamatergic neurons derive energy from increases in CBF and glucose utilization, relative to GABAergic neurons that are more significantly supported by increases in oxidative phosphorylation [30]. Second, the signal changes are not necessarily compartmentalized to the tissue or capillaries, but arise in both small and large vessels and extravascular tissue in a complex manner that varies with imaging parameter choice and static magnetic field strength [31, 32]. More specifically, in conventional gradient-echo BOLD scans, contrast is approximately 70% intravascular at low field strengths of 1.5 T, yet nearly 100% extravascular at the higher field strength of 7.0 T. Therefore, it is not straightforward to draw quantitative physiological conclusions from BOLD fMRI data acquired in isolation, or at separate facilities or field strengths, and it is difficult to interpret the spatial relationship between the BOLD activation maps and the underlying neuronal activity.

Additionally, BOLD fMRI is most commonly performed by acquiring long echo time (TE) gradient echo images (TE = 30–45 ms for typical field strengths of 1.5–3 T) during periods of both baseline activity and task performance. A long TE is required to achieve an adequate sensitivity to magnetic susceptibility changes in blood, and the TE is generally chosen to be near the effective relaxation time (T_2^*) of the tissue. However, the long TE required with BOLD, while increasing BOLD sensitivity, reduces the overall SNR and leads to specific regions of signal loss near air–tissue interfaces. An additional problem encountered in these brain areas is geometric distortion that is most pronounced near regions of magnetic field heterogeneity, such as in frontal and temporal lobe, cerebellum, and brainstem. This is a

Table 7.1. Typical blood oxygenation level-dependent (BOLD) and arterial spin labeling (ASL) information for static magnetic field strengths of 1.5–3 T

	Contrast origin	MR contrast parameter	Voxel size (mm)	Temporal resolution (s)	Contrast-to-noise ratio	Signal change (%)	Typical variations
BOLD	Capillary and venous blood oxygenation	T_2^* or T_2	3–4	2–3	4–5	1–4	Gradient echo, spin echo
ASL	Perfusion	Labeled blood	3–5	4–8	2–3	20–80	Pulsed, continuous, pseudo-continuous

result of the sensitivity of echo-planar imaging (EPI), which is invariably used as the readout sequence, to local field inhomogeneities, leading to distortions that frequently complicate interpretation of BOLD contrast and registration approaches. Finally, BOLD contrast is sensitive to low-frequency drift, largely owing to small hardware instabilities and gradient heating over the duration of the experiment, and to gradual head motion. This complication generally requires that the BOLD data be low-frequency filtered prior to statistical analysis, and thus BOLD is generally insensitive to very low-frequency fluctuations (e.g., < 0.01 Hz).

Thus, while BOLD fMRI has revolutionized the field of cognitive neuroscience, largely owing to its non-invasive nature, ease of implementation, and general availability of post-processing packages, it possesses several noticeable shortcomings. Alternative functional neuroimaging approaches are being developed and implemented with the aim of addressing some of these issues.

Functional neuroimaging with arterial spin labeling (ASL) MRI

Perfusion imaging in conjunction with, or in substitution for, conventional BOLD imaging can be useful for providing additional insight, for example, to help disentangle the complexities of the BOLD signal origin. This strategy for understanding brain function has become increasingly popular since the development of non-invasive perfusion contrast and ASL. Furthermore, ASL scans, which can be applied in sequence [19, 24] or parallel [33, 34] to BOLD fMRI, can provide additional contrast to better understand the ensemble BOLD response. As with BOLD, a functional ASL experiment can be performed by acquiring ASL images over a period of baseline and task conditions, and corresponding activation maps can be generated by applying statistical tests to the ASL difference images (Table 7.1).

Labeling in functional ASL experiments has most commonly been performed using short (5–15 ms) labeling pulses (saturation or inversion), after which a delay is allowed for the labeled blood water spins to flow to the capillary exchange site and exchange with tissue water. This sort of pulsed ASL (PASL) experiment provides an effective temporal resolution of 4–5 s, once the accompanying control acquisition is included. Alternatively, continuous ASL (CASL) and more recently pseudo-continuous ASL (pCASL) labeling approaches have gained popularity, in which blood water is labeled with a single long pulse or train of short pulses, respectively [35–37] (see Chapter 3). These labeling strategies reduce slightly the temporal resolution of the perfusion measurement to 6–8 s owing to the longer labeling duration. However, they can significantly add to the SNR of a single measurement. For instance, SNR has been shown to increase by as much as 50% when using pCASL approaches, compared with PASL approaches [36]. For most current ASL sequences, perfusion-weighted maps can be obtained with sufficiently high temporal resolution to facilitate the acquisition of multiple images over a relatively short scan session of a few minutes and to assess temporal dynamics in perfusion patterns.

Advantages of ASL fMRI

There are several components of the ASL experiment that make it distinct and potentially advantageous relative to BOLD fMRI. First, the ASL signal is derived from CBF only, rather than from multiple competing hemodynamic sources as is the case for BOLD. The ASL perfusion-weighted map is obtained by subtracting an image in which inflowing blood water is magnetically labeled from an image in which such inflowing blood water is not labeled, and therefore the resulting difference image contains visible perfusion information. This is in contrast to the BOLD image, which is fundamentally a T_2- or T_2^*-weighted image, from which information regarding blood flow or metabolism can only be inferred during activation experiments or after complex post-processing. Furthermore, the evoked BOLD hemodynamic response is in the order of 2–3% at 1.5–3 T. ASL provides CBF-weighted maps from which both baseline perfusion and perfusion changes can be quantified. Perfusion changes in response to strong neuronal stimulation (e.g., flashing checkerboards, finger tapping, etc.) are in the order of 20–80%, and therefore the measured ASL change is much larger than the measured BOLD signal change. It should be noted, however, that the SNR of the ASL data itself is poorer than the equivalent BOLD data, since the T_1 decay of the label during transit from the labeling location, and the relatively low blood volume in brain tissue, means that the ASL signal itself is never more than 1–2% of the available tissue signal, notwithstanding the large changes in perfusion that can accompany activation. These effects in combination result in ASL-based fMRI having an appreciably lower contrast-to-noise ratio (CNR) than BOLD fMRI (Table 7.1). Second, as ASL contrast is fundamentally derived from perfusion, the contrast is in principle better localized to tissue and capillaries that are expected to be more closely related to spatial regions of brain activity than draining veins. A comparison of BOLD and ASL during a memory-encoding task [38] showed better localization and stronger group activation maps for ASL relative to BOLD in the hippocampus and mesial temporal lobe for comparable spatial resolutions (3–4 mm isotropic voxel dimensions). Third, while the temporal resolution with ASL is generally poorer than with BOLD, the pairwise subtraction in ASL makes the ASL maps less sensitive to low-frequency noise relative to the BOLD fMRI scan. This allows for improved sensitivity during longer experiments. Fourth, it has been reported that intra-subject variability in BOLD responses is smaller compared with ASL; however, greater inter-subject BOLD variability relative to ASL has been reported in regimes of long task/control periods where the stability advantages of ASL become decisive [39].

Disadvantages of ASL fMRI

There are several considerations involved when interpreting ASL changes in response to task-evoked activity as well. While it is generally assumed that the ASL signal change reflects a pure physiological CBF response, influences from BOLD effects, as well as changes in the arterial arrival time (AAT) between baseline and activation, can further complicate quantification, particularly during periods of CBF transition. BOLD effects may become most pronounced for long TE acquisitions, and can be reduced using both alternative subtraction procedures [40], ultra-short TE acquisitions enabled by spiral-out readout methods [37], and post-processing modeling approaches [41]. These complications are most pronounced at transition periods in the paradigm, for instance where the control and label ASL image may have different blood oxygenation levels, leading to incomplete cancelation of BOLD effects when the label image is subtracted from the control image. If such differences in oxygenation level are not accounted for, the perfusion-weighted ASL time course may be contaminated by BOLD artifacts, which could complicate the temporal interpretation of the BOLD time course. Additionally, it has been found that fractional reductions in the AATs are approximately as large as the CBF increase associated with activation [42–44]. Therefore, if blood water is labeled in ASL, a different fraction of water may reach the imaging slice in a baseline vs. task period (where perfusion is increased and transit time decreased). Failure to account for changes in the AAT between baseline and task periods will lead to incorrect perfusion quantification [43, 44] Finally, ASL can be complicated by transit time discrepancies between slices. For instance, scans that have 2D readouts will have a slice timing discrepancy of generally 20–80 ms depending on spatial resolution. This will lead to different post-labeling delays for different slices. This complication will alter the ASL contrast, and thus CBF, in a slice-dependent way. New approaches which utilize 3D readouts have been developed to eliminate this complication [45], and current pCASL and CASL sequences are much less sensitive to small variations in AAT.

BOLD vs. ASL fMRI

Figure 7.3 shows BOLD activation maps of the visual and motor cortex, as well as ASL activation maps acquired in the same subject with an identical task paradigm. As can be seen, the ASL activation maps appear to be more specific to the functionally eloquent regions for identical statistical thresholds, a finding that is consistently observed and has been

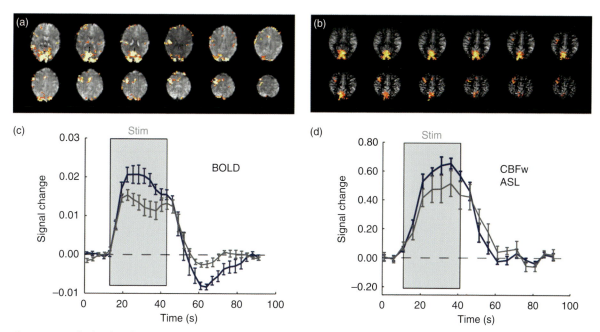

Figure 7.3 Multi-slice fMRI for simultaneous flashing (8 Hz) checkerboard and unilateral finger tapping (1 Hz) tasks. (a) BOLD and (b) CBF-weighted (CBFw) ASL activation maps. Time courses are shown for visual (blue) and motor (gray) voxels below (c, d). Time courses are averages over eight healthy volunteers; error bars represent standard deviation over all subjects. Adapted from Donahue *et al.* (24).

attributed to the spatial specificity of ASL for arterioles, capillaries, microvasculature, and tissue compared to BOLD contrast, which is additionally derived from draining veins. The time courses for these tasks are shown in the lower panels. In this study [24], as in the majority of combination BOLD and ASL investigations, the ASL data were acquired separately (e.g., either directly before or after) the BOLD contrast data. While this still gives a reasonable estimation of the CBF contribution to BOLD signal changes, any differences in task performance between the BOLD and ASL acquisitions could complicate interpretation. Additionally, this strategy doubles the time of the exam. An alternative strategy is to acquire the BOLD and ASL data simultaneously in the same scan [33]. This is achieved by taking advantage of the fact that most ASL readout modules use a gradient echo sequence, and hence the ASL control acquisition is fundamentally a T_2^*-weighted scan with some BOLD sensitivity. This BOLD sensitivity can be increased by acquiring a second, longer TE echo in the ASL acquisition, with the longer echo having a TE that is close to the inherent T_2^* of the tissue. Therefore, the subtraction of the labeled scan from the short TE control scan yields the desired CBF-weighted ASL map, whereas the long TE

control scans yield a BOLD time course. The main advantage of this approach is that both BOLD and ASL data can be acquired in the same scan without the need for a separate experiment which adds time and complications owing to variations in paradigm compliance. The disadvantage of the combined approach is that the temporal resolution of the BOLD scan is reduced, as BOLD images are only acquired in every other repetition time (TR). Thus, whereas a stand-alone BOLD scan would have a temporal resolution of 2–4 s, a BOLD-ASL combination approach would yield a BOLD temporal resolution of 4–8 s, depending on the choice of TR. Additionally, owing to the need to acquire two volumes of data (each corresponding to a different TE), the number of slices and volume coverage may be reduced relative to a stand-alone BOLD scan. Therefore, the advantages and disadvantages of each approach must be weighed in the context of the desired application and scientific question of interest. A final complication of the dual-echo approach is that it precludes the use of tissue background suppression [46], which can improve the cancelation of static tissue in the label and control images, and thereby improves the CNR of the ASL difference signal. If BOLD data are desired then it becomes

109

Table 7.2. Comparison of ASL MRI measures of CBF with more established PET and/or SPECT approaches

Author	Year	Reference technique (Parameter)	Population	N	Findings
Liu et al. [115]	2011	SPECT (CBF)	Gulf war illness and controls	47	ASL provided similar CBF trends as SPECT (SPECT trends measured in a separate study)
Noguchi et al. [49]	2011	SPECT (CBF)	Moyamoya patients	12	Hemispherical CBF values correlated between ASL and SPECT
Bokkers et al. [116]	2010	PET (CBF)	Carotid artery occlusion patients	14	ASL at multiple labeling delays depicted areas of low CBF similar to PET. A systematic overestimation of CBF in ASL relative to PET
Qiu et al. [117]	2010	PET (CBF)	Controls	14	Variations in AAT influence regional ASL CBF quantification compared with PET
Wissmeyer et al. [118]	2010	PET (CBF)	Epilepsy patients	3	CBF correlation between ASL and PET
Xu et al. [119]	2010	PET (CBF)	Elderly controls	9	Global and regional CBF agreement between ASL and PET
Lüdemann et al. [120]	2009	PET (CBF)	Brain tumor patients	12	CBF measured most reliably with ASL compared with other methods.
Chen et al. [121]	2008	PET (CBF)	Controls	10	Correlation between CBF in ASL and PET, yet with ASL providing slightly lower CBF values
Kimura et al. [122]	2005	PET (CBF)	Carotid artery occlusion patients	11	Correlation between ASL and PET CBF, yet with CBF underestimation in the occluded hemisphere
Newberg et al. [123]	2005	PET (CMR_{Glc})	Controls	5	Concordance between ASL CBF and cerebral metabolic rate of glucose (CMR_{Glc}) as measured by PET
Liu et al. [124]	2001	PET (CBF)	Temporal lobe epilepsy patients	8	Correlation between ASL and PET hypoperfusion
Ye et al. [47]	2000	PET (CBF)	Controls	12	Gray matter CBF similar between ASL and PET. White matter CBF underestimated with ASL

impossible to deploy the static signal suppression, with a consequent degradation in the quality of the ASL data.

Methods for ASL functional brain activation experiments: expectations and limitations

Before using ASL for the study of brain function, it is useful to know the limits of the technique, and existing validation studies that have been performed. CBF measurements using ASL have been validated against $H_2^{15}O$-PET, both for baseline [47] and activation-related changes in CBF [48]. Additional validation studies have been performed for ASL CBF measurements and perfusion SPECT [49], perfusion CT (pCT) [50], dynamic susceptibility contrast (DSC)-MRI [51], and Doppler ultrasound [52]; however, certain minor variations between techniques do exist (Table 7.2) [8, 13].

Recent studies using pCASL CBF sequences in the same subjects spaced 2–4 weeks apart demonstrated high precision (intra-class correlation, ICC = 0.62) and accuracy (ICC = 0.77) for the CBF-weighted contrast [53]. The same study outlined the sensitivity limits of ASL; for instance, detecting a 15% change in CBF with 90% power, given the measured 15% variation between repeated measurements, requires approximately 20 subjects. Finally, a large test-retest study recently measured a mean gray matter CBF of $47.4 \pm 7.5 \, ml/100 \, g/min$ for a between-subject standard variation of $5.5 \, ml/100 \, g/min$ and a within-subject standard deviation of $4.7 \, ml/100 \, g/min$. The corresponding repeatability from this study including 284 subjects scanned four times each in 28 centers around the world was $13.0 \, ml/100 \, g/min$, which was found to be within the range of previous studies [54].

Important sequence and analysis strategies have been developed over the past several years that have greatly improved the reliability of ASL, and in turn this has made it a reasonable approach for distinguishing volunteer populations based on CBF variations, as well as for measuring CBF changes in response to neuronal or pharmacologically induced changes. Specifically, as explained in more detail in Chapter 3, SNR benefits obtainable from pCASL labeling schemes [36], 3D readouts [45], and background suppression techniques [46, 55] have increased the SNR of the ASL image several fold. Additional improvements such as Quantitative Imaging of Perfusion using a Single Subtraction (QUIPSS) II [33] for PASL or long labeling schemes for CASL and pCASL reduce the sensitivity of the resulting measurement to unknown inflowing blood water bolus sizes, thereby further improving the specificity for CBF changes.

Applications

ASL and neurovascular coupling

The relationship between neuronal activity and the hemodynamic response continues to be an area of active research and debate [16, 19, 24, 56–62]. However, a thorough understanding of this relationship would greatly improve the interpretability of BOLD fMRI contrast and would be valuable for making inferences regarding neurovascular coupling. One active area of research pertaining to this topic relates to carefully identifying the specific hemodynamic (e.g., CBF and CBV) and metabolic (e.g., cerebral rate of oxygen metabolism ($CMRO_2$)) sources to the BOLD fMRI response, and their corresponding temporal dynamics. Fundamentally, since the BOLD effect arises from the mismatch in the increase of CBF and $CMRO_2$, independent measurements of CBF can be used to better characterize the sources of BOLD signal variability, and to understand how hemodynamic, metabolic, and neuronal activity are related.

Two general pathways have been debated regarding the relationship between neuronal activity and the hemodynamic response. In the *metabolic pathway*, hemodynamic changes are induced by vasodilatory metabolites (carbon dioxide [CO_2] and H^+) released during increased aerobic metabolism; changes in CBF and CBV are thus a direct reflection of local tissue energy demands and are coupled to changes in $CMRO_2$. Alternatively, the *neurotransmitter pathway* proposes that molecules released at the synapse during neuronal activity, such as glutamate, trigger the release of vasodilatory mediators (e.g., nitric oxide), which then increase CBF and CBV [1]; according to this view, changes in CBF and CBV are not directly coupled to changes in $CMRO_2$.

Efforts to understand which of these pathways provides the best account of hemodynamic responses to brain activation have proven difficult. The fundamental reason for this is because changes in neuronal activity, oxygen metabolism, neurotransmitter release, and CBF are often in the same direction and proportional. One approach is to compare the time-dependent changes in CBF, CBV, and $CMRO_2$ induced during and following cortical activation. Early optical studies reported a "pre-stimulus" blood oxygenation undershoot occurring before the positive hemodynamic response, but this has been found difficult to reproduce in MRI studies at more coarse spatial resolutions [18]. Recent work using two-photon microscopy at high spatial resolution (200–600 mm) in conjunction with BOLD fMRI in anesthetized rats and somatosensory stimulation demonstrated that the initial dip is dependent on cortical depth [63]. Specifically, the fastest BOLD response was observed in the deep layers of cortex, whereas the most delayed response, and largest initial dip, was observed in layer I. This observation is consistent with the hypothesis that there is upstream propagation of vasodilatation toward the cortical surface along arterioles, and also downstream propagation into capillaries. Therefore, variations in the BOLD onset and dip magnitude will depend on the precise spatial location along the cortical ribbon, and the somewhat coarse spatial resolution (3–5 mm) where most human BOLD fMRI experiments are conducted is not sufficient to reproducibly detect the initial dip. Consequently, much BOLD research has focused on the post-stimulus response. Specifically, following this elusive initial dip, the typical BOLD fMRI time course consists of an increase in signal intensity corresponding to increases in capillary and venous blood oxygenation, followed by a decrease in MR signal to sub-baseline intensity.

The origin of this latter phase of reduced oxygenation, referred to as the post-stimulus undershoot, is still under discussion and could have relevance for better understanding neurovascular coupling mechanisms, as well as for improving spatial specificity in BOLD analysis. Initially, it was hypothesized that the undershoot resulted from continued oxygen metabolism in the absence of changes in CBF [64]. Subsequent experiments on anesthetized mammals [58, 65] suggested that the BOLD undershoot could be due to continued elevated venular CBV, described by the so-called delayed venular/venous compliance balloon model [23] and the Windkessel model [58]. Additional evidence for the delayed compliance model has been provided using monocrystalline iron oxide nanoparticles (MION) contrast-enhanced CBV MRI [65, 66], and using optical imaging approaches [67] in anesthetized rats. More recently, initial fMRI experiments using ultrasmall superparamagnetic iron oxide (USPIO) particles have been performed [68]. These experiments, which are highly weighted to CBV changes, suggest that the CBV signal recovers more slowly than the traditional BOLD signal as measured without contrast.

Other recent studies using the vascular space occupancy (VASO) (see Chapter 6) and bolus-tracking (i.e., DSC) techniques (see Chapter 2) in awake humans have provided evidence for an uncoupling of CBV, CBF, and BOLD responses during the post-stimulus undershoot period [19, 56, 69], which, under the assumption of negligible changes in hematocrit, point to a persisting increase in tissue oxygen metabolism as the source of the undershoot. In support of this possibility, another study using near-infrared spectroscopy in conjunction with BOLD fMRI reported that dHb concentration remained elevated during the BOLD post-stimulus undershoot, providing evidence for persisting tissue hypermetabolism following neuronal stimulation [70]. Recently, using BOLD and DSC, it was shown that the BOLD post-stimulus undershoot persisted after CBV had returned to baseline [56]. Collectively, these data suggest that activity-elicited changes in $CMRO_2$ can occur in the absence of changes in CBF and CBV, with the preserved coupling of responses during stimulus onset being coincidental rather than causal. Moreover, the uncoupling of metabolic and hemodynamic activity during the post-stimulus undershoot would tend to refute the metabolic account of the neurovascular relationship, and indirectly support the neurotransmitter account.

Finally, it is also possible that a CBF reduction below baseline could account for the BOLD post-stimulus undershoot. This hypothesis has been suggested to arise owing to an autoregulatory feedback mechanism [71]. Additionally, electrophysiological recordings have demonstrated a reduction in neuronal activity following visual stimulation [72], which could be accompanied by a CBF reduction. However, such findings have been somewhat difficult to reproduce, and may vary heavily with brain region and stimulus type [73, 74].

CBF-weighted ASL sequences, as well as CBV-weighted sequences, are being used in sequence with BOLD fMRI to better understand these pathways. For example, BOLD, CBV-weighted, and CBF-weighted fMRI were performed using both visual stimulation and a mild hypercapnic stimulus (breath-hold), under normoxic conditions [75]. In both of these physiological perturbations, CBV and CBF increase; however, contrary to visual activation where $CMRO_2$ increases, $CMRO_2$ is known to remain largely unchanged during a brief breath-hold [76–78]. Therefore, the comparison of breath-hold and visual stimulation may yield insight concerning the relationship between CBF, CBV, and $CMRO_2$. In the experiment by Donahue et al., a BOLD undershoot was observed following periods of visual stimulation, but was not evident following periods of breath-hold, providing some evidence for the undershoot being due to persisting oxygen metabolism, hypothesized to be required for restoring ion gradients [75]. However, in that study $CMRO_2$ was not specifically measured and changes in $CMRO_2$ can only be inferred from the measured BOLD, CBF, and CBV time courses.

The above explanation was in direct conflict with the explanation of the BOLD undershoot as a component of passive, delayed vascular compliance and persisting elevated venous CBV. The elevated CBV theory was based on observations using injected CBV contrast agents (reporting on total CBV) in anesthetized rats that, contrary to the human CBV-weighted studies using the VASO technique, provided a different CBV trend. The post-stimulus BOLD undershoot has more recently been investigated using newer approaches with arterial CBV weighting in

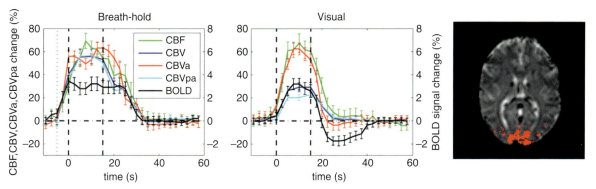

Figure 7.4 An example of a neurovascular coupling study using multi-modality fMRI. On the left, the BOLD time course is shown in response to a breath-hold, along with the ASL time course (CBF), and CBV time courses for total CBV (CBV), arterial CBV (CBVa) and post-arterial (CBVpa). CBV measurements were made using the VASO approach. On the right, the time courses are shown in response to a visual stimulus, in which CBF, CBV, and $CMRO_2$ are all known to change. Note that the BOLD post-stimulus undershoot is present in the visual stimulus, but not in the breath-hold, suggesting that the undershoot may have a metabolic origin. This study found that both CBF and CBV return to baseline during this undershoot, suggesting an uncoupling of CBF and CBV from $CMRO_2$ during this period. Adapted from Hua *et al.* (79).

awake humans [79]. Here (Figure 7.4), it was similarly observed that the BOLD undershoot disappeared following the largely isometabolic task of breath-hold. Furthermore, the relative contributions of post-arterial CBV and $CMRO_2$ to the post-stimulus undershoot were estimated to be approximately 20% and 80%, respectively. This work provides support for both delayed venular compliance and persisting elevated $CMRO_2$ contributing to the BOLD undershoot; however, the dominant contributions come from $CMRO_2$. Such findings were partly based on a newer inflow VASO (iVASO) approach [80]. This approach is believed to have contrast derived primarily from arterial CBV changes; however, it may also suffer from blood inflow and CBF effects.

However, not all recent work supports the above findings. Very recently, BOLD neurovascular coupling experiments were conducted in anesthetized rats for varying levels of intracranial pressure; it was demonstrated that a reduction in the undershoot magnitude was associated with increased intracranial pressure, suggesting a mechanical rather than metabolic origin for the undershoot [60]. Additionally, studies by Kim *et al.* and Drew *et al.* have found that the temporal dynamics of arteries and veins may vary quite substantially for short vs. long stimuli [61, 62], suggesting that much of the discord in experimental results may be due to stimulation duration, as optical measurements generally use very short durations, whereas fMRI experiments with more coarse temporal resolution employ longer stimulus durations.

A third explanation for the undershoot, which has historically been less rigorously investigated, is that it could be due to a post-stimulus CBF undershoot, which has been reported using both ASL and optical imaging approaches [73, 81, 82] (Figure 7.5). Interestingly, a very small CBF reduction below baseline of only a few percent could explain the BOLD undershoot. Such a small change is generally difficult to distinguish from noise in the ASL signal, and therefore has not always been reported. However, recent studies of CBF contributions to BOLD contrast have found small CBF post-stimulus undershoots [83] and ongoing measurements are being conducted to assess the possibility of a CBF undershoot providing some explanation for the BOLD undershoot [84].

The above distinctions may seem inconsequential; however, accurately characterizing the BOLD hemodynamic response is of great importance to studies that aim to use BOLD as a tool for quantitatively understanding brain function. For, if a post-stimulus undershoot could be accurately attributable to a specific physiologic process (e.g., CBF or $CMRO_2$), then this may represent a better indicator of brain activity than the ensemble positive response, reflective of venous blood oxygenation changes. Additionally, the positive BOLD response may appear normal in some patient studies where neurovascular coupling relationships are impaired, owing to competing abnormal contributions from CBF, CBV, and $CMRO_2$. Indeed, this has been reported in certain clinical studies of cerebrovascular disease [85]. Therefore, complementing BOLD fMRI studies with CBF-weighted ASL

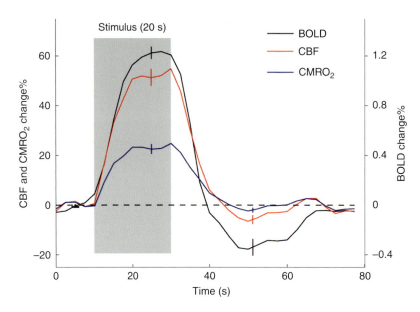

Figure 7.5 The relationship between BOLD and CBF, using ASL for the CBF measurement. Here, a small reduction in ASL signal below baseline is observed, suggesting that the BOLD post-stimulus undershoot may be due to a reduction in CBF below baseline. Note that if either a CBF reduction, as shown here, or an elevated $CMRO_2$ contribution, is the source of the BOLD undershoot, the undershoot may provide a more specific (e.g., $CMRO_2$ or CBF) marker for neuronal activity than simply the positive BOLD response, which is generally localized to draining veins at field strengths of 1.5–3.0 T. Adapted from Griffeth *et al.* (84).

approaches and CBV-weighted approaches is becoming increasingly popular in order to more reliably identify the physiological and hemodynamic sources of BOLD signal variability. To successfully accomplish this however, it is necessary that the CBF-weighted and CBV-weighted approaches are responsibly implemented and the contrast mechanisms of different techniques are thoroughly understood. We direct the readers to the respective chapters of this book (Chapters 3 and 6 in particular) for a description of the ideal parameters to be used in these circumstances. While CBF-weighted ASL is quite widely accepted as a good indicator of perfusion (Table 7.2), CBV-weighted measurements using exogenous USPIO contrast in awake humans and anesthetized animals, VASO using endogenous blood water in awake humans, and gadolinium bolus-tracking CBV measurements in humans and animals have all provided somewhat conflicting reports of CBV dynamics, which are likely due to small differences in the contrast mechanisms of these techniques, as well as to different physiological neurovascular coupling relationships between awake and anesthetized subjects. Thus, this is an active, yet unresolved area of research.

Pharmacological ASL

ASL has been used as a tool to understand perfusion changes in response to pharmacological manipulation of cerebral hemodynamics. This ability is useful for gauging the physiological response to drug therapies.

Such studies of vascular responses to vasodilatory drugs may have use for non-invasively measuring vessel compliance, and for assessing cerebrovascular reserve.

While PET imaging and BOLD fMRI have more commonly been applied to study drug effects, ASL possesses several additional advantages. Compared with PET, ASL is completely non-invasive and is therefore preferable from a patient safety and comfort perspective. BOLD fMRI, which has been successfully applied to study a range of pharmacological agents, is prone to uncertainties in interpreting the complex contrast that is measured, and is not quantitative. Additionally, noise properties and signal drift in the BOLD signal reduce the sensitivity to low-frequency fluctuations, rendering BOLD less useful for many pharmacological paradigms where only a single drug epoch may be possible. ASL provides an absolute measure of CBF and provides a relatively flat frequency spectrum compared to BOLD and is thus potentially better suited to studying slow changes in hemodynamics. Therefore, the ASL contrast is particularly promising for pharmacological studies [53, 86].

For instance, CBF and AAT maps during rest and infusion of remifentanil, an opioid analgesic drug, demonstrated an increase in CBF from 57 ± 2.0 to 77 ± 18.4 ml/100 g tissue/min and a reduction in AAT from 0.73 ± 0.07 s to 0.64 ± 0.08 s in healthy volunteers (Figure 7.6) [87]. In a separate study, healthy

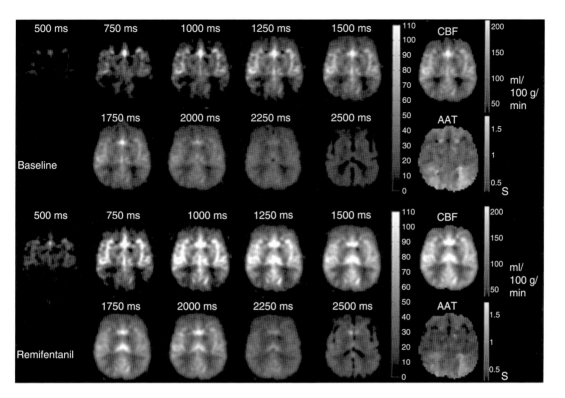

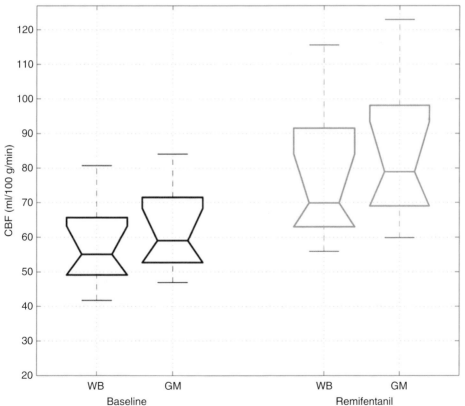

Figure 7.6 An example of measuring changes in CBF using ASL in response to a pharmacological agent. Above, ASL and arterial arrival time (AAT) maps are shown at baseline, whereas below they are shown following infusion of remifentanil. Note the clear increase in CBF and reduction in AAT following remifentanil administration. Below, CBF is quantified in whole brain (WB) and gray matter (GM) before and after remifentanil in ten healthy volunteers. Adapted from MacIntosh *et al.* (87).

volunteers received remifentanil infusion with an increasing dose (0–2 µg/kg/min) and CBF values were measured using a PASL approach [88]. Regional CBF values in the amygdala, hippocampus, cingulate, insula, and thalamus were normalized by global CBF. Following this normalization, increased CBF was found in the cingulate, whereas decreased CBF was observed in the hippocampus and amygdala. The authors further observed that these trends were reversed in volunteers with the ApoE4 polymorphism, a genetic risk factor for Alzheimer's disease.

Caffeine, an adenosine antagonist and vasoconstrictor, has been one of the most popular drug targets of pharmacological MRI studies. Importantly, as the most widely used psychostimulant and with its well-known effect of lowering CBF, variations in caffeine consumption can contribute to large inter-subject variations in evoked BOLD responses. Using BOLD and ASL together, in conjunction with a popular calibration approach involving the administration of 5% CO_2 [89], it was demonstrated that the $CBF:CMRO_2$ coupling ratio reduced slightly from 2.53 ± 2.33 in the motor cortex to 2.45 ± 2.23 in the visual cortex upon caffeine administration (not significant) [90]. In a separate study [91], ASL and BOLD data were collected before and after intravenous infusion of saline or caffeine (1–5 mg/kg doses) and the magnitude of evoked responses were recorded during visual and motor stimulation. This study found that the maximum BOLD response occurred for a caffeine dose of 2.5 mg/kg, whereas the maximum CBF response occurred at 5 mg/kg (highest dose studied). This finding was attributed to different adenosine receptors (A_1 and A_{2A}, respectively). Of importance, therefore, for longitudinal ASL studies is attention to control for the effects of caffeine. Caffeine is present in many sources (coffee, tea, soft drinks, energy drinks, etc.) and has a significant potential confounding effect due to its ability to decrease CBF by as much as 30%, which may be similar to, or greater than, the effect on CBF of the treatment or intervention being studied.

Similar combined BOLD and ASL studies have been carried out using indomethacin, a common non-steroidal anti-inflammatory drug and inhibitor of cyclooxygenase and prostaglandin synthesis. Here, a reduction in CBF was observed during neuronal stimulation [92], yet $CMRO_2$ was observed not to change. However, it is also possible that indomethacin may alter the baseline $CMRO_2$ [93], and this would alter the trend of the evoked $CMRO_2$ response.

The cerebral autoregulatory status of brain tissue in patients with symptomatic stenosis of the internal carotid artery (ICA) has been assessed using ASL. For instance, in patients with symptomatic stenosis of the ICA, the flow territory (i.e., volume of tissue perfused) of the symptomatic ICA was smaller than that of the asymptomatic ICA [94]. After administration of acetazolamide, a carbonic anhydrase inhibitor and vasodilator, a significant increase in CBF was observed in both control subjects and patients ($n = 23$) in all perfusion territories. Mean cerebrovascular reactivity values were $35.9 \pm 3.0\%$ and $44.6 \pm 3.5\%$ in the flow territories of the patients with symptomatic ICAs and those with asymptomatic ICAs, respectively, compared with $47.9 \pm 3.1\%$ in the control subjects. The results of this study indicate that in patients with symptomatic stenosis of the ICA, vasodilatory capacity in the flow territories of the major cerebral arteries can be visualized and quantified at the brain tissue level with ASL MRI.

ASL studies are also frequently conducted during administration of 4–5% CO_2, which causes vasodilatation and CBF increase in gray matter parenchyma. This approach has been used to evaluate the effects of diabetes on CBF regulation. Baseline CBF ($p = 0.006$) and CO_2 reactivity ($p = 0.005$) were found to be reduced in the diabetic volunteers, and, furthermore, reductions in CBF in frontal brain regions were closely associated with gray matter atrophy ($p < 0.0001$) [95].

Additionally, ASL in conjunction with CO_2 administration is frequently used to calibrate BOLD responses. As mentioned earlier, the BOLD response has a complex dependence on underlying modulations in CBF, CBV, and $CMRO_2$, in addition to baseline levels of these parameters within the brain, which are known to vary spatially, as well as between volunteers. A range of commonly administered medications and even foods may raise or lower baseline CBF, resulting in substantially different BOLD responses between individuals. For example, for a dose of caffeine (a vasoconstrictor) of 2.5 mg/kg, approximately that found in a typical cup of coffee, the BOLD response increases by approximately 30–35% [91]. To account for differences in basal levels of CBF and metabolism, it has been hypothesized that a calibration experiment can be performed, whereby BOLD and ASL measurements are made for both a vascular stimulus (e.g., 5% CO_2 administration) as well as a neuronal stimulus (e.g., visual for motor task). For the vascular stimulus, CBF and CBV both increase, whereas for the neuronal stimulus CBF, CBV, and $CMRO_2$ all increase. Thus, by comparing signal changes from the isometabolic vascular task with those from the neuronal task, it is possible to quantify the $CBF/CMRO_2$ coupling ratios and in principle to compare more accurately inter-subject BOLD responses. While this approach has been frequently employed, it relies on the assumption that $CMRO_2$ does not change during CO_2 administration, as well as the assumption that neuronal and vascular stimuli elicit similar CBF and CBV responses, both of which have been questioned recently [44, 79, 96].

Another approach that has been used to provide a method of inter-subject calibration is to use baseline venous oxygenation via measurements in the sagittal sinus vein [97]. Using the so-called "TRUST" method (see Chapter 5), venous blood in the main draining vein from the brain is isolated using ASL subtraction principles, and this signal is then acquired at various TEs in order to measure its T_2 value. The blood oxygen level can then be inferred from the known relationship between blood T_2 and oxygenation, giving an indication of the systemic oxygen extraction fraction for the brain (in turn inversely proportional to the resting CBF). This information can then be used as a normalization for baseline physiological state, and has been demonstrated to improve inter-subject variability in BOLD fMRI studies [98].

Finally, it is additionally possible to measure in vivo neurotransmitter concentrations in humans using ^1H magnetic resonance spectroscopy (MRS) and spectral editing [99–101], and robust techniques for measuring GABA and Glu from multiple brain regions have been demonstrated [102]. Using this approach, it has been shown that basal GABA concentration can explain variations in the magnitude of the positive stimulus-evoked BOLD response in human visual cortex, as well as variations in CBF and CBV responses (Figure 7.7) [20]. Interestingly, a positive trend has been observed between CBF-weighted ASL signal changes and baseline GABA concentration. Since ASL measurements are sensitive to both CBF as well as AAT, it is possible that AAT, not CBF, is positively correlated with basal GABA levels and this underlies the direct ASL-GABA correlation. This would provide support for blood velocity, likely at the arteriolar level, being correlated with basal GABA concentration. Alternatively, the positive correlation between ASL and GABA could be driven by CBF. Thus, the inverse correlation between BOLD

and baseline GABA is likely due to a positive correlation between $CMRO_2$ reactivity and GABA. This hypothesis is consistent with recent suggestions that energy supply in GABAergic neurons arises predominately from increases in oxidative phosphorylation [30]. Additionally, voxels with large amounts of GABAergic neurons may require a larger increase in glutamatergic activity in response to stimulus to overcome an elevated basal state of inhibition.

In other investigations, synaptic inhibition, as similarly measured by baseline GABA concentration on MRS, has been shown to correlate inversely with the BOLD fMRI signal change in human visual cortex [103] and rat somatosensory cortex [104], and directly with negative BOLD responses in the anterior cingulate cortex [105]. These findings suggest that hemodynamic fMRI variations are linked to measurable excitation–inhibition balance and cortical network activity. Furthermore, the link between neurotransmission and fMRI responses can be probed non-invasively in vivo using MRI and MRS together. These recent findings carry great potential for investigating a variety of pharmacological applications where neurotransmitter imbalance may be addressed, as well as for a range of clinical applications in schizophrenia, epilepsy, behavior control disorders, post-stroke plasticity, and dementia-related excitotoxicity. Perfusion imaging, in conjunction with neurotransmitter quantification, may play an important role in these fields in the future.

Baseline CBF and functional connectivity

Spontaneous low-frequency BOLD signal fluctuations, in the absence of specific cognitive tasks, are increasingly being used to identify spatial regions of functional connectivity [106]. This so-called "resting-state fMRI" (rs-fMRI) approach is especially promising in clinical scenarios where inadequate patient compliance prevents the administration of many tasks or stimuli. Already, altered BOLD connectivity has successfully been observed in a variety of neurological disorders [107].

Recently, ASL has also been applied to the study of baseline brain activity. As the ASL experiment requires pair-wise subtraction with a resultant overall reduction in temporal resolution, the sampling frequency at which such experiments are performed is generally lower than in BOLD experiments. However, coherent fluctuations observed with BOLD are most

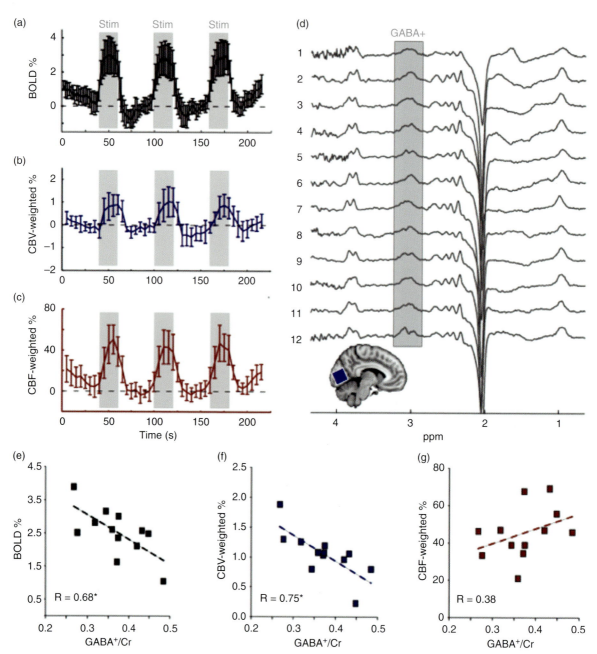

Figure 7.7 Hemodynamics and cortical inhibition. (a) Mean evoked BOLD responses in the visual cortex in response to a flashing (8 Hz) checkerboard stimulus, with error bars representing standard deviation over 12 volunteers. The hemodynamic contributions to the BOLD effect can be independently estimated with (b) CBV-weighted VASO and (c) CBF-weighted ASL fMRI. Notice the large inter-subject variation in BOLD response (2–4%) between healthy volunteers. (d) Edited spectroscopy measurements in the visual cortex of the same volunteers reveal inter-subject variations in the GABA peak at 3 ppm (gray). (e–g) The magnitude of stimulus-evoked BOLD and CBV-weighted responses correlate inversely ($p < 0.05$) with baseline GABA concentration (GABA$^+$ macromolecules normalized by creatine, Cr). Alternatively, a trend ($p > 0.05$) for a positive correlation between CBF-weighted reactivity and GABA is observed. These findings demonstrate that variations in hemodynamic responses can be partly explained by baseline GABA concentration. Adapted from Donahue *et al.* (20).

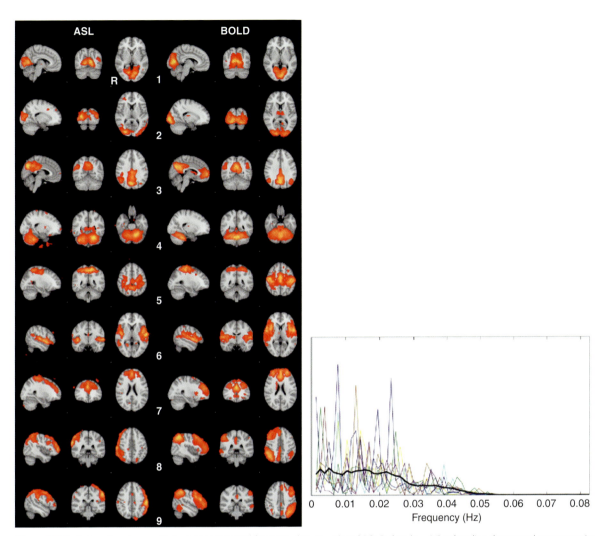

Figure 7.8 Left: Functional connectivity maps calculated from ASL data (n = 8) and BOLD data (n = 36) at baseline show good agreement in the nine (representative) networks. Right: Power spectra of the low-frequency ASL signals within the primary visual network. Each color represents a different subject. The mean of all subjects is shown in black. It is apparent from the ASL data that below 0.02 Hz, the power spectrum is relatively flat. This supports the notion that resting-state networks are broadband processes, spanning a wide range of frequencies to as low as 0.001 Hz. Adapted from Xie *et al.* (108).

frequently reported at very low frequencies (e.g., < 0.1 Hz), and thus it is in principle possible to detect much of this coherence within the Nyquist sampling requirement when using a more coarse temporal resolution of 4–8 s (0.13–0.25 Hz) as generally required by ASL.

Using a multi-slice CASL sequence with short TE and thus reduced BOLD sensitivity, in sequence with standard BOLD fMRI, a comparison between functional networks detectable by ASL and BOLD has recently been demonstrated [108]. Figure 7.8 shows nine representative networks identified in separate

ASL and BOLD experiments. As can be seen, there is good visual comparison between the modalities. However, the ASL networks are fundamentally derived from coherent CBF-weighted fluctuations, whereas the BOLD maps are derived from composite hemodynamic (CBF, CBV, $CMRO_2$) fluctuations. All hemodynamic fluctuations are frequently interpreted as being secondary to neuronal activity. Interestingly, BOLD data are particularly insensitive to very low-frequency fluctuations, owing to signal drift and hardware instabilities. However, ASL data are less sensitive to this effect owing to the subtraction

119

procedure. A view of the power spectrum of the ASL signal shows a relatively flat dependence between power and frequency in the low range of the spectrum (< 0.02 Hz), which supports the hypothesis that resting-state networks span a large range of frequencies, possibly as low as 0.001 Hz. Thus, ASL may be useful, and indeed better suited than BOLD, for probing functional connectivity in these very low-frequency regimes.

Additional studies have also been conducted that exploit ASL to better understand resting networks. A considerable emphasis of this work is on understanding the so-called "default mode network" (DMN) [109], which contains regions of prefrontal, anterior and posterior cingulate, lateral parietal, and inferior/middle temporal gyri; cerebellar areas; and thalamic nuclei. The DMN has been observed to be characterized by coherent oscillations at a rate < 0.1 Hz, and is hypothesized to be involved in task-independent activity and self-referential thought, and is known to reduce in coherence upon activation of various task-specific networks. Clinically, the DMN coherence has been shown to be altered in a variety of disorders, including autism, schizophrenia, and Alzheimer's disease [110–112]. In a study of individuals genetically predisposed for Alzheimer's disease, functional connectivity within the DMN was found to be altered decades (third and fourth decade of life) before clinical symptoms would be expected to manifest [112]. Therefore, DMN research is gaining momentum as a promising avenue for brain research; however, the precise role of this network, and its deviation in disease, remain incompletely understood.

Using ASL, it was observed that CBF-weighted images acquired at baseline show significantly higher CBF in the posterior cingulate cortex, thalamus, insula/superior temporal gyrus, and medial prefrontal cortex compared with other regions of the brain [113]. Furthermore, increased synchrony was observed between these brain regions, suggesting again that ASL may be useful for functional connectivity studies. Using ASL in conjunction with interleaved periods of baseline and memory encoding, deactivation patterns within the DMN have been observed during periods of memory encoding [114].

Thus, ASL has been applied, although somewhat sparsely, to study functional connectivity. Additionally, the majority of baseline ASL studies merely quantify baseline perfusion (an important parameter in its own right), and do not generally focus on CBF connectivity. Perhaps one of the main reasons that BOLD functional connectivity has taken precedence to date over ASL functional connectivity studies pertains to the historically poorer volume coverage with ASL relative to BOLD, which precludes the ability in many cases to assess functional connectivity in different brain regions. Additionally, the subtraction approach required in ASL, while preserving low-frequency information, essentially degrades the temporal resolution of the experiment by a factor of two. Therefore, as the data are more sparsely sampled in ASL (4–8 s compared with 2–3 s for BOLD), the frequencies that one can reliably detect are downshifted. However, given the initial demonstrations that ASL can be used to detect functional connectivity, together with the increased volume coverage available with ASL, it is likely that ASL approaches will become more heavily used to study functional connectivity patterns.

Conclusions

In conclusion, MR measurements of cerebral perfusion can be performed non-invasively using ASL, and such measurements are being used in an increasing number of clinical, neuroscience, and pharmacological applications to better understand brain function. Since the requirement for exogenous contrast agents is eliminated, ASL is a good candidate for longitudinal and clinical studies of perfusion, though control for potential global CBF confounders, particularly caffeine consumption, is critical to the success of such endeavors. In terms of neuroscience applications, the composite BOLD effect, which is most frequently exploited in functional neuroimaging studies, has a complex dependence on changes in CBF, CBV, and $CMRO_2$, and therefore independent measures of CBF are useful in identifying the hemodynamic source of BOLD modulations. In pharmacological fMRI, where assessments of drug efficacy and changes in brain state are desired over hours or days, CBF measurements may be preferable, owing to good stability and quantitative capability (when correctly normalized and modeled). Increases in magnetic field strength and related technical advances in ASL approaches are continuing to improve the quality of ASL data and corresponding CBF measurements, and both clinical and basic neuroscience applications of ASL are likely to continue to increase in the future.

References

1. Attwell D, Iadecola C. The neural basis of functional brain imaging signals. *Trends Neurosci* 2002;**25**(12):621–5.

2. Logothetis NK. The neural basis of the blood-oxygen-level-dependent functional magnetic resonance imaging signal. *Philos Trans R Soc Lond B Biol Sci* 2002;**357**(1424):1003–37.

3. Gjedde A. Brain energy metabolism and the physiological basis of the haemodynamic response. In: Jezzard P, Matthews PM, Smiths SM, editors. *Functional MRI: An Introduction to Methods*. New York: Oxford University Press, 2001; 37–65.

4. Ogawa S, Lee TM, Kay AR, Tank DW. Brain magnetic resonance imaging with contrast dependent on blood oxygenation. *Proc Natl Acad Sci U S A* 1990;**87**(24): 9868–72.

5. Iadecola C. Neurovascular regulation in the normal brain and in Alzheimer's disease. *Nat Rev Neurosci* 2004;**5**(5):347–60.

6. Powers WJ, Grubb RL, Jr., Darriet D, Raichle ME. Cerebral blood flow and cerebral metabolic rate of oxygen requirements for cerebral function and viability in humans. *J Cereb Blood Flow Metab* 1985;**5**(4):600–8.

7. Raichle ME, Martin WR, Herscovitch P, Mintun MA, Markham J. Brain blood flow measured with intravenous H2 (15)O. II. Implementation and validation. *J Nucl Med* 1983;**24**(9):790–8.

8. Wintermark M, Sesay M, Barbier E, *et al.* Comparative overview of brain perfusion imaging techniques. *J Neuroradiol* 2005;**32**(5):294–314.

9. Kuo PH, Kanal E, Abu-Alfa AK, Cowper SE. Gadolinium-based MR contrast agents and nephrogenic systemic fibrosis. *Radiology* 2007;**242**(3):647–9.

10. Huang B, Law MW, Khong PL. Whole-body PET/CT scanning: estimation of radiation dose and cancer risk. *Radiology* 2009; **251**(1):166–74.

11. Williams DS, Detre JA, Leigh JS, Koretsky AP. Magnetic resonance imaging of perfusion using spin inversion of arterial water. *Proc Natl Acad Sci U S A* 1992;**89**(1): 212–16.

12. Lu H, Clingman C, Golay X, van Zijl PC. Determining the longitudinal relaxation time (T1) of blood at 3.0 Tesla. *Magn Reson Med* 2004;**52**(3):679–82.

13. Donahue MJ, Lu H, Jones CK, Pekar JJ, van Zijl PC. An account of the discrepancy between MRI and PET cerebral blood flow measures. A high-field MRI investigation. *NMR Biomed* 2006;**19**(8):1043–54.

14. Ogawa S, Tank DW, Menon R, *et al.* Intrinsic signal changes accompanying sensory stimulation: functional brain mapping with magnetic resonance imaging. *Proc Natl Acad Sci U S A* 1992;**89**(13):5951–5.

15. Kwong KK, Belliveau JW, Chesler DA, *et al.* Dynamic magnetic resonance imaging of human brain activity during primary sensory stimulation. *Proc Natl Acad Sci U S A* 1992;**89**(12):5675–9.

16. Buxton RB, Uludag K, Dubowitz DJ, Liu TT. Modeling the hemodynamic response to brain activation. *Neuroimage* 2004;**23** Suppl 1:S220–33.

17. van Zijl PC, Eleff SM, Ulatowski JA, *et al.* Quantitative assessment of blood flow, blood volume and blood oxygenation effects in functional magnetic resonance imaging. *Nat Med* 1998;**4**(2):159–67.

18. Buxton RB. The elusive initial dip. *Neuroimage* 2001;**13**(6 Pt 1):953–8.

19. Lu H, Golay X, Pekar JJ, Van Zijl PC. Sustained poststimulus elevation in cerebral oxygen utilization after vascular recovery. *J Cereb Blood Flow Metab* 2004;**24**(7):764–70.

20. Donahue MJ, Near J, Blicher JU, Jezzard P. Baseline GABA concentration and fMRI response. *Neuroimage* 2010;**53**(2):392–8.

21. Kannurpatti SS, Motes MA, Rypma B, Biswal BB. Non-neural BOLD variability in block and event-related paradigms. *Magn Reson Imaging* 2011;**29**(1):140–6.

22. Lu H, Zhao C, Ge Y, Lewis-Amezcua K. Baseline blood oxygenation modulates response amplitude: physiologic basis for intersubject variations in functional MRI signals. *Magn Reson Med* 2008;**60**(2):364–72.

23. Buxton RB, Wong EC, Frank LR. Dynamics of blood flow and oxygenation changes during brain activation: the balloon model. *Magn Reson Med* 1998;**39**(6): 855–64.

24. Donahue MJ, Blicher JU, Ostergaard L, *et al.* Cerebral blood flow, blood volume, and oxygen metabolism dynamics in human visual and motor cortex as measured by whole-brain multi-modal magnetic resonance imaging. *J Cereb Blood Flow Metab* 2009;**29**(11):1856–66.

25. Sotero RC, Trujillo-Barreto NJ. Modelling the role of excitatory and inhibitory neuronal activity in the generation of the BOLD signal. *Neuroimage* 2007;**35**(1): 149–65.

26. Chatton JY, Pellerin L, Magistretti PJ. GABA uptake into astrocytes is not associated with significant metabolic cost: implications for brain imaging of inhibitory transmission. *Proc Natl Acad Sci U S A* 2003;**100**(21): 12456–61.

27. Hyder F, Patel AB, Gjedde A, *et al.* Neuronal-glial glucose oxidation and glutamatergic-GABAergic function. *J Cereb Blood Flow Metab* 2006;**26**(7): 865–77.

28. Patel AB, de Graaf RA, Mason GF, *et al*. The contribution of GABA to glutamate/glutamine cycling and energy metabolism in the rat cortex *in vivo*. *Proc Natl Acad Sci U S A* 2005;**102**(15): 5588–93.

29. Sibson NR, Dhankhar A, Mason GF, *et al*. *In vivo* 13C NMR measurements of cerebral glutamine synthesis as evidence for glutamate-glutamine cycling. *Proc Natl Acad Sci U S A* 1997;**94**(6):2699–704.

30. Buzsaki G, Kaila K, Raichle M. Inhibition and brain work. *Neuron* 2007;**56**(5):771–83.

31. Duong TQ, Yacoub E, Adriany G, *et al*. Microvascular BOLD contribution at 4 and 7 T in the human brain: gradient-echo and spin-echo fMRI with suppression of blood effects. *Magn Reson Med* 2003;**49**(6):1019–27.

32. Donahue MJ, Hoogduin H, van Zijl PC, *et al*. Blood oxygenation level-dependent (BOLD) total and extravascular signal changes and DeltaR(2)* in human visual cortex at 1.5, 3.0 and 7.0 T. *NMR Biomed* 2011;**24**(1):25–34.

33. Wong EC, Buxton RB, Frank LR. Implementation of quantitative perfusion imaging techniques for functional brain mapping using pulsed arterial spin labeling. *NMR Biomed* 1997;**10**(4–5):237–49.

34. Chiarelli PA, Bulte DP, Wise R, Gallichan D, Jezzard P. A calibration method for quantitative BOLD fMRI based on hyperoxia. *Neuroimage* 2007;**37**(3):808–20.

35. Detre JA, Alsop DC. Perfusion magnetic resonance imaging with continuous arterial spin labeling: methods and clinical applications in the central nervous system. *Eur J Radiol* 1999;**30**(2):115–24.

36. Wu WC, Fernandez-Seara M, Detre JA, Wehrli FW, Wang J. A theoretical and experimental investigation of the tagging efficiency of pseudocontinuous arterial spin labeling. *Magn Reson Med* 2007;**58**(5):1020–7.

37. Dai W, Garcia D, de Bazelaire C, Alsop DC. Continuous flow-driven inversion for arterial spin labeling using pulsed radio frequency and gradient fields. *Magn Reson Med* 2008;**60**(6):1488–97.

38. Fernandez-Seara MA, Wang J, Wang Z, *et al*. Imaging mesial temporal lobe activation during scene encoding: comparison of fMRI using BOLD and arterial spin labeling. *Hum Brain Mapp* 2007;**28**(12):1391–400.

39. Wang J, Aguirre GK, Kimberg DY, *et al*. Arterial spin labeling perfusion fMRI with very low task frequency. *Magn Reson Med* 2003;**49**(5):796–802.

40. Lu H, Donahue MJ, van Zijl PC. Detrimental effects of BOLD signal in arterial spin labeling fMRI at high field strength. *Magn Reson Med* 2006;**56**(3):546–52.

41. Woolrich MW, Chiarelli P, Gallichan D, Perthen J, Liu TT. Bayesian inference of hemodynamic changes in functional arterial spin labeling data. *Magn Reson Med* 2006;**56**(4):891–906.

42. Gonzalez-At JB, Alsop DC, Detre JA. Cerebral perfusion and arterial transit time changes during task activation determined with continuous arterial spin labeling. *Magn Reson Med* 2000;**43**(5): 739–46.

43. Ho YC, Petersen ET, Golay X. Measuring arterial and tissue responses to functional challenges using arterial spin labeling. *Neuroimage* 2010;**49**(1):478–87.

44. Ho YC, Petersen ET, Zimine I, Golay X. Similarities and differences in arterial responses to hypercapnia and visual stimulation. *J Cereb Blood Flow Metab* 2011;**31**(2):560–71.

45. Günther M, Oshio K, Feinberg DA. Single-shot 3D imaging techniques improve arterial spin labeling perfusion measurements. *Magn Reson Med* 2005;**54**(2): 491–8.

46. Ye FQ, Frank JA, Weinberger DR, McLaughlin AC. Noise reduction in 3D perfusion imaging by attenuating the static signal in arterial spin tagging (ASSIST). *Magn Reson Med* 2000;**44**(1): 92–100.

47. Ye FQ, Berman KF, Ellmore T, *et al*. H(2)(15)O PET validation of steady-state arterial spin tagging cerebral blood flow measurements in humans. *Magn Reson Med* 2000;**44**(3):450–6.

48. Feng CM, Narayana S, Lancaster JL, *et al*. CBF changes during brain activation: fMRI vs. PET. *Neuroimage* 2004;**22**(1): 443–6.

49. Noguchi T, Kawashima M, Irie H, *et al*. Arterial spin-labeling MR imaging in moyamoya disease compared with SPECT imaging. *Eur J Radiol* 2011;**80**(3):e557–62.

50. Koziak AM, Winter J, Lee TY, Thompson RT, St Lawrence KS. Validation study of a pulsed arterial spin labeling technique by comparison to perfusion computed tomography. *Magn Reson Imaging* 2008;**26**(4):543–53.

51. Knutsson L, van Westen D, Petersen ET, *et al*. Absolute quantification of cerebral blood flow: correlation between dynamic susceptibility contrast MRI and model-free arterial spin labeling. *Magn Reson Imaging* 2010;**28**(1): 1–7.

52. He J, Devonshire IM, Mayhew JE, Papadakis NG. Simultaneous laser Doppler flowmetry and arterial spin labeling MRI for measurement of functional perfusion changes in the cortex. *Neuroimage* 2007;**34**(4):1391–404.

53. Wang DJ, Chen Y, Fernandez Seara MA, Detre JA. Potentials and challenges for arterial spin labeling (ASL) in pharmacological MRI (phMRI). *J Pharmacol Exp Ther* 2011; **337**(2):359–66.

54. Mouridsen K, Golay X; all named co-authors of the QUASAR test-retest study. The QUASAR reproducibility study, Part II: Results from a multi-center Arterial Spin Labeling test-retest study. *Neuroimage* 2010;**49**(1): 104–13.

55. Talagala SL, Ye FQ, Ledden PJ, Chesnick S. Whole-brain 3D perfusion MRI at 3.0 T using CASL with a separate labeling coil. *Magn Reson Med* 2004;**52**(1): 131–40.

56. Frahm J, Baudewig J, Kallenberg K, *et al.* The post-stimulation undershoot in BOLD fMRI of human brain is not caused by elevated cerebral blood volume. *Neuroimage* 2008;**40**(2):473–81.

57. Yacoub E, Ugurbil K, Harel N. The spatial dependence of the poststimulus undershoot as revealed by high-resolution BOLD- and CBV-weighted fMRI. *J Cereb Blood Flow Metab* 2006; **26**(5):634–44.

58. Mandeville JB, Marota JJ, Ayata C, *et al.* Evidence of a cerebrovascular postarteriole windkessel with delayed compliance. *J Cereb Blood Flow Metab* 1999;**19**(6):679–89.

59. Hillman EM, Devor A, Bouchard MB, *et al.* Depth-resolved optical imaging and microscopy of vascular compartment dynamics during somatosensory stimulation. *Neuroimage* 2007;**35**(1):89–104.

60. Fuchtemeier M, Leithner C, Offenhauser N, *et al.* Elevating intracranial pressure reverses the decrease in deoxygenated hemoglobin and abolishes the post-stimulus overshoot upon somatosensory activation in rats. *Neuroimage* 2010;**52**(2):445–54.

61. Kim T, Kim SG. Temporal dynamics and spatial specificity of arterial and venous blood volume changes during visual stimulation: implication for BOLD

quantification. *J Cereb Blood Flow Metab* 2011;**31**(5):1211–22.

62. Drew PJ, Shih AY, Kleinfeld D. Fluctuating and sensory-induced vasodynamics in rodent cortex extend arteriole capacity. *Proc Natl Acad Sci U S A* 2011; **108**(20):8473–8.

63. Tian P, Teng IC, May LD, *et al.* Cortical depth-specific microvascular dilation underlies laminar differences in blood oxygenation level-dependent functional MRI signal. *Proc Natl Acad Sci U S A* 2010;**107**(34): 15246–51.

64. Frahm J, Kruger G, Merboldt KD, Kleinschmidt A. Dynamic uncoupling and recoupling of perfusion and oxidative metabolism during focal brain activation in man. *Magn Reson Med* 1996;**35**(2):143–8.

65. Mandeville JB, Marota JJ, Kosofsky BE, *et al.* Dynamic functional imaging of relative cerebral blood volume during rat forepaw stimulation. *Magn Reson Med* 1998;**39**(4):615–24.

66. Kida I, Rothman DL, Hyder F. Dynamics of changes in blood flow, volume, and oxygenation: implications for dynamic functional magnetic resonance imaging calibration. *J Cereb Blood Flow Metab* 2007;**27**(4): 690–6.

67. Jones M, Berwick J, Johnston D, Mayhew J. Concurrent optical imaging spectroscopy and laser-Doppler flowmetry: the relationship between blood flow, oxygenation, and volume in rodent barrel cortex. *Neuroimage* 2001;**13**(6 Pt 1):1002–15.

68. Qiu D, Zaharchuk G, Christen T, Ni WW, Moseley ME. Contrast-enhanced functional blood volume imaging (CE-fBVI): enhanced sensitivity for brain activation in humans using the ultrasmall superparamagnetic iron oxide agent ferumoxytol. *Neuroimage* 2012;**62**:1726–31.

69. Tuunanen PI, Vidyasagar R, Kauppinen RA. Effects of mild hypoxic hypoxia on poststimulus undershoot of blood-oxygenation-level-dependent fMRI signal in the human visual cortex. *Magn Reson Imaging* 2006;**24**(8):993–9.

70. Schroeter ML, Kupka T, Mildner T, Uludag K, von Cramon DY. Investigating the post-stimulus undershoot of the BOLD signal–a simultaneous fMRI and fNIRS study. *Neuroimage* 2006;**30**(2):349–58.

71. Friston KJ, Mechelli A, Turner R, Price CJ. Nonlinear responses in fMRI: the Balloon model, Volterra kernels, and other hemodynamics. *Neuroimage* 2000;**12**(4):466–77.

72. Shmuel A, Augath M, Oeltermann A, Logothetis NK. Negative functional MRI response correlates with decreases in neuronal activity in monkey visual area V1. *Nat Neurosci* 2006;**9**(4): 569–77.

73. Hoge RD, Atkinson J, Gill B, *et al.* Stimulus-dependent BOLD and perfusion dynamics in human V1. *Neuroimage* 1999;**9**(6 Pt 1): 573–85.

74. Kruger G, Kleinschmidt A, Frahm J. Stimulus dependence of oxygenation-sensitive MRI responses to sustained visual activation. *NMR Biomed* 1998; **11**(2):75–9.

75. Donahue MJ, Stevens RD, de Boorder M, *et al.* Hemodynamic changes after visual stimulation and breath holding provide evidence for an uncoupling of cerebral blood flow and volume from oxygen metabolism. *J Cereb Blood Flow Metab* 2009;**29**(1): 176–85.

76. Fox PT, Raichle ME. Stimulus rate dependence of regional cerebral blood flow in human striate cortex, demonstrated by positron emission tomography. *J Neurophysiol* 1984;**51**(5): 1109–20.

77. Mintun MA, Lundstrom BN, Snyder AZ, *et al.* Blood flow and oxygen delivery to human brain during functional activity: theoretical modeling and experimental data. *Proc Natl Acad Sci U S A* 2001;**98**(12):6859–64.

78. Siesjö BK. *Brain Energy Metabolism.* Chichester (Eng.); New York: Wiley, 1978.

79. Hua J, Stevens RD, Huang AJ, Pekar JJ, van Zijl PC. Physiological origin for the BOLD poststimulus undershoot in human brain: vascular compliance versus oxygen metabolism. *J Cereb Blood Flow Metab* 2011;**31**(7): 1599–611.

80. Hua J, Qin Q, Donahue MJ, *et al.* Inflow-based vascular-space-occupancy (iVASO) MRI. *Magn Reson Med* 2011;**66**(1):40–56.

81. Huppert TJ, Hoge RD, Diamond SG, Franceschini MA, Boas DA. A temporal comparison of BOLD, ASL, and NIRS hemodynamic responses to motor stimuli in adult humans. *Neuroimage* 2006; **29**(2):368–82.

82. Uludag K, Dubowitz DJ, Yoder EJ, *et al.* Coupling of cerebral blood flow and oxygen consumption during physiological activation and deactivation measured with fMRI. *Neuroimage* 2004;**23**(1): 148–55.

83. Griffeth VE, Perthen JE, Buxton RB. Prospects for quantitative fMRI: investigating the effects of caffeine on baseline oxygen metabolism and the response to a visual stimulus in humans. *Neuroimage* 2011;**57**(3):809–16.

84. Griffeth VE, Perthen AB, Buxton RB. Quantitative combined ASL/BOLD imaging: implications for the interpretation of the BOLD post-stimulus undershoot. *Proc Intl Soc Magn Reson Med*, Honolulu, Hawai'i, USA, 2009.

85. Rossini PM, Altamura C, Ferretti A, *et al.* Does cerebrovascular disease affect the coupling between neuronal activity and local haemodynamics? *Brain* 2004;**127**(Pt 1):99–110.

86. Iannetti GD, Wise RG. BOLD functional MRI in disease and pharmacological studies: room for improvement? *Magn Reson Imaging* 2007;**25**(6):978–88.

87. MacIntosh BJ, Pattinson KT, Gallichan D, *et al.* Measuring the effects of remifentanil on cerebral blood flow and arterial arrival time using 3D GRASE MRI with pulsed arterial spin labelling. *J Cereb Blood Flow Metab* 2008;**28**(8):1514–22.

88. Kofke WA, Blissitt PA, Rao H, *et al.* Remifentanil-induced cerebral blood flow effects in normal humans: dose and ApoE genotype. *Anesth Analg* 2007;**105**(1):167–75.

89. Davis TL, Kwong KK, Weisskoff RM, Rosen BR. Calibrated functional MRI: mapping the dynamics of oxidative metabolism. *Proc Natl Acad Sci U S A* 1998;**95**(4):1834–9.

90. Chen Y, Parrish TB. Caffeine's effects on cerebrovascular reactivity and coupling between cerebral blood flow and oxygen metabolism. *Neuroimage* 2009;**44**(3):647–52.

91. Chen Y, Parrish TB. Caffeine dose effect on activation-induced BOLD and CBF responses. *Neuroimage* 2009;**46**(3):577–83.

92. St Lawrence KS, Ye FQ, Lewis BK, Frank JA, McLaughlin AC. Measuring the effects of indomethacin on changes in cerebral oxidative metabolism and cerebral blood flow during sensorimotor activation. *Magn Reson Med* 2003;**50**(1):99–106.

93. Uludag K, Buxton RB. Measuring the effects of indomethacin on changes in cerebral oxidative metabolism and cerebral blood flow during sensorimotor activation. *Magn Reson Med* 2004;**51**(5): 1088–9; author reply 1090.

94. Bokkers RP, van Osch MJ, van der Worp HB, *et al.* Symptomatic carotid artery stenosis: impairment of cerebral autoregulation measured at the brain tissue level with arterial spin-labeling MR imaging. *Radiology* 2010;**256**(1):201–8.

95. Last D, Alsop DC, Abduljalil AM, *et al.* Global and regional effects of type 2 diabetes on brain tissue volumes and cerebral vasoreactivity. *Diabetes Care* 2007;**30**(5):1193–9.

96. Zappe AC, Uludag K, Oeltermann A, Ugurbil K, Logothetis NK. The influence of moderate hypercapnia on neural activity in the anesthetized nonhuman primate. *Cereb Cortex* 2008;**18**(11):2666–73.

97. Lu H, Ge Y. Quantitative evaluation of oxygenation in venous vessels using T2-relaxation-under-spin-tagging MRI. *Magn Reson Med* 2008;**60**(2):357–63.

98. Lu H, Yezhuvath US, Xiao G. Improving fMRI sensitivity by normalization of basal physiologic state. *Hum Brain Mapp* 2010;**31**(1):80–7.

99. Mescher M, Merkle H, Kirsch J, Garwood M, Gruetter R. Simultaneous *in vivo* spectral editing and water suppression. *NMR Biomed* 1998;**11**(6):266–72.

100. Edden RA, Barker PB. Spatial effects in the detection of gamma-aminobutyric acid: improved sensitivity at high fields using inner volume saturation. *Magn Reson Med* 2007;**58**(6):1276–82.

101. Waddell KW, Avison MJ, Joers JM, Gore JC. A practical guide to robust detection of GABA in human brain by J-difference spectroscopy at 3 T using a standard volume coil. *Magn Reson Imaging* 2007;**25**(7): 1032–8.

102. Waddell KW, Zanjanipour P, Pradhan S, *et al.* Anterior

cingulate and cerebellar GABA and Glu correlations measured by (1)H J-difference spectroscopy. *Magn Reson Imaging* 2011; **29**(1):19–24.

103. Muthukumaraswamy SD, Edden RA, Jones DK, Swettenham JB, Singh KD. Resting GABA concentration predicts peak gamma frequency and fMRI amplitude in response to visual stimulation in humans. *Proc Natl Acad Sci U S A* 2009;**106**(20): 8356–61.

104. Chen Z, Silva AC, Yang J, Shen J. Elevated endogenous GABA level correlates with decreased fMRI signals in the rat brain during acute inhibition of GABA transaminase. *J Neurosci Res* 2005;**79**(3):383–91.

105. Northoff G, Walter M, Schulte RF, *et al.* GABA concentrations in the human anterior cingulate cortex predict negative BOLD responses in fMRI. *Nat Neurosci* 2007; **10**(12):1515–17.

106. Fox MD, Raichle ME. Spontaneous fluctuations in brain activity observed with functional magnetic resonance imaging. *Nat Rev Neurosci* 2007;**8**(9):700–11.

107. He BJ, Shulman GL, Snyder AZ, Corbetta M. The role of impaired neuronal communication in neurological disorders. *Curr Opin Neurol* 2007;**20**(6):655–60.

108. Xie J, Jezzard P, Li L, *et al.* Identification of resting state networks using whole-brain CASL. *Proc Intl Soc Mag Reson Med*, Stockholm, Sweden, 2010;3424.

109. Raichle ME, MacLeod AM, Snyder AZ, *et al.* A default mode of brain function. *Proc Natl Acad Sci U S A* 2001;**98**(2):676–82.

110. Garrity AG, Pearlson GD, McKiernan K, *et al.* Aberrant "default mode" functional

connectivity in schizophrenia. *Am J Psychiatry* 2007;**164**(3):450–7.

111. Assaf M, Jagannathan K, Calhoun VD, *et al.* Abnormal functional connectivity of default mode sub-networks in autism spectrum disorder patients. *Neuroimage* 2010;**53**(1):247–56.

112. Greicius MD, Srivastava G, Reiss AL, Menon V. Default-mode network activity distinguishes Alzheimer's disease from healthy aging: evidence from functional MRI. *Proc Natl Acad Sci U S A* 2004;**101**(13):4637–42.

113. Zou Q, Wu CW, Stein EA, Zang Y, Yang Y. Static and dynamic characteristics of cerebral blood flow during the resting state. *Neuroimage* 2009;**48**(3):515–24.

114. Pfefferbaum A, Chanraud S, Pitel AL, *et al.* Cerebral blood flow in posterior cortical nodes of the default mode network decreases with task engagement but remains higher than in most brain regions. *Cereb Cortex* 2011;**21**(1):233–44.

115. Liu P, Aslan S, Li X, *et al.* Perfusion deficit to cholinergic challenge in veterans with Gulf War Illness. *Neurotoxicology* 2011;**32**(2):242–6.

116. Bokkers RP, Bremmer JP, van Berckel BN, *et al.* Arterial spin labeling perfusion MRI at multiple delay times: a correlative study with H(2)(15)O positron emission tomography in patients with symptomatic carotid artery occlusion. *J Cereb Blood Flow Metab* 2010;**30**(1):222–9.

117. Qiu M, Paul Maguire R, Arora J, *et al.* Arterial transit time effects in pulsed arterial spin labeling CBF mapping: insight from a PET and MR study in normal human subject. *Magn Reson Med* 2010; **63**(2): 374–84.

118. Wissmeyer M, Altrichter S, Pereira VM, *et al.* Arterial

spin-labeling MRI perfusion in tuberous sclerosis: correlation with PET. *J Neuroradiol* 2010; **37**(2):127–30.

119. Xu G, Rowley HA, Wu G, *et al.* Reliability and precision of pseudo-continuous arterial spin labeling perfusion MRI on 3.0 T and comparison with ^{15}O-water PET in elderly subjects at risk for Alzheimer's disease. *NMR Biomed* 2010;**23**(3): 286–93.

120. Lüdemann L, Warmuth C, Plotkin M, *et al.* Brain tumor perfusion: comparison of dynamic contrast enhanced magnetic resonance imaging using T1, T2, and T2* contrast, pulsed arterial spin labeling, and H2(15)O positron emission tomography. *Eur J Radiol* 2009;**70**(3):465–74.

121. Chen JJ, Wieckowska M, Meyer E, Pike GB. Cerebral blood flow measurement using fMRI and PET: a cross-validation study. *Int J Biomed Imaging* 2008;**2008**: 516359.

122. Kimura H, Kado H, Koshimoto Y, *et al.* Multislice continuous arterial spin-labeled perfusion MRI in patients with chronic occlusive cerebrovascular disease: a correlative study with CO_2 PET validation. *J Magn Reson Imaging* 2005;**22**(2):189–98.

123. Newberg AB, Wang J, Rao H, *et al.* Concurrent CBF and CMRGlc changes during human brain activation by combined fMRI-PET scanning. *Neuroimage* 2005;**28**(2):500–6.

124. Liu HL, Kochunov P, Hou J, *et al.* Perfusion-weighted imaging of interictal hypoperfusion in temporal lobe epilepsy using FAIR-HASTE: comparison with H(2)(15)O PET measurements. *Magn Reson Med* 2001;**45**(3): 431–5.

Chapter

8

MR perfusion imaging in neurovascular disease

Greg Zaharchuk

Key points

- Perfusion abnormalities are the underlying cause of symptoms in primary neurovascular diseases.
- Knowledge of the tissue perfusion status can improve the characterization and treatment of stroke and vasospasm.
- Perfusion deficits in patients with reversible neurological deficits can help distinguish vascular transient ischemic attack from non-vascular mimics.
- Perfusion imaging can determine the severity of chronic cerebrovascular disease such as carotid occlusion and Moyamoya disease.
- The sensitivity to detect small arteriovenous malformations (AVMs) and dural arteriovenous fistulas can be improved by looking for venous ASL signal.
- Visualization of bilateral ASL signal dropout in the vascular borderzones may point to the presence of low cardiac output or small vessel disease.

Introduction: Clinical background: what are the diagnostic issues?

A wide variety of vascular diseases can affect the central nervous system. These include acute ischemic stroke, the third most common cause of death in the developed world. The key diagnostic question for acute stroke patients is to determine whether they will benefit from therapies aimed at vessel recanalization and tissue reperfusion [1]. Intravenous (IV) tissue plasminogen activator (tPA) is the only US Food and Drug Administration (FDA)-approved treatment

for acute stroke, but must be administered within the 3–4.5-hr time period. However, most stroke victims miss this window or do not have a clearly defined time of onset. In this large group of patients, the presence of a significant mismatch between the volume of under-perfused but not yet infarcted tissue identified by MR imaging may identify patients who may still benefit from tPA [2, 3]. This so-called "diffusion-perfusion mismatch" approach is the dominant paradigm for stroke imaging. Of paramount importance for acute stroke triage is a short MR protocol and near-immediate post-processing such that information regarding large vessel status, ischemic damage, and tissue perfusion is available within minutes [4].

Transient ischemic attack (TIA) is known to be a precursor to subsequent stroke in 5–10% of patients. Since patients are asymptomatic at the time of evaluation, it can be difficult to distinguish "true" vascular TIAs from non-vascular mimics. This separation is useful to triage patients to appropriate treatments as well as to identify patients that might respond to experimental therapies in clinical trials. Unlike acute stroke, the time window for intervention is likely in the order of days rather than hours, enabling initiation of treatment strategies in a larger number of patients.

Chronic hypoperfusion states, such as those associated with carotid stenosis or Moyamoya disease, also represent a significant diagnostic challenge, particularly given the negative results of surgical bypass trials. Arteriovenous shunt lesions, such as arteriovenous malformation (AVM) and dural arteriovenous fistula (dAVF), can cause headaches, tinnitus, seizures, and intracranial hemorrhage. Large lesions are generally not difficult to diagnose with routine MRI, but diagnosis of smaller or recurrent lesions following surgery or embolization continues to be

Clinical Perfusion MRI: Techniques and Applications, ed. Peter B. Barker, Xavier Golay, and Greg Zaharchuk. Published by Cambridge University Press. © Peter B. Barker, Xavier Golay, and Greg Zaharchuk 2013.

challenging using tomographic techniques. Perfusion-based techniques might improve diagnostic accuracy, thereby refining triage to conventional catheter-based angiography. Aneurysms are common, and MR angiography (MRA) does an excellent job at identifying *de novo* lesions; however, the most common cause of morbidity and mortality following aneurysmal subarachnoid hemorrhage is vasospasm, an alteration of tissue perfusion due to reduced caliber of large feeding arteries. This chapter will address the current role of MR perfusion imaging in the diagnosis and treatment of these neurovascular diseases.

Perfusion studies in different neurovascular diseases

Acute ischemic stroke

In acute ischemic stroke, it is said that time is brain; indeed, the current guidelines for IV tPA cite a 3-hr time window from last seen normal for administration. Recent stroke trials in Europe have suggested benefit out to 4.5 hrs. Such guidelines ignore the possible impact of individual hemodynamic and tissue factors, such as the degree and duration of cerebral blood flow (CBF) reduction, the state of collateral flow, the possibility of spontaneous reperfusion, and ultimately, the amount of viable but at-risk tissue within the brain. More recently, studies have shown that it is possible to achieve high recanalization rates even outside the traditional IV tPA window using intra-arterial (IA) approaches (such as IA tPA, clot retrievers, and vacuum devices); despite this, the rates of good outcome remain low. Part of this is clearly that these patients have large vessel occlusions and are predisposed to poor outcomes. However, it has been also hypothesized that despite recanalization, there is poor tissue-level perfusion due to inflammatory changes at the small vessel level, the so-called "flow–no-reflow" phenomenon [5]. Furthermore, there is no consistent triage practice for such patients; some treat based on time windows (such as up to 6 or 9 hrs), while others propose neglecting time, instead relying on individual imaging studies to select patients. Patients with unclear or unknown time of onset, such as "wake-up" strokes, may particularly benefit from image-based triage.

Perfusion-diffusion mismatch concept

Decreased CBF is the root cause of acute stroke. The brain typically has some reserve and can maintain its normal CBF level (about 50 ml/100 g/min) despite decreases in cerebral perfusion pressure (CPP) down to about 50 mmHg in most people [6, 7]. This is known as cerebral autoregulation, which is thought to occur via arteriolar vasodilatation. However, decreased CPP below this range will result in a CBF drop.

Studies using different modalities suggest that there exist CBF thresholds for ischemia and infarction. Roughly, it appears that gray matter CBF above about 18–22 ml/100 g/min or about 40% of contralateral can be tolerated indefinitely, and this flow range has been termed benign oligemia [8, 9]. The lower CBF threshold that predicts infarction (i.e., irreversible damage) appears to be time-dependent. If sustained for 3 hrs or more, any tissue below the above-mentioned threshold appears to become infarcted; however, if reperfusion can be accomplished earlier, it appears that regions with lower CBF may yet be salvageable, with some authors suggesting that CBF in the 8–12 ml/100 g/min range (and lower) may best depict the irreversibly damaged tissue within the 0–3-hr period. This has given rise to the idea of a "penumbra" of ischemic tissue with milder CBF decreases surrounding a "core" of irreversible infarction with even lower CBF. This model also suggests that if the CBF decreases are sustained, more tissue (i.e., that with slightly higher CBF) will be progressively recruited into the irreversible core of the lesion. This is the rationale behind the "time-is-brain" mentality that surrounds acute ischemic stroke therapy.

Identifying irreversibly infarcted tissue using MRI is usually straightforward using the high signal on diffusion-weighted images (DWI). This represents reduced water diffusion signifying impaired tissue metabolism. This is a good marker of irreversible damage, provided that the apparent diffusion coefficient (ADC) falls below the level of about 550–650×10^{-6} mm^2/s. While rare examples of rapid DWI reversal immediately following reperfusion have been documented in the literature, it appears that very little of this tissue ultimately is excluded from the final infarct based on T$_2$-weighted images acquired at later time points [10]. For this reason, a thresholded ADC map appears to give a reasonable indication of the size of the infarct core. The real challenge is defining the borders of the penumbra, where the perfusion abnormality is still severe enough to result in irreversible damage if no subsequent reperfusion occurs.

Which perfusion marker best shows the penumbra?

While DWI as a marker of irreversible damage is generally accepted, multiple potential hemodynamic biomarkers for the penumbra can be obtained from MRI, the most common of which are CBF, cerebral blood volume (CBV), mean transit time (MTT), T_{max} (the time to peak of the residue function, a delay time corrected for the timing and broadening of the arterial input function [AIF]), and time to peak (TTP). Furthermore, multiple different software methods can be used, which are not all equivalent. The question naturally arises: What is the best way of defining the penumbra?

In theory, based on the above discussion of CBF, it would seem that a gray matter flow threshold of about 20 ml/100 g/min or about 40% of contralateral should provide this missing information in most patients. However, such a measurement with MRI has its problems. First, there is a 2-fold difference between gray and white matter CBF under normal conditions, making it difficult to detect small regions with CBF decreases. Also, it appears that gray and white matter may have different CBF thresholds. Next, the most common MRI perfusion method applied to stroke studies has been bolus dynamic susceptibility contrast (DSC). As discussed in earlier chapters, unless advanced methods are used, the absolute CBF values obtained are not quantitative. This limits analysis to relative (i.e., lesion to contralateral) CBF measurements. This is particularly problematic in stroke patients, because one cannot always assume that the contralateral side is normal. Arterial spin labeling (ASL) has also been applied to stroke, and it has been shown that it can depict regions of decreased CBF in most patients [11, 12]. However, ASL is prone to underestimate true CBF in ischemic and infarcted regions due to increased arterial arrival times. This leads to the risk of overestimating the size of the perfusion lesion. More recent methods, such as the bookend/quantitative CBF (qCBF) technique [13] or the combined ASL-DSC method [14], may overcome some of these limitations and enable MRI comparisons with the extensive positron emission tomography (PET) literature on CBF thresholds and ischemia. The last challenge with existing MR-based CBF measurements is the limited signal-to-noise ratio (SNR) of the measurement and the relatively narrow CBF range that is thought to separate ischemic from infarcted tissue [15].

Given the above-mentioned challenges with MR-based CBF methods, various indirect markers of reduced perfusion have been evaluated to outline the penumbra. In particular, researchers have seized upon time-based parameters, such as MTT, TTP, and T_{max}, for this purpose. Early studies suggested that MTT was a good marker, as the lesions were quite conspicuous, given that the MTTs in normal gray and white matter are similar. Many of these studies failed to use delay-insensitive post-processing and some element of arrival delay likely contaminated the results. It was found that while there might be growth of the infarction into the region of the MTT abnormality, MTT tended to overestimate the penumbra, including some tissue with benign oligemia [16].

More recent stroke studies have focused on measures of arterial arrival delay (TTP and T_{max}) [2, 3, 17]. These parameters also share the nice feature that the lesions are conspicuous due to the similarity of the delay times in gray and white matter, at least at the temporal resolution of DSC. Multi-time point ASL techniques allow the opportunity to distinguish of primary perfusion territories from borderzones, even in healthy individuals [18]. However, one potential concern is that the measurement yields no information about the brain tissue voxel itself, but is instead a measure of the time it took the blood to get there. In theory, as long as the CBF is adequate, the delay should not matter; adequate CBF provided by collaterals, for example, might show up as a lesion on TTP or T_{max} maps. In practice, however, it appears that there is a correlation between delay and reduced CBF in acute ischemic stroke. One study compared xenon computed tomography (CT) CBF measurements with MRI-based T_{max}, and found that there was a significant relationship between decreasing CBF and increasing T_{max} [19]. It was found that $T_{max} > 4$ s was a good threshold to detect CBF values below 20 ml/100 g/min, and that T_{max} performed better in this respect than MTT (using delay-insensitive processing methods). Similarly, a PET study demonstrated that T_{max} in the range of 4–6 s was optimal to detect such regions of low flow [20]. Another study used receiver operating characteristic (ROC) analysis to determine that a delay measure (TTP) had the best performance among various MRI perfusion measures to identify critically hypoperfused CBF values as identified by PET [21]. Finally, a study of ten different perfusion metrics in a retrospective group of patients with early perfusion imaging and

> 5 day follow-up [22] found that time-based measures performed well, with delay-insensitive T_{max}, and non-deconvolution-based TTP, having the highest predictive value. CBV, in particular, performed poorly in this study. Because of these considerations, and because the SNR of the delay measurements is better than the SNR of the CBF measurements, most recent image-based stroke trials have used a thresholded TTP or T_{max} map to outline the penumbra. More sophisticated models have been developed to determine "infarct probability" maps which evaluate all available MR measures (including anatomical, DWI, and perfusion-weighted imaging (PWI) measures) with a tissue outcome gold standard [23, 24]. This approach has shown utility in small studies, but has yet to be applied in a large-scale clinical trial.

What kind of post-processing should be used?

There are many potential ways to process and interpret PWI parameters. Software methodology has not yet been standardized, and different parameters are available from different software packages, which vary in terms of deconvolution methods and the level of automation. Beyond this, there remains a question of whether quantitative processing of core and penumbra size adds value over qualitative visual inspection.

The differences between AIF-based deconvolution techniques are described in Chapters 1 and 2. From a physiological standpoint, it would appear logical that delay-insensitive methods should be used if at all possible, despite the strong correlation between delay metrics and CBF in human stroke, as mentioned previously. Interestingly, in the study mentioned earlier [22], the metric in their study that performed best was the first moment of the tissue concentration curve, which is a metric that does not require deconvolution. The authors hypothesize that the reason for this is that it is a "composite" measure that includes elements of delay and reduced CBF in a complex fashion. Ultimately, this question will have to be answered by large prospective clinical trials.

It should be noted that while automated methods for identifying perfusion defects are becoming more common [4], they are not yet perfect [25]. For this reason, if an automated algorithm for the assessment of perfusion volume deficits is used, it remains important to observe the spatial location of the at-risk tissue to be sure that it makes physiological sense and corresponds with the expected clinical deficits. The need for this step has led some to advocate visual inspection of PWI maps rather than automated volumes to determine mismatch status. While expert readers in academic medical centers may be able to use this approach consistently, it is ultimately arbitrary, and does not yield an approach that can be implemented across a broad range of care levels, where experience with PWI may be more limited.

Basics of using PWI-DWI mismatch to triage acute stroke patients

The basic idea is that reperfusion will be efficacious in patients who have a large difference in the size between their perfusion and diffusion lesions, and that this represents hypoperfused tissue that has not yet become irreversibly infarcted (based on DWI). Beyond the compelling physiological evidence, it has been noted that patients with small initial DWI lesions and larger PWI lesions who do not reperfuse tend to have growth of the DWI lesion into the PWI region.

A flow chart (Figure 8.1) may be used to classify acute stroke patients into those in whom reperfusion therapies, particularly IV or IA tPA, are either not indicated, likely to harm, likely to not impact patient outcome, or likely to improve the chances of a good outcome. This chart describes a reasonable triage pattern for patients outside of the standard tPA window of 3–4.5 hrs. Finally, it is possible in some circumstances to consider IA mechanical clot retraction therapies, such as stent retrievers, in patients with coexisting intracranial hemorrhage (ICH). In addition to imaging criteria, any other contraindications to thrombolytic therapy need to be taken into account as well. A rapid protocol for acute stroke imaging at both 1.5 T and 3 T is provided at the end of this section.

Figure 8.2 shows an example of an 88-year-old woman with acute onset of aphasia and right-sided weakness, and an NIH stroke scale (NIHSS) of 22. She received IV tPA, but had no clinical improvement after 1 hr. An MRI was obtained, and demonstrated a left M1 middle cerebral artery (MCA) occlusion and a mismatch based on DWI and PWI. Based on these findings, she was taken to IA therapy, where she had her clot removed using the MERCI clot retriever, with restoration of anterograde flow and perfusion. The patient demonstrated significant clinical improvement following the procedure. A follow-up MRI study 5 days later demonstrated only a small region of infarct in the left basal ganglia, with sparing of most of the cortex.

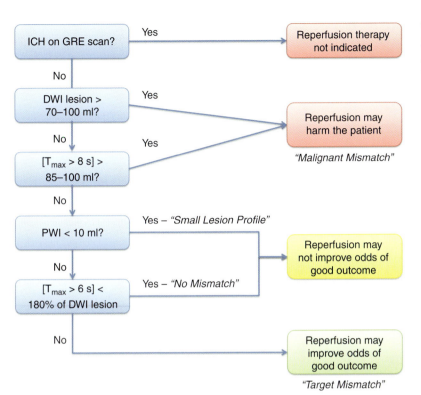

Figure 8.1 Flow chart to classify patients using MR perfusion imaging. This is usually most applicable beyond the 3–4.5-hr time period, since before this, most patients will receive IV tPA as long as they do not show evidence of ICH.

A contrary example is shown in Figure 8.3. This 53-year-old man experienced fluctuating symptoms of aphasia, with an NIHSS of 8, and arrived too late to be treated with IV tPA. MR imaging demonstrated a left internal carotid artery (ICA) occlusion and a target mismatch based on DWI-PWI analysis within the left MCA territory. Given the left ICA occlusion, it was decided to administer IA tPA to the left MCA via the right circulation, which failed. There was no recanalization or reperfusion on follow-up imaging, and the DWI lesion increased in size from 33 ml to 94 ml on follow-up imaging.

A further example shows that not all mismatches respond to successful reperfusion therapy. Figure 8.4 shows images from a 70-year-old woman with left-sided weakness and sensory deficits compatible with a right MCA stroke, with an NIHSS of 22. She received IV tPA at 3.5 hrs, but had a persistent clinical deficit and right M1 occlusion. She had a relatively small DWI lesion (52 ml), but a large region of severe T_{max} > 8 s (91 ml), compatible with a malignant mismatch. She was sent to the catheterization laboratory, where partial recanalization of the right M1 segment of the

MCA was achieved, with a reduction in the volume of severely under-perfused tissue. Despite this, she had no clinical improvement and her infarct grew in size to involve the entire territory of the perfusion abnormality on follow-up imaging. Additionally, she developed a small region of hemorrhage in the right basal ganglia.

ASL offers the potential to identify regions of abnormal perfusion without the need for IV contrast. Compared with DSC, there is relatively little experience with ASL in acute stroke. Even if ASL is performed, acquiring DSC perfusion images is recommended if possible, since these methodologies are often complementary, as exemplified in the following two cases shown. Of particular concern is that ASL may overestimate the size of a CBF deficit in a patient with a large region of delayed (but otherwise adequate) flow. Such a situation is usually evident by comparing ASL with CBF and T_{max} maps obtained from DSC. Figure 8.5 shows a 74-year-old man who was imaged 6 hrs following right eye deviation, left facial droop, and dysarthria. This patient had a right M1 occlusion and large perfusion deficit by T_{max}.

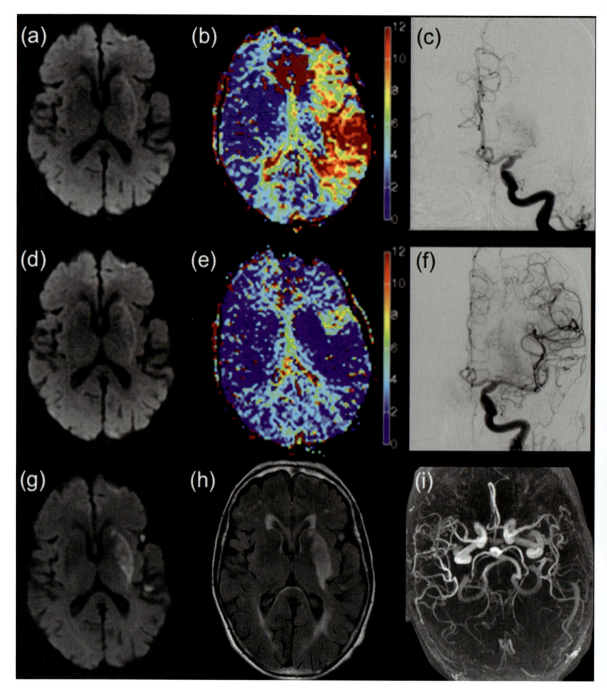

Figure 8.2 An 88-year-old woman with aphasia and right-sided weakness (NIHSS 22), post IV tPA with no improvement in symptoms. Initial (a) DWI and (b) DSC T_{max} demonstrated a PWI-DWI target mismatch. She was taken for emergent angiography and IA therapy, which confirmed occlusion of the M1 segment of the left MCA (c). The clot was removed using the MERCI clot retriever, with restoration of anterograde flow and perfusion (f). Immediately following the procedure, the patient demonstrated significant clinical improvement. MRI 2 hrs later (d, e) confirmed reperfusion to the ischemic territory with no growth in the DWI lesion size. A follow-up MRI study 5 days later (g–i) demonstrated only a small region of infarct in the left basal ganglia, with sparing of the cortex.

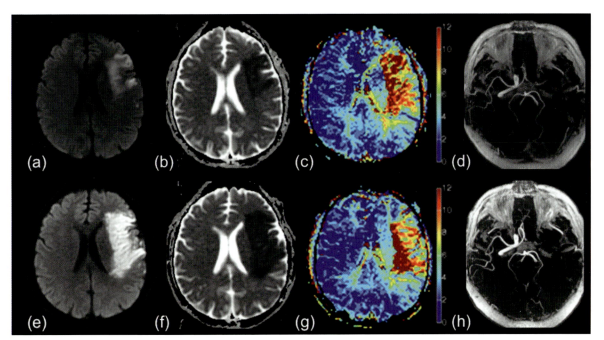

Figure 8.3 A 53-year-old man with fluctuating symptoms of aphasia (NIHSS 8), who arrived too late to be treated with IV tPA. (a) DWI and (b) ADC showed a smaller lesion when compared with the (c) DSC T_{max} lesion. (d) MRA demonstrated a left ICA occlusion. Since the left ICA was occluded, it was attempted to deliver IA tPA to the left MCA through the right circulation. However, there was no change seen on angiography. Imaging several hours later showed growth of the (e) DWI and (f) ADC lesion size into the region of persistent reduced perfusion (g). (h) MRA confirmed absence of flow in the left MCA.

Similar findings are noted on his ASL examination, where there is a large region of signal dropout. Another example is shown in Figure 8.6, which shows acute imaging in another 74-year-old man with a mild left facial droop. DWI demonstrates small regions of infarct with a much larger region of perfusion abnormality. On DSC, the majority of the perfusion lesion has a T_{max} less than 6 s, suggesting benign oligemia, and consistent with the patient's mild presentation. ASL shows a small core of reduced signal, but a great deal of arterial transit artifact, which likely represents robust collateral flow.

Several recent studies comparing ASL with PWI as the perfusion methodology for an acute stroke study demonstrated that ASL and PWI agreed frequently regarding the distinction between mismatch and no mismatch [26, 27]. When the two methods disagreed, typically the ASL would overestimate the degree of mismatch due to its dependency on arterial arrival times. Another recent ASL study demonstrated that ASL and PWI gave similar quantitative information, and, in particular, highlighted the value of ASL for detecting reperfusion hyperemia

("luxury perfusion") [28]. Finally, pseudo-continuous ASL (pCASL) was shown to be as capable of measuring different CBF levels within the core, penumbra, and normal tissues as DSC [29]. This spate of recent studies suggests that ASL perfusion imaging will likely play an important role in future stroke studies. Advantages of ASL include the absence of need to administer a contrast agent, and its relative ease of quantifying CBF values. Disadvantages of ASL compared with DSC, however, include its relative motion sensitivity (because it is inherently a subtraction technique), longer scan time, lower spatial resolution and SNR ratio. Unlike DSC, it also does not provide information on blood–brain barrier permeability, which also may be useful in evaluating acute stroke patients.

What have we learned from MR imaging-based stroke trials?

Multiple trials have either focused on the use of perfusion imaging in acute stroke or used diffusion-perfusion mismatch as an entry criterion. Most large trials completed to date evaluated the use of IV tPA, such as DEFUSE, EPITHET, DIAS, and DEDAS.

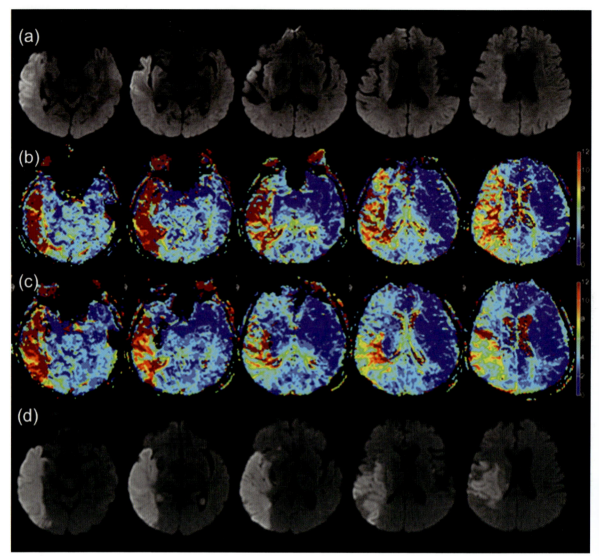

Figure 8.4 A-70 year-old woman with left-sided weakness and sensory deficits (NIHSS 22). She received IV tPA at 3.5 hrs, but had a persistent clinical deficit and right M1 occlusion. She had a relatively small (a) DWI lesion (52 ml), but a large region of severe (b) $T_{max} > 8$ s (91 ml), compatible with a malignant mismatch. She was sent to the catheterization laboratory, where they were able to achieve partial recanalization on the right M1, with a reduction in the volume of severely under-perfused tissue (c). Despite this, she had no clinical improvement and her (d) DWI lesion grew in size to involve the entire territory of the perfusion abnormality on follow-up imaging. Additionally, she developed a small region of hemorrhage in the right basal ganglia (not shown).

The DEFUSE-2 trial evaluated whether MR perfusion patterns can predict who will benefit from endovascular therapy (intra-arterial tPA and mechanical thrombectomy approaches) [30].

The DEFUSE trial examined whether DWI-PWI analysis could predict the response of patients to IV tPA in the 3–6-hr period [3]. All 74 patients received IV tPA as well as imaging at enrollment, in the 3–6-hr time period following tPA, and at 90 days.

PWI lesions were defined as $T_{max} > 2$ s, and a mismatch was defined as a PWI lesion that was 20% greater than the DWI lesion and had to have an absolute volume of 10 ml.

Using these criteria, it was found that 54% of patients had a DWI-PWI mismatch on initial imaging. Clinical outcomes were assessed not only based on the presence/absence of mismatch, but also on whether reperfusion was achieved. It was found

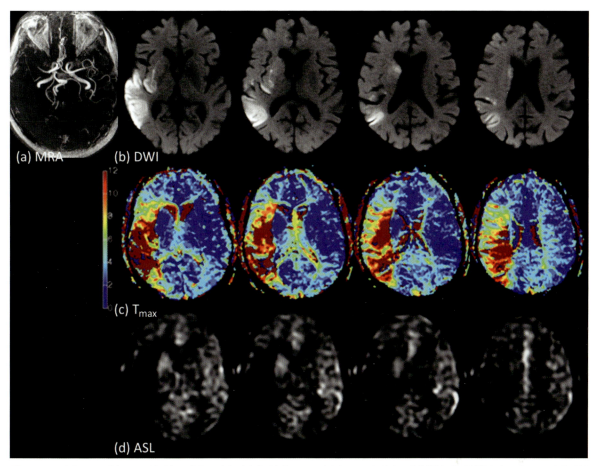

Figure 8.5 A 74-year-old man with 6 hrs of dysarthria, left facial droop, and right eye deviation (NIHSS 3–5). (a) MRA demonstates right M1 occlusion. (b) DWI shows a moderately sized region of irreversible damage in the right MCA territory. Both (c) DSC T_{max} and (d) ASL show evidence of a larger perfusion deficit. This patient received no therapy as the mild clinical findings matched the DWI rather than PWI lesion. In fact on DSC CBF imaging (not shown), the anterior portion of the lesion showed only mild CBF decrease. This case demonstrates the challenges of ASL imaging in acute stroke, which may demonstrate loss of signal in the setting of CBF decrease as well as due to prolonged arterial arrival time.

that if reperfusion occurred, patients with a mismatch were about five times more likely to have a good outcome than those without a mismatch. It was also found that very large lesions with severe imaging abnormalities (i.e., > 100 ml DWI lesion and/or > 100 ml severe PWI lesion defined as $T_{max} > 8$ s) appeared more likely to develop symptomatic ICH, and poor outcome, an imaging pattern dubbed a "malignant mismatch." Mismatch patients who did not fall into this "malignant" category were termed "target mismatch" patients. To date, this remains the only mismatch-based study to meet its prespecified endpoints. However, since all patients received tPA, the study only demonstrated that a DWI-PWI mismatch increases the odds of a good outcome if reperfusion occurs. It did not test whether patients with mismatch treated with tPA would have better outcomes than those treated with placebo, since patients can also spontaneously reperfuse. Further post-hoc analyses suggested that the relative benefit for mismatch patients was greater in those with larger percentage mismatches [31], and a trial evaluating IA tPA therapy, using a criterion of 80% or greater PWI volume compared with DWI to define the mismatch, is currently being performed.

The goal of the EPITHET trial was to determine whether IV tPA led to smaller infarct growth compared with placebo in the 3–6-hr time period [2]. Imaging of 101 patients was performed at enrollment, in the 3–5-day time period, and at 90 days.

135

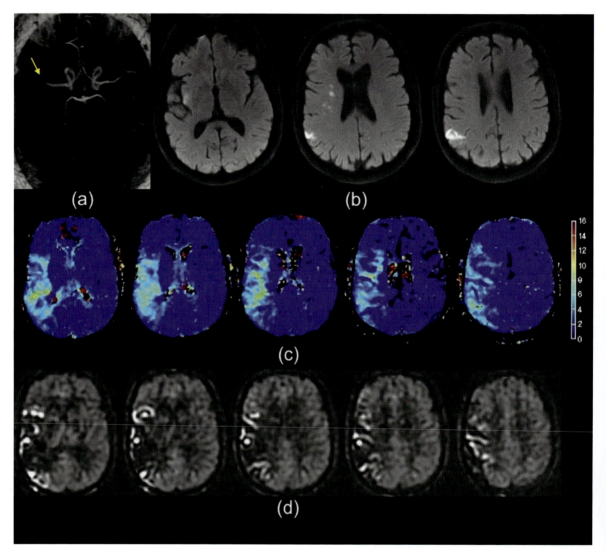

Figure 8.6 A 74-year-old man with left facial droop. (a) MRA shows a right M1 occlusion. (b) DWI demonstrates tiny acute infarcts scattered throughout the right MCA territory. (c) DSC T_{max} shows a much larger region with mild T_{max} abnormality (<6 s). This is compatible with benign oligemia rather than tissue at risk, and is consistent with the mild symptoms experienced by the patient. (d) ASL shows a small region of low signal, but a much larger region of high signal in the feeding arteries, which has been termed arterial transit artifact (ATA). In this setting, the findings are most compatible with robust collateral flow. This interpretation is supported by the lack of progression of the patient's symptoms.

The primary endpoint was to show less infarct growth between the initial and 3–5-day scans in patients who received tPA, with other endpoints that included reperfusion on the late scan as well as good functional and neurological outcome. It was found that the infarct growth was indeed less in patients who received IV tPA, by a factor of about 30–35%, but this was not statistically significant. It was found that reperfusion was more frequent in the patients who received tPA, and that reperfusion led to better neurological and

functional outcomes. Limitations of the study included lack of an early time point to assess reperfusion, a mild definition of T_{max} (≥ 2 s) as a criterion for the penumbra, and a 20% difference in size between DWI and PWI as a definition of DWI-PWI mismatch. Because of these latter factors, the overwhelming majority of the patients enrolled (86%) had a mismatch, which limited the ability to compare the mismatch and nonmismatch groups. Overall, no differences were seen in rates of good outcome between the group that received tPA and the group that received placebo. This was true for the overall cohort as well as the patients with DWI-PWI mismatch. The conclusion was that the sample size was too small to assess the primary functional endpoints, and a new larger trial with similar overall design and questions, known as EXTEND, is currently under way.

Analysis has also been performed using automated software and mismatch definitions with the combined DEFUSE and EPITHET datasets [32, 33]. One significant difference between the PWI methods used in the original studies and the combined analysis was a more stringent criterion for a perfusion lesion, namely T_{max} > 6 s, which is thought to better exclude benign oligemia; this resulted in smaller PWI lesion sizes. It was found that a target mismatch pattern was common in the 3–6-hr time period (52% of cases), and this led to better outcomes if the patient subsequently reperfused. The combined analysis found 18% of cases had malignant mismatches, and confirmed the finding of the original DEFUSE study that these patients did not benefit from reperfusion. Also, optimal thresholds for DWI and PWI lesions that defined the malignant pattern for predicting poor outcome were determined: it was found that a DWI lesion of greater than 80 ml and a T_{max} > 8 s lesion size of greater than 85 ml were the optimal thresholds, and that PWI appeared to have greater predictive accuracy than did DWI.

The recently completed DEFUSE-2 trial extended the group's prior results showing that a DWI-PWI mismatch profile could also identify patients likely to benefit from intra-arterial stroke therapy [30]. A favorable mismatch profile was defined as (1) a ratio between the volumes of T_{max} > 6 s lesion volume and the DWI lesion ≥ 1.8, with an absolute difference ≥ 15 ml; (2) DWI volume < 70 ml; and (3) volume of tissue with a severe delay in bolus arrival (T_{max} > 10 s) < 100 ml. Like in DEFUSE, patients with this pattern showed benefit from early perfusion, while those without the pattern (which included patients without a mismatch and those who already had large infarcts or very severe perfusion deficits) did not. All of these trials together suggest a central role for MR perfusion imaging in acute stroke patients.

Ultimately, large shared datasets will be required with standardized PWI acquisition, post-processing, and imaging and clinical follow-up, to help answer this question using a phenomenological approach. In particular, assessment of early reperfusion/recanalization in the immediate aftermath of treatment appears important for determining the efficacy of treatments and the potential of spontaneous reperfusion.

Challenges to the DWI-PWI mismatch model

It should be noted that the perfusion-diffusion mismatch model is not without its detractors. Some studies have shown that "penumbral" tissue appears to be more stable than one might expect based on animal experiments. For instance, one study showed that mismatches were common even after 9 hrs of proximal artery occlusion [34], and another study showed that in some patients without reperfusion the penumbra was stable over a 4-hr period [35]. This has led to the idea that regardless of time, a small DWI lesion coupled with a proximal artery occlusion on MRA will result in a mismatch pattern, and for this reason PWI does not provide additional information, and only "wastes time" before implementing treatment. Despite the fact that the penumbra as defined by MRA and PWI T_{max} appears to differ within individual patients, the use of an MRA-DWI mismatch model appears to be able to identify patients who will benefit from reperfusion, supporting this theory [36]. This most likely reflects the fact that patients with a major vessel occlusion or high-grade stenosis in the context of a sudden onset of neurological symptoms almost certainly have a fairly large area of clinically significant hypoperfusion.

Because of these types of issues, other approaches have been suggested for identifying patients who might respond favorably to reperfusion; besides the MRA-DWI mismatch, there is interest in the "good scan-occlusion" paradigm, in which a small DWI lesion (or region of CT hypointensity) is present in the face of a large vessel arterial occlusion. Such patients are likely to have a DWI-PWI mismatch, with the exception of those with chronic well-compensated vessel occlusion. Furthermore, it has been recently suggested that there may be different kinds of mismatch (e.g., target vs. malignant mismatch). Several future clinical trials that use imaging as an entry criterion, such as DIAS-3 and MR-WITNESS, will use proximal large artery occlusion or stenosis as a marker of a large at-risk territory, rather than PWI [37].

While the mismatch model is intuitively attractive, it may be too simple to explain the myriad situations that occur in human stroke. First, it is important to remember that MRI yields a snapshot of the brain at the time of imaging; stroke is a dynamic disease and hemodynamics may not be stable over time. Second, stroke is a spatially heterogeneous disease and the final determinant of patient outcome depends not only on the severity but also on the location of ischemia. Patients with large infarcts in the non-dominant hemisphere, for example, can have better quality of life following their stroke than others with smaller lesions localized to eloquent regions such as motor and language. It is possible that "atlas-based" techniques may be useful for future stroke perfusion trials [38, 39]. Finally, it is important to recognize that most large trials of the mismatch hypothesis are performed only for anterior circulation stroke, and that it is not clear whether similar methods can be applied to stroke in the posterior circulation.

Assessing recanalization versus reperfusion: the flow–no-reflow phenomenom

One striking observation from the IA mechanical thrombolysis trials is that despite very high rates of recanalization of large arteries, patient outcome was not very good [40–42]. Part of the reason for this is likely due to the fact that the initial deficits were quite severe and size of the initial DWI lesion is the best predictor of outcome regardless of therapy. However, another potential reason is that reperfusion, rather than recanalization, is the most relevant factor to salvage tissue [43]. For example, even if the large vessel is opened, distal migration of thrombus in the vascular territory of previously viable tissue may actually exacerbate ischemic severity. A more general concept of large vessel patency combined with small vessel occlusions, due to clot or inflammatory cells, has been described as the flow–no-reflow phenomenom [5]. One manifestation of this is increased AV shunting following reperfused ischemia. MR perfusion imaging may be uniquely suited to image these distinctions; ASL can identify the AV shunting while spin-echo-based DSC perfusion imaging is believed to be more heavily weighted towards vessels in the capillary range [44, 45]. Pulse sequences that combine multiple spin and gradient echoes enable evaluation of total brain hemodynamics using the gradient-echo images and hemodynamics weighted towards capillary-sized vessels using the spin-echo images [45, 47]. An example of subacute stroke demonstrating differential large and small vessel hemodynamics using multiple gradient-echo and spin-echo perfusion imaging as well as AV shunting using ASL imaging is shown in Figure 8.7.

Assessing collaterals with perfusion imaging

The idea that time is brain and that the penumbra in acute stroke shrinks with time is a dogmatic principle of the perfusion-diffusion mismatch approach to acute stroke. However, there is some evidence that the size of the penumbra does not depend on time, but rather is fixed at the time of the acute event, and largely determined by the presence and intensity of flow delivered through collateral routes [35]. Collateral blood flow is defined as that which arrives through non-anterograde pathways, such as that re-routed around the circle of Willis and via leptomeningeal (or pial) anastomoses. Many qualitative scales have been developed to grade the quality of collateral flow, most of which are based on conventional angiography [48–50]. Using such grading schemes, various small studies have suggested that the degree of collateral supply to the ischemic territory is a better predictor of outcome than even reperfusion itself [49, 51, 52].

Therefore, it would be tremendously helpful to have a non-invasive, tomographic method to assess the presence of collateral flow and quantify its amount. The challenge in this case is that the two main methods of assessing perfusion, DSC and ASL, suffer from errors in the setting of arterial arrival time delay and bolus dispersion. These problems have been extensively addressed in the setting of Moyamoya disease for bolus DSC [53], though delay invariant deconvolution methods have ameliorated this problem to some degree. One study attempted to address this issue by examining delay gradients to measure local direction (or wavefronts) of perfusion [54]. It was found that T_{max}, as determined by delay-insensitive deconvolution, was too noisy, and instead, that the normalized first moment of the contrast concentration–time curve showed the expected patterns of collateral flow from neighboring vascular territories. But delay measures alone cannot assess whether the flow to a region is adequate. A more recent abstract described the use of thresholded maps of CBF, MTT, and T_{max} to segment DSC images into regions supplied by collaterals, and showed basic correspondence between these maps and a digital subtraction angiography (DSA)-based collateral grading scale in patients with MCA occlusions [55].

Several studies have examined whether ASL could be used in a similar fashion. ASL does not typically yield information about delay times, although multi-delay

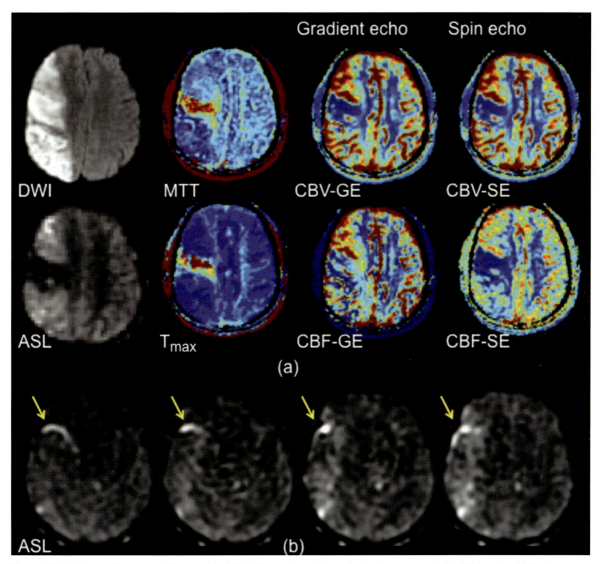

Figure 8.7 A 48-year-old woman with acute right MCA infarct with partial reperfusion demonstrated with ASL imaging. (a) Simultaneous spin- and gradient-echo (SAGE) bolus DSC perfusion was performed, yielding CBV and CBF maps corresponding to the total vascular compartment (gradient echo (GE)) and the microvascular compartment (spin echo [SE]). Note that the SNR of the SE maps is not markedly degraded compared with the GE maps. Also, the perfusion lesion on the microvascular CBF maps in the region without reperfusion appears more conspicuous, compatible with the flow–no-reflow phenomenon. (b) ASL images also showed evidence of AV shunting in this patient, with ASL signal seen in the sphenoparietal venous sinus (arrows).

and vessel-selective ASL may have some utility in this respect. One study showed that collateral scores using vessel-selective ASL agreed substantially with those determined by DSA [56]. Using a single post-label delay time (2000 ms), another study showed that identification of arterial transit artifact (ATA) and its characteristics had similarly good concordance to DSA [57]. Also, this study demonstrated that the agreement between readers for the ASL-based collateral score

was higher than that for the DSA-based score, and that higher collateral scores corresponded with increasing CBF measured using the "gold standard" of xenon CT. An example of ASL imaging to assess perfusion territory using vessel-selective ASL in a patient with stroke is shown in Figure 8.8. In this patient, it is clear that the region of the infarct in the right anterior cerebral artery (ACA) territory is perfused by blood arising from the left ICA, due to a variant in the circle of Willis.

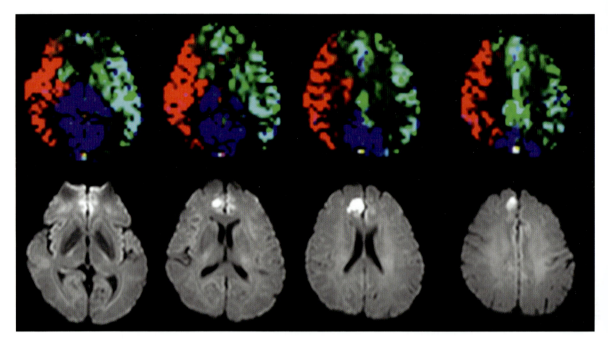

Figure 8.8 Perfusion territory ASL images and corresponding DWI images in a patient with an acute infarct of the right anterior cerebral artery perfusion territory. Colors represent the perfusion territory of the right ICA (red), left ICA (green), and the vertebrobasilar arteries (blue). Unexpectedly, the area of ischemia is within the perfusion territory of the left ICA, as in 11% of cases [109]. Note also the mixed perfusion origin in the basal ganglia of this patient, which has been shown to vary widely from one patient to the next [110].

One issue that plagues all of these approaches is that it is difficult to assess the directionality of flow (i.e., slow anterograde flow around a high-grade stenosis versus true collateral flow). However, it remains unclear whether such information is of clinical value. From a physiological viewpoint, the only important measure is CBF, which when coupled with evidence of delayed flow, suggests that non-physiological pathways are (at that moment) successful in delivering adequate flow. In this case, the highest priority is to make accurate qCBF measurements in such regions. This implies that approaches that minimize errors with delay, such as velocity-selective ASL (VS-ASL) among the ASL techniques and various quantitative DSC methods (such as the bookend approach [13] or the combined ASL-DSC approach [14]), may have utility under these circumstances. Please see Chapters 2 and 3 for a description of delay-insensitive methods existing within each of the techniques.

Other perfusion techniques in acute stroke (oxygenation, flow heterogeneity, permeability)

In acute stroke, CBF reductions have two main effects: (1) they reduce the delivery of oxygen and other substrates to the brain and (2) they reduce the ability of the

brain to remove waste products. The direct measurement of oxygenation levels in the brain tissue is an area of intense interest. Combining biophysical models with the well-known blood oxygenation level-dependent (BOLD) effect has suggested that it is possible to make quantitative measurements of oxygen saturation using MRI [58, 59]. More detail in this area is described in Chapter 5. Even the relatively simple approach of just measuring T_2^* or T_2' has been shown to be sensitive to penumbral tissue [60, 61], though the SNR of such techniques has limited their applicability in acute stroke studies. It has been suggested that images of oxygen extraction fraction may allow a more accurate assessment of the penumbra (Figure 8.9).

Other information can be extracted from DSC perfusion measurements, including flow heterogeneity [62, 63]. This is defined as the width of the residue function, and corresponds physiologically to a wider range of voxel transit times. Some theoretical data suggest that as the flow heterogeneity increases, the efficiency of extracting oxygen decreases.

Permeability to small molecules is limited in the brain by the presence of tight epithelial junctions, the so-called blood–brain barrier (BBB). Increased permeability related to the opening of the BBB under

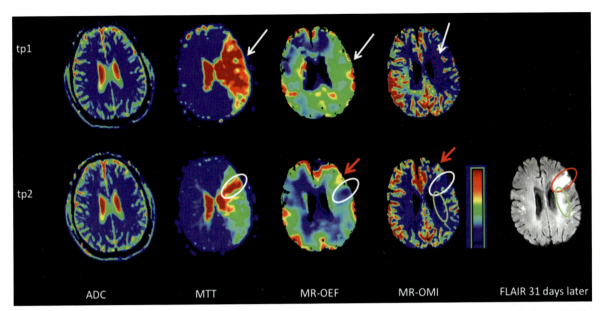

Figure 8.9 A 64-year-old man with a left MCA syndrome (NIHSS 12), treated with IV tPA within 2 hrs. Top row: 3 hrs, at which time NIHSS was 11; Bottom row: 6 hrs, at which time the NIHSS was 5. Elevated oxygen extraction fraction (OEF) was observed at the first time point consistent with region of hypoperfusion (white arrow), but the oxygen metabolic image (OMI), which is a surrogate marker of cerebral rate of oxygen metabolism ($CMRO_2$), appears confined to the subcortical region. Following tPA, the tissue perfusion status improves with normalization of OEF following 6 hrs. Nevertheless, a small region (white circles) remains severely hypoperfused, and has a low OEF and OMI, and subsequently goes on to infarction (red circle on the 31 day FLAIR image). A small region anterior to the severely hypoperfused area exhibits an elevated OEF and normal OMI (red arrows) at 6 hrs, and this tissue is not infarcted on the follow-up images. However, the subcortical region (green circles) which continues to have high OEF and low OMI does become part of the final infarct. Images courtesy of Weili Lin; Hongyu An; William Powers (University of North Carolina, Chapel Hill, USA), and Andria Ford; Katie Vo; Jin-Moo Lee (Washington University, Washington, USA).

pathological conditions is the physiological basis of contrast enhancement in the brain. Measurement of permeability, using markers such as K^{trans}, has been suggested as a method of quantifying BBB integrity, as explained in Chapter 4. In acute stroke, most work has focused on the value of permeability measurements to detect regions at risk of hemorrhagic transformation in acute stroke, usually following the administration of tPA [64]. Another clinical study suggested that qualitative evidence of BBB leakage during the recirculation phase of bolus DSC images had some utility to predict hemorrhagic transformation [65]. It is likely that measures of permeability using both methods are highly correlated with each other [66].

Transient ischemic attack

TIA is a risk factor for subsequent stroke, with 6–14% of TIA patients subsequently suffering a completed stroke within the next 90 days [67]. Half of these occur during the first week. Purely clinical scales, such as the $ABCD^2$ score, can help risk stratify patients.

Recognizing TIA allows the opportunity for interventions, both surgical (such as carotid endarterectomy) and medical (aspirin, statins, or other agents). Rapid access to these therapies has been shown to improve outcomes [68].

TIA is presumed to result most often from an embolus that causes a transient CBF decrease. This is followed by early spontaneous lysis, and the tissue is reperfused before permanent functional loss can occur. About a third of patients with classical TIA have small DWI lesions; these patients are at particularly high risk of subsequent clinically evident stroke [69]. However, such DWI-positive TIA cases are being classified differently, using the term "transient symptoms with infarct." Because of this decision, the importance of perfusion imaging in DWI-negative TIA will likely increase.

The challenge with TIA patients is that transient neurological symptoms are common, experienced by about 20% of patients over 45 years of age. Not all of these are due to vascular causes; TIA mimics include migraine, post-ictal syndromes, carpal tunnel disease, multiple sclerosis, and vasovagal reactions. Including these patients in a TIA treatment trial is suboptimal, as it exposes those without vascular symptoms to potentially deleterious interventions, and increases the number of patients needed to see an effect of intervention. Identifying a vascular or hemodynamic lesion increases the confidence in the diagnosis, particularly among non-neurologists. It has been shown that patients who were deemed to have a vascular cause of their neurological symptoms were 18 times more likely to have a stroke within the next 90 days [70].

TIA perfusion lesions are expected to be milder than those of stroke. Additionally, they may be reverting to normal or be well compensated by collateral flow. For these reasons, earlier imaging, preferably less than 24 hrs after symptom onset and ideally less than 6 hrs, is likely to be important to increase the yield of perfusion imaging. While there have been many reports of the presence of DWI lesions in TIA patients, the number of MR-based studies of vascular or perfusion abnormalities is more limited [71–75]. Only one of these studies, focusing on cine phase-contrast velocity-encoded measurements of bulk blood flow in the large cerebral arteries, failed to show abnormalities [71]. The remainder found alterations of bolus PWI hemodynamic markers, including the MTT and TTP of the contrast bolus. In these studies, PWI lesions were seen in approximately 33% of patients, with 3–16% demonstrating abnormality on PWI only. At 1.5 T, one study analyzed TTP maps in 22 patients with TIA and found 68% with either a DWI or PWI abnormality, 32% with a perfusion lesion (with or without DWI), and 14% with a perfusion lesion only [73]. Using a 3 T scanner, another study used MTT to assess perfusion [72], and found similar results: 34% with perfusion lesions, but only 3% (2/62) with isolated perfusion lesions. Part of the discrepancy may relate to field strength, but could also be related to the differences in the hemodynamic marker assessed. A prospective study performed at 1.5 T demonstrated 33% yield for perfusion imaging (again using MTT) and 16% with a perfusion lesion only [75]. Markers of arterial arrival delay such as TTP and T_{max} outline the milder deficits of TIA better than CBV and CBF [76, 77], similar as seen in acute stroke. No large studies have been performed to examine whether patients with isolated PWI lesions have an increased rate of subsequent stroke, as has been shown for DWI. It is possible that the mismatch model that has been proposed for acute ischemic

stroke may be applicable to TIA patients in a modified form [78]. An example of a PWI-DWI mismatch in a TIA patient who subsequently had a stroke one day later is shown in Figure 8.10.

More recently, ASL imaging has been applied to TIA. One study demonstrated asymmetry between hemispheres that was greater in TIA and minor stroke patients than in normals, using a multi-delay ASL sequence [79]. Another study found that abnormalities on a single post-label delay (PLD) time (2000 ms) pCASL sequence without application of vascular crushers were about twice as frequent compared with PWI, with about 50–60% sensitivity [77]. An example of increased sensitivity to mild arterial arrival delays using ASL is shown in Figure 8.11. The most common abnormality was bilateral hypoperfusion with arterial transit delay in the vascular watershed regions, a finding termed the "borderzone sign" [80]. Given that this finding is non-focal and seen in many older patients without acute ischemia, it may not reflect the presumed focal event associated with TIA, but rather reduced cardiac output, small vessel disease, and the overall vulnerability of the brain to stroke and TIA. An example of the borderzone sign in a patient with TIA is shown in Figure 8.12.

Chronic hypoperfusion and the role of surgical bypass

High-grade stenosis or occlusion of the major feeding arteries of the brain can cause focal hypoperfusion either at rest or under stressed conditions. Perfusion imaging can be useful for documenting the "tissue level" effect caused by proximal arterial lesions, which may range from mild or no effect to severe symptomatic cerebrovascular compromise. Given the overall increase in imaging, more patients are being identified with vascular lesions that cause relatively mild or no symptoms related to ischemia.

Treatments do exist for some of these lesions. Carotid endarterectomy and stenting can be used in the setting of non-occlusive carotid bifurcation disease. Direct and indirect extracranial-to-intracranial (EC-IC) bypass can be used to revascularize carotid occlusions or more distal lesions. Large studies have suggested benefits for treating carotid bifurcation disease (NASCET, CREST). However, given improvements in medical therapy, it is possible that perfusion imaging might help direct this therapy to those at highest risk of ipsilateral stroke. On the other

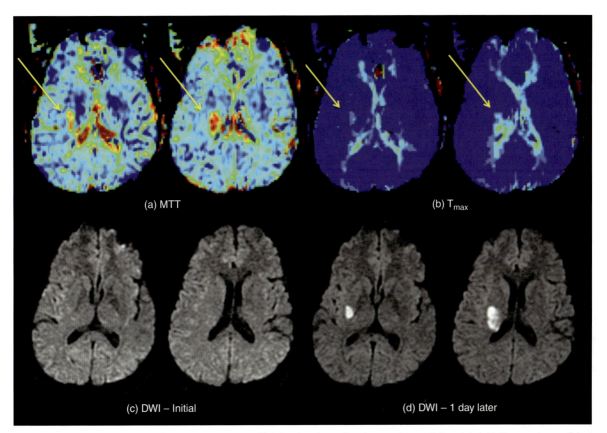

Figure 8.10 A 48-year-old man with transient symptoms of left facial weakness, hemisensory loss, and dysarthria. Initial images demonstrated prolonged (a) MTT and (b) T_{max} in a small region within the right putamen. (c) DWI was normal at this time, but a new infarct (d) corresponding to the region of the initial perfusion abnormality was seen on follow-up imaging one day later when the patient's symptoms returned. TIA patients with a PWI-DWI mismatch may be at higher risk of subsequent completed stroke.

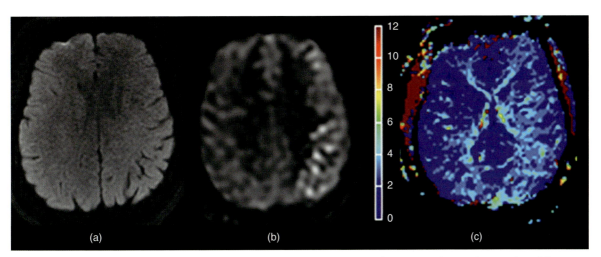

Figure 8.11 A 41-year-old woman with 1 hr of right-sided weakness, which resolved before imaging. (a) DWI does not show definite infarction. (b) ASL demonstrates a region within the left frontoparietal lobe with arterial transit artifact representing slow flow. (c) DSC T_{max} demonstrates a similar, but more subtle, prolongation. Subsequent cerebral angiogram showed 65% stenosis of the M1 segment of the left MCA. This example illustrates that ASL is more sensitive to mild perfusion alterations than DSC, due to its exquisite sensitivity to arrival time.

143

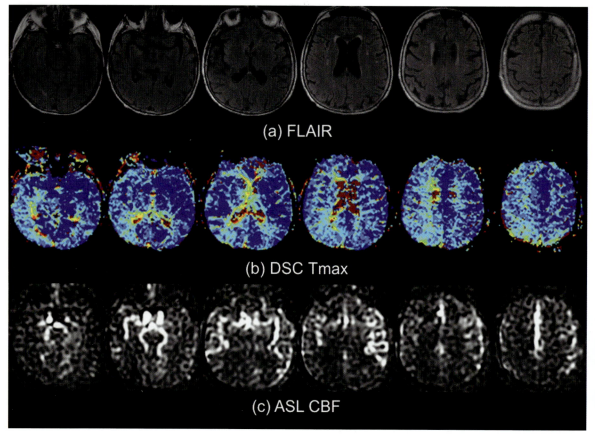

(a) FLAIR

(b) DSC Tmax

(c) ASL CBF

Figure 8.12 A 87-year-old woman with transient ataxia. (a) FLAIR images show only scattered high signal in the MCA-ACA watershed regions without DWI or MRA abnormalities (not shown). (b) DSC T_{max} images show mild, right greater than left, arterial delay. (c) ASL CBF shows very prominent vascular signal (severe bilateral borderzone sign), again right greater than left. This is likely related to a combination of reduced CBF and increased arrival time, possibly due to reduced overall cardiac output and/or small vessel disease.

hand, EC-IC bypass trials have been largely negative [81, 82]. In these patients, there has been much interest in whether perfusion imaging, including measurement of reserve and oxygenation, can improve the selection of this treatment to those most likely to benefit. To date, however, no prospective studies have used MR-based methods to triage patients to therapy.

Many patients have brain hypoperfusion that is either global or focal, but which does not cause classic DWI-positive stroke. These patients are often able to maintain adequate CBF levels through maximal vasodilatation, which should manifest itself as a focal increase on CBV maps. An example of this in a patient with Moyamoya disease is shown in Figure 8.13. Patients with maximal vasodilatation may also show impaired cerebrovascular reactivity, which is the ability to increase CBF during a vasodilator challenge, such as breath-hold, carbon dioxide (CO_2) inhalation, or acetazolamide. This inability to transiently increase

CBF under stressful conditions can lead to acute infarcts, usually in the vascular watershed regions. It is likely that a percentage of "small vessel ischemic disease," or FLAIR hyperintensities in the subcortical and periventricular regions, are actually small watershed infarcts due to the poor washout and removal of small emboli that lodge in the cerebrovascular borderzone regions.

Global hypoperfusion may be caused by poor cardiac output due to cardiomyopathy, arrhythmias such as atrial fibrillation, or systemic vasodilatation in the setting of sepsis. Focal hypoperfusion is usually a result of large vessel occlusion or high-grade stenosis, either in the great vessels or intracranially. This can be caused most often by atherosclerosis or dissection, but a small number of patients have progressive vasculopathies, such as Moyamoya disease. Moyamoya disease is a well-recognized vasculopathy of unknown etiology affecting young adults, primarily affecting

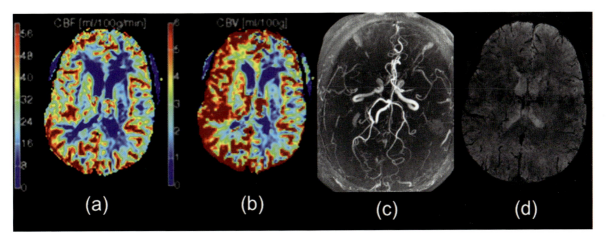

Figure 8.13 A 57-year-old man with bilateral Moyamoya disease, right worse than left. (a) DSC CBF maps demonstrate mildly reduced CBF bilaterally. (b) CBV image shows markedly increased CBV in the right hemisphere, consistent with maximal vasodilatation. (c) MRA demonstrates a similar appearance of bilateral supraclinoid ICA occlusion, but does not capture the relatively more disrupted tissue hemodynamics in the right hemisphere. (d) SWI demonstrates increased conspicuity of hypointense draining veins in the right hemisphere, compatible with increased oxygen extraction in the right hemisphere.

the carotid terminus region. It is progressive, and leads to the development of the characteristic collateral "moyamoya pattern," which resembles a puff of smoke (Moyamoya in Japanese, where the disease has a higher prevalence). These collaterals are imperfect and patients are at risk of stroke and hemorrhage. DSC perfusion imaging is known to be challenging in Moyamoya disease due to the long arterial delays and dispersion caused by proximal stenoses and the challenges in selecting an appropriate AIF [53]. In these patients, the use of delay-insensitive post-processing is important. ASL is also suboptimal, because the long delays can often result in apparent lack of flow in patients who are clinically asymptomatic. If ASL is to be used, very long PLD times (on the order of 2.5 s or greater) are recommended; despite the lower SNR associated with long PLD, one can often get a better idea of the true perfusion using these parameters. VS-ASL, which in theory eliminates the impact of arrival time, may have particular utility in these patients. An example of improved CBF visualization in a patient with Moyamoya disease using long PLD pCASL and VS-ASL is shown in Figure 8.14. Insights from Moyamoya patients are likely applicable to patients with a wide range of cerebrovascular disease.

Shunt lesions (AVMs and dAVF)

AVMs and dAVFs are characterized by an abnormal connection between the arterial and venous circulation. They can cause seizures and lead to catastrophic hemorrhages. Large AVMs are also thought to "steal" blood flow from the surrounding parenchyma. A dAVF is an abnormal connection between dural arteries and the venous system. They can be associated with debilitating symptoms, including headache and tinnitus. High risk of hemorrhage is associated with cortical venous drainage. Potential treatments for these shunt lesions include surgical resection, IA embolization, and radiation.

Large AVMs are fairly easy to diagnose with either CT or MRI, while small AVMs can be occult on all cross-sectional imaging. They can even occasionally be difficult to visualize using cerebral angiography in the acute setting due to mass effect from hemorrhage. AVMs are graded using the Spetzler-Martin criteria [83], which assign points for nidus size, eloquent location, and venous drainage. AVMs are largely graded based on cerebral angiography, although recent advances in time-resolved MRA may enable a non-invasive staging.

Bolus PWI has been applied to the study of AVMs. It is most suited to examine lesions that have not bled, since the artifacts from the presence of blood in the region of the nidus can result in a severe loss of signal due to dephasing on gradient-echo EPI images (Figure 8.15). Spin echo-based images may ameliorate these problems. One study demonstrated the feasibility of ASL imaging in seven AVM patients using continuous ASL imaging [84], and found high ASL signal in the region of the nidus and draining veins. The signal difference ΔM between the label and

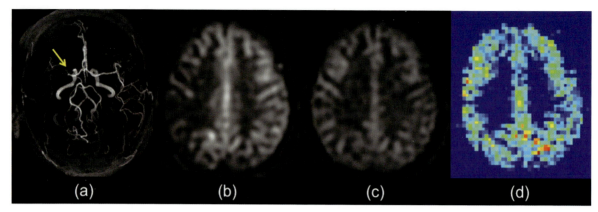

Figure 8.14 A 68-year-old woman with high-grade stenosis of the M1 segment of the right MCA as demonstrated by (a) MRA. pCASL using a labeling time of 1.5 s was performed with two different post-label delay (PLD) times. A region within the right MCA territory shows low ASL signal on (b) the early PLD (1 s) image, which fills in on (c) the long PLD (2.5 s) image. (d) VS-ASL demonstrates normal CBF in this region. Long PLD conventional pCASL or VS-ASL should be considered to improve quantitative CBF measurements in patients expected to have long arterial transit delays.

control ASL images for the nidus and draining veins as well as a whole brain average were measured, and used to calculate a shunt fraction, which ranged from 0% to 30% of total CBF. Peri-nidal steal in the neighboring white matter was not detected and, in fact, a tendency towards increased CBF with increasing shunt fraction was observed. There was a statistically significant negative correlation between ipsilateral thalamic CBF and shunt fraction, which might be related to steal. These analyses were limited due to the small number of patients.

Another study in 29 patients showed that pulsed ASL could be used to follow changes in AVM perfusion following radiosurgery [85]. It was found that the CBF in the ipsilateral vascular territory surrounding the AVM was 25–27 ml/100 g/min lower when compared with a similar region on the contralateral side, evidence of peri-nidal steal phenomenon. There was no evidence that this difference changed with treatment time, instead both ipsilateral and contralateral peri-nidal gray matter CBF increased following treatment, with no change in the ratio. More importantly, the shunt fraction (ASL signal within the shunt compared with contralateral gray matter) decreased with time following treatment. While relatively few of the patients in this study had pre-radiosurgery scans, the general conclusion was that quantitative ASL will prove to be a useful way of following response to treatment in this group, which is otherwise challenging.

It has also been shown that the information of venous signal on ASL improved the diagnostic accuracy and confidence of clinicians to determine the presence of a small AVM (< 2 cm) or dAVF, using conventional digital subtraction angiography as a gold standard test [86]. Three clinicians were asked to grade the likelihood of a shunt lesion after reviewing either just the conventional MR images, or the conventional images with the addition of the ASL, in 26 patients, 15 of who had shunt lesions. There was significant improvement in the ROC area under the curve following ASL review, indicating that this improved performance. When the readers saw venous ASL signal, they were more likely to rate the possibility of a shunt lesion higher, and because venous ASL signal had a high association with shunt lesions, it led to higher diagnostic accuracy. If confirmed in a prospective trial, such an approach may enable a more scientific basis for triaging patients with suspected vascular malformations to more invasive tests, such as conventional angiography. An example of a patient with unilateral tinnitus and normal conventional imaging is shown in Figure 8.16; in this case, a bright focus of ASL signal in the region of the petrous apex was identified, which corresponded to a small dAVF on cerebral angiography. Figure 8.17 shows another example of venous ASL signal in a patient with an intraparenchymal hemorrhage and a new high-risk dAVF with cortical venous drainage.

Aneurysms and vasospasm

While MRA can be used to identify aneurysms in a non-invasive fashion, conventional X-ray angiography remains the gold standard for this diagnosis.

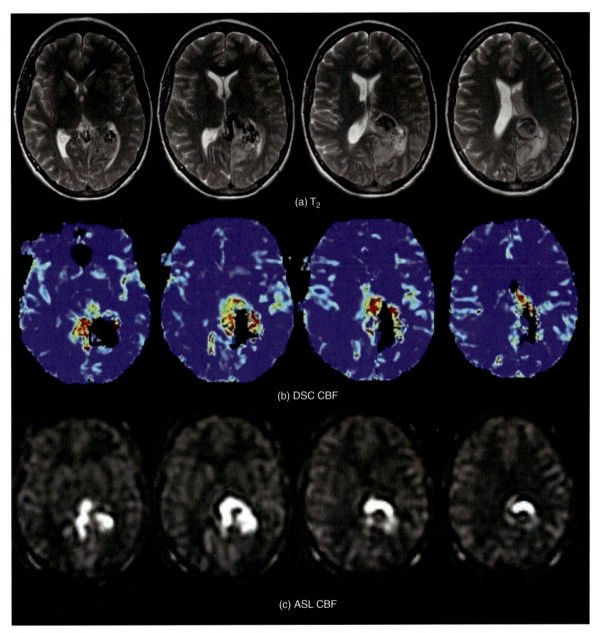

(a) T$_2$

(b) DSC CBF

(c) ASL CBF

Figure 8.15 A 49-year-old man with a large residual AVM despite recent embolization therapy. (a) T$_2$-weighted images show signal dropout in the embolization regions. (b) DSC CBF maps are marred by artifacts in the same regions due to susceptibility effects from the embolization material. (c) ASL performed using a fast-spin-echo 3D readout has minimal sensitivity to the embolization material, and depicts the high flow associated with the AVM nidus. It is possible that using spin-echo DSC techniques could mitigate the problems shown in this example.

Many patients receive brain imaging without MRA, and clinically unsuspected unruptured aneurysms may be detected based on high signal on ASL perfusion imaging (Figure 8.18). The physiological reason for the high signal seen in aneurysms in ASL is the visualization of the labeled spins due to the relative stasis of flow and recirculation within the aneurysm itself. Often, the presence of an aneurysm can be verified on T$_2$-weighted images, which will show an abnormal flow void (if large enough), or a pulsation

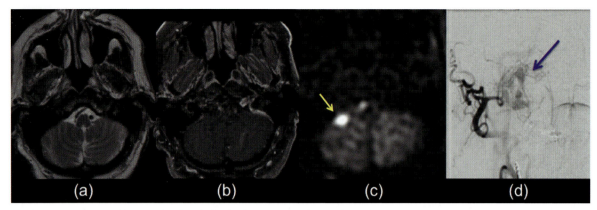

Figure 8.16 A 76-year-old man with right-sided pulsatile tinnitus. No abnormalities were seen on conventional MR imaging, such as (a) T_2-weighted and (b) T_1-weighted post-contrast images. (c) ASL demonstrates focal high signal in the region of the right petrous apex, compatible with a shunt lesion. (d) Cerebral angiography confirmed the presence of a dAVF in this region, which was treated by embolization. The patient's symptoms resolved. While not used as a perfusion technique in this case, ASL was the only MR imaging modality that identified a treatable lesion through its sensitivity to AV shunting.

artifact in the phase encode direction. Thus, ASL may have a role identifying aneurysms in patients not clinically suspected and who do not undergo MRA; also, it may offer a way to follow residual or recanalized aneurysms.

The largest source of morbidity following subarachnoid hemorrhage (SAH) due to aneurysm rupture is large artery vasospasm, which usually occurs during the first two weeks following rupture. Current methods of assessing vasospasm include clinical examination (which is often limited) and transcranial Doppler (TCD) of the intracranial arteries. TCD, in particular, is challenging and prone to many problems, such as being impossible in a significant portion of the population (about 20%) due to the lack of the so-called "acoustical temporal window" [87]. Treatment for vasospasm is also somewhat limited, but frequently will involve angiography (to confirm the diagnosis), angioplasty, or IA infusion of vasodilators, such as calcium channel blockers.

Perfusion imaging in theory permits visualization of the tissue consequences due to the narrowing of the large arteries at the base of the brain. This is relevant because angiographic evidence of vasospasm is more common than symptomatic vasospasm or DWI changes. Some of the first evidence of the utility of PWI in a series of symptomatic SAH patients demonstrated that small DWI lesions could be seen which were surrounded by larger regions with PWI lesions, particularly on MTT maps [88]. Another report suggested that PWI was more sensitive than either TCD or the clinical examination [89], and also found that

MTT and TTP were the most sensitive DSC indices for this purpose. However, this was a retrospective study which was limited by both small numbers of subjects, and the variable treatments that they received. It was suggested that a "baseline" PWI measurement at the time of SAH before the occurrence of vasospasm might be useful, to better understand the significance of changes that might occur in the setting of clinical vasospasm. A prospective study of PWI and angiography in aneurysmal SAH patients at high risk of vasospasm found a good correlation between increased cerebral circulation time (CCT), as determined from angiography, and the perfusion deficit, as measured by TTP. In particular, a significant TTP delay of 6.5 s in patients with severe vasospasm based on CCT was found, as well as watershed infarcts associated with severe vasospasm angiographically, while lacunar or territorial strokes could be additionally seen in the setting of moderate vasospasm.

More recently, an extension of the PWI-DWI mismatch model was applied to vasospasm patients [90]. The brain was divided into 19 segments for analysis, and "segments-at-risk" defined based on whether there was a PWI-DWI mismatch within the region (with a PWI lesion defined as TTP > 2 s compared with contralateral presumed normal regions). Angioplasty was primarily used as a treatment, but vasodilators were also used in some cases. A repeat MRI 48 hrs later was used to assess for possible infarction. While the study was limited in that DWI may transiently reverse during this time period, it was found that despite treatment, 37% of regions deemed

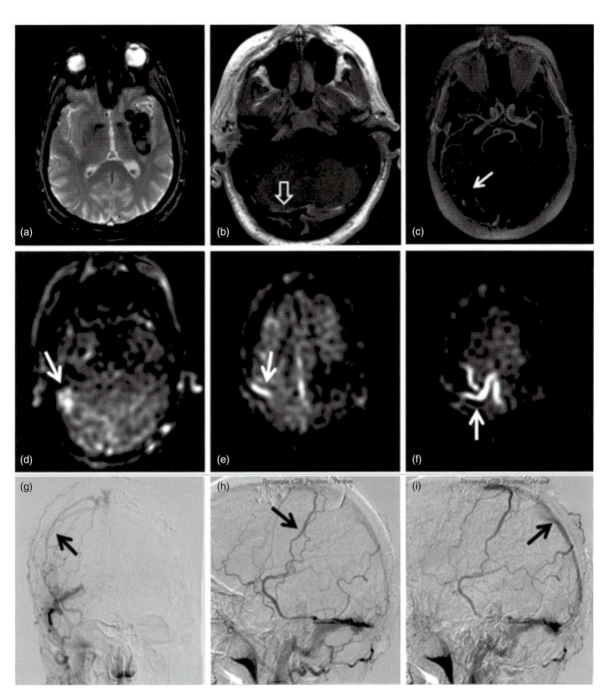

Figure 8.17 A 57-year-old man with a history of left frontoparietal AVM, status post endovascular embolization and surgical resection. He presented with new left insular hemorrhage. (a) Gradient echo image shows new left insular parenchymal hemorrhage. (b) T_1-weighted post-contrast image shows an occluded right transverse sinus with prominent perivenous enhancement (open arrow). (c) MRA shows abnormal vasculature in the right posterior fossa (arrow). (d–f) ASL images demonstrate venous shunting with high signal intensity labeled spins within the right transverse-sigmoid sinus (arrow in d) and multiple cortical veins (arrows in e and f). Findings were suspicious for presence of right transverse-sigmoid dAVF with retrograde cortical venous drainage. Frontal (g) and lateral (h, i) angiograms from the right external carotid artery injection show a right transverse-sigmoid sinus dAVF, with main arterial supplies from the right middle meningeal and right occipital arteries. The fistula drains directly into the right transverse sinus, with additional retrograde venous filling into the right veins of Labbe's and Trolard (black arrows in g and h) and superior sagittal sinus (black arrow in i).

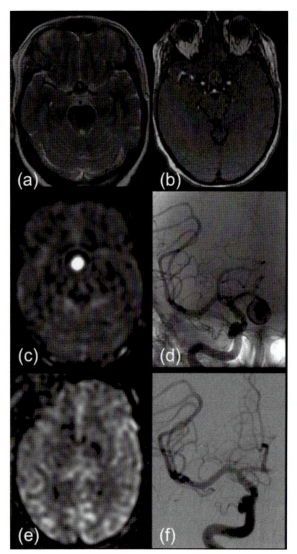

Figure 8.18 A 55-year-old woman with an unruptured anterior communicating artery aneurysm. (a) T$_2$-weighted image shows a rounded abnormality in the suprasellar cistern. (b) Source image from MRA shows only mild flow-related enhancement surrounding the rim of the mass, due presumably to the very slow flow within the aneurysm itself. (c) ASL shows a marked focal region of increased signal, compatible with labeled spins pooling within the aneurysm. (d) Cerebral angiography confirms the presence of the aneurysm. Post-operatively, (e) ASL and (f) angiography confirm the exclusion of the aneurysm by the surgical clip.

at risk went on to infarction, compared with 4% of regions without mismatch. It was also suggested that there was a lower rate of subsequent infarction in patients in whom the treatment was thought to be successful (i.e., led to increased caliber of the affected vessels at the conclusion of the procedure). To date, however, there has not been a clinical trial in which

DWI-PWI imaging has been applied in a rigorous fashion to patients with vasospasm. An example of a DWI-PWI mismatch in a patient with vasospasm is shown in Figure 8.19.

Cerebrovascular reactivity

Cerebrovascular reactivity is defined as the response of brain perfusion to a physiological challenge. As with cardiac stress testing, the goal is to visualize the ability of the brain to increase CBF; it is thought that patients with better reserve are better able to withstand temporary fluctuations in systemic blood pressure or oxygenation compared with those with poor reserve. In fact, poor reserve was used as an entry criterion for the Japanese EC-IC bypass trial (JET). This trial reported positive results with improved outcomes in bypass patients, but the main data have yet to be translated into the English-language literature [91].

Many agents have been suggested as stress agents, including balloon test occlusion, breath-hold, CO$_2$ inhalation, and acetazolamide (trade name: Diamox). Acetazolamide is a carbonic anhydrase inhibitor that causes a 30–70% CBF increase in normal animal or human brain [92, 93]. The typical dose is 1 mg (approximately 15 mg/kg) administered IV. The peak effect occurs within about 10 min and lasts for several hours. Cerebrovascular reserve measurements are typically performed 20 min after injection. While it is somewhat controversial, it has been reported that there is a high correlation between patients with poor cerebrovascular reserve (CVR) as measured by acetazolamide, and those with resting elevated OEF (e.g., as measured by PET). If so, this is important because MRI methods of measuring CBF change are less expensive and cumbersome than the use of H$_2$^{15}O-PET, and would thus be available to a large number of patients.

The two most common approaches to measure CVR using MRI are bolus PWI and ASL. An example of both perfusion-based methodologies applied in the same patient is shown in Figure 8.20. Bolus PWI has the advantage of enabling the concurrent measurement of changes in other hemodynamic variables, such as CBV, MTT, and T$_{max}$. The disadvantage of bolus PWI for this purpose is the need to administer either two doses or to split a single dose, with concomitant reduction in the SNR of each individual measurement. Also, since bolus PWI is typically

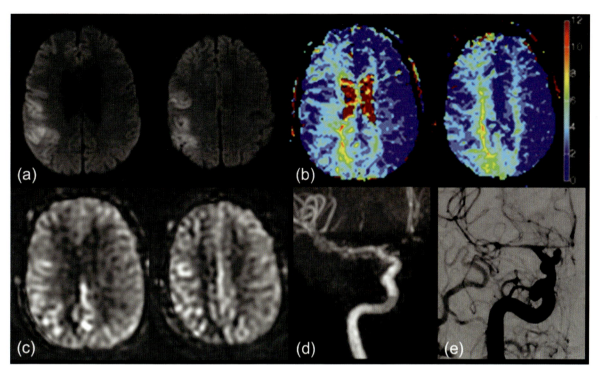

Figure 8.19 A 59-year-old woman with a ruptured right posterior communicating artery aneurysm and clinical signs of left hemiparesis. (a) DWI shows early infarct in the right MCA territory. The ACA territory has normal diffusion. (b) DSC T_{max} demonstrates increased arterial delay in the right ACA territory, worse than the right MCA territory. The band of severe delay is along the MCA-ACA borderzone. This is compatible with a PWI-DWI mismatch. (c) ASL shows similar findings of prolonged arterial delay in the right MCA and ACA territories. (d) MRA and (e) cerebral angiography show severe narrowing of the right M1 and A1 segments, consistent with vasospasm. The role of perfusion imaging is to assess the tissue consequences of proximal arterial stenosis in vasospasm.

considered a qualitative method, comparison between healthy and diseased regions is required; this obviously has its drawbacks in patients with bilateral or global disease. For example, a patient with good CVR may be indistinguishable from one with globally poor CVR. Also, if this approach is desired, it is suggested that the selection of the AIF and venous output function be the same between the two measurements, and preferably in the "normal" hemisphere if such a hemisphere exists [94].

ASL might be considered more ideal for this application, since it does not require multiple contrast administration and offers in theory a quantitative CBF measurement. However, one must be aware that both absolute arrival time and changes in arrival time following acetazolamide can lead to measurement errors. Multi-delay ASL may mitigate some of these methodological errors. However, in many patients with cerebrovascular disease, particularly those with severe stenosis or occlusion, transit delays are extremely long, far longer than can be accommodated

using multi-delay or even long PLD conventional ASL. In such patients, VS-ASL may offer an alternative, given that the labeling occurs closer to the site of imaging, which should mitigate the effects of transit delay. However, such transit time effects do exist with VS-ASL [95] as well, yet less pronounced, and to date there are little data that demonstrate the advantage of VS-ASL in patients with long transit delays [96].

MRI measurements of CVR have been performed in normal subjects and patients with carotid occlusion. One study measured CBF pre- and post-acetazolamide in 12 normal subjects on two separate occasions using a single-slice FAIR ASL method [97]. It was found that acetazolamide produced an approximately 40% increase in CBF in both gray and white matter. Importantly, both the pre-acetazolamide baseline CBF and the degree of augmentation varied in the order of 2–4% and 5–10%, respectively, meaning that the reproducibility of measurements over a period of days was satisfactory. Another study examined CVR in 14 patients with

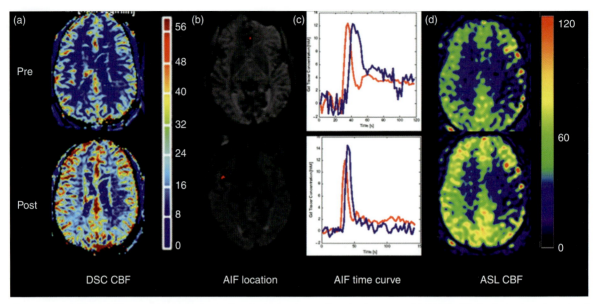

DSC CBF   AIF location   AIF time curve   ASL CBF

Figure 8.20 A 57 year-old man with repeated episodes of aphasia who was found to have a small left MCA diffusion lesion (not shown) and focal occlusion of an M2 branch of the left MCA. Acetazolamide study was requested to evaluate CVR in the affected territory. DSC was performed pre- and post- 1 g IV acetazolamide (on separate days). (a) Pre- and post-acetazolamide DSC CBF maps are shown. Overall CBF appears to increase, but to a lesser extent in the left M2 territory. (b) Automated software found different locations for the AIF during the two sessions (shown in red). (c) Perhaps because of this, the AIF concentration–time curve is different between the two acquisitions. These factors can lead to variability in DSC CBF maps of CVR. (d) ASL images at the same level demonstrate a similar CBF increase outside the affected territory, but no change in the affected M2 region. Because ASL does not require an AIF, post-processing is simplified. However, CBF assessment in the lesion is limited by possible changes in arterial arrival time.

symptomatic large vessel stenosis, and found a 35% and 37% CBF increase in the unaffected and affected hemispheres [98].

Finally, BOLD-based approaches have also been pursued, yet present the additional challenge of lack of possible quantification and need to resort to simple description of reactivity as "normal," "reduced" or "negative" CVR, as compared with normative controls [99]. In addition, because of its non-quantitative nature, BOLD CVR calculations cannot be done with baseline and stress measurements performed on separate days. This limits its ability to follow therapeutic interventions which might occur over days to months, but it can be used in a single session, for example with CO_2 manipulation or acetazolamide [100].

Other considerations: comparison with other modalities, limitations, pitfalls, etc.

Beyond the question of what parameters to use and how (and if) to determine the penumbra, one must be cognizant that there is a debate in the field as to whether CT or MRI is the best modality to evaluate acute ischemic stroke and other neurovascular diseases. Since time is important, some practioners advocate CT, which is fast, widely available, and which does not have as many contraindications as MRI. A non-contrast CT is required before treatment with tPA to exclude hemorrhagic stroke. CT angiography (CTA) has been shown to have high specificity to determine proximal arterial occlusions, which are the cause of most high-morbidity strokes. A debate surrounds the value of CT perfusion (CTP). While it yields similar hemodynamic information to that obtained with MRI, there is much debate whether CT-based methods can determine the core of an infarct, with various groups reporting different metrics [101, 102]. Other groups have advocated acute stroke MRI, which can be performed quickly (< 10 min exam times), but which requires more logistical support than CT [103]. Selection of patients for thrombolysis can be improved using acute MRI as compared with CT, probably due to the value of acute DWI to detect irreversible lesions.

More generally, diffusible tracer methods, such as $H_2^{15}O$-PET, 133-xenon single-photon emission computed tomography (SPECT), and stable xenon CT, are usually taken as gold standards for perfusion (see Chapter 1) [104]. It should be recognized that all of these techniques also make assumptions and have limited efficacy in patients with severe cerebrovascular disease. One difficulty comparing techniques is that CBF fluctuations occur based on time of day and diet, and can be in the order of 10–15% [105]. This makes it difficult to prove that an MR-based technique is any more accurate than this. Future technologies, particularly simultaneous MR-PET, are likely to be useful for the accurate validation of MR-based perfusion techniques against $H_2^{15}O$-PET, widely considered to be the "gold standard" for imaging CBF quantitatively.

Recommended protocols/analysis techniques for specific indications

The combination of bolus PWI and ASL affords a rich picture of cerebrovascular dynamics. In particular, since the artifacts of these two methodologies are different, it often helps clarify the difference between a true cerebrovascular disturbance and an artifact. Also, by combining the two methods in a straightforward manner, it is possible to improve the quantitation of CBF and CBV above and beyond that which could be accomplished by either technique alone [14]. Of course, in patients with contraindications to gadolinium contrast agents, only ASL can be used. In patients in whom one expects significant susceptibility artifacts, one should consider using spin-echo rather than gradient-echo techniques. Dual gradient-echo and spin-echo bolus DSC techniques may prove to be ideal for such indications.

In patients with a focal lesion, the technique can be optimized to focus on this region. For ASL, this might mean a limited number of slices (for 2D techniques) or more averages (for 3D techniques). For bolus DSC, this might entail fewer slices acquired at higher temporal or spatial resolution.

Protocols for rapid stroke MRI

MR imaging for acute stroke can be performed using a rapid protocol that takes less than 10 min (Figure 8.21). The exam focuses on the four "Ps": parenchyma, plumbing, perfusion, and penumbra [106]. The first sequence to acquire is isotropic DWI using a b-value of 1000 s/mm^2. ADC maps are created from

these to identify acute infarcts. It is important to remember that acute arterial infarcts are not the only cause of DWI bright lesions; particularly in the presence of lesions that cross arterial vascular territories, one must consider venous ischemia and cerebritis. An ADC threshold of around $550–650 \times 10^{-6}$ mm^2/s is specific for irreversibly damaged tissue; more mild ADC regions may still be viable. B_0 images from the DWI sequence can be used to visualize T_2-bright regions, which indicate subacute or chronic ischemia. Following this, non-contrast 3D time-of-flight MRA should be acquired, covering the intracranial circulation. If a head-and-neck vascular array coil is available, and neck imaging is desired, it can be performed with a 2D time-of-flight method.

Next, gradient-echo or "hemosiderin" images are acquired to identify hemorrhage, which is a contra-indication to tPA treatment. Gradient-echo imaging has been show to be more sensitive than CT for the identification of acute hemorrhage [107]. Often, small microhemorrhages are identified on gradient echo; it has been suggested that patients with such lesions are at higher risk of ICH following thrombolytics, although this has not been borne out in studies (including the BRASIL trial [108]), so this should not exclude patients from therapy if they are otherwise eligible.

Finally, if the patient can tolerate gadolinium, bolus DSC using gradient-echo readout should be performed. In patients who cannot receive gadolinium, which is usually due to reduced renal function, ASL perfusion images might be acquired instead. The entire protocol as shown in Figure 8.21 requires less than 10 min of scanner time, though this will be longer if neck MRA and ASL are included. A method for rapid processing of perfusion images to create maps of hemodynamic parameters, particularly time-based parameters such as MTT, TTP, and T_{max}, is essential if the perfusion images are to be interpreted in a timely fashion in order to impact decision-making. While "eyeballing" the lesion acutely has been suggested to be adequate to make treatment decisions, objective quantitative methods of measuring DWI and PWI volumes may lead to better outcomes. T_{max} in the 4–6 s region should be used to identify critically hypoperfused tissue with DSC.

Chronic ischemia and TIA protocols

There is less time urgency for most studies of chronic cerebrovascular disease. Under these circumstances, additional imaging sequences can be added to the

Sequence	Parameters	Time	Comments
Scouts	3-plane GRE + parallel imaging cal	0:40	
DWI	Spin-echo EPI; TR/TE 7600/70 ms; 128 × 128 matrix; FOV 24 cm; ST 5 skip 0 mm; 25–30 slices; 8 nex (2 B_0, 2 b = 1000 s/mm^2 in each of three directions)	1:01	B_0 maps used to exclude chronic infarcts
MRA	TR/TE 30/2 ms; 256 × 192 matrix; FOV 22 cm; ST 1.4 overlapping 0.7 mm; PI reduction factor 2	3:12	Cover from below sella to 1 cm above MCA bifurcation
GRE	2D fast GRE; TR/TE 900/30 ms; 256 × 192 matrix; FOV 24 cm; ST 5 skip 1.5 mm; BW 150 kHz	2:13	
ASL*	Pseudo-continuous labeling; TR/TE/TL/PLD 5500/2/1500/2000 ms; 3 × 3 × 4–6 mm; 3D-FSE readout. Background suppression	4:00-6:00	Time varies based on implementation and field strength
DSC	Gradient-echo EPI; TR/TE 1800/40 ms; 96 × 128 matrix; FOV 24 cm; ST 5 skip 1.5 mm; 14–20 slices; 60 time points	2:24	0.1 mmol/kg Gd, 3–5 ml/s followed by saline flush (20 ml) at same rate
Total		**9:30**	**13:30–15:30 with ASL**

* Optional, always performed if patient cannot receive Gd.

Figure 8.21 Typical rapid protocol for acute ischemic stroke. BW, bandwidth; FOV, Field of view; FSE, fast spin echo; Gd, gadolinium; GRE, gradient echo; PI, parallel imaging; PLD, post-label delay; ST, slice thickness; TL, label time; TR/TE, repetition time/echo time.

core rapid stroke protocol outlined above. These should include ASL (often with short and long PLD), VS-ASL, FLAIR, T_2, and T_1 post-contrast imaging.

Conclusions

It is perhaps no surprise that perfusion imaging is relevant to, and has been brought to bear on, a wide variety of neurovascular diseases. While much information can be gleaned from angiographic sequences alone, perfusion yields added information about the tissue microenvironment. In acute ischemic stroke, it has been shown to better identify patients that either benefit from or may be harmed by thrombolytic therapy. Perfusion imaging of TIA is a new field, but may have great clinical impact for management of these at-risk and challenging patients. Patients with chronic hypoperfusion, such as carotid occlusions/ stenosis and Moyamoya disease, show different patterns of perfusion deficits, and these may be helpful for patient management, such as selection for surgical bypass. Relatively little work has been done so far in the area of vasospasm, but perfusion imaging has been shown to detect tissue consequences. Qualitative findings on ASL imaging, such as venous ASL signal, appear to be sensitive to detect both large and small AV shunt lesions and aneurysms. Finally, the ability to map cerebrovascular reactivity, perfusion territories, and collaterals points to a rich future and a better understanding of both the healthy and pathological brain.

References

1. Powers WJ. Imaging preventable infarction in patients with acute ischemic stroke. *AJNR Am J Neuroradiol* 2008;**29**(10): 1823–5.

2. Davis SM, Donnan GA, Parsons MW, *et al.* Effects of alteplase beyond 3 h after stroke in the Echoplanar Imaging Thrombolytic Evaluation Trial (EPITHET): a placebo-controlled

randomised trial. *Lancet Neurol* 2008;**7**(4):299–309.

3. Albers GW, Thijs VN, Wechsler L, *et al*. Magnetic resonance imaging profiles predict clinical response to early reperfusion: the diffusion and perfusion imaging evaluation for understanding stroke evolution (DEFUSE) study. *Ann Neurol* 2006; **60**(5):508–17.

4. Straka M, Albers GW, Bammer R. Real-time diffusion-perfusion mismatch analysis in acute stroke. *J Magn Reson Imaging* 2010;**32**(5):1024–37.

5. del Zoppo G. Microvascular changes during cerebral ischemia and reperfusion. *Cerebrovasc Brain Metab Rev* 1994;**6**:47–96.

6. Powers WJ. Cerebral hemodynamics in ischemic cerebrovascular disease. *Ann Neurol* 1991;**29**(3): 231–40.

7. Zaharchuk G, Bogdanov AA, Jr., Marota JJ, *et al*. Continuous assessment of perfusion by tagging including volume and water extraction (CAPTIVE): a steady-state contrast agent technique for measuring blood flow, relative blood volume fraction, and the water extraction fraction. *Magn Reson Med* 1998;**40**(5):666–78.

8. Astrup J, Siesjö BK, Symon L. Thresholds in cerebral ischemia – the ischemic penumbra. *Stroke* 1981;**12**(6):723–5.

9. Jones TH, Morawetz RB, Crowell RM, *et al*. Thresholds of focal cerebral ischemia in awake monkeys. *J Neurosurg* 1981;**54**:773–82.

10. Campbell BC, Purushotham A, Christensen S, Desmond PM, Nagakane Y, Parsons MW, *et al*. The infarct core is well represented by the acute diffusion lesion: sustained reversal is infrequent. *J Cereb Blood Flow Metab* 2012;**32**: 50–6.

11. Siewert B, Schlaug G, Edelman RR, Warach S. Comparison of EPISTAR and T2*-weighted gadolinium-enhanced perfusion imaging in patients with acute cerebral ischemia. *Neurology* 1997;**48**(3):673–9.

12. Chalela JA, Alsop DC, Gonzalez-Atavales JB, *et al*. Magnetic resonance perfusion imaging in acute ischemic stroke using continuous arterial spin labeling. *Stroke*. 2000 Mar;**31**(3):680–7.

13. Sakaie KE, Shin W, Curtin KR, *et al*. Method for improving the accuracy of quantitative cerebral perfusion imaging. *J Magn Reson Imaging* 2005;**21**(5):512–19.

14. Zaharchuk G, Straka M, Marks MP, *et al*. Combined arterial spin label and dynamic susceptibility contrast measurement of cerebral blood flow. *Magn Reson Med* 2010;**63**(6):1548–56.

15. Zaro-Weber O, Moeller-Hartmann W, Heiss WD, Sobesky J. The performance of MRI-based cerebral blood flow measurements in acute and subacute stroke compared with ^{15}O-water positron emission tomography: identification of penumbral flow. *Stroke* 2009;**40**(7):2413–21.

16. Sorensen AG, Copen WA, Ostergaard L, *et al*. Hyperacute stroke: simultaneous measurement of relative cerebral blood volume, relative cerebral blood flow, and mean tissue transit time. *Radiology* 1999; **210**(2):519–27.

17. Hacke W, Furlan AJ, Al-Rawi Y, *et al*. Intravenous desmoteplase in patients with acute ischaemic stroke selected by MRI perfusion-diffusion weighted imaging or perfusion CT (DIAS-2): a prospective, randomised, double-blind, placebo-controlled study. *Lancet Neurol* 2009;**8**(2):141–50.

18. Hendrikse J, Petersen ET, van Laar PJ, Golay X. Cerebral border zones between distal end branches of intracranial arteries:

MR imaging. *Radiology* 2008; **246**(2):572–80.

19. Olivot JM, Mlynash M, Zaharchuk G, *et al*. Perfusion MRI (Tmax and MTT) correlation with xenon CT cerebral blood flow in stroke patients. *Neurology* 2009; **72**(13):1140–5.

20. Zaro-Weber O, Moeller-Hartmann W, Heiss WD, Sobesky J. Maps of time to maximum and time to peak for mismatch definition in clinical stroke studies validated with positron emission tomography. *Stroke* 2010; **41**(12):2817–21.

21. Zaro-Weber O, Moeller-Hartmann W, Heiss WD, Sobesky J. MRI perfusion maps in acute stroke validated with ^{15}O-water positron emission tomography. *Stroke* 2010;**41**(3):443–9.

22. Christensen S, Mouridsen K, Wu O, *et al*. Comparison of 10 perfusion MRI parameters in 97 sub-6-hour stroke patients using voxel-based receiver operating characteristics analysis. *Stroke* 2009;**40**(6):2055–61.

23. Wu O, Koroshetz WJ, Ostergaard L, *et al*. Predicting tissue outcome in acute human cerebral ischemia using combined diffusion- and perfusion-weighted MR imaging. *Stroke* 2001;**32**(4):933–42.

24. Gottrup C, Thomsen K, Locht P, *et al*. Applying instance-based techniques to prediction of final outcome in acute stroke. *Artif Intell Med* 2005;**33**(3): 223–36.

25. Galinovic I, Brunecker P, Ostwaldt AC, *et al*. Fully automated postprocessing carries a risk of substantial overestimation of perfusion deficits in acute stroke magnetic resonance imaging. *Cerebrovasc Dis* 2011;**31**(4):408–13.

26. Zaharchuk G, El Mogy IS, Fischbein NJ, Albers GW. Comparison of arterial spin labeling and bolus perfusion-weighted imaging for detecting

mismatch in acute stroke. *Stroke* 2012;**43**(7):1843–8.

27. Bokkers RP, Hernandez DA, Merino JG, *et al.* Whole-brain arterial spin labeling perfusion MRI in patients with acute stroke. *Stroke* 2012;**43**(5):1290–4.

28. Wang D, Alger J, Qian J, *et al.* The value of arterial spin-labeled perfusion imaging in acute ischemic stroke – comparison with dynamic susceptibility contrast enhanced MRI. *Stroke* 2012;**43**(4):1018–24.

29. Hernandez DA, Bokkers RP, Mirasol RV, *et al.* Pseudocontinuous arterial spin labeling quantifies relative cerebral blood flow in acute stroke. *Stroke* 2012;**43**(3):753–8.

30. Lansberg M, Straka M, Kemp S, *et al.* Magnetic resonance imaging profile and response to endovascular reperfusion: results of the DEFUSE-2 prospective cohort study. *Lancet Neurol* 2012;**11**:860–7.

31. Kakuda W, Lansberg MG, Thijs VN, *et al.* Optimal definition for PWI/DWI mismatch in acute ischemic stroke patients. *J Cereb Blood Flow Metab* 2008; **28**(5):887–91.

32. Mlynash M, Lansberg MG, De Silva DA, *et al.* Refining the definition of the malignant profile: insights from the DEFUSE-EPITHET pooled data set. *Stroke* 2011; **42**(5):1270–5.

33. Lansberg MG, Lee J, Christensen S, *et al.* RAPID automated patient selection for reperfusion therapy: a pooled analysis of the Echoplanar Imaging Thrombolytic Evaluation Trial (EPITHET) and the Diffusion and Perfusion Imaging Evaluation for Understanding Stroke Evolution (DEFUSE) Study. *Stroke* 2011; **42**(6):1608–14.

34. Copen WA, Rezai Gharai L, Barak ER, *et al.* Existence of the diffusion-perfusion mismatch within 24 hours after onset of acute stroke: dependence on proximal arterial occlusion. *Radiology* 2009;**250**(3):878–86.

35. Gonzalez RG, Hakimelahi R, Schaefer PW, *et al.* Stability of large diffusion/perfusion mismatch in anterior circulation strokes for 4 or more hours. *BMC Neurol* 2010;**10**:13.

36. Lansberg MG, Thijs VN, Bammer R, *et al.* The MRA-DWI mismatch identifies patients with stroke who are likely to benefit from reperfusion. *Stroke* 2008; **39**(9):2491–6.

37. Paciaroni M, Medeiros E, Bogousslavsky J. Desmoteplase. *Expert Opin Biol Ther* 2009; **9**(6):773–8.

38. Menezes NM, Ay H, Wang Zhu M, *et al.* The real estate factor: quantifying the impact of infarct location on stroke severity. *Stroke* 2007;**38**(1):194–7.

39. Kosior RK, Lauzon ML, Steffenhagen N, *et al.* Atlas-based topographical scoring for magnetic resonance imaging of acute stroke. *Stroke* 2010; **41**(3):455–60.

40. Smith WS, Sung G, Saver J, *et al.* Mechanical thrombectomy for acute ischemic stroke: final results of the Multi MERCI trial. *Stroke* 2008;**39**(4):1205–12.

41. Smith WS, Sung G, Starkman S, *et al.* Safety and efficacy of mechanical embolectomy in acute ischemic stroke: results of the MERCI trial. *Stroke* 2005; **36**(7):1432–8.

42. Grunwald IQ, Walter S, Papanagiotou P, *et al.* Revascularization in acute ischaemic stroke using the penumbra system: the first single center experience. *Eur J Neurol* 2009;**16**(11):1210–16.

43. Soares BP, Chien JD, Wintermark M. MR and CT monitoring of recanalization, reperfusion, and penumbra salvage: everything that recanalizes does not necessarily reperfuse! *Stroke* 2009;**40**(3 Suppl):S24–7.

44. Boxerman JL, Hamberg LM, Rosen BR, Weisskoff RM. MR contrast due to intravascular magnetic susceptibility perturbations. *Magn Reson Med* 1995;**34**:555–66.

45. Speck O, Chang L, DeSilva NM, Ernst T. Perfusion MRI of the human brain with dynamic susceptibility contrast: gradient-echo versus spin-echo techniques. *J Magn Reson Imaging* 2000; **12**(3):381–7.

46. Donahue KM, Krouwer HG, Rand SD, *et al.* Utility of simultaneously acquired gradient-echo and spin-echo cerebral blood volume and morphology maps in brain tumor patients. *Magn Reson Med* 2000;**43**(6):845–53.

47. Vonken EJ, van Osch MJ, Bakker CJ, Viergever MA. Measurement of cerebral perfusion with dual-echo multi-slice quantitative dynamic susceptibility contrast MRI. *J Magn Reson Imaging* 1999;**10**(2):109–17.

48. Kim JJ, Fischbein NJ, Lu Y, Pham D, Dillon WP. Regional angiographic grading system for collateral flow: correlation with cerebral infarction in patients with middle cerebral artery occlusion. *Stroke* 2004;**35**(6):1340–4.

49. Christoforidis GA, Mohammad Y, Kehagias D, Avutu B, Slivka AP. Angiographic assessment of pial collaterals as a prognostic indicator following intra-arterial thrombolysis for acute ischemic stroke. *AJNR Am J Neuroradiol* 2005;**26**(7):1789–97.

50. Higashida RT, Furlan AJ, Roberts H, *et al.* Trial design and reporting standards for intra-arterial cerebral thrombolysis for acute ischemic stroke. *Stroke* 2003; **34**(8):e109–37.

51. Kucinski T, Koch C, Eckert B, *et al.* Collateral circulation is an

independent radiological predictor of outcome after thrombolysis in acute ischaemic stroke. *Neuroradiology* 2003; **45**(1):11–18.

52. Bang OY, Saver JL, Buck BH, *et al*. Impact of collateral flow on tissue fate in acute ischaemic stroke. *J Neurol Neurosurg Psychiatry* 2008;**79**(6):625–9.

53. Calamante F, Ganesan V, Kirkham FJ, *et al*. MR perfusion imaging in Moyamoya Syndrome: potential implications for clinical evaluation of occlusive cerebrovascular disease. *Stroke* 2001;**32**(12):2810–16.

54. Christensen S, Calamante F, Hjort N, *et al*. Inferring origin of vascular supply from tracer arrival timing patterns using bolus tracking MRI. *J Magn Reson Imaging* 2008;**27**(6):1371–81.

55. Eldeniz C, Lee Y, Smith JK, *et al*., editors. Determination of collateral supply patterns using conventional dynamic susceptibility contrast perfusion imaging. *Proc Intl Soc Magn Reson Med*, Montreal, Canada, 2011;1977.

56. Chng SM, Petersen ET, Zimine I, *et al*. Territorial arterial spin labeling in the assessment of collateral circulation: comparison with digital subtraction angiography. *Stroke* 2008; **39**(12):3248–54.

57. Zaharchuk G, Do HM, Marks MP, *et al*. Arterial spin-labeling MRI can identify the presence and intensity of collateral perfusion in patients with moyamoya disease. *Stroke* 2011;**42**(9):2485–91.

58. An H, Lin W. Quantitative measurements of cerebral blood oxygen saturation using magnetic resonance imaging. *J Cereb Blood Flow Metab* 2000;**20**(8):1225–36.

59. He X, Yablonskiy DA. Quantitative BOLD: mapping of human cerebral deoxygenated blood volume and oxygen extraction fraction: default state.

Magn Reson Med 2007;**57**(1): 115–26.

60. Wardlaw JM, von Heijne A. Increased oxygen extraction demonstrated on gradient echo (T2*) imaging in a patient with acute ischaemic stroke. *Cerebrovasc Dis* 2006;**22** (5–6):456–8.

61. Siemonsen S, Fitting T, Thomalla G, *et al*. T2′ imaging predicts infarct growth beyond the acute diffusion-weighted imaging lesion in acute stroke. *Radiology* 2008;**248**(3): 979–86.

62. Ostergaard L, Sorensen AG, Chesler DA, *et al*. Combined diffusion-weighted and perfusion-weighted flow heterogeneity magnetic resonance imaging in acute stroke. *Stroke* 2000; **31**(5):1097–103.

63. Perkio J, Soinne L, Ostergaard L, *et al*. Abnormal intravoxel cerebral blood flow heterogeneity in human ischemic stroke determined by dynamic susceptibility contrast magnetic resonance imaging. *Stroke* 2005;**36**(1):44–9.

64. Kassner A, Roberts T, Taylor K, Silver F, Mikulis D. Prediction of hemorrhage in acute ischemic stroke using permeability MR imaging. *AJNR Am J Neuroradiol* 2005;**26**(9):2213–17.

65. Bang OY, Buck BH, Saver JL, *et al*. Prediction of hemorrhagic transformation after recanalization therapy using T2*-permeability magnetic resonance imaging. *Ann Neurol* 2007; **62**(2):170–6.

66. Kassner A, Mandell DM, Mikulis DJ. Measuring permeability in acute ischemic stroke. *Neuroimaging Clin N Am* 2011; **21**(2):315–25, x–xi.

67. Johnston SC, Rothwell PM, Nguyen-Huynh MN, *et al*. Validation and refinement of scores to predict very early stroke risk after transient ischaemic

attack. *Lancet* 2007;**369** (9558):283–92.

68. Rothwell PM, Giles MF, Chandratheva A, *et al*. Effect of urgent treatment of transient ischaemic attack and minor stroke on early recurrent stroke (EXPRESS study): a prospective population-based sequential comparison. *Lancet* 2007;**370** (9596):1432–42.

69. Ay H, Arsava EM, Johnston SC, *et al*. Clinical- and imaging-based prediction of stroke risk after transient ischemic attack: the CIP model. *Stroke* 2009; **40**(1):181–6.

70. Josephson SA, Sidney S, Pham TN, Bernstein AL, Johnston SC. Higher ABCD2 score predicts patients most likely to have true transient ischemic attack. *Stroke* 2008;**39**(11):3096–8.

71. Bisschops RH, Kappelle LJ, Mali WP, van der Grond J. Hemodynamic and metabolic changes in transient ischemic attack patients: a magnetic resonance angiography and (1)H-magnetic resonance spectroscopy study performed within 3 days of onset of a transient ischemic attack. *Stroke* 2002;**33**(1):110–15.

72. Krol AL, Coutts SB, Simon JE, *et al*. Perfusion MRI abnormalities in speech or motor transient ischemic attack patients. *Stroke* 2005;**36**(11):2487–9.

73. Restrepo L, Jacobs MA, Barker PB, Wityk RJ. Assessment of transient ischemic attack with diffusion- and perfusion-weighted imaging. *AJNR Am J Neuroradiol* 2004;**25**(10):1645–52.

74. Coutts SB, Eliasziw M, Hill MD, *et al*. An improved scoring system for identifying patients at high early risk of stroke and functional impairment after an acute transient ischemic attack or minor stroke. *Int J Stroke* 2008; **3**(1):3–10.

75. Mlynash M, Olivot JM, Tong DC, *et al*. Yield of combined perfusion

and diffusion MR imaging in hemispheric TIA. *Neurology* 2009;72(13):1127–33.

76. Zaharchuk G. Arterial spin label imaging of acute ischemic stroke and transient ischemic attack. *Neuroimaging Clin N Am* 2011; 21(2):285–301, x.

77. Zaharchuk G, Olivot J-M, Fischbein NJ, *et al.* Arterial spin label imaging findings in transient ischemic attack patients: comparison with diffusion- and bolus perfusion-weighted imaging. *Cerebrovasc Dis* 2012; 34(3):221–8.

78. Olivot JM, Albers GW. Diffusion-perfusion MRI for triaging transient ischemic attack and acute cerebrovascular syndromes. *Curr Opin Neurol* 2011; 24(1):44–9.

79. Macintosh BJ, Lindsay AC, Kylintireas I, *et al.* Multiple inflow pulsed arterial spin-labeling reveals delays in the arterial arrival time in minor stroke and transient ischemic attack. *AJNR Am J Neuroradiol* 2010;31(10):1892–4.

80. Zaharchuk G, Bammer R, Straka M, *et al.* Arterial spin-label imaging in patients with normal bolus perfusion-weighted MR imaging findings: pilot identification of the borderzone sign. *Radiology* 2009;252(3): 797–807.

81. Failure of extracranial-intracranial arterial bypass to reduce the risk of ischemic stroke. Results of an international randomized trial. The EC/IC Bypass Study Group. *N Engl J Med* 1985; 313(19):1191–200.

82. Grubb RL, Jr., Powers WJ, Derdeyn CP, Adams HP, Jr., Clarke WR. The Carotid Occlusion Surgery Study. *Neurosurg Focus* 2003;14(3):e9.

83. Spetzler R, Martin N. A proposed grading system for arteriovenous malformations. *J Neurosurg* 1986;65:476–83.

84. Wolf RL, Wang J, Detre JA, Zager EL, Hurst RW. Arteriovenous shunt visualization in arteriovenous malformations with arterial spin-labeling MR imaging. *AJNR Am J Neuroradiol* 2008; 29(4):681–7.

85. Pollock JM, Whitlow CT, Simonds J, *et al.* Response of arteriovenous malformations to gamma knife therapy evaluated with pulsed arterial spin-labeling MRI perfusion. *AJR Am J Roentgenol* 2011;196(1):15–22.

86. Le TT, Fischbein NJ, Andre JB, *et al.* Identification of venous signal on arterial spin labeling improves diagnosis of dural arteriovenous fistulas and small arteriovenous malformations. *AJNR Am J Neuroradiol* 2012; 33(1):61–8.

87. Wijnhoud AD, Franckena M, van der Lugt A, Koudstaal PJ, Dippel ED. Inadequate acoustical temporal bone window in patients with a transient ischemic attack or minor stroke: role of skull thickness and bone density. *Ultrasound Med Biol* 2008; 34(6):923–9.

88. Rordorf G, Koroshetz WJ, Copen WA, *et al.* Diffusion- and perfusion-weighted imaging in vasospasm after subarachnoid hemorrhage. *Stroke* 1999; 30(3):599–605.

89. Hertel F, Walter C, Bettag M, Morsdorf M. Perfusion-weighted magnetic resonance imaging in patients with vasospasm: a useful new tool in the management of patients with subarachnoid hemorrhage. *Neurosurgery* 2005;56(1):28–35; discussion 35.

90. Vatter H, Guresir E, Berkefeld J, *et al.* Perfusion-diffusion mismatch in MRI to indicate endovascular treatment of cerebral vasospasm after subarachnoid haemorrhage. *J Neurol Neurosurg Psychiatry* 2011;82(8):876–83.

91. Ogasawara K, Ogawa A. [JET study (Japanese EC-IC Bypass Trial)]. *Nihon Rinsho* 2006;64 Suppl 7:524–7.

92. Laux BE, Raichle ME. The effect of acetazolamide on cerebral blood flow and oxygen utilization in the rhesus monkey. *J Clin Invest* 1978;62(3):585–92.

93. Vorstrup S, Henriksen L, Paulson OB. Effect of acetazolamide on cerebral blood flow and cerebral metabolic rate for oxygen. *J Clin Invest* 1984;74(5):1634–9.

94. Mukherjee P, Kang HC, Videen TO, *et al.* Measurement of cerebral blood flow in chronic carotid occlusive disease: comparison of dynamic susceptibility contrast perfusion MR imaging with positron emission tomography. *AJNR Am J Neuroradiol* 2003; 24(5):862–71.

95. Wu WC, Wong EC. Intravascular effect in velocity-selective arterial spin labeling: the choice of inflow time and cutoff velocity. *Neuroimage* 2006;32(1):122–8.

96. Qiu D, Straka M, Zun Z, *et al.* CBF measurements using multidelay pseudocontinuous and velocity-selective arterial spin labeling in patients with long arterial transit delays: Comparison with xenon CT CBF. *J Magn Reson Imaging* 2012; 36(1):110–19.

97. Yen Y-F, Field AS, Martin EM, *et al.* Test-retest reproducibility of quantitative CBF measurements using FAIR perfusion MRI and acetazolamide challenge. *Magn Reson Med* 2002;47:921–8.

98. Detre JA, Samuels OB, Alsop DC, *et al.* Noninvasive magnetic resonance imaging evaluation of cerebral blood flow with acetazolamide challenge in patients with cerebrovascular stenosis. *J Magn Reson Imaging* 1999;10(5):870–5.

99. Mandell DM, Han JS, Poublanc J, et al. Quantitative measurement of cerebrovascular reactivity by blood oxygen level-dependent MR imaging in patients with intracranial stenosis: preoperative cerebrovascular reactivity predicts the effect of extracranial-intracranial bypass surgery. *AJNR Am J Neuroradiol* 2011; **32**(4):721–7.

100. Mikulis DJ, Krolczyk G, Desal H, et al. Preoperative and postoperative mapping of cerebrovascular reactivity in moyamoya disease by using blood oxygen level-dependent magnetic resonance imaging. *J Neurosurg* 2005;**103**(2): 347–55.

101. Wintermark M, Reichhart M, Thiran JP, et al. Prognostic accuracy of cerebral blood flow measurement by perfusion computed tomography, at the time of emergency room admission, in acute stroke patients. *Ann Neurol* 2002; **51**(4):417–32.

102. Schaefer PW, Barak ER, Kamalian S, et al. Quantitative assessment of core/penumbra mismatch in acute stroke: CT and MR perfusion imaging are strongly correlated when sufficient brain volume is imaged. *Stroke* 2008; **39**(11):2986–92.

103. Schellinger PD, Thomalla G, Fiehler J, et al. MRI-based and CT-based thrombolytic therapy in acute stroke within and beyond established time windows: an analysis of 1210 patients. *Stroke* 2007;**38**(10):2640–5.

104. Wintermark M, Sesay M, Barbier E, et al. Comparative overview of brain perfusion imaging techniques. *Stroke* 2005;**36**(9):e83–99.

105. Petersen ET, Mouridsen K, Golay X. The QUASAR reproducibility study, Part II: Results from a multi-center Arterial Spin Labeling test-retest study. *Neuroimage* 2010;**49**(1):104–13.

106. Rowley HA. The four Ps of acute stroke imaging: parenchyma, pipes, perfusion, and penumbra.

AJNR Am J Neuroradiol 2001;**22** (4):599–601.

107. Kidwell CS, Chalela JA, Saver JL, et al. Comparison of MRI and CT for detection of acute intracerebral hemorrhage. *JAMA* 2004;**292**(15):1823–30.

108. Fiehler J, Albers GW, Boulanger JM, et al. Bleeding risk analysis in stroke imaging before thromboLysis (BRASIL): pooled analysis of T2*-weighted magnetic resonance imaging data from 570 patients. *Stroke* 2007; **38**(10):2738–44.

109. Hendrikse J, Petersen ET, Chèze A, et al. Relationship between cerebral perfusion teritories and location of cerebral infarcts. *Stroke* 2009;**40**(5):1617–22.

110. Hendrikse J, Petersen ET, Chng SM, Venketasubramanian N, Golay X. Distribution of cerebral blood flow in the nucleus caudatus, nucleus lentiformis, and thalamus: a study of territorial arterial spin-labeling MR imaging. *Radiology* 2010;**254**(3):867–75.

History

An 82-year-old woman, last seen normal 1 hr prior, now mute and with right hemiparesis, NIHSS 22.

Technique

Diffusion and perfusion imaging using bolus DSC imaging.

Imaging findings

See Figure 8.22.

Discussion

This represents a target mismatch, thought to be associated with improved response if thrombolysis can be achieved. The patient received IV tPA without improvement. She was then taken to the catheterization laboratory, where her M1 was recanalized at 4 hrs using the MERCI clot retriever. Initial follow-up images suggest acute DWI reversal; however, subsequent images demonstrate that the infarcted region is FLAIR-positive. Despite this, the patient had an NIHSS score of 0 at this time.

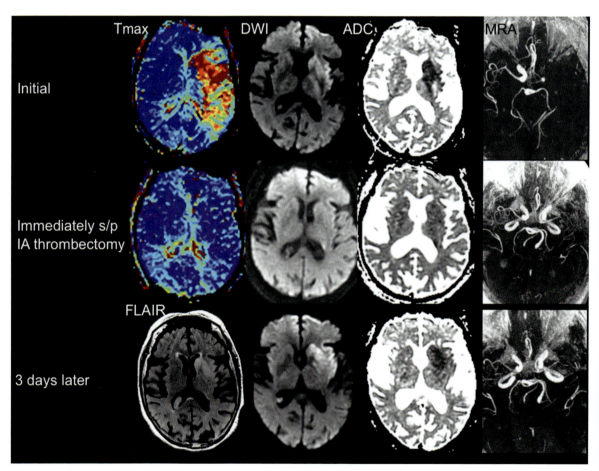

Figure 8.22 There is occlusion of the left M1 segment of the MCA with a small acute infarct of the left basal ganglia. A larger perfusion abnormality is noted on T_{max} maps that involves most of the MCA territory. The sizes of the acute DWI and critically hypoperfused PWI regions are 9 ml and 90 ml, respectively.

- Early reperfusion of patients with a target DWI-PWI mismatch can lead to improved clinical and imaging outcome.
- DWI reversal may be seen on early post-reperfusion images, but this tissue rarely demonstrates a normal appearance on later follow-up.

- Clinical and imaging findings may differ based on the location of tissue damage.

Bibliography

Albers GW, Thijs VN, Wechsler L, *et al.* Magnetic resonance imaging profiles predict clinical response to early reperfusion: the diffusion and perfusion imaging evaluation for understanding stroke evolution (DEFUSE) study. *Ann Neurol* 2006;**60**(5):508–17.

PWI and ASL in transient ischemic attack

History

A 64 year-old man with atrial fibrillation and transient left-sided hemiparesis.

Technique

Diffusion and perfusion imaging using bolus DSC and ASL imaging.

Imaging findings

See Figure 8.23.

Discussion

This is an example of a PWI-DWI mismatch in a TIA patient who later had a completed infarct in a region of perfusion abnormality.

- A perfusion abnormality in a DWI-negative TIA patient confirms the vascular etiology of the patient's symptoms.
- ASL is more sensitive than PWI to detect minor perfusion abnormalities associated with TIA.
- Perfusion abnormalities in TIA may be transient, and early imaging is essential.
- TIA patients with a DWI-PWI mismatch may be at higher risk of stroke.

Bibliography

Mlynash M, Olivot JM, Tong DC, *et al.* Yield of combined perfusion and diffusion MR imaging in hemispheric TIA. *Neurology* 2009;**72**(13):1127–33.

Olivot JM, Albers GW. Diffusion-perfusion MRI for triaging transient ischemic attack and acute cerebrovascular syndromes. *Curr Opin Neurol* 2011;**24**(1):44–9.

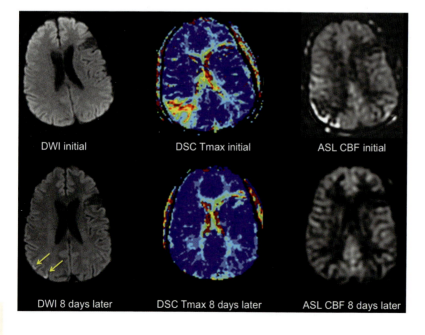

DWI initial   DSC Tmax initial   ASL CBF initial

DWI 8 days later   DSC Tmax 8 days later   ASL CBF 8 days later

Figure 8.23 There is no diffusion lesion. A wedge-shaped region of T_{max} prolongation and arterial transit artifact representing slow flow on ASL imaging is noted in the right parietal region. This patient had a DWI-positive region (arrows) on follow-up imaging 8 days later, at which time the perfusion studies had normalized.

ASL in subtle arteriovenous malformation

History

A 60-year-old woman with 10/10 headache.

Technique

FLAIR, T2, ASL, and MRA pre- and post-contrast.

Imaging findings

See Figure 8.24.

Discussion

This case shows that high ASL signal in the veins can be associated with small vascular malformations, such as micro AVM in this case. Anatomic imaging was normal and the MRA findings were subtle and noted only in retrospect. This patient underwent cerebral angiography for confirmation and treatment planning.

- Venous ASL signal may point to the presence of an AV shunt lesion, such as AVM or dAVF.
- Venous shunting on ASL can be seen in children generally as well as in the setting of subacute stroke, hyperperfusion syndrome, and vascular tumors, such as hemangioblastoma. However, outside of these conditions, it is rarely seen in adults with normal ASL parameters.

Bibliography

Le T, Fischbein NJ, Andre JB, *et al*. Identification of venous signal on arterial spin labeling improves diagnosis of dural arteriovenous fistulae and small arteriovenous malformations. *AJNR Am J Neuroradiol* 2012;**33**(1): 61–8.

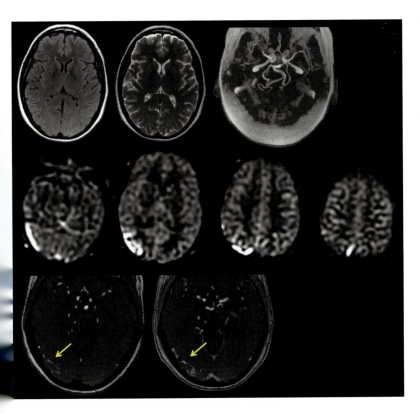

Figure 8.24 Anatomic imaging was normal, as was a first overview of the MRA (shown here as a collapsed maximum intensity projection image). ASL demonstrates high signal within the superior sagittal and right transverse sinuses, as well as a region overlying the cortex of the right parietal lobe. Closer inspection of the source images of the MRA shows several conspicuous vessels in this region. Post-contrast MRA improves conspicuity of the vascular lesion, which was confirmed on angiography to represent a micro AVM.

Chapter

9

MR perfusion imaging in neurodegenerative disease

Norbert Schuff

Key points

- Most neurodegenerative diseases exhibit a characteristic regional pattern of altered brain perfusion.
- These perfusion patterns generally provide complementary information to patterns of brain atrophy; Alzheimer's disease (AD) shows reduced flow in the posterior cingulate gyri and parietal association cortices; in contrast, frontotemporal dementia (FTD) shows frontal lobe hypoperfusion, both compared with normal aging (controls) and AD.
- ASL-MRI provides an attractive approach to measure the abnormal perfusion patterns in neurodegenerative diseases.
- The perfusion patterns based on ASL-MRI exhibit similar features to those based on functional PET and SPECT scans.
- ASL-MRI-based perfusion imaging has clinical potential for aiding an early diagnosis of neurodegenerative diseases and for assessing potential treatment interventions; however, it remains to be determined if changes are robust enough to be detected with confidence in individual patients.

Introduction

Neurodegenerative diseases, such as Alzheimer's disease (AD), frontotemporal lobar degeneration (FTLD), Lewy body dementia (DLB), and other forms of dementia, are characterized pathologically by slowly progressive dysfunction and loss of neurons. The risk for neurodegenerative diseases usually increases dramatically with advancing age, although familial variants of these conditions exist but occur at much lower frequency than the sporadic versions. Many of these diseases also share a common neuropathology associated with the malicious accumulation of misfolded protein aggregates in the brain [1]. On structural brain MRI, however, most neurodegenerative diseases do not show characteristic lesions that are readily identifiable by a radiologist's eye. Accordingly, the diagnostic value of structural MRI for neurodegenerative diseases has been limited (except to rule out the presence of other brain pathologies, such as tumors and stroke). Aside from brain structure, the importance of perfusion to maintain brain viability is well documented [2] and there is substantial evidence for alterations of brain perfusion in neurodegenerative diseases from radioactive labeled tracer studies using positron emission tomography (PET) or single-photon computed emission tomography (SPECT) [3]. There is also broad agreement that functional alterations in the brain generally precede neuronal/synaptic loss. Accordingly, perfusion imaging in general holds great promise for detecting neurodegeneration at an early stage, before advanced neuronal loss. Perfusion imaging should also be useful for the assessment of potentially disease-modifying treatments. Finally, by mapping brain perfusion researchers hope to learn more about the physiological and functional underpinnings of neurodegenerative diseases, thereby uncovering the biometric fingerprints of these devastating conditions.

Arterial spin labeling (ASL)-MRI – as described in detail in Chapter 3 of this book – has gained particular interest for studying brain perfusion in neurodegenerative disease, largely because of its ability to measure cerebral blood flow (CBF) both quantitatively and completely non-invasively. Aside from its non-significant risk, the non-invasiveness of

ASL-MRI also permits repeating perfusion measurements virtually indefinitely, thereby enabling studies of cerebral blood circulation at an unprecedented temporal resolution. ASL-MRI also has an edge over PET and SPECT studies due to its quicker (more convenient) examination time, lack of radiation, and higher spatial resolution. While there have been some studies of neurodegeneration using dynamic susceptibility contrast (DSC)-MRI [4], these are much fewer than ASL. Recently, resting-state (rs)-fMRI has also been applied to neurodegeneration [5], but this is a topic that is beyond the scope of the current chapter. The goal of this chapter is to provide an update of ASL-MRI findings in neurodegenerative diseases and to discuss the potential clinical application of this MRI modality. Other considerations, such as the added value of ASL-MRI for studies of neurodegenerative diseases, limitations, and pitfalls, as well as new emerging and promising developments in ASL-MRI will also be addressed.

Applications

Alzheimer's disease (AD)

AD is associated with progressive decline of cognitive function, resulting in dementia. AD is also by far the most frequent cause of age-related neurodegeneration, affecting about 20% of the population over 80 years of age [6]. As people around the globe live longer, the impact of the disease is expected to increase further, with dire social and economical consequences for societies if no effective treatment is developed soon. There is also growing concern that once individuals show clinical symptoms of AD, it could be too late for treatments to be effective, as neuronal damage may have reached already an advanced stage. Early detection of the disease and better knowledge about the natural course of disease progression are therefore paramount for early interventions when treatment is likely most effective (and once treatment for AD becomes available).

Many ASL-MRI studies have focused on detecting brain perfusion alterations in AD. One of the first ASL-MRI studies compared a small group of patients diagnosed with AD with cognitively normal elder subjects [7]. A significantly lower ASL signal in parieto-occipital and tempero-occipital lobe regions was found in the AD patients, consistent with diminished cerebral perfusion in these regions. Later, another study demonstrated that ASL-MRI captures

a characteristic profile of regional hypoperfusion in AD, similar to the profile known from PET and SPECT studies [8], namely hypoperfusion primarily affecting the temporal, parietal, and posterior cingulate cortices. Moreover, hypoperfusion in these cortical regions correlated with increased severity of AD symptoms, providing further evidence that ASL-MRI can capture the disease stage. However, these initial ASL-MRI studies, lacking adequate spatial resolution to obtain perfusion separately of gray matter and white matter, were difficult to interpret because variable contributions from white and gray matter can induce artificial variations in perfusion via partial volume effects. In particular, since AD is also associated with substantial cortical atrophy, a concern is that the observations of cortical hypoperfusion may simply mirror atrophy, without other useful complementary information. In a subsequent study, this issue was addressed specifically by correcting ASL-MRI for partial volume effects [9]. Previously reported patterns of hypoperfusion in AD were replicated, and furthermore, the perfusion abnormalities in AD were found to further extend to the superior and middle frontal gyri. Importantly, the extent of regional hypoperfusion in AD was found to change little when applying partial volume corrections. Consequently, the findings of hypoperfusion in AD could no longer be explained simply as an "artifact" associated with underlying brain atrophy. For illustration, clusters of voxels with significant hypoperfusion from a group analysis of AD versus normal aging are depicted in Figure 9.1. The parametric maps indicate that the most significant perfusion reductions in AD affect the posterior cingulate gyri and parietal association cortices. Results from the original uncorrected ASL-MRI data are shown in Figure 9.1a. Results from the same ASL-MRI data corrected for atrophy and gray/white matter partial volume effects are depicted in Figure 9.1b. This demonstrates that the pattern of regional hypoperfusion in AD remains largely unchanged after correction. The disentanglement of regional variations in cerebral perfusion from underlying structural changes is important for a better understanding of the onset and progression of dementia, since structural and perfusion processes can differ in temporal as well as spatial extent. However, a major limitation of this study was that inferior and mesial temporal lobe regions, especially the hippocampus (a prominent target of AD pathology), were not sampled for technical reasons. Subsequently,

(a) Not atrophy corrected   (b) Corrected

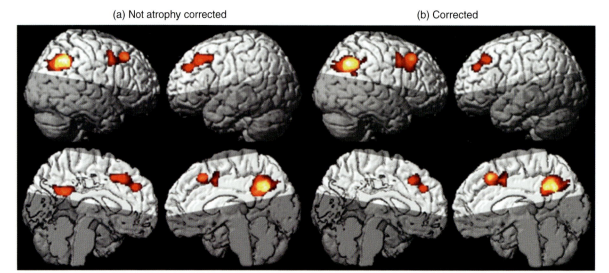

Figure 9.1 Statistical parametric maps of regional hypoperfusion in Alzheimer's disease relative to normal aging. All colored voxels are contained within clusters with a corrected cluster-level $p = 0.05$. Yellow voxels are regions of greatest group differences. The most significant region of hypoperfusion involves the posterior cingulate gyri and parietal association cortices. (a) Data not corrected for local brain atrophy and partial volume effects. (b) Data corrected. The regional pattern of hypoperfusion changes little after the corrections, suggesting that the pattern of hypoperfusion in AD is not simply an artifact of underlying variations in brain structure.

several other ASL-MRI studies [10–12], utilizing improved ASL methodology or modern higher magnetic field (3 T) MRI systems, did measure perfusion within the temporal lobes and the rest of the brain. In particular, one study replicated previous ASL findings in AD, and found additional brain regions with systematic hypoperfusion, including the superior temporal, parahippocampal, and fusiform gyri, as well as the thalamus, insula cortex, and hippocampus [12]. Moreover, by evaluating perfusion in these regions simultaneously using multivariate statistics, it was shown that the perfusion differences between AD patients and control subjects were very robust, not only at the group level, but also on a subject-by-subject basis. Surprisingly, some of the new ASL-MRI investigations found an increase of cerebral perfusion in AD in various brain regions, including the hippocampus [10], the anterior cingulate cortex [11], and more broadly in frontal lobe regions [13]. All studies, however, found consistent hypoperfusion in posterior brain regions in AD, in agreement with autopsy findings of high concentration of amyloid β deposits in these regions, one of the hallmarks of AD [14]. While the phenomenon of increased perfusion in AD has rarely been reported before, the finding is not irreconcilable. Hyperperfusion is consistent with fMRI data in AD that revealed increased activation

in mesial temporal lobe regions with advancing cognitive impairment [15]. The observation that regional variations of hyperperfusion and hypoperfusion can coexist in AD has been interpreted as a compensatory response to local neuronal damage that leads elsewhere in the brain to increased neuronal activity, resulting in hyperperfusion [10]. However, observations of hyperperfusion in AD are not entirely consistent across these studies. While one study reported hyperperfusion in the hippocampus [10] without alterations in the frontal cortex, other studies reported hyperperfusion in the frontal cortex without changes in the hippocampus [11, 13].

It should be noted that several biological factors may potentially skew perfusion measurements, especially in the presence of pathology. One of the factors is variation in perfusion hemodynamics that is not yet fully understood in AD. To shed light on variations in hemodynamics (which would impact pulsed ASL more than continuous ASL), one study measured simultaneous variations in regional arterial blood flow, blood volume, and transit time of the spin labels in a group of AD patients and control subjects, by acquiring ASL-MRI series with multiple post-labeling delay times [16]. It was found that there was neither a significant difference in blood volume, nor in transit time, between the groups, despite substantial regional

CBF reductions in the AD patients compared with controls. The investigators concluded that variations in perfusion hemodynamics in AD do not play a major role. Likewise, discrepant findings of hypo- or hyperperfusion in AD may not be due to differences in hemodynamics. However, this study employed a simplistic single-compartment model of cerebral perfusion in which the transfer of labels from the vasculature to the brain is instantaneous and spatially homogeneous. Another ASL-MRI study of perfusion hemodynamics in AD obtained results that supported a different conclusion [17]. Adapting a more realistic model for perfusion in which the labels have finite transfer rates to the brain and the labels are spatially distributed, it was found that the transfer time of spin labels through arteries and arterioles before reaching the capillary bed was significantly longer in AD than in normal aging. Interestingly, reduced CBF and prolonged transit time were partially unrelated in AD. The finding implies that other pathological processes, e.g., cerebrovascular disease, may also contribute to regional variations of perfusion in AD. This raises the possibility that some of the diverse findings of hypo- versus hyperperfusion in AD may reflect the level of pathological heterogeneity in the AD population. More studies on larger groups of patients and control subjects are warranted to replicate findings of simultaneous hypo- and hyperperfusion in AD and also to determine if hyperperfusion could potentially provide an index for staging disease severity.

The finding of simultaneous hypo- and hyperperfusion in AD is also interesting from the perspective of the relationship between perfusion and neurodegeneration. It is generally thought that reduced perfusion is a consequence of reduced energy demand of the brain in AD due to extensive synaptic and neuronal loss [18]. Likewise, increased perfusion might reflect compensatory or pathological neuronal hyperactivity or inflammation, as argued by Alsop and colleagues [10]. Alternatively, the perfusion alterations in AD could reflect also cerebrovascular aberrations that ASL-MRI may be able to detect. From this perspective, reduced perfusion in AD could be a secondary effect of diminished brain activity rather than its cause. ASL-MRI studies together with studies of brain metabolic activity (e.g., using ^{18}F-fluorodeoxyglucose (FDG)-PET) should help elucidate the relationship between altered perfusion and neurodegeneration in AD.

Mild cognitive impairment (MCI)

MCI is a clinical term used to characterize elderly subjects whose cognitive performance falls between that of normal aging and dementia [19]. On average, MCI subjects progress toward AD at a much higher rate than cognitively normal elderly [20]. MCI is therefore considered a transitional state between normal aging and AD. In recent years, studies of MCI subjects have become a major focus of investigations aiming to identify early markers of AD.

ASL-MRI in MCI revealed hypoperfusion in the right parietal lobe and precuneus, similar to but less prominent than the perfusion changes seen in AD, and also similar to findings using PET or SPECT [9]. A few ASL-MRI studies also found hyperperfusion in MCI. Specifically, increased perfusion in the hippocampus [10] and amygdala and basal ganglia [11] have been reported. However, the prognostic value of ASL-MRI for the progression of MCI to AD is currently unclear, largely due to lack of prospective ASL-MRI studies. On the other hand, ASL-MRI seems to capture fairly sensitively the clinical diversity of MCI with respect to the affected cognitive domains. In an ASL-MRI study that compared one group of MCI subjects with primarily memory deficits (also known as amnestic MCI) with another MCI group with primarily executive dysfunctions, striking differences in regional perfusion levels were found [21]. Namely, amnestic MCI patients exhibited hypoperfusion in the posterior cingulate cortex relative to controls, whereas MCI patients with executive dysfunctions showed hypoperfusion in the middle frontal gyrus and precuneus. MCI patients with executive dysfunctions further had hypoperfusion in primarily the left middle frontal gyrus, posterior cingulate gyrus, and precuneus relative to amnestic MCI patients. Moreover, hypoperfusion of the posterior cingulate cortex correlated with increased memory deficits, whereas hypoperfusion of predominantly frontal brain regions correlated with increased executive deficits, indicating that the magnitude of perfusion changes reflects disease severity. The finding that amnestic and executive dysfunctional MCI patients show different patterns of hypoperfusion also supports the existence of distinct pathological subgroups in MCI. Taken together, the results suggest that ASL-MRI has potential in differentiating between MCI subtypes, which vary in the risks for progression toward AD. However, more work is needed on this field to obtain definitive answers on the power of ASL in differentiating between MCI subtypes.

Frontotemporal lobar degeneration (FTLD)

Once considered a rare disorder, FTLD is now recognized as a common cause of early-onset dementia. Patients with this condition are typically between 50 and 60 years old, several decades younger than most patients with sporadic AD. They typically present with severe behavioral problems. Nonetheless, the differential diagnosis between AD and FTLD is often difficult to achieve on clinical grounds alone, because some FTLD variants, such as the behavioral-variant of frontotemporal dementia (bvFTD) or the variant of progressive non-fluent aphasia (PNFA), can also have memory impairments that mimic AD. Structural MRI has been used to differentiate between FTLD and AD but the patterns of structural atrophy often merge across diseases as impairments become more severe [22, 23]. On the other hand, studies have shown functional PET and SPECT improve the differential diagnoses between FTLD and AD [24] over anatomical MRI alone, and the same has been demonstrated for ASL-MRI.

One of the first ASL-MRI studies of the FTLD complex compared 21 patients with FTD and 24 patients with AD [25] (Figure 9.2). It was found that FTD patients had regional hypoperfusion in the right superior and middle frontal gyri compared with normal subjects, while normal perfusion levels were found in parietal and occipital brain regions. This pattern of regional hypoperfusion on ASL-MRI also agrees with the typical distribution of disease pathology seen at autopsy. Hypoperfusion of the frontal cortex in bvFTD patients also correlated with deficits in judgment and problem solving. Overall, these perfusion findings from ASL-MRI in bvFTD are consistent with results from PET and SPECT [24]. Furthermore, since the ASL-MRI data were corrected for atrophy and partial volume effects, the ASL-MRI findings are likely more robust than the results from PET and SPECT, which were largely uncorrected, indicating that the regional pattern of hypoperfusion in bvFTD is not simply due to underlying variations in brain structure. Another interesting finding was that perfusion was markedly higher in bvFTD patients than in AD patients in some regions, especially in the precuneus and posterior cingulate cortex. In another ASL-MRI focusing on FTLD in general, it was also found that the frontal lobe bilaterally showed significantly reduced perfusion [13]. In addition, it was reported that FTLD patients had hyperperfusion in posterior cingulate and medial parietal/precuneus regions. Interestingly, the two separate ASL-MRI studies both found evidence for a functional dissociation between bvFTD and AD based on ASL-MRI perfusion when the patient groups were compared directly. One study found bvFTD was associated with hyperperfusion in the parietal lobe relative to perfusion in AD, whereas the other observed a double dissociation of hypoperfusion in inferior, medial, and dorsolateral regions in FTLD and hypoperfusion in lateral temporo-parietal brain regions in AD. More recently, another study replicated the ASL-MRI results in bvFTD, exploiting the benefits of a higher magnetic field strength (4 T) [26]. Further hypoperfusion extending to the anterior cingulate cortex and thalamus in bvFTD was found. The anterior cingulate cortex is known for its role in problem solving and emotional control, two cognitive domains frequently affected in bvFTD. The thalamus is a major hub for processing sensory and movement information and is thought to be compromised in bvFTD. Taken together, the results suggest that ASL-MRI captures a pattern of regional perfusion abnormalities in AD and FTLD that is consistent with the known distribution of each pathology typically seen at autopsy. ASL-MRI could therefore have use for a differential diagnosis between AD and FTLD types of dementia.

Other neurodegenerative diseases

ASL-MRI applications to more rare forms of neurodegenerative diseases so far are limited. In patients with Parkinson's disease, a slowly progressive movement disorder, who also showed symptoms of dementia, hypoperfusion in a bilateral posterior cortical region including both occipital and parietal lobes was found, in line with previous PET and SPECT studies [27]. Interestingly, Parkinson's patients without any symptoms of dementia also showed some level of hypoperfusion on ASL-MRI in the same brain region, though of lower magnitude than in the Parkinson's patients with dementia. It remains to be seen whether posterior hypoperfusion is a general index of Parkinson's pathology (although Parkinson's patients with dementia rarely have neuropathological lesions in this brain region at autopsy) or hypoperfusion represents a potential marker of incipient dementia

(a)

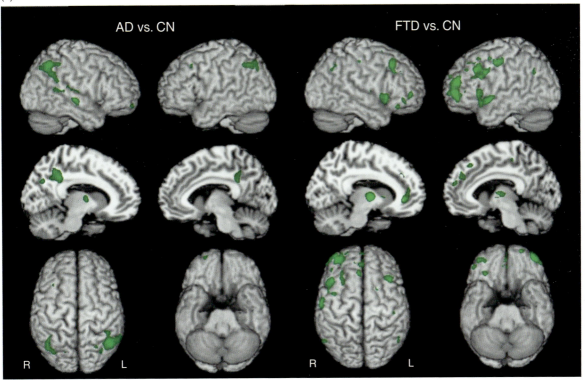

(b)

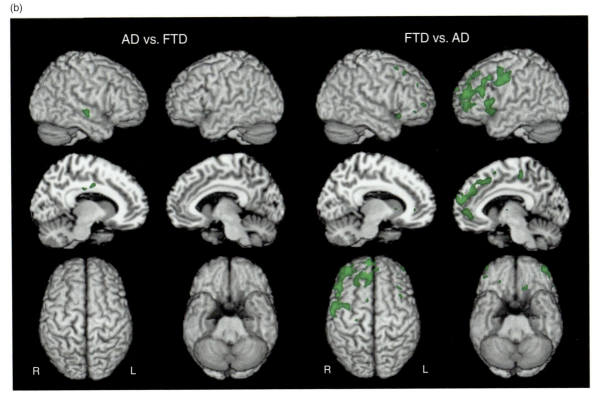

Figure 9.2 Statistical parametric maps of characteristic patterns of hypoperfusion in Alzheimer's disease (AD) and frontotemporal dementia (FTD), superimposed on a surface rendered brain template. Significant voxels are contained within clusters at an uncorrected cluster-level p = 0.001. Light green indicates more hypoperfusion. (a) Hypoperfusion in AD and FTD relative to cognitive normal (CN) subjects; (b) Comparisons of hypoperfusion between AD and FTD; Hypoperfusion in AD relative to FTD is illustrated in the left panel, hypoperfusion in FTD relative to AD is shown in the right panel.

in connection to Parkinson's disease. The clarification requires prospective perfusion studies where patients are followed over time.

Finally, ASL-MRI has also been applied to study cerebral perfusion in mild dementia with Lewy bodies (DLB), a progressive degenerative form of dementia that is frequently accompanied by hallucinations and parkinsonian motor features, yet which is difficult to differentiate from AD because cognitive deficits can overlap [28]. In a group of 14 patients diagnosed with DLB, hypoperfusion in DLB patients relative to control subjects was observed, most notably in the frontal, parietal, and occipital lobes but also in the precuneus. When compared with AD patients, DLB patients showed lower perfusion levels bilaterally in the frontal lobe and precuneus and in right temporal lobe regions. In addition to the regional pattern of hypoperfusion, DLB patients also showed a markedly greater reduction of perfusion than the AD patients, although matching disease severity across these conditions is not without complication. Therefore, the extent to which perfusion differences between AD and DLB reflect different pathological processes, or mainly reflect disease severity, remains to be determined.

Differential diagnosis

ASL-MRI studies that attempted differentiating among the various neurodegenerative diseases based on cerebral perfusion are still sparse. Of particular clinical interest is the differential diagnosis between AD and neurodegenerative diseases with an entirely different etiology than AD, notably FTLD and subcortical ischemic vascular dementia (SIVD). Specifically SIVD, a syndrome associated with cerebrovascular origins for neurodegeneration and therefore with practical treatment options in contrast to AD or FTLD, can be difficult to differentiate from the dementias based on clinical assessment alone. In contrast to AD and FTLD, however, brain imaging studies have not found coherent regional patterns of brain atrophy or perfusion alterations in SIVD, although changes in frontal lobe regions have been reported. It is conceivable that ASL-MRI might aid in the differential diagnosis between all three major forms of dementias (AD, FTLD, SIVD).

Aiming to distinguish AD and FTLD, one study investigated differences in the regional perfusion pattern between AD and the bvFTD variant of FTLD

[25]. ASL-MRI revealed reduced perfusion in the frontal cortex in bvFTD, whereas perfusion in parietal and occipital brain regions remained normal, in contrast to perfusion changes in AD. Imaging measures of frontal perfusion and gray matter atrophy together significantly improved accuracy in classifying correctly bvFTD patients and control subjects over classifications using each measure alone. Using these measures 74% of the subjects could be correctly classified. Similarly, the differential classification between patients with bvFTD and those with AD improved when parietal perfusion and gray matter atrophy were used together, reaching 75% accuracy. The addition of frontal and parietal lobe perfusion further improved classification between patients with bvFTD and those with AD, reaching 87% accuracy.

A study aiming to distinguish between SIVD and AD compared regional perfusion variations using ASL-MRI [29]. This study also aimed to determine the relationship between reduced perfusion in cortical regions and SIVD, indicated by white matter lesions on MRI. Both SIVD and AD generally exhibit various amounts of white matter pathology. Previous PET and SPECT studies in SIVD reported a patchy pattern of regional reduction in cerebral perfusion, in contrast to AD, though more characteristic alterations of perfusion in SIVD have been reported [30–34]. It was found that there were marked reductions in perfusion in both frontal and parietal brain regions in SIVD patients compared with controls. Furthermore, reduced perfusion of the cortex strongly correlated with the extent of subcortical white matter lesions in agreement with PET findings in SIVD [35, 36]. However, the difference in regional perfusion patterns between SIVD and AD was difficult to interpret, because many patients diagnosed with SIVD can have mixed AD/SIVD pathology and diagnosis was not confirmed by autopsy in this study.

In summary, ASL-MRI studies capture patterns of abnormal regional brain perfusion that may sometimes be helpful in the differentiation of different neurodegenerative diseases. The abnormal patterns seen with ASL-MRI are generally similar to those seen on functional PET and SPECT scans. ASL-MRI also improved differentiation between patients and control subjects, as well as between different neurodegenerative diseases compared to classifications based on structural MRI alone. Although more studies involving a large number of subjects are warranted to validate and generalize these results, the preliminary results suggest perfusion MRI has clinical value in the diagnosis of neurodegenerative disorders.

Additional considerations

Added value of ASL-MRI

An important consideration for clinical applications of ASL-MRI is the value added by perfusion imaging to characterizing neurodegenerative diseases relative to the value of other image modalities, specifically structural MRI. Although there is not yet a definite outcome in this regard, joint studies analyzing ASL-MRI and structural MRI together have provided valuable information about the benefit of perfusion imaging. One investigation [37] aimed to determine if ASL-MRI and structural MRI provide complementary or simply redundant information. To address this issue, a non-parametric statistical framework was developed that allowed testing voxel-wise dissociations between perfusion and structural imaging data. Findings of dissociations (as well as concordance) between changes in brain structure and perfusion in AD are illustrated in Figure 9.3. Results from a separate analysis of structural MRI and ASL-MRI data are shown in panel (a) of Figure 9.3. Clusters of significant structural and perfusion changes in the brain can overlap, but the overlap is difficult to interpret since separate analyses provide no information on how variations in one image modality relate to variations in the other. More information can be obtained by analyzing the data together. Testing for dissociations, it was found that in AD perfusion reduction without significant gray matter loss in frontal brain regions was observed, as illustrated in Figure 9.3c. In contrast, gray matter loss without perfusion reduction occurred primarily in parietal brain regions in AD, including the posterior cingulate cortex, as seen in Figure 9.3d. The results are consistent with studies comparing structural MRI and perfusion SPECT data [38]. More importantly, the results demonstrate that ASL-perfusion provides complementary information to that from structural MRI. For comparison, the distribution of concordant gray matter loss and hypoperfusion in AD is shown in Figure 9.3b. More studies are warranted to determine the clinical relevance of dissociations between brain structure and perfusion.

Another study extended observations of perfusion/structural dissociation/concordance to bvFTD patients [39]. Using the same statistical methods as

before [37], it was found that gray matter loss without significant perfusion reduction occurred in premotor regions in bvFTD and concordant alterations occurred in frontal lobe regions. No regions with reduced perfusion in absence of gray matter loss were found. This contrasts with the dissociation pattern seen in AD. Whether gray matter loss without perfusion reduction is a characteristic observation for bvFTD or simply the result of limited power to detect perfusion alterations is currently a matter of debate and more studies are needed for clarification.

More recently, an alternative approach was used to determine the joint contribution of structural and perfusion imaging for group classifications [40]. In a cross-sectional study that included 24 patients diagnosed with AD and 38 cognitively normal subjects, an integrated multimodality MRI processing framework for the joint evaluation of structural and perfusion MRI data was used. Changes of cortical thickness and perfusion were mapped to a cortical surface, thereby simplifying computations for statistics [41]. Logistic regressions were employed to determine sequentially the classification power of cortical thickness, cortical perfusion, and the interaction between the two measures. In this particular population sample, cortical thinning dominated the correct classification of AD patients and controls, with only moderate contributions from perfusion data. However, in the superior temporal sulcus there was a significant positive interaction between reduced perfusion and cortical thinning in AD, consistent with the idea that alterations in structure and perfusion provide complementary information. The main results from this study are illustrated in Figure 9.4. The parametric maps on the left side of Figure 9.4 show the contribution of regional variations in perfusion to the classification of AD patients versus controls, while the maps on the right side show the statistical significance of the contributions for solving the classification problem. It can be seen that hypoperfusion bilaterally in posterior brain regions, including the precuneus and posterior cingulate, made significant contributions to the classification. One might expect that when brain atrophy is less severe than in AD, perfusion might play an even greater role for the classification of neurodegenerative diseases.

Another study combining analysis of structural MRI, ASL-MRI, and diffusion tensor MRI was used in order to separate the contributions of each modality for the differentiation of AD and bvFTD

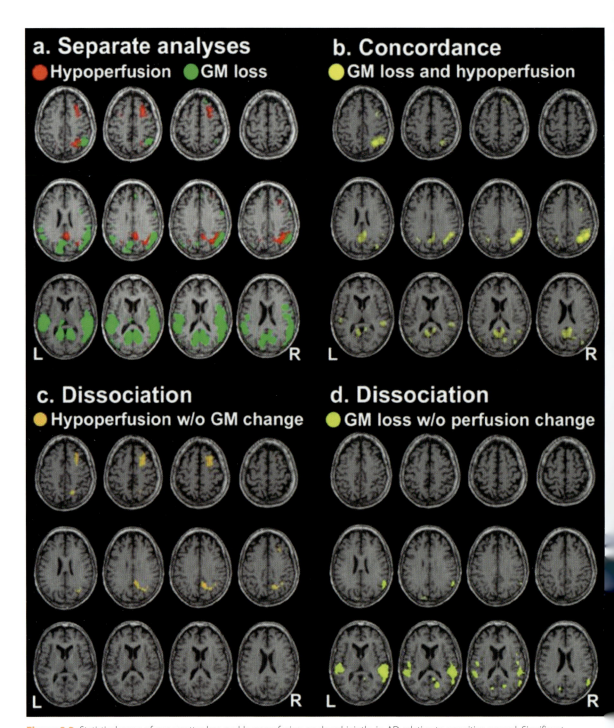

Figure 9.3 Statistical maps of gray matter loss and hypoperfusion, analyzed jointly, in AD relative to cognitive normal. Significant voxels are contained within clusters at a cluster level of $p = 0.05$ after permutation tests. (a) For reference, results from conventional separate analysis of gray matter (GM) loss (green) and hypoperfusion (red) in AD. (b) Analysis of concordant alterations in gray matter loss and hypoperfusion in AD. (c) Analysis of dissociation between significant hypoperfusion without gray matter loss in AD. (d) Analysis of dissociation between significant gray matter loss without hypoperfusion in AD. Reproduced from Hayasaka *et al.* [37] with permission from Elsevier Inc.

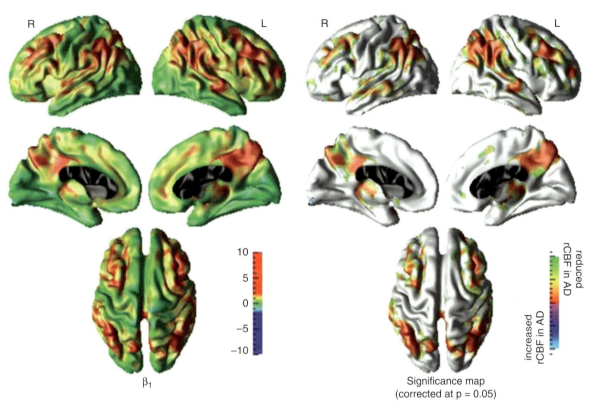

Figure 9.4 Statistical maps of the power of perfusion to correctly classify AD patients and control subjects using voxel-wise logistic regression. The contribution of perfusion (β_1) to the classification is shown region by region in the left panel. Warmer colors indicate more contributions. The statistical significance of the contributions is shown in the right panel. Regions with highly significant contributions are shown in green to red, with non-significant regions left transparent. rCBF, regional cerebral blood flow.

patients [26]. The study included 20 patients with AD, 20 patients with bvFTD, and 20 control subjects. A joint analysis of structural, perfusion, and diffusion MRI data provided several interesting results. First, it was found that AD and bvFTD differ with respect to relative damage of white matter to the damage in gray matter, aside from the different regional patterns of brain atrophy and perfusion. Specifically, bvFTD was associated overall with greater white matter damage than AD relative to the same amount of gray matter damage for each disease. This was also reflected by varying contributions of each MRI modality (structural, perfusion, and diffusion MRI) to the characterization of each disease. In bvFTD, for example, where white matter damage was more prominent than in AD, ASL-MRI was less relevant than the other two MRI modalities for the characterization of disease than in AD. However, this picture also changed with disease severity and perfusion measurements generally gained relevance for the characterization of mild stages of disease.

New developments and future directions

ASL is still a field of rapid new developments in data acquisition, image reconstruction, and analysis. Technical improvements from which ASL-MRI studies in neurodegenerative diseases would particularly benefit are gains in sensitivity from more efficient labeling strategies [42, 43], gains from higher magnetic fields (3 T and above), reduction in sensitivity to motion artifacts, as well as from improvements in image reconstruction. Especially, improvements to boost resolution of low-resolution ASL-MRI data at image reconstruction by utilizing information from high-resolution structural MRI [44] are expected to benefit perfusion imaging when brain atrophy is substantial. An example of the level of ASL-MRI quality that is possible today with the co-analysis of structural MRI is illustrated in Figure 9.5. The images from left to right are representative individual ASL perfusion maps from a young control subject (33 years, male), an older control subject (74 years, male), a subject

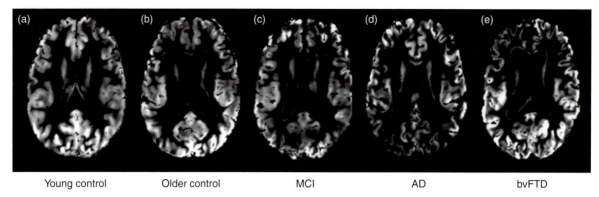

(a)	(b)	(c)	(d)	(e)
Young control	Older control	MCI	AD	bvFTD

Figure 9.5 Individual perfusion maps from ASL-MRI at 4 T after post-processing. The perfusion maps have been corrected for gray matter density and interpolated to the resolution of structural MRI. CBF maps of (a) a young normal volunteer, (b) a cognitively normal older subject, (c) a subject diagnosed with mild cognitive impairment (MCI), (d) a patient with Alzheimer's disease (AD), and (e) a patient with the behavioral variant of frontotemporal dementia (bvFTD) are shown.

classified as having MCI (75 years, male), an AD patient (73 years, male), and a bvFTD patient (63 years, male). Hypoperfusion in parietal brain regions in the AD patient and hypoperfusion in frontal lobe regions in the bvFTD patient are readily visible.

Benefits for MRI perfusion are also expected from more advanced statistical approaches to analyzing the perfusion images. Multivariate statistical approaches, which evaluate variations across brain regions simultaneously as opposed to conventional voxel-by-voxel approaches, are well suited to neurodegenerative diseases, as their abnormalities typically are spread out across the brain. An interesting example performed multivariate statistics to evaluate correlation/covariance of perfusion variations across a large number of brain regions [12]. It was found that there was a significant covariance pattern of regional perfusion reductions in AD patients relative to control subjects that involved the posterior cingulate, parahippocampal, and fusiform gyri as well as the thalamus, hippocampus, and insula. Results based on covariance patterns are also easier to interpret than voxel-wise tests in terms of a signature of functional brain networks [45].

Lastly, the possibility to distinguish with high confidence an abnormal perfusion pattern based on ASL-MRI in a single subject is especially interesting in the context of diagnosis. So far, such attempts have failed for neurodegenerative diseases. However, studies are under way comparing the consistency of radiological readings based on ASL-MRI with those based on PET data for diagnosis. For quantitative image assessments, advances in machine learning and pattern recognition methods, such as support vector machine algorithms [46, 47], which have been used successfully for classifications of AD and MCI at the single subject level based on structural MRI, are expected to be also useful for the analysis of perfusion images.

Conclusion

In summary, most neurodegenerative diseases exhibit a characteristic pattern of abnormal regional perfusion variations, which can be captured using ASL-MRI. Furthermore, the abnormal perfusion patterns based on ASL-MRI are similar to the patterns obtained using functional PET and SPECT scans. Since ASL is a relatively rapid add-on to a conventional MRI scan and is completely non-invasive and does not involve radiation, it compares favorably to these nuclear medicine studies in terms of cost and risks. The perfusion patterns also provide complementary information to imaging of brain atrophy, thereby improving the classification of neurodegenerative diseases. Taken together, ASL-MRI provides an attractive approach to study brain perfusion in neurodegenerative diseases. ASL-MRI has potential clinical applications for aiding early diagnosis of neurodegenerative diseases, monitoring disease progression, and evaluating treatment interventions, once treatment becomes available.

Acknowledgements

I am indebted to Dr. Gil Rabinovici of the Memory and Aging Center of the University of California in San Francisco for providing the case study of ASL in behavioral variant FTD.

The work was financially supported in part by a grant from the National Center for Research Resources (P41 RR 023953) and by a grant from the Department of Defense and by the Michael J. Fox Foundation for Parkinson's Research. This material is the result of work supported with resources and the use of facilities at the Veterans Affairs Medical Center in San Francisco, with administrative support by the Northern California Institute of Research and Education (NCIRE).

References

1. Matus S, Glimcher LH, Hetz C. Protein folding stress in neurodegenerative diseases: a glimpse into the ER. *Curr Opin Cell Biol* 2011;**23**(2):239–52.

2. Raichle ME. Behind the scenes of functional brain imaging: a historical and physiological perspective. *Proc Natl Acad Sci U S A* 1998;**95**(3):765–72.

3. Szymanski P, Markowicz M, Janik A, Ciesielski M, Mikiciuk-Olasik E. Neuroimaging diagnosis in neurodegenerative diseases. *Nucl Med Rev Cent East Eur.* 2010;**13**(1):23–31.

4. Harris GJ, Lewis RF, Satlin A, *et al.* Dynamic susceptibility contrast MR imaging of regional cerebral blood volume in Alzheimer disease: a promising alternative to nuclear medicine. *AJNR Am J Neuroradiol* 1998;**19**(9):1727–32.

5. Agosta F, Pievani M, Geroldi C, *et al.* Resting state fMRI in Alzheimer's disease: beyond the default mode network. *Neurobiol Aging* 2012;**33**(8):1564–78. Epub 2011/08/03.

6. Ferri CP, Prince M, Brayne C, *et al.* Global prevalence of dementia: a Delphi consensus study. *Lancet* 2005;**366**(9503):2112–17.

7. Sandson TA, O'Connor M, Sperling RA, Edelman RR, Warach S. Noninvasive perfusion MRI in Alzheimer's disease: a preliminary report. *Neurology* 1996;**47**(5):1339–42.

8. Alsop DC, Detre JA, Grossman M. Assessment of cerebral blood flow in Alzheimer's disease by spin-labeled magnetic resonance imaging. *Ann Neurol* 2000;**47**(1):93–100.

9. Johnson NA, Jahng GH, Weiner MW, *et al.* Pattern of cerebral hypoperfusion in Alzheimer disease and mild cognitive impairment measured with arterial spin-labeling MR imaging: initial experience. *Radiology* 2005;**234**(3):851–9.

10. Alsop DC, Casement M, de Bazelaire C, Fong T, Press DZ. Hippocampal hyperperfusion in Alzheimer's disease. *Neuroimage* 2008;**42**(4):1267–74.

11. Dai W, Lopez OL, Carmichael OT, *et al.* Mild cognitive impairment and alzheimer disease: patterns of altered cerebral blood flow at MR imaging. *Radiology* 2009;**250**(3):856–66.

12. Asllani I, Habeck C, Scarmeas N, *et al.* Multivariate and univariate analysis of continuous arterial spin labeling perfusion MRI in Alzheimer's disease. *J Cereb Blood Flow Metab* 2008;**28**(4):725–36.

13. Hu WT, Wang Z, Lee VM, *et al.* Distinct cerebral perfusion patterns in FTLD and AD. *Neurology* 2010;**75**(10):881–8.

14. Braak H, Braak E. Neuropathological staging of Alzheimer-related changes. *Acta Neuropathol* 1991;**82**(4):239–59.

15. Sperling R. Functional MRI studies of associative encoding in normal aging, mild cognitive impairment, and Alzheimer's disease. *Ann N Y Acad Sci* 2007;**1097**:146–55.

16. Yoshiura T, Hiwatashi A, Yamashita K, *et al.* Simultaneous measurement of arterial transit time, arterial blood volume, and cerebral blood flow using arterial spin-labeling in patients with Alzheimer disease. *AJNR Am J Neuroradiol* 2009;**30**(7):1388–93.

17. Liu Y, Rosen H, Miller BL, Weiner MW, Schuff N, editors. Cerebral Blood Perfusion Dynamics in Alzheimer's Disease and Mild Cognitive Impairment Using Discrete Modeling of Arterial Spin Labeling MRI. *Proc Intl Soc Magn Reson Med*, Montreal, Canada, 2011.

18. Scheff SW, Price DA, Schmitt FA, Mufson EJ. Hippocampal synaptic loss in early Alzheimer's disease and mild cognitive impairment. *Neurobiol Aging* 2006;**27**(10):1372–84.

19. Petersen RC, Doody R, Kurz A, *et al.* Current concepts in mild cognitive impairment. *Arch Neurol* 2001;**58**(12):1985–92.

20. Geslani DM, Tierney MC, Herrmann N, Szalai JP. Mild cognitive impairment: an operational definition and its conversion rate to Alzheimer's disease. *Dement Geriatr Cogn Disord* 2005;**19**(5–6):383–9.

21. Chao LL, Pa J, Duarte A, *et al.* Patterns of cerebral hypoperfusion in amnestic and dysexecutive MCI. *Alzheimer Dis Assoc Disord* 2009;**23**(3):245–52.

22. Young K, Du AT, Kramer J, *et al.* Patterns of structural complexity in Alzheimer's disease and frontotemporal dementia. *Hum Brain Mapp* 2009;**30**(5):1667–77.

23. Rosen HJ, Allison SC, Schauer GF, *et al.* Neuroanatomical correlates of behavioural disorders in dementia. *Brain* 2005;**128**(Pt 11):2612–25.

24. Laforce R, Jr., Buteau JP, Paquet N, et al. The value of PET in mild cognitive impairment, typical and atypical/unclear dementias: a retrospective memory clinic study. *Am J Alzheimers Dis Other Demen* 2010;**25**(4):324–32.

25. Du AT, Jahng GH, Hayasaka S, et al. Hypoperfusion in frontotemporal dementia and Alzheimer disease by arterial spin labeling MRI. *Neurology* 2006;**67**(7):1215–20.

26. Zhang Y, Schuff N, Ching C, et al. Joint assessment of structural, perfusion, and diffusion MRI in Alzheimer's disease and frontotemporal dementia. *Int J Alzheimers Dis* 2011;**2011**: 546–871.

27. Kamagata K, Motoi Y, Hori M, et al. Posterior hypoperfusion in Parkinson's disease with and without dementia measured with arterial spin labeling MRI. *J Magn Reson Imaging* 2011;**33**(4):803–7.

28. Fong T, Inouye S, Dai W, Press D, Alsop D. Association cortex hypoperfusion in mild dementia with Lewy bodies: a potential indicator of cholinergic dysfunction? *Brain Imaging Behav* 2011;**5**(1):25–35.

29. Schuff N, Matsumoto S, Kmiecik J, et al. Cerebral blood flow in ischemic vascular dementia and Alzheimer's disease, measured by arterial spin-labeling magnetic resonance imaging. *Alzheimers Dement* 2009;**5**(6):454–62.

30. Deutsch G, Tweedy JR. Cerebral blood flow in severity-matched Alzheimer and multi-infarct patients. *Neurology* 1987;**37**(3):431–8.

31. Tohgi H, Yonezawa H, Takahashi S, et al. Cerebral blood flow and oxygen metabolism in senile dementia of Alzheimer's type and vascular dementia with deep white matter changes. *Neuroradiology* 1998;**40**(3):131–7.

32. Nagata K, Maruya H, Yuya H, et al. Can PET data differentiate Alzheimer's disease from vascular dementia? *Ann N Y Acad Sci* 2000;**903**:252–61.

33. Hanyu H, Shimuzu S, Tanaka Y, et al. Cerebral blood flow patterns in Binswanger's disease: a SPECT study using three-dimensional stereotactic surface projections. *J Neurol Sci* 2004;**220**(1–2):79–84.

34. Shim YS, Yang DW, Kim BS, Shon YM, Chung YA. Comparison of regional cerebral blood flow in two subsets of subcortical ischemic vascular dementia: statistical parametric mapping analysis of SPECT. *J Neurol Sci* 2006;**250**(1–2): 85–91.

35. Tullberg M, Fletcher E, DeCarli C, et al. White matter lesions impair frontal lobe function regardless of their location. *Neurology* 2004;**63**(2):246–53.

36. Kraut MA, Beason-Held LL, Elkins WD, Resnick SM. The impact of magnetic resonance imaging-detected white matter hyperintensities on longitudinal changes in regional cerebral blood flow. *J Cereb Blood Flow Metab* 2008;**28**(1):190–7.

37. Hayasaka S, Du AT, Duarte A, et al. A non-parametric approach for co-analysis of multi-modal brain imaging data: application to Alzheimer's disease. *Neuroimage* 2006;**30**(3):768–79.

38. Matsuda H, Kitayama N, Ohnishi T, et al. Longitudinal evaluation of both morphologic and functional changes in the same individuals with Alzheimer's disease. *J Nucl Med* 2002;**43**(3):304–11.

39. Shimizu S, Zhang Y, Laxamana J, et al. Concordance and discordance between brain perfusion and atrophy in frontotemporal dementia. *Brain Imaging Behav* 2010;**4**(1):46–54.

40. Tosun D, Mojabi P, Weiner MW, Schuff N. Joint analysis of structural and perfusion MRI for cognitive assessment and classification of Alzheimer's disease and normal aging. *Neuroimage* 2010;**52**(1):186–97.

41. Tosun D, Schuff N, Weiner M. An integrated multimodality MR brain imaging study: gray matter tissue loss mediates the association between cerebral hypoperfusion and Alzheimer's disease. *Conf Proc IEEE Eng Med Biol Soc* 2009;**1**:6981–4.

42. Dai W, Garcia D, de Bazelaire C, Alsop DC. Continuous flow driven inversion for arterial spin labeling using pulsed radiofrequency and gradient fields. *Magn Reson Med* 2008;**60**(6):1488–97.

43. Nezamzadeh M, Matson GB, Young K, Weiner MW, Schuff N. Improved pseudo-continuous arterial spin labeling for mapping brain perfusion. *J Magn Reson Imaging* 2010;**31**(6):1419–27.

44. Kornak J, Young K, Schuff N, et al. K-Bayes reconstruction for perfusion MRI. I: concepts and application. *J Digit Imaging* 2009;**23**(3):277–86.

45. Habeck C, Rakitin BC, Moeller J, et al. An event-related fMRI study of the neural networks underlying the encoding, maintenance, and retrieval phase in a delayed-match-to-sample task. *Brain Res Cogn Brain Res* 2005;**23**(2–3): 207–20.

46. Davatzikos C, Resnick SM, Wu X, Parmpi P, Clark CM. Individual patient diagnosis of AD and FTD via high-dimensional pattern classification of MRI. *Neuroimage* 2008;**41**(4):1220–7.

47. Stonnington CM, Chu C, Kloppel S, et al. Predicting clinical scores from magnetic resonance scans in Alzheimer's disease. *Neuroimage* 2010;**51**(4):1405–13.

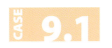

ASL in behavioral variant of frontotemporal dementia

History

A 67-year-old right-handed man with a 5-year history of behavioral changes including impulsivity, disinhibition, disorganization, poor judgment, apathy, poor self-hygiene, loss of empathy, craving for sweets, and compulsive behaviors. His neurologic examination revealed poor insight, perseveration, echolalia, stereotypy of speech, repetitive motor behaviors, and utilization behaviors. Neuropsychological testing showed marked impairment in executive function.

Technique

Continuous ASL with multi-slice single-shot echo-planar imaging, acquired at 4 T. 10 mm labeling slab, 2 s labeling time with 1 s post-label delay.

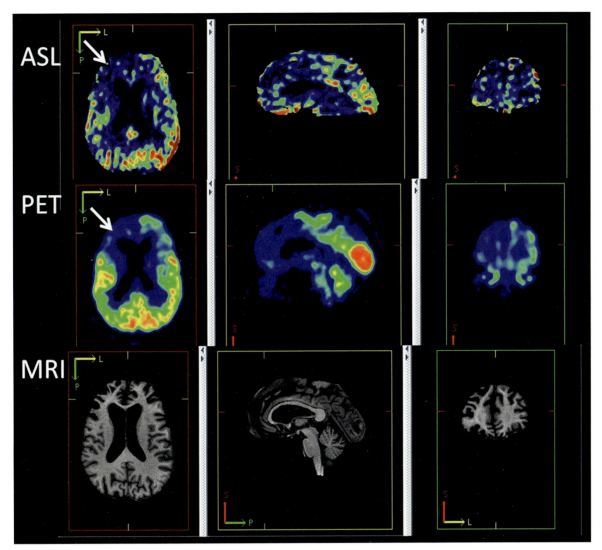

Figure 9.6 ASL-MRI showed marked hypoperfusion of the right lateral and mesial frontal cortex (arrow, top row). Perfusion of the parietal cortex was normal. Only a mild degree of atrophy was present on structural MRI in the frontal regions (bottom row). The FDG-PET glucose metabolic map (middle row) mirrors the pattern of hypoperfusion seen on ASL.

177

Imaging findings

See Figure 9.6.

Discussion

Selective unilateral hypoperfusion of the frontal lobe with normal perfusion of parietal lobe regions reflects the characteristic pattern of abnormal perfusion for the behavioral variant of frontotemporal dementia (bvFTD). Lack of major brain atrophy and normal perfusion of parietal lobe regions makes AD less likely. The mirroring of the hypoperfusion pattern with FDG-PET, showing diminished glucose metabolism in regions of hypoperfusion, further supports the diagnosis of bvFTD.

Key points

- Unilateral frontal lobe hypoperfusion is characteristic for bvFTD.
- The similarity between ASL-MRI perfusion and FDG-PET supports the use of ASL-MRI for clinical assessments of dementia.

MR perfusion imaging in clinical neuroradiology

Blake E. McGehee, Joseph A. Maldjian, and Jonathan Burdette

Key points

- Radiological pattern recognition aids with characterization when MR perfusion imaging is incorporated into routine clinical neuroimaging.
- Perfusion imaging is useful to categorize perfusion changes into either global or focal and either hypo- or hyperperfusion.
- More than one pattern can be present in a given patient.
- Several of the more common clinical entities can display patterns of both hypo- and hyperperfusion, and the patterns often vary temporally.
- Artifact should always be considered in the differential diagnosis of a perfusion abnormality.

Introduction

While the earliest uses of MR perfusion imaging were primarily in oncological and neurovascular imaging, increasingly MR perfusion has shown its utility both in research and clinical practice in a large range of both normal physiological states and pathological conditions. MR perfusion improves disease characterization, and with the growing number of entities studied, it becomes useful and at times necessary to categorize perfusion patterns. Changes in brain perfusion parameters can loosely be grouped into either global or focal, and either hypo- or hyperperfusion (Table 10.1). Though it is useful to employ such a categorization scheme, several of the more common disease states can demonstrate both hypo- and hyperperfusion patterns, which can be seen synchronously or vary temporally (reflective of the underlying

pathophysiology). This chapter will describe the typical perfusion patterns in the more commonly encountered physiological states and pathological conditions, primarily with an emphasis on the use of arterial spin labeling (ASL) techniques. Oncological and stroke imaging will only be discussed for completeness where appropriate, but are otherwise detailed in dedicated chapters (Chapters 11 and 8, respectively).

Global hypoperfusion

Brain death

Accurate diagnosis of brain death is paramount. A false positive in the setting of a patient with a chance of reasonable recovery is a disastrous outcome. For this reason and others, brain death criteria have been in existence for some time. There is institutional variation, but the primary criteria are based on clinical data, physical and neurological examination, apnea testing, period of observation, and ancillary testing [1]. Accordingly, neuroimaging studies fall in the category of "ancillary testing."

It is accepted that an absence of brain perfusion equates to brain death. Imaging confirmation of absent perfusion has traditionally been performed using nuclear medicine techniques, which remain the gold standard [2, 3]. Small studies have indicated that MRI and MR angiography (MRA) are sensitive tests for the diagnosis of brain death, based on morphological changes from brain edema and absence of intracranial arterial signal on MRA [4, 5]. Loss of flow-related enhancement on MRA occurs when the intracranial pressure exceeds mean arterial pressure (usually due to cerebral edema) and perfusion to the brain ceases. Also, no contrast will be seen in the brain following

Table 10.1. Non-oncological, neurological conditions which may involve either global or focal perfusion abnormalities. Some conditions may exhibit either hypo- or hyperperfusion.

	Global	Focal
Hypoperfusion	<ul><li>Brain death</li><li>Decreased cardiac output</li><li>Cerebral volume loss/atrophy</li></ul>	<ul><li>Stroke</li><li>Vasculitis/vasospasm</li><li>Seizures</li><li>PRES</li><li>Migraine</li><li>Infection</li><li>Hematoma</li><li>Remote insult</li><li>Neurodegenerative disorders</li></ul>
Hyperperfusion	<ul><li>Pediatrics</li><li>Hyperdynamic cardiac states</li><li>Anoxic brain injury</li><li>Hypercapnia</li></ul>	<ul><li>Stroke</li><li>Seizures</li><li>PRES</li><li>Post carotid endarterectomy</li><li>Multiple sclerosis</li><li>Infection and inflammation</li></ul>

PRES, posterior reversible encephalopathy syndrome.

gadolinium administration. With these changes in mind, it is not unexpected that perfusion changes will be seen with MR perfusion techniques. Given that dynamic susceptibility contrast (DSC)-MRI perfusion relies on passage of a gadolinium bolus – and as outlined, the transit of contrast is absent in brain death – this technique has limited utility in the context of brain death. It may provide ancillary evidence supporting brain death in that the time–signal curves should be flat, but in isolation, this is not enough to support brain death as a final diagnosis. ASL techniques, on the other hand, are useful primarily because of the ability to quantify cerebral blood flow (CBF). Reductions of CBF below various thresholds can result in neuronal dysfunction (< 20 ml/100 g/min) and subsequently death (< 10–12 ml/100 g/min) [6, 7]. ASL can graphically depict absent blood flow as well as quantify the flow expected to result in brain death (Figure 10.1).

Decreased cardiac output

With the difficulties inherent in quantifying CBF using DSC perfusion techniques, global changes in cerebral perfusion may be difficult to detect using tracer-kinetic model approaches. Furthermore, while ASL can quantify CBF, one of its major limitations in clinical use arises from the wide range of transit times of arterial blood. Therefore, both techniques are suboptimal when considering the wide range of

pathologies – heart failure, arrhythmias, valvular disease, etc. – that may reduce global cerebral perfusion. It is likely that the common clinical ASL applications underestimate CBF in such scenarios. Utilizing a tagging plane near the brain or velocity-selective ASL techniques may reduce the bulk flow effects in these conditions [8]. Alternatively, combined DSC and ASL techniques, in which the ASL measurement is used to provide a patient-specific scaling factor for the DSC CBF maps, may enable more quantitative CBF measurements in such patients [9].

Cerebral volume loss/atrophy

Cerebral volume loss and subsequent enlargement of the subarachnoid spaces, whether age-related or secondary to neurodegenerative disorders, is a common cause of globally decreased cerebral perfusion in a typical clinical population. Age-related reductions of gray matter perfusion in the order of 0.45–0.7% per year are well known [10–12]. Studies have also shown gender discrepancies, with average CBF values in female subjects typically between 10% and 40% higher for both whole-brain and gray matter perfusion values relative to age-matched men; a study using continuous arterial spin labeling (CASL) demonstrated a 13% difference between genders [12]. With the various neurodegenerative disorders, which typically occur in a more elderly

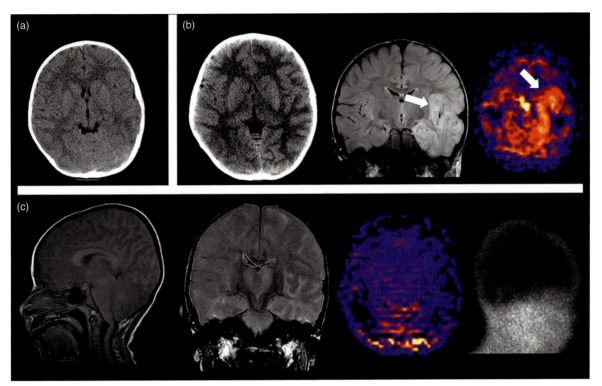

Figure 10.1 A 7-year-old boy presenting with persistent fever and generalized tonic-clonic seizures two weeks following IV antibiotic treatment for pneumonia. (a) Head CT on admission is normal. (b) One day after admission, repeat head CT (left), coronal FLAIR (center), and ASL CBF perfusion map (right). The head CT demonstrates marked generalized edema throughout the white matter. Similar changes are seen on FLAIR imaging involving the left temporal lobe and hippocampus. There is focal hyperperfusion in the left temporal lobe (arrow) but perfusion is otherwise normal. (c) Studies obtained on admission day 3, from left to right – sagittal T1, coronal FLAIR, ASL CBF map, and technetium 99m-ECD brain scintigraphy. The sagittal T1 image demonstrates marked generalized cerebral edema with T1 prolongation and tonsillar herniation. Progressive edema is also identified on the coronal FLAIR imaging within the subcortical white matter and thalami. These areas showed restricted diffusion on diffusion-weighted imaging (DWI) (not shown). There is a marked decrease in CBF as evaluated using ASL, with absolute CBF of < 5 ml/100 g/min. The nuclear medicine study confirms brain death. The final diagnosis was auto-immune necrotizing encephalitis.

population, areas of focal hypoperfusion may be superimposed on a background of generally decreased cerebral perfusion, as would be expected with aging (Figure 10.2). More specific patterns of perfusion imaging in neurodegenerative disorders are detailed in Chapter 9.

Focal hypoperfusion

Stroke

The use of MR perfusion in neurovascular disease and stroke is comprehensively described in Chapter 8 and is mentioned here simply for completeness. Completed infarcts can appear as focal or regional hypoperfusion, but often exhibit a mixed pattern, combining regions of persistent hypoperfusion with other regions of hyperperfusion (sometimes called

"luxury perfusion"). For areas of focal hypoperfusion in stroke, DSC perfusion will typically show matched relative CBV (rCBV) decrease (although sometimes CBV increases occur with compensatory vasodilatation) and increase in transit times. Similarly, with ASL, areas of focally decreased CBF can be seen, which might originate in part from transit time effects. A diffusion abnormality confirms an acute infarction in either case.

Vasculitis/vasospasm

Whether primary or secondary, with its protean manifestations, the diagnosis of central nervous system (CNS) vasculitis can be difficult. Secondary CNS vasculitis can result from systemic vasculitides (such as polyarteritis nodosa, Behçet's disease, Wegner's granulomatosis, or cryoglobulinemic

181

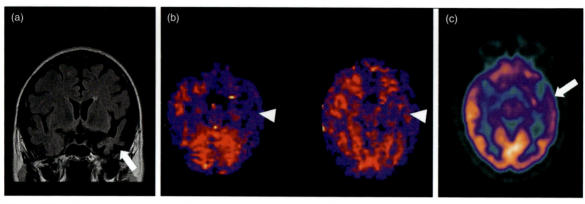

Figure 10.2 A 60-year-old man with several years of slowly progressive word-finding difficulty. His clinical diagnosis following neuropsychological testing and neuroimaging was progressive fluent aphasia, also known as semantic dementia or the temporal variant. (a) FLAIR demonstrates marked asymmetric volume loss within the left temporal lobe without signal abnormality (arrow). (b) ASL images show focal hypoperfusion within the left temporal lobe (arrowheads). (c) Axial ^{18}F-fluorodeoxyglucose (FDG) PET image shows corresponding focal hypometabolism in the same region (arrow). These imaging findings are consistent with the clinical diagnosis of primary fluent aphasia.

vasculitis), connective tissue diseases (such as systemic lupus erythematosus, rheumatoid arthritis, Sjogren's syndrome, mixed connective tissue disease, or dermatomyositis/polymyositis), and infections (neurosyphilis, Lyme disease, HIV, etc.). In the primary form, vasculitis patients often present with diffuse neurologic dysfunction; other common symptoms include decreased cognition, headache, seizure, and stroke [13]. An important consideration in the patient with suspected vasculitis is the reversible cerebral vasoconstrictive syndrome (RCVS, Figure 10.3). RCVS is typically distinguished from CNS vasculitis based on patient demographics, symptomatology, absence of inflammatory markers in the cerebrospinal fluid (CSF), and reversibility (usually) of angiographic findings [14]. Vasculitis and RCVS often involves regions of focal hypoperfusion in multiple vascular territories. A working differential for the vasculitis/RCVS patient may include CNS neoplasm, metastatic disease, and infection, entities that are often associated with at least mild hyperperfusion. Thus, perfusion imaging may help formulate a more reasonable differential diagnosis for the patient ultimately suffering from vasculitis or RCVS.

It is critical to note, that for ASL techniques, these perfusion patterns assume the use of crusher gradients to null residual tagged signal in vessels (as from slow-flow states) as already discussed in Chapters 3 and 8. Many ASL implementations, however, do not use crusher gradients. As such, areas with delayed arterial arrival times – such as in stroke,

Moyamoya disease, and presumably vasculitides – can show peripheral areas of high signal representing slow flow in cortical vessels.

Following intracranial aneurysm rupture, prognosis is related to the presenting neurologic (Hunt and Hess) grade, patient age, and the amount and distribution of blood on admission CT (Fisher scale), among other factors [15]. Vasospasm with associated stroke during hospitalization is present in 20–30% of patients with ruptured aneurysms, and is associated with significant morbidity [16]. As such, much effort has been invested in its early detection and treatment. A consolidated imaging approach for post-subarachnoid hemorrhage vasospasm does not currently exist, but with increased recognition of CT-related radiation exposures, often further augmented by diagnostic and interventional X-ray catheter angiographic procedures, MR perfusion approaches will likely increase in importance. Prior studies have demonstrated perfusion changes following subarachnoid hemorrhage [17]. The role of perfusion data in the management of the asymptomatic vasospasm patient is not established, but it may one day allow a more aggressive treatment strategy, perhaps based on the same diffusion-weighted imaging-perfusion-weighted imaging (DWI-PWI) mismatch paradigm as in acute ischemic stroke. More detail regarding perfusion changes in vasospasm can be found in Chapter 8. Finally, it should be recognized that global perfusion can be further reduced if intracranial pressure rises in the setting of intra-ventricular hemorrhage and hydrocephalus.

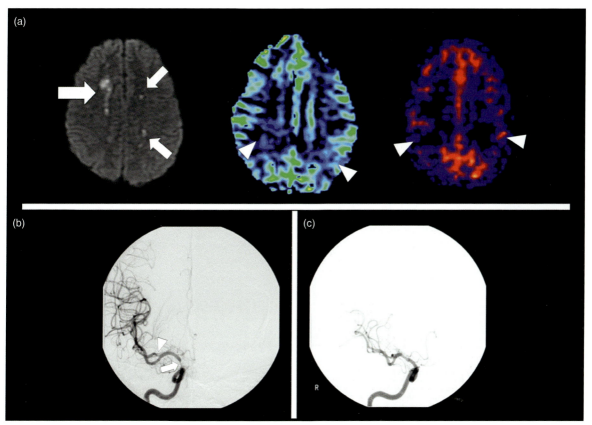

Figure 10.3 A 37-year-old woman presenting with headache, multiple focal neurologic symptoms, delirium, and chorea. She had a small amount of right frontal subarachnoid hemorrhage on initial CT (not shown). (a) Diffusion imaging (left) demonstrates infarcts in multiple vascular territories, several of which are within watershed regions. DSC perfusion relative cerebral blood volume (CBV) map (center) and ASL CBF map (right) both depict focal areas of decreased perfusion (arrowheads). B) AP projection digital subtraction angiography (DSA) image from a right internal carotid artery (ICA) injection shows multiple areas of high-grade concentric vessel stenosis, including the ICA terminus (arrow), right A1, and a proximal M2 branch (arrowhead). Note the severely diminished opacification of the arterior cerebral artery (ACA) territories. (c) Follow-up angiogram 4 months later shows marked improvement in these areas. There is, however, persistent diminished flow in the ACA territories. The patient reported heavy marijuana use. Erythrocyte sedimentation rate, HIV testing, viral hepatitis panel, rapid plasma reagent testing for syphilis, and CSF studies were negative. Based on the presentation, laboratory testing, and significant improvement angiographically, the patient was diagnosed with RCVS.

Seizures

The typical imaging workup for seizure includes structural brain MRI with contrast, inter-ictal single-photon emission computed tomography (SPECT) or positron emission tomography (PET), and ictal SPECT. As SPECT brain imaging is a surrogate marker of perfusion, MR perfusion is correlative. Since all seizure patients should receive brain MRI, it is extremely useful to include routine perfusion imaging, which can yield functional information without ionizing radiation.

During the inter-ictal phase, focal hypoperfusion has been observed in epileptogenic foci and adjacent territories (Figure 10.4). This observation has been well established through investigations of inter-ictal SPECT. Whether inter-ictal hypoperfusion or ictal/peri-ictal hyperperfusion is better in predicting a seizure focus has not been conclusively established [18]. While hypoperfusion can be demonstrated in the post-ictal period, it is more difficult to diagnose cases of established mesial temporal sclerosis with MR perfusion. This is because of susceptibility artifact and the proximity of the hippocampal formations to the skull base.

The simultaneous use of blood oxygenation level-dependent (BOLD) and MR perfusion techniques has allowed the investigation of neurovascular coupling in seizures patients. Decreases in BOLD signal within

183

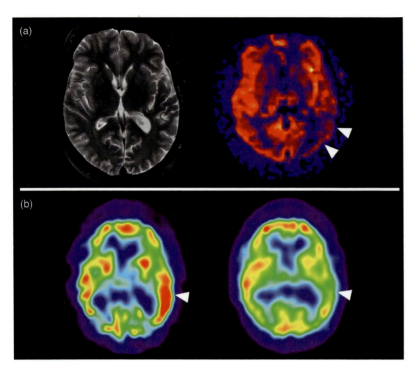

Figure 10.4 MR perfusion imaging in a patient with medically refractory seizures. EEG testing localized the seizure activity to the left temporal lobe. (a) T2 image (left) demonstrates subtle volume loss in the left hemisphere with enlargement of the subarachnoid spaces and atrium of the left lateral ventricle. The left hippocampus was also small (not pictured). Inter-ictal ASL CBF map (right) demonstrates focal hypoperfusion in the posterior left temporal lobe (arrowheads). (b) Ictal SPECT (left) and inter-ictal SPECT (right) demonstrate hyperperfusion and hypoperfusion, respectively (arrowheads), in the posterior left temporal lobe, correlating with the focally decreased perfusion on ASL.

regions of the brain may reflect a decrease in brain metabolic activity simultaneously with decreases in blood flow (coupling) or an increase in oxygen consumption without a corresponding CBF increase (abnormal coupling). Recent research suggests that seizure patients with general spike wave background activity on electroencephalography (EEG) exhibit coupling [19]. Negative BOLD responses correlate well with CBF decreases measured by ASL. This reinforces the notion that inter-ictal regions of brain typically reflect hypoperfusion, and when coupled, ultimately reflects decreased neuronal metabolism.

Posterior reversible encephalopathy syndrome (PRES)

Many etiologies have been linked to the clinical entity of PRES, including hypertension, pre-eclampsia/eclampsia, auto-immune syndromes, renal disease, and drugs (tacrolimus, cyclosporine, etc.). Patients commonly present with encephalopathy, headache, seizure, or visual disturbances [20].

The pathogenesis of PRES has not been fully elucidated and various theories have been proposed. Loss of autoregulation within the posterior circulation is likely present to some extent in all cases, regardless of the exact mechanism. Other proposed mechanisms and/or contributing factors to the pathophysiology include cerebral ischemia and endothelial dysfunction. With less perivascular sympathetic neurons relative to the anterior circulation, the posterior circulation may be more vulnerable to autoregulatory dysfunction. The perfusion changes in PRES mimic pathophysiological observations, and as with other disorders involving the cerebral vasculature, the radiological appearance of PRES can vary with time. Initially, vasoconstriction occurs in response to progressive loss in autoregulation. This can manifest itself as focal hypoperfusion, though this is likely to occur in only severe cases. However, the clinical symptoms that prompt medical attention typically occur later, during the hyperperfused stage of the syndrome. After the initial attempts to maintain perfusion pressures, rebound vasodilatation with focal hyperperfusion can occur, which is associated with reversible vasogenic edema (Figure 10.5). Finally, patients suffering from severe cases of PRES imaged in the subacute phase may progress to show areas of focal hypoperfusion in the occipital and posterior frontal lobes. If the subacute hypoperfusion exceeds

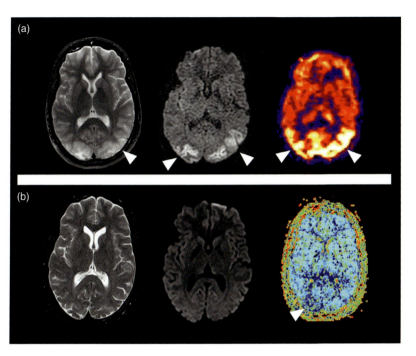

Figure 10.5 A 19-year-old woman with headache several days following elective uterine dilatation and curettage. (a) T2 image (left) demonstrates symmetric T2 prolongation consistent with edema in the parieto-occipital regions (arrowhead). Diffusion image (center) shows moderate reduced diffusion in the areas of edema (arrowheads). ASL CBF image (right) demonstrates marked hyperperfusion in the affected areas of the brain (arrowheads). Average gray matter CBF was 99 ml/100 g/min, which is significantly higher than expected for age. (b) 6 months later, the patient was asymptomatic. The T2 (left) and diffusion (center) images have normalized. DSC-based relative time-to-peak (TTP) map demonstrates subtle but persistent decreased transit times in the right parieto-occipital region (arrowhead). The clinical and imaging findings are consistent with the diagnosis of PRES.

thresholds for neuronal metabolism, either by the duration or magnitude, infarcts can occur.

Aside from the perfusion changes outlined above, there are many "atypical" features of PRES on conventional imaging that are not uncommon, including enhancement; involvement of the basal ganglia, brainstem, and cerebellum; diffusion reduction; hemorrhage [21]. Work has been performed to establish the predictors of reversibility in PRES [22]. Several factors seem to contribute to a poor prognosis, including the extent of T_2 and diffusion abnormalities [23], brainstem involvement, and elevated serum creatinine levels.

Migraine

Migraine is a common ailment, with an estimated incidence of up to 12% in the United States [24]. The classical migraine presents with unilateral headache, phonophobia, photophobia, nausea, and vomiting. Of migraine sufferers, approximately 30% may present with an aura (focal neurologic deficits) prior to headache onset. Auras may be motor, sensory, or both; and in the extreme example may include hemiplegia ("hemiplegic migraine"). With such acute neurologic deficits, neuroimaging is often employed

in evaluation of the sentinel migraine, primarily to exclude acute stroke. If imaged in the aura phase of the migraine, focal hypoperfusion can be seen in the involved cortex using both DSC and ASL [25–27].

Though the exact pathophysiological mechanism of migraine auras is unknown, there are two dominant theories. The first, the vascular theory, proposes that the aura phase is secondary to vasoconstriction, whereas the headache phase is a result of rebound vasodilatation [28]. The alternative theory involves a wave of neuronal depression that spreads through the cortex, generating the aura [29]. The neuronal depression theory suggests that the perfusion changes are reactive to the neuronal changes and not the underlying mechanism of the migraine.

Infection

CNS infections are yet another example of pathology which can demonstrate variable perfusion. There is some evidence that indicates that the majority of infections exhibit more hypoperfusion than hyperperfusion [30]. In the instance of intracranial abscess, the extensive surrounding vasogenic edema will be focally hypoperfused whereas the enhancing rim can demonstrate hyperperfusion. However, mildly increased perfusion can sometimes be seen in the inflammatory region immediately surrounding the abscess.

Spongiform encephalopathy or Creuzfeldt–Jakob disease (CJD) is an infection secondary to prion infiltration of the CNS. The perfusion patterns of CJD have been variable with nuclear medicine studies [31, 32]. A subtype of CJD known as the Heidenhain variant preferentially involves the occipital lobes, parieto-occipital regions, and basal ganglia and cases have been described where perfusion decreases in affected regions precede diffusion or FLAIR signal abnormalities [33]. Most of the work in the perfusion changes with CJD is in nuclear medicine and MR perfusion data are scarce. Nevertheless, case examples exist of MR perfusion changes that mimic findings from nuclear medicine studies (Figure 10.6).

Hematoma

A focus of "hypoperfusion" seen on ASL or DSC-MRI secondary to parenchymal intracranial hematoma (ICH) typically represents an artifact, since most perfusion imaging sequences are acquired using fast imaging techniques such as gradient-echo echo-planar imaging (EPI), which are very sensitive to variations in magnetic susceptibility. In the presence of a large clot, the local signal is spoiled and the tagged or bolus-related decline in signal intensity can often not be detected. Despite this, peri-hematoma regions may often be evaluable using DSC imaging, and it has been concluded that there is prolonged T_{max} surrounding the hematoma, and that this is more common in patients with some degree of diffusion abnormality surrounding the

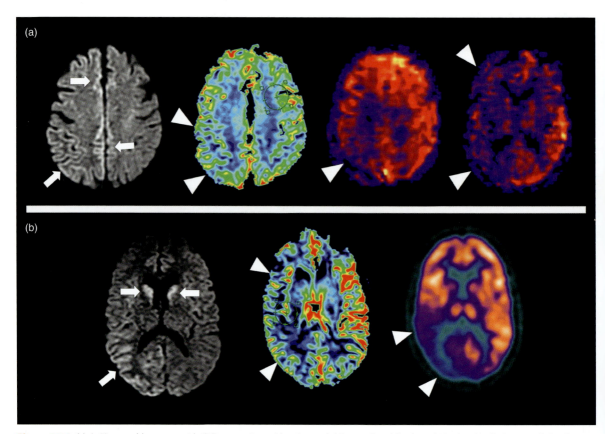

Figure 10.6 (a) A 68-year-old woman with CJD presenting with a 1-month history of rapidly progressive ataxia, dizziness, and visual hallucinations. From left to right, axial diffusion, rCBV map from DSC perfusion study, and two ASL CBF images show areas of, respectively, reduced diffusion throughout the right hemispheric cortex (arrows) with corresponding decreased perfusion (arrowheads). The perfusion changes are more dramatic on ASL imaging. (b) A 51-year-old man with ataxia, balance problems, and "brain fog." His EEG was consistent with prion disease. Diffusion (left), rCBV DSC perfusion map (center), and brain PET (right) demonstrate reduced diffusion in the posterior hemispheres, right greater than left, and the caudate heads bilaterally (arrows). There is corresponding reduced perfusion on both MRI and PET (arrowheads). This distribution and the clinical presentation are consistent with the Heidenhain variant of CJD.

hematoma [34]. It has also been suggested that this hypoperfusion may be related to aggressive blood pressure reduction following ICH. ASL techniques also using EPI or other gradient-echo readouts (Chapter 3) may give erroneously low flow values in hematomas. ASL techniques that use spin-echo or fast-spin-echo readouts may give more accurate perfusion measurements in such settings (Figure 10.7).

Remote insult

Areas of prior brain injury (i.e., gliosis or encephalomalacia), whether from trauma, ischemia, infection, surgery, or other mechanism, will exhibit focal hypoperfusion. In the context of ischemia, it is important to correlate anatomical data with perfusion findings for infarct aging. This is particularly critical for interpreting acute stroke DWI-PWI studies, so as not to overestimate the amount of tissue at risk.

Global hyperperfusion

Pediatrics

Most recently with ASL studies, CBF changes during normal childhood have been demonstrated in multiple studies [35, 36]. CBF typically increases from birth and peaks in early childhood (ranging from 5 to 12 years of age), after which there is a decline in CBF to adult levels (Figure 10.8 and Chapter 16). Recent ASL studies show that the decline from preadolescent peak to adult levels is fairly rapid, but this has not been validated with other techniques. Normal physiological global hyperperfusion in a pediatric patient should not be misinterpreted as pathology. After a long plateau, whole-brain and gray matter CBF declines at a predictable rate in the adult. Also, some of the hyperperfusion seen in pediatric populations might be related to slightly misaligned values for blood and tissue relaxation rates, for example, if a general perfusion analysis package is used, as in the case of Figure 10.8. More details regarding the use of perfusion imaging in pediatric patients can be found in Chapter 16.

Hyperdynamic cardiovascular states (including sickle cell anemia)

The range of normal gray matter CBF for a healthy adult is between 40 and 70 ml/100 g/min [37]. Higher CBF values have been observed clinically in the absence of pathologies such as those discussed below. This may be seen in patients with inherently robust CBF as a consequence of high cardiac index, such as the young patient population or well-conditioned athletes. There are, however, pathological states that generate increased CBF as a consequence of a hyperdynamic cardiovascular state. The prototypical example is sickle cell anemia. Conventional and perfusion MRI studies are both valuable in the management of these patients. Brain infarcts (symptomatic and clinically silent) and perfusion disturbances all complicate the care of these patients. Perfusion imaging can demonstrate focal hypoperfusion within infarcts, typically with a background of global hyperperfusion that is related to the underlying sickle cell disease. Furthermore, in sickle cell patients, there is an inverse relationship between CBF and neurocognitive function [38, 39]. Though not validated, there is some indication that the degree of anemia and CBF values can be used to monitor treatment efficacy, with the ultimate goal of delaying neurocognitive decline (Figure 10.9) [40].

Anoxic brain injury

Varied and serious alterations in cerebral metabolism occur following significant reduction of CBF in the setting of hypoxic-ischemic insult. Brain regions with increased metabolic demand, such as the basal ganglia and cerebral cortex, may infarct [41]. Various techniques have been employed to study CBF following anoxic brain injury (ABI), including CT perfusion, SPECT, and PET, with mixed results [42, 43]. Since these patients typically receive brain MRI studies, the incorporation of MR perfusion into the evaluation of ABI is not only convenient, but also helpful for establishing the diagnosis. Studies have been performed investigating the physiology of autoregulation and the mechanism by which autoregulation is lost in brain anoxia [44, 45]. The central premise of autoregulation is that CBF = CPP / CVR, where CPP is the perfusion pressure and CVR is cerebral vascular resistance. In the setting of brain edema, the CPP can be expressed as the difference between the mean arterial pressure (MAP) and the intracranial pressure (ICP); thus, CBF = (MAP – ICP) / CVR. If the brain arterioles remain capable of dilatation and constriction, thus modulating CVR, then a wide range of MAP/ICP combinations can be counteracted, and a physiological range of CBF can be maintained.

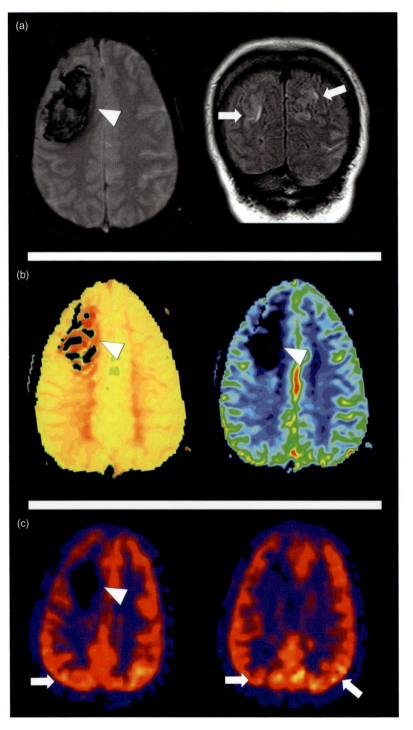

Figure 10.7 (a) Gradient-echo sequence (left) demonstrates susceptibility artifact in the right frontal lobe in a patient with intraparenchymal hemorrhage. Coronal FLAIR (right) image demonstrates focal areas of increased signal, consistent with edema in the posterior parieto-occipital lobe. (b) DSC-based TTP (left) and rCBV (right) images show focal hypoperfusion surrounding the hematoma. This is secondary to signal loss from the paramagnetic blood products. (c) Two ASL CBF images similarly show decreased perfusion in the area of hematoma. Also, note the focal hyperperfusion in the parieto-occipital regions, corresponding to the areas of FLAIR signal abnormality (arrows). These parieto-occipital perfusion changes are more apparent on ASL images compared with DSC. This patient was three days post-operative from emergent Cesarean section for eclampsia. Following surgery, she was markedly hypertensive and presented with a severe headache. Her clinical data and imaging are consistent with spontaneous intraparenchymal hemorrhage and PRES.

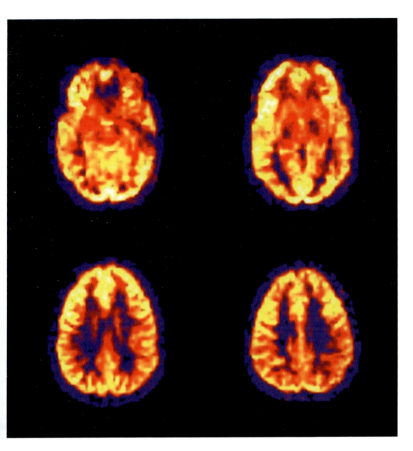

Figure 10.8 A 10-year-old boy imaged for diplopia. No abnormality was detected on the MRI. ASL CBF images show symmetric global "hyperperfusion." The average gray matter CBF was 124 ml/100 g/min. This would be a high level for an adult, but is within the normal range for the patient's age.

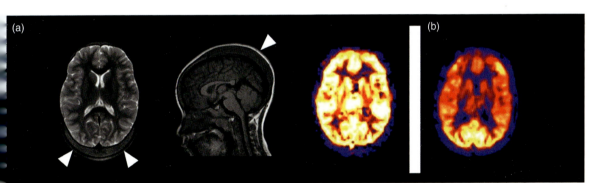

Figure 10.9 (a) This adolescent sickle cell disease patient inconsistently received medical care at the time of this scan. T_2 (left) and sagittal T_1 (center) images depict marked enlargement of the marrow-containing spaces of the calvarium. There is marked symmetric global hyperperfusion on the ASL CBF image (right). The average gray matter CBF was 181 ml/100 g/min. The patient's hemoglobin was 7.1 g/dl with 11% reticulocytes. (b) 21 months later, after regular medical care and hydroxyurea treatment, the ASL CBF image shows less intense global perfusion. The average gray matter CBF decreased to 103 ml/100 g/min. Hemoglobin was 9.6 g/dl with 8% reticulocytes. The ability of ASL to document global changes in perfusion is particularly helpful in such patients to monitor the efficacy of therapies.

Whether the loss of autoregulation is from a myogenic response, neurogenic factors, local metabolites, or a combination thereof, following ABI the CVR falls such that CPP drives the CBF, thus accounting for the super-physiological CBF [46]. While little information on perfusion changes in ABI has been reported, one observational study suggested that CBF was usually high, except in the setting of brain edema and

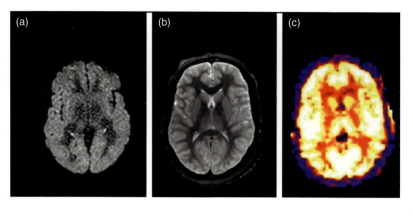

Figure 10.10 A 49-year-old woman who was an unrestrained passenger in a significant motor vehicle collision. She was pulseless at the scene and received CPR. Brain MRI was obtained one day after the accident. (a) No focal signal abnormality is detected on diffusion. (b) T_2-weighted image demonstrates possible subtle diffuse cortical edema, but is otherwise normal. (c) There is marked symmetric global hyperperfusion consistent with anoxic brain injury. The average gray matter CBF was 156 ml/100 g/min. Even more striking, the average white matter CBF was 103 ml/100 g/min.

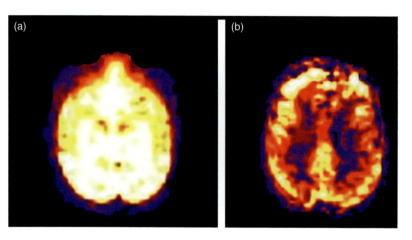

Figure 10.11 (a) An 18-month-old boy with history of premature birth and bronchopulmonary dysplasia. He had elevated pCO_2 levels near the time of the scan, peaking at 64 mmHg (normal range: 35–45 mmHg). The average gray matter CBF measured by ASL was 240 ml/100 g/min. The elevation is likely compounded by the patient's age. (b) A 73-year-old man with chronic obstructive pulmonary disease and heart failure. His pCO_2 at the time of the exam was 73 mmHg. The average gray matter CBF was 109 ml/100 g/min, well above the normal range for an adult man. There were no clinical events in either patient that may have caused a hypoxic/anoxic brain injury.

herniation, in which low or absent CBF was observed [47]. Of eight patients in whom DSC perfusion imaging was performed, only one patient (who had relatively normal CBF) was alive 6 months following the event. Of course, knowledge of the "normal" age values of CBF is extremely helpful for making these distinctions (Figure 10.10).

Hypercapnia

It is well established that hypercapnia is a stimulator of CBF due to the vasodilatory effects of carbon dioxide (CO_2) on the cerebral vasculature [48, 49]. Induction of hypercapnia has been used to evaluate cerebrovascular reserve, which can be useful in the workup of stenotic lesions [50]. Previous studies have demonstrated a wide range of increased CBF when pCO_2 was elevated experimentally. Observations during these studies include a blunted response in the elderly and a slightly greater response in men

[51, 52]. A predictable rise in CBF per mmHg has been derived, ranging from 5.8% to 6.7% CBF increase/mmHg [37, 53, 54]. Given the ability of ASL to measure absolute CBF, it may be better suited than gadolinium bolus DSC techniques in the assessment of such patients (Figure 10.11). Hypercapnia is often an unsuspected diagnosis in patients who present with altered mental status. A simple rule of thumb is that hypercapnia should be considered in patients who are over 80 years of age if their gray matter CBF is above 80 ml/100 g/min.

Focal hyperperfusion

Seizures

Commonly, seizure patients are imaged in the "peri-ictal" phase, that is, usually several hours after presenting with seizure activity. In this peri-ictal state, focal hyperperfusion can be observed in the seizure focus and within adjacent territories. This has been demonstrated with both DSC and ASL MR perfusion techniques [55, 56]. Specifically with ASL, hyperperfusion has been demonstrated for up to 1 hr post-ictus [57]. The mechanism of hyperperfusion with seizures is not completely understood, but may relate to loss of autoregulation, excitatory neurotransmitter release, or as a response to increased metabolic demand due to seizure activity [58]. Following prolonged seizures or status epilepticus, extensive cortical T_2 prolongation, reduced diffusion, and hyperperfusion can be demonstrated (Figure 10.12). Subsequent scans will often demonstrate complete reversal of these findings.

Another important consideration with MR perfusion imaging in the setting of seizures is that seizure activity can mimic stroke. In the acute setting, a patient presenting with focal neurologic signs without a diffusion abnormality may be experiencing seizures or epiphenomena of stroke (clot lysis with reperfusion or transient ischemic attack), or may be in the very earliest stages of stroke evolution. Either seizures or stroke epiphenomena could exhibit a focal hyperperfusion pattern, which can often be differentiated by risk factors for stroke and with clinical history. One helpful finding that can suggest a diagnosis of peri-ictal seizure is hyperperfusion in the presence of lesions involving or crossing multiple vascular territories, though this is not always present.

PRES

As discussed above, the vasodilatory/vasogenic edema phase of PRES typically demonstrates focal hyperperfusion (see Figure 10.5). Whether due to autoregulatory perturbation, endothelial dysfunction, or both, the ensuing vasogenic edema represents an inability to contain the intravascular contents, with extravasation of fluid and sometimes blood products into the brain parenchyma. If severe blood–brain barrier (BBB) breakdown occurs, parenchymal enhancement can also be seen.

Migraine

As alluded to previously, migraine sufferers are more likely to be imaged during the headache phase of the syndrome. This is not surprising given that the majority of migraine patients do not experience aura and their headache dominates their clinical picture.

In general, if perfusion abnormalities are present during the headache phase, cortical focal hyperperfusion will be seen (Figure 10.13). With patients who do experience aura, the subsequent hyperperfusion is often demonstrated in the cortex, and thought to be responsible for the clinical symptoms. Subtle cortical edema (T_2 prolongation and cortical thickening) can also be seen in hyperperfused areas. When DSC and ASL techniques are employed conjointly, the perfusion disturbance can be more striking on ASL, which may reflect the quantitative properties of CBF as measured by ASL. Again, it is sometimes challenging to distinguish the perfusion imaging characteristics of migraine from peri-ictal changes in seizure, and in these cases, history and EEG findings can be helpful.

Post carotid endarterectomy syndrome

The management of patients with carotid atherosclerotic disease is difficult and controversial. Appropriate management hinges on the degree of stenosis and whether the patient is symptomatic. Further factors influencing surgical/interventional outcomes include gender, age, and expertise of the center/surgeon [59–62]. Carotid endarterectomy (CEA) and more recently carotid artery stenting (CAS) are the options for surgical intervention in the setting of hemodynamically significant carotid stenosis. A syndrome of cerebral hyperperfusion can occur following either revascularization technique. The syndrome typically presents with ipsilateral headache, hypertension, seizures, and focal neurological signs (commonly vision changes) [63]. The reported incidence of hyperperfusion following CEA is variable, but can occur in up to 3% of treated patients [64]. The incidence of hyperperfusion after CAS may be higher than with CEA [65, 66].

Conventional imaging can demonstrate cerebral edema, petechial hemorrhage, or frank parenchymal hemorrhage in the affected hemisphere in post-CEA syndrome. Perfusion imaging demonstrates a wide range of absolute CBF increases following revascularization (Figure 10.14). Many cases of revascularization hyperperfusion demonstrate marked increases relative to pre-procedural values [63]. With bolus perfusion DSC-MRI, the clinical hyperperfusion syndrome has been observed even after modest increases in ipsilateral perfusion relative to the contralateral hemisphere [67]. As patients experiencing

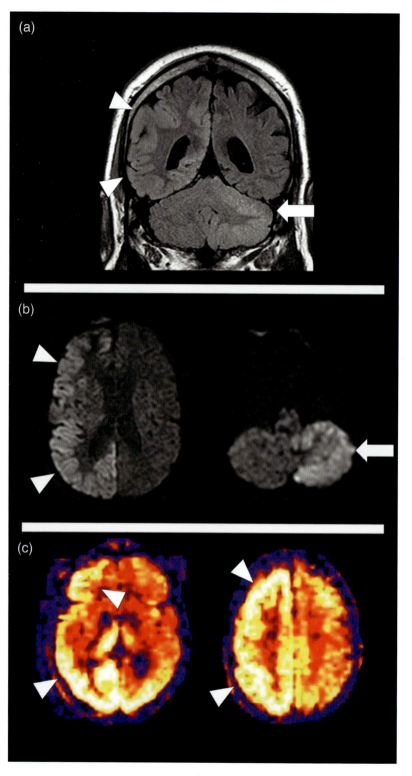

Figure 10.12 This man was found in his home, unconscious, in status epilepticus of unknown duration. (a) Coronal FLAIR image demonstrates increased T2 signal and cortical edema involving the right hemisphere (arrowheads). There is crossed cerebellar diaschisis, with similar changes in the left cerebellum (arrow). (b) The areas of abnormal FLAIR signal exhibit reduced diffusion, indicative of neuronal injury. (c) ASL CBF images show hyperperfusion involving the right hemisphere (arrowheads). The cerebellum was not included in the ASL slice planes. This example shows that focal high CBF can be seen in the peri-ictal period following sustained seizure activity.

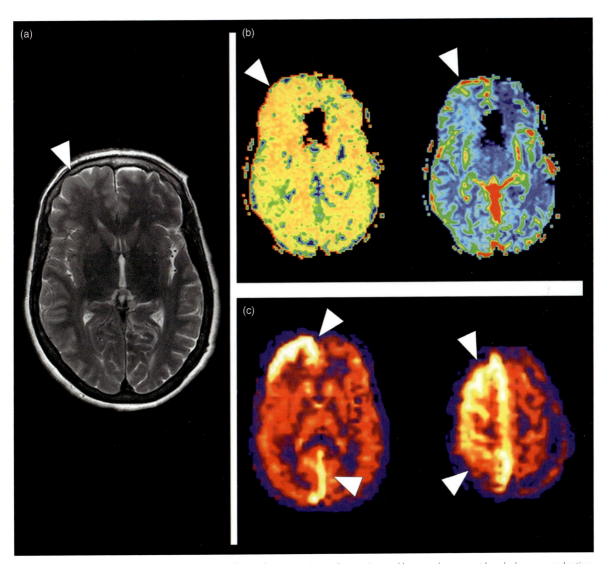

Figure 10.13 A 55-year-old woman with a history of hemiplegic migraines, who was imaged because her current headache was unrelenting. (a) T_2-weighted image shows subtle increased T_2 signal and cortical swelling of the right frontal lobe (arrowhead). (b) DSC-based relative TTP (left) and rCBV (right) images show respective decreased transit time and increased CBV in the right frontal lobe (arrowhead). (c) ASL demonstrates increased CBF within the right hemisphere (arrowheads), involving a larger territory than visually apparent on conventional imaging and DSC perfusion. Diffusion imaging at the time was normal (not shown), excluding infarct. EEG showed no evidence of seizure activity.

revascularization hyperperfusion are at greater risk of hemorrhage, prediction of patients at risk for hyperperfusion is valuable. Work with CT perfusion suggests that pre-procedural transit time elevation correlates with risk; that is, the greater the elevation in MTT ipsilateral to the stenosis of interest, the greater the likelihood of developing hyperperfusion [68]. Prediction using MR perfusion has not been thoroughly investigated.

Multiple sclerosis

Multiple sclerosis (MS) is the most common autoimmune demyelinating inflammatory disorder of the CNS. Women of child-bearing age and Northern European descent are most commonly affected. Presenting symptoms include vision loss (optic neuritis), double vision, limb sensory deficit, motor dysfunction/weakness, and gait disturbance among other

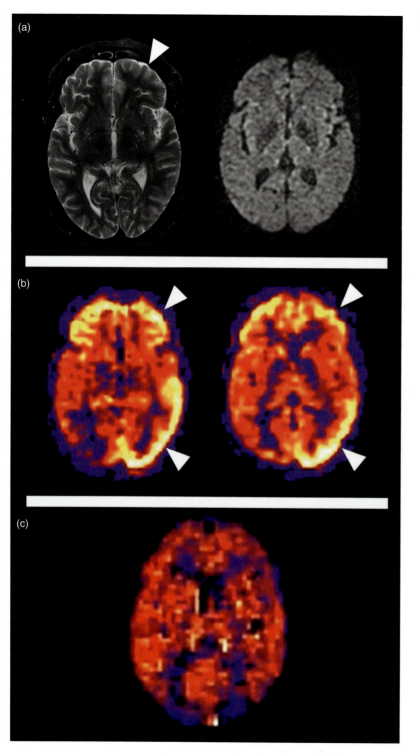

Figure 10.14 A 68-year-old woman who underwent left-sided CEA for a 95% ICA stenosis. She was recovering well at home but then developed left-sided headache and right arm heaviness. She was imaged on post-operative day 4. (a) The T_2 (left) image depicts subtle edema in the left frontal lobe (arrowhead). The diffusion (right) image is normal. (b) ASL CBF map on post-operative day 4 shows left hemispheric hyperperfusion (arrowheads), consistent with post-CEA syndrome. (c) Single image from an ASL CBF study obtained 6 weeks later demonstrates CBF normalization.

neurological findings. The diagnosis is complex and largely based on clinical criteria, the so-called McDonald criteria [69]. The unifying factor in the diagnosis of MS is neurological deficits separated in space and time. With an increasing role for MR brain imaging in the diagnosis and treatment of MS patients, separate neuroimaging requirements were emphasized in revisions to the McDonald criteria in 2005 [70]. The imaging findings that support the diagnosis of MS are based largely on conventional sequences. A large amount of work has been done to improve MS lesion detection, provide more accurate prognosis, and monitor treatments, including recently with diffusion tensor imaging sequences and anisotropy mapping [71].

Absent from the imaging criteria for MS are MR perfusion findings. Several perfusion changes have been observed, however. Intracranial lesions that enhance following gadolinium administration have created some degree of BBB breakdown, but studies with MS patients have shown that the extent of enhancement does not correlate with clinical disability and that plaque formation begins long before BBB breakdown. Similarly, perfusion changes occur prior to plaque enhancement, with regional increases of CBF and CBV several weeks prior to gadolinium enhancement [72]. The perfusion increases are noted to precede changes in diffusivity, suggesting a physiological response prior to pathological apparent diffusion coefficient (ADC) changes. Other studies have shown decreased gray matter perfusion in MS patients relative to normal subjects, which may be secondary to cerebral atrophy. Interestingly, the perfusion values in so-called areas of "normal-appearing white matter (NAWM)" are often elevated [73, 74]. Finally, enhancing MS plaques can demonstrate focally increased CBV values, even when corrected for BBB leakage [75]. This finding can be seen in cases of tumefactive MS (Figure 10.15), where the enhancing rim can be focally mildly hyperperfused, with hypoperfusion in the surrounding vasogenic edema. This pattern of mildly increased perfusion in the rim surrounded by decreased perfusion is also seen in cerebral abscesses. Diffusion and post-contrast imaging, which usually show a characteristic incomplete rim, can help distinguish the two. Usually, the degree of hyperperfusion of the rim is significantly lower than would be found in high-grade enhancing brain neoplasms (and this is more thoroughly discussed in Chapter 11).

Encephalitis/meningoencephalitis

Little has been published to date regarding the MR perfusion findings in cases of encephalitis or meningoencephalitis, both of which are typically viral in origin. Anecdotal clinical experience has shown that the perfusion pattern can be variable both at a single point in time and over a time interval. In clinical experiences with ASL, cases of encephalitis such as from herpes simplex virus tend to be hyperperfused in areas of brain demonstrating T_2 prolongation and/or enhancement. As discussed above, the enhancing rim of abscesses can also exhibit mild hyperperfusion, but again, this finding is variable.

Other considerations

One must be careful when interpreting MR perfusion images. Numerous artifacts can mimic perfusion abnormalities on both DSC and ASL techniques. As such, no matter the MR perfusion technique used, the perfusion images must be interpreted in conjunction with conventional MR sequences. Specific limitations for MR perfusion in the various clinical conditions are discussed under the respective clinical sections in this chapter.

Recommended protocols/analysis techniques for specific indications

MR perfusion patterns in the myriad clinical scenarios have been discussed under each section in this chapter. For each physiological state or pathological condition, discussions of specific MR perfusion techniques that may prove more useful have been given, including the choice between ASL and DSC.

For the purposes of screening, the MR perfusion technique used often becomes a question of practicality. There are inherent benefits to the ASL technique, which does not require gadolinium, which include no need for IV access and no risk of nephrogenic systemic fibrosis. As ASL techniques have improved over the last few years, scan times have decreased. However, ASL is more sensitive to motion degradation than DSC, which is a consideration when incorporating perfusion imaging into routine protocols, particularly for relatively non-compliant patients. Newer ASL sequences that incorporate background suppression and motion-correction may alleviate some of these concerns (see Chapter 3). DSC perfusion has been well validated and is widely available. DSC scan

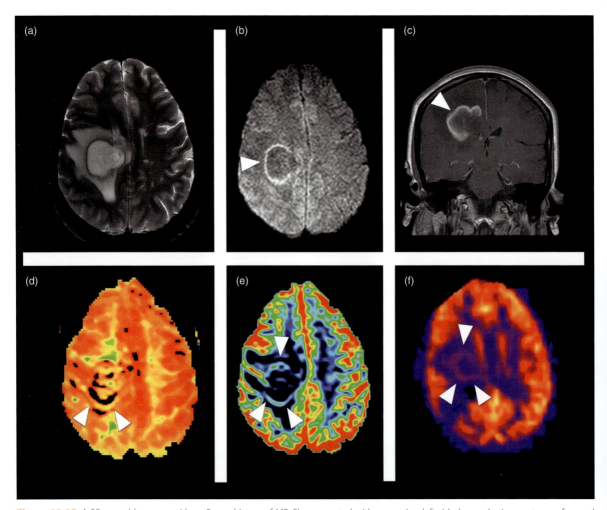

Figure 10.15 A 38-year-old woman with an 8-year history of MS. She presented with worsening left-sided neurologic symptoms of several weeks duration. (a) T_2-weighted image demonstrates a mass-like lesion in the posterior right frontal lobe with surrounding vasogenic edema. (b) DWI shows increased signal in the rim of the lesion (arrowhead), confirmed on ADC mapping (not shown). (c) Following contrast administration, T_1 imaging shows an incomplete ring of enhancement (arrowhead). (d) DSC TTP, (e) CBV, and (f) ASL CBF maps demonstrate mild hyperperfusion in the rim of the lesion (arrowheads). Collectively, these characteristics suggest the diagnosis of tumefactive MS, which was confirmed with biopsy.

times are relatively short, and generation of perfusion maps is either simple to perform or largely automated (see Chapter 2). Either technique will typically suffice for screening purposes. However, in general, ASL appears to be more efficacious in pediatric patients or patients with either difficult IV access or poor renal function; while DSC perfusion may be more appropriate for uncooperative patients or those more likely to move during acquisition. DSC perfusion also has the advantage of providing access to CBV, which cannot be measured using ASL. It can also be performed in the case of longer arterial delays, for which conventional ASL would not show any signal.

Conclusions

This chapter highlights the growing role of routine MR perfusion techniques in clinical neuroimaging, beyond that of stroke and oncology. The spectrum of pathology that may disturb cerebral perfusion underscores the need for perfusion imaging in all patients, when feasible, as this better allows radiologists to become familiar with the spectrum of normal and the identification of pathology. With the expanding list of pathologies, radiological pattern recognition and classification is useful and the scheme presented above functions well in clinical practice. However, the interpreter must not forget that perfusion patterns can change over time and that a single patient can exhibit multiple patterns simultaneously.

References

1. Wijdicks EF, Varelas PN, Gronseth GS, Greer DM. Evidence-based guideline update: determining brain death in adults: report of the Quality Standards Subcommittee of the American Academy of Neurology. *Neurology* 2010;**74**:1911–18.

2. Wieler H, Marohl K, Kaiser KP, Klawki P, Frossler H. Tc-99m HMPAO cerebral scintigraphy. A reliable, noninvasive method for determination of brain death. *Clin Nucl Med* 1993;**18**:104–9.

3. Munari M, Zucchetta P, Carollo C, *et al.* Confirmatory tests in the diagnosis of brain death: comparison between SPECT and contrast angiography. *Crit Care Med* 2005;**33**:2068–73.

4. Karantanas AH, Hadjigeorgiou GM, Paterakis K, Sfiras D, Komnos A. Contribution of MRI and MR angiography in early diagnosis of brain death. *Eur Radiol* 2002;**12**:2710–16.

5. Ishii K, Onuma T, Kinoshita T, *et al.* Brain death: MR and MR angiography. *AJNR Am J Neuroradiol* 1996;**17**:731–5.

6. Powers WJ, Grubb RL, Jr., Darriet D, Raichle ME. Cerebral blood flow and cerebral metabolic rate of oxygen requirements for cerebral function and viability in humans. *J Cereb Blood Flow Metab* 1985;**5**:600–8.

7. Astrup J, Siesjo BK, Symon L. Thresholds in cerebral ischemia – the ischemic penumbra. *Stroke* 1981;**12**:723–5.

8. Wong EC, Cronin M, Wu WC, *et al.* Velocity-selective arterial spin labeling. *Magn Reson Med* 2006;**55**:1334–41.

9. Zaharchuk G, Straka M, Marks MP, *et al.* Combined arterial spin label and dynamic susceptibility contrast measurement of cerebral blood flow. *Magn Reson Med* 2010;**63**:1548–56.

10. Meyer JS. Improved method for noninvasive measurement of regional cerebral blood flow by 133Xenon inhalation. Part II: measurements in health and disease. *Stroke* 1978;**9**:205–10.

11. Leenders KL, Perani D, Lammertsma AA, *et al.* Cerebral blood flow, blood volume and oxygen utilization. Normal values and effect of age. *Brain* 1990;**113** (Pt 1):27–47.

12. Parkes LM, Rashid W, Chard DT, Tofts PS. Normal cerebral perfusion measurements using arterial spin labeling: reproducibility, stability, and age and gender effects. *Magn Reson Med* 2004;**51**:736–43.

13. Calabrese LH, Duna GF, Lie JT. Vasculitis in the central nervous system. *Arthritis Rheum* 1997;**40**:1189–201.

14. Ducros A, Boukobza M, Porcher R, *et al.* The clinical and radiological spectrum of reversible cerebral vasoconstriction syndrome. A prospective series of 67 patients. *Brain* 2007;**130**:3091–101.

15. Rosengart AJ, Schultheiss KE, Tolentino J, Macdonald RL. Prognostic factors for outcome in patients with aneurysmal subarachnoid hemorrhage. *Stroke* 2007;**38**:2315–21.

16. Kassell NF, Sasaki T, Colohan AR, Nazar G. Cerebral vasospasm following aneurysmal subarachnoid hemorrhage. *Stroke* 1985;**16**:562–72.

17. Leclerc X, Fichten A, Gauvrit JY, *et al.* Symptomatic vasospasm after subarachnoid haemorrhage: assessment of brain damage by diffusion and perfusion-weighted MRI and single-photon emission computed tomography. *Neuroradiology* 2002;**44**:610–16.

18. Oommen KJ, Saba S, Oommen JA, *et al.* The relative localizing value of interictal and immediate postictal SPECT in seizures of temporal lobe origin. *J Nucl Med* 2004;**45**:2021–5.

19. Hamandi K, Laufs H, Noth U, *et al.* BOLD and perfusion changes during epileptic generalised spike wave activity. *Neuroimage* 2008;**39**:608–18.

20. Fugate JE, Claassen DO, Cloft HJ, *et al.* Posterior reversible encephalopathy syndrome: associated clinical and radiologic findings. *Mayo Clin Proc* 2010;**85**:427–32.

21. McKinney AM, Short J, Truwit CL, *et al.* Posterior reversible encephalopathy syndrome: incidence of atypical regions of involvement and imaging findings. *AJR Am J Roentgenol* 2007;**189**:904–12.

22. Pande AR, Ando K, Ishikura R. Clinicoradiological factors influencing the reversibility of posterior reversible encephalopathy syndrome: a multicenter study. *Radiat Med* 2006;**24**:659–68.

23. Covarrubias DJ, Luetmer PH, Campeau NG. Posterior reversible encephalopathy syndrome: prognostic utility of quantitative diffusion-weighted MR images. *AJNR Am J Neuroradiol* 2002;**23**:1038–48.

24. Diamond S, Bigal ME, Silberstein S, *et al*. Patterns of diagnosis and acute and preventive treatment for migraine in the United States: results from the American Migraine Prevalence and Prevention study. *Headache* 2007;**47**:355–63.

25. Friberg L, Olesen J, Lassen NA, Olsen TS, Karle A. Cerebral oxygen extraction, oxygen consumption, and regional cerebral blood flow during the aura phase of migraine. *Stroke* 1994;**25**:974–9.

26. Pollock JM, Deibler AR, Burdette JH, *et al*. Migraine associated cerebral hyper-perfusion with arterial spin-labeled MR imaging. *AJNR Am J Neuroradiol* 2008;**29**:1494–7.

27. Kapinos G, Fischbein NJ, Zaharchuk G, Venkatasubramanian C. Migraine-like headache with visual deficit and perfusion abnormality on MRI. *Neurology* 2010;**74**:1743–5.

28. Oberndorfer S, Wober C, Nasel C, *et al*. Familial hemiplegic migraine: follow-up findings of diffusion-weighted magnetic resonance imaging (MRI), perfusion-MRI and [99mTc] HMPAO-SPECT in a patient with prolonged hemiplegic aura. *Cephalalgia* 2004;**24**:533–9.

29. Leone M, Proietti Cecchini A, Mea E, *et al*. Functional neuroimaging and headache pathophysiology: new findings and new prospects. *Neurol Sci* 2007;**28** Suppl 2:S108–13.

30. Pollock JM, Tan H, Kraft RA, *et al*. Arterial spin-labeled MR perfusion imaging: clinical applications. *Magn Reson Imaging Clin N Am* 2009;**17**:315–38.

31. Frazzitta G, Grampa G, La Spina I, *et al*. SPECT in the early diagnosis of Creutzfeldt-Jakob disease. *Clin Nucl Med* 1998;**23**:238–9.

32. Miller DA, Vitti RA, Maslack MM. The role of 99m-Tc HMPAO SPECT in the diagnosis of Creutzfeldt-Jacob disease.

33. Mathews D, Unwin DH. Quantitative cerebral blood flow imaging in a patient with the Heidenhain variant of Creutzfeldt-Jakob disease. *Clin Nucl Med* 2001;**26**:770–3.

34. Olivot JM, Mlynash M, Kleinman JT, *et al*. MRI profile of the perihematomal region in acute intracerebral hemorrhage. *Stroke* 2010;**41**:2681–3.

35. Wintermark M, Lepori D, Cotting J, *et al*. Brain perfusion in children: evolution with age assessed by quantitative perfusion computed tomography. *Pediatrics* 2004;**113**:1642–52.

36. Wang Z, Fernandez-Seara M, Alsop DC, *et al*. Assessment of functional development in normal infant brain using arterial spin labeled perfusion MRI. *Neuroimage* 2008;**39**:973–8.

37. Ito H, Kanno I, Ibaraki M, Hatazawa J, Miura S. Changes in human cerebral blood flow and cerebral blood volume during hypercapnia and hypocapnia measured by positron emission tomography. *J Cereb Blood Flow Metab* 2003;**23**:665–70.

38. Oguz KK, Golay X, Pizzini FB, *et al*. Sickle cell disease: continuous arterial spin-labeling perfusion MR imaging in children. *Radiology* 2003;**227**:567–74.

39. Strouse JJ, Cox CS, Melhem ER, *et al*. Inverse correlation between cerebral blood flow measured by continuous arterial spin-labeling (CASL) MRI and neurocognitive function in children with sickle cell anemia (SCA). *Blood* 2006;**108**:379–81.

40. Helton KJ, Paydar A, Glass J, *et al*. Arterial spin-labeled perfusion combined with segmentation techniques to evaluate cerebral blood flow in white and gray matter of children with sickle cell anemia. *Pediatr Blood Cancer* 2009;**52**:85–91.

41. Arbelaez A, Castillo M, Mukherji SK. Diffusion-weighted MR imaging of global cerebral anoxia. *AJNR Am J Neuroradiol* 1999;**20**:999–1007.

42. Inoue Y, Shiozaki T, Irisawa T, *et al*. Acute cerebral blood flow variations after human cardiac arrest assessed by stable xenon enhanced computed tomography. *Curr Neurovasc Res* 2007;**4**:49–54.

43. Giubilei F, Lenzi GL, Di Piero V, *et al*. Predictive value of brain perfusion single-photon emission computed tomography in acute ischemic stroke. *Stroke* 1990;**21**:895–900.

44. Cohan SL, Mun SK, Petite J, *et al*. Cerebral blood flow in humans following resuscitation from cardiac arrest. *Stroke* 1989;**20**:761–5.

45. Sundgreen C, Larsen FS, Herzog TM, *et al*. Autoregulation of cerebral blood flow in patients resuscitated from cardiac arrest. *Stroke* 2001;**32**:128–32.

46. Pollock JM, Whitlow CT, Deibler AR, *et al*. Anoxic injury-associated cerebral hyper-perfusion identified with arterial spin-labeled MR imaging. *AJNR Am J Neuroradiol* 2008;**29**:1302–7.

47. Jarnum H, Knutsson L, Rundgren M, *et al*. Diffusion and perfusion MRI of the brain in comatose patients treated with mild hypothermia after cardiac arrest: a prospective observational study. *Resuscitation* 2009;**80**:425–30.

48. Madden JA. The effect of carbon dioxide on cerebral arteries. *Pharmacol Ther* 1993;**59**:229–50.

49. Brian JE, Jr. Carbon dioxide and the cerebral circulation. *Anesthesiology* 1998;**88**:1365–86.

50. de Boorder MJ, Hendrikse J, van der Grond J. Phase-contrast magnetic resonance imaging measurements of cerebral autoregulation with a breath-hold

challenge: a feasibility study. *Stroke* 2004;**35**:1350–4.

51. Ito H, Kanno I, Ibaraki M, Hatazawa J. Effect of aging on cerebral vascular response to Paco2 changes in humans as measured by positron emission tomography. *J Cereb Blood Flow Metab* 2002;**22**:997–1003.

52. Robertson JW, Debert CT, Frayne R, Poulin MJ. Variability of middle cerebral artery blood flow with hypercapnia in women. *Ultrasound Med Biol* 2008;**34**:730–40.

53. Noth U, Meadows GE, Kotajima F, *et al.* Cerebral vascular response to hypercapnia: determination with perfusion MRI at 1.5 and 3.0 Tesla using a pulsed arterial spin labeling technique. *J Magn Reson Imaging* 2006;**24**:1229–35.

54. Pollock JM, Deibler AR, Whitlow CT, *et al.* Hypercapnia-induced cerebral hyper-perfusion: an underrecognized clinical entity. *AJNR Am J Neuroradiol* 2009; **30**:378–85.

55. Warach S, Levin JM, Schomer DL, Holman BL, Edelman RR. Hyper-perfusion of ictal seizure focus demonstrated by MR perfusion imaging. *AJNR Am J Neuroradiol* 1994;**15**:965–8.

56. Wolf RL, Alsop DC, Levy-Reis I, *et al.* Detection of mesial temporal lobe hypo-perfusion in patients with temporal lobe epilepsy by use of arterial spin labeled perfusion MR imaging. *AJNR Am J Neuroradiol* 2001;**22**:1334–41.

57. Pollock JM, Deibler AR, West TG, *et al.* Arterial spin-labeled magnetic resonance imaging in hyperperfused seizure focus: a case report. *J Comput Assist Tomogr* 2008;**32**:291–2.

58. Lee SK, Lee SY, Yun CH, *et al.* Ictal SPECT in neocortical epilepsies: clinical usefulness and factors affecting the pattern of hyper-perfusion. *Neuroradiology* 2006;**48**:678–84.

59. Beneficial effect of carotid endarterectomy in symptomatic patients with high-grade carotid stenosis. North American Symptomatic Carotid Endarterectomy Trial Collaborators. *N Engl J Med* 1991;**325**: 445–53.

60. Endarterectomy for asymptomatic carotid artery stenosis. Executive Committee for the Asymptomatic Carotid Atherosclerosis Study. *JAMA* 1995;**273**:1421–8.

61. Brott TG, Hobson RW, 2nd, Howard G, *et al.* Stenting versus endarterectomy for treatment of carotid-artery stenosis. *N Engl J Med* 2010;**363**:11–23.

62. Yadav JS, Wholey MH, Kuntz RE, *et al.* Protected carotid-artery stenting versus endarterectomy in high-risk patients. *N Engl J Med* 2004;**351**:1493–501.

63. Sundt TM, Jr., Sharbrough FW, Piepgras DG, *et al.* Correlation of cerebral blood flow and electroencephalographic changes during carotid endarterectomy: with results of surgery and hemodynamics of cerebral ischemia. *Mayo Clin Proc* 1981;**56**:533–43.

64. Coutts SB, Hill MD, Hu WY. Hyper-perfusion syndrome: toward a stricter definition. *Neurosurgery* 2003;**53**:1053–8; discussion 1058–60.

65. Meyers PM, Higashida RT, Phatouros CC, *et al.* Cerebral hyper-perfusion syndrome after percutaneous transluminal stenting of the craniocervical arteries. *Neurosurgery* 2000;**47**:335–43; discussion 343–5

66. Morrish W, Grahovac S, Douen A, *et al.* Intracranial hemorrhage after stenting and angioplasty of extracranial carotid stenosis. *AJNR Am J Neuroradiol* 2000;**21**:1911–16.

67. Karapanayiotides T, Meuli R, Devuyst G, *et al.* Postcarotid endarterectomy hyper-perfusion or reperfusion syndrome. *Stroke* 2005;**36**:21–6.

68. Tseng YC, Hsu HL, Lee TH, Hsieh IC, Chen CJ. Prediction of cerebral hyperperfusion syndrome after carotid stenting: a cerebral perfusion computed tomography study. *J Comput Assist Tomogr* 2009;**33**:540–5.

69. McDonald WI, Compston A, Edan G, *et al.* Recommended diagnostic criteria for multiple sclerosis: guidelines from the International Panel on the diagnosis of multiple sclerosis. *Ann Neurol* 2001;**50**:121–7.

70. Polman CH, Reingold SC, Edan G, *et al.* Diagnostic criteria for multiple sclerosis: 2005 revisions to the "McDonald Criteria". *Ann Neurol* 2005;**58**:840–6.

71. Kealey SM, Kim Y, Provenzale JM. Redefinition of multiple sclerosis plaque size using diffusion tensor MRI. *AJR Am J Roentgenol* 2004;**183**: 497–503.

72. Wuerfel J, Bellmann-Strobl J, Brunecker P, *et al.* Changes in cerebral perfusion precede plaque formation in multiple sclerosis: a longitudinal perfusion MRI study. *Brain* 2004;**127**:111–19.

73. Rashid W, Parkes LM, Ingle GT, *et al.* Abnormalities of cerebral perfusion in multiple sclerosis. *J Neurol Neurosurg Psychiatry* 2004;**75**:1288–93.

74. De Keyser J, Steen C, Mostert JP, Koch MW. Hypo-perfusion of the cerebral white matter in multiple sclerosis: possible mechanisms and pathophysiological significance. *J Cereb Blood Flow Metab* 2008;**28**:1645–51.

75. Ge Y, Law M, Johnson G, *et al.* Dynamic susceptibility contrast perfusion MR imaging of multiple sclerosis lesions: characterizing hemodynamic impairment and inflammatory activity. *AJNR Am J Neuroradiol* 2005;**26**: 1539–47.

History

A 43-year-old woman was found unresponsive with agonal breaths. She was diagnosed with sepsis and disseminated intravascular coagulation (DIC) secondary to intestinal ischemia and bowel perforation.

Technique

Conventional MRI and pulsed ASL perfusion imaging was obtained. Due to acute renal failure and the risk of nephrogenic systemic fibrosis, gadolinium contrast could not be administered to perform DSC perfusion imaging.

Imaging findings

See Figure 10.16.

Discussion

This case illustrates the value of perfusion imaging in refining diagnoses in complex patients, who often have coexistent cerebral pathologies. The CBF maps confirm completed MCA territory infarcts bilaterally, which justifies withholding aggressive thrombolytic therapies. With the increased T_2 signal of the globus pallidus nuclei on conventional MRI alone, one might suggest a global hypoxic/anoxic brain injury. The elevated absolute global CBF (in the absence of hypercapnia) makes the diagnosis more certain. This case also highlights the general utility of ASL techniques, which do not require gadolinium. ASL can easily be performed in patients with difficult IV access, pediatric patients (thereby foregoing IV access attempts), and in patients with renal dysfunction.

Key points

- Matched diffusion-perfusion defects typically represent completed infarcts.
- Hypoxic/anoxic brain injury should be considered in cases of global hyperperfusion.
- Multiple perfusion patterns can be present on a single exam.
- ASL techniques are useful in patients with renal dysfunction.

Bibliography

Pollock JM, Whitlow CT, Deibler AR, *et al*. Anoxic injury-associated cerebral hyperperfusion identified with arterial spin-labeled MR imaging. *AJNR Am J Neuroradiol* 2008;**29**(7):1302–7.

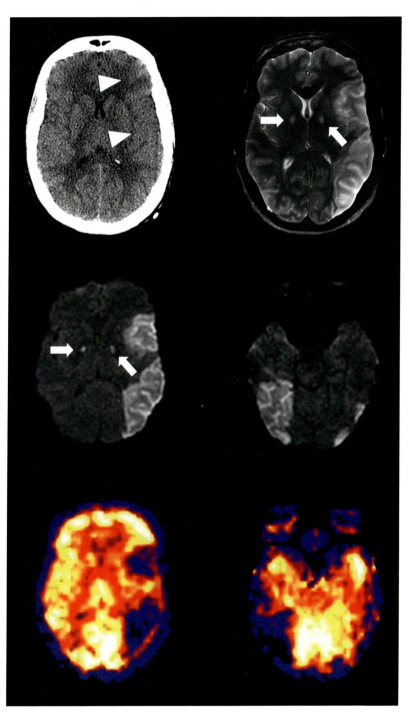

Figure 10.16 The stroke-windowed CT exam shows subtle loss of gray–white matter differentiation in the frontal and temporal regions on the left (arrowheads). At the time of MRI (4 days later), there is marked cortical edema and diffusion reduction within multiple regions of the middle cerebral artery (MCA) territory bilaterally. The globus pallidus nuclei also shown increased T_2 signal and diffusion reduction (arrows), suggesting a more global injury. The CBF maps from ASL imaging depict matched defects in the areas of reduced diffusion, which represent completed infarcts presumably thromboembolic related to DIC. Also shown on the CBF images is a background of global symmetric hyperperfusion. This finding, along with infarction of the deep gray nuclei, is very suspicious for hypoxic/anoxic brain injury in addition to the MCA infarcts. The pCO_2 at the time of the MRI was normal, excluding hypercapnia as a source of global hyperperfusion. The average gray matter CBF was 125 ml/100 g/min.

History

This 80-year-old female presented with abrupt onset of left-sided facial droop and extremity weakness. Subsequent imaging workup revealed a critical right ICA stenosis, for which she underwent CEA. Soon after discharge, she developed left extremity weakness and was unable to ambulate.

Technique

Conventional MRI with DSC perfusion was obtained at initial presentation. Neck MRA without and with gadolinium contrast was obtained the following day. Post-operatively, conventional MRI and pulsed ASL perfusion imaging were performed.

Imaging findings

See Figure 10.17.

Discussion

The case emphasizes the role of perfusion imaging in routine clinical practice. Strong consideration should be given to adding perfusion MR imaging to standard protocols. The small watershed infarcts in the right hemisphere at presentation are subtle clues to a potentially life-threatening problem elsewhere. With the perfusion imaging, there is no doubt the cerebral perfusion parameters are abnormal. When such a large perfusion disturbance is encountered, the interpreter should suggest additional vascular imaging. Further emphasizing

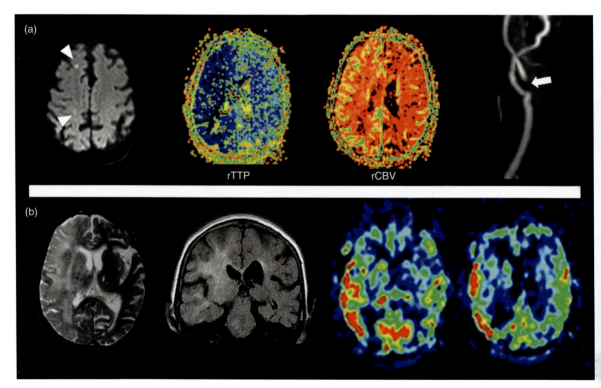

Figure 10.17 (a) at the time of presentation, several punctate watershed infarcts were observed in the right hemisphere borderzone region (arrowheads). On the DSC perfusion, there is right hemispheric prolonged TTP and increased rCBV. Based on these observations, evaluation of the neck was recommended to evaluate for proximal stenosis. The contrast-enhanced neck MRA shows a signal gap at the origin of the right ICA (arrow). Subsequent carotid ultrasound confirmed a critical stenosis, with peak systolic velocity in excess of 700 cm/s. (b) approximately 1 week post-operative from CEA, there is edema throughout the right hemisphere on T$_2$ and FLAIR imaging. The ASL CBF images show right hemispheric hyperperfusion. The patient was treated for post-CEA syndrome, and in spite of several small parenchymal hemorrhages, she eventually recovered.

the value of this recommendation, in this case, is the fact that this patient has a fetal right posterior cerebral artery (not shown). This explains why the perfusion changes affect the entire hemisphere, rather than just the anterior circulation. Should the carotid occlude, a severe hemispheric infarct would ensue. Perfusion imaging also plays a role in post-operative evaluation. The perfusion pattern shown corroborates the diagnosis of post-CEA syndrome.

Key points

- Large vascular territory perfusion abnormalities in the brain often indicate a proximal vessel stenosis, for which further imaging is needed.
- Including MR perfusion imaging into routine clinical exams can improve detection of pathologies that may be subtle or remain occult on conventional imaging.

Bibliography

Karapanayiotides T, Meuli R, Devuyst G, *et al.* Postcarotid endarterectomy hyperperfusion or reperfusion syndrome. *Stroke* 2005;**36**(1):21–6.

11

MR perfusion imaging in oncology: neuro applications

Ramon Francisco Barajas Jr. and Soonmee Cha

Key points

- The three most-commonly used perfusion techniques for the evaluation of intracranial mass lesions are DSC, DCE, and ASL.
- The limitations of histopathology to assess tumor angiogenesis have led to the development of imaging-based methods for the non-invasive quantification of angiogenic processes.
- Among high-grade gliomas, glioblastoma multiforme (GBM) tends to demonstrate elevated CBV, high vascular permeability (K^{trans}), and increased CBF compared with anaplastic astrocytomas.
- Low-grade gliomas exhibit significantly lower CBV, K^{trans}, and CBF when compared with higher-grade gliomas.
- Oligodendrogliomas, regardless of grade, tend to demonstrate elevated CBV when compared with low-grade astrocytomas.
- Contrast-enhancing intra-axial metastases and meningiomas typically demonstrate significantly reduced percentage of signal intensity recovery (PSR), elevated K^{trans}, and increased CBF when compared with treatment-naïve high-grade gliomas.
- Relative CBV, peak height, and PSR tend to be significantly elevated within enhancing recurrent gliomas when compared with similar appearing regions of radiation necrosis.
- Enhancing recurrent metastatic lesions tend to demonstrate elevated PSR when compared with regions of progressively enhancing radiation necrosis.

- Tumefactive demyelinating lesions demonstrate mild, if any, elevation of CBV.
- ASL imaging of CBF and DSC imaging of CBV appear to show significant concordance in the evaluation of intracranial neoplasms.

Introduction

The application of perfusion MRI in clinical neuro-oncology hinges upon the differential expression of angiogenic processes within neoplastic tissues when compared with surrounding normal brain. All neoplastic tissues rely upon the formation of new blood vessels, a biological process known as angiogenesis, to constantly supply nutrients and remove metabolic waste materials. Angiogenesis is a complex biological process that is upregulated by a number of cytokines, including vascular endothelial growth factor (VEGF), which is released within tumors, endothelial cells, and surrounding immune cells [1–5]. As tumor growth occurs beyond its existing blood supply, regional cellular hypoxic and hypoglycemic conditions ensue. This change within the cellular microenvironment promotes the transcription of VEGF that ultimately results in endothelial mitosis, cellular migration, and the formation of new microvasculature, thereby improving tumor nutrient supply that is essential to continued tumor growth and development [1–7].

VEGF expression and angiogenesis is known to vary by tumor type and grade. VEGF expression within gliomas and meningiomas has been associated with increased tumor grade and expression of histologically aggressive vascular features [8–11]. Tumor-related VEGF expression ultimately leads to the abnormal development of microvasculature, resulting in elevated vascular density with disrupted flow characteristics

Clinical Perfusion MRI: Techniques and Applications, ed. Peter B. Barker, Xavier Golay, and Greg Zaharchuk. Published by Cambridge University Press. © Peter B. Barker, Xavier Golay, and Greg Zaharchuk 2013.

[12–14]. The observation that angiogenesis plays a critical role in tumor growth has led to the development of therapeutic agents which directly inhibit angiogenic activity. The clinical implementation of anti-angiogenic chemotherapeutics has necessitated histological and imaging-based quantification of angiogenic activity.

Histopathological techniques that quantify tumor angiogenic activity have many clinical limitations. The pathological assessment of tumors relies on an invasive procedure for tissue sampling; however, many tumors demonstrate considerable heterogeneity in their expression of angiogenic processes. The assessment of tumor-wide angiogenic processes based on isolated regional tissue biopsies often leads to sampling error, resulting in under-grading in up to 30% of glioma cases [15, 16]. Aside from regional tumor heterogeneity, angiogenic activity also demonstrates a significant temporal heterogeneity that can influence the clinical assessment. Intra-tumor angiogenesis significantly varies based upon when the sampled tissue is assessed; therefore, reliance on an infrequent, invasive technique to acquire tissue samples does not lend itself to reliable clinical information in the setting of ongoing administration of anti-angiogenic therapies. The inherent limitations of histological techniques to actively assess tumor angiogenesis have led to the development of imaging-based methods [8].

In addition to the formation of new microvasculature, regional tumor VEGF expression results in increased blood–brain barrier (BBB) permeability. The increase in local capillary endothelial permeability results in an immediate increase in the interstitial nutrient supply that facilitates tumor growth. Capillary permeability is also the mechanism by which intravascular contrast material passes into the tumor interstitial space, resulting in enhancement on T_1-weighted MRI sequences, and providing the foundation by which dynamic contrast-enhanced (DCE) sequences may quantify tumor angiogenesis (see Chapter 4).

Recent advances in MR imaging allow for the acquisition of physiological maps of perfusion in the cerebral microcirculation. These added data complement the standard information provided by traditional morphological T_1- and T_2-weighted techniques. As mentioned earlier, physiologically, cerebral perfusion (or cerebral blood flow [CBF]) is defined as the steady-state delivery of blood to brain parenchyma. However, on an informal basis, the term "perfusion" is often broadly applied to include other tissue microcirculatory hemodynamic parameters, such as cerebral blood volume (CBV), mean transit time (MTT), and vascular permeability. These parameters can be derived from the passage of either endogenously labeled blood or contrast agents, through the cerebrovascular system. Such tracers can evaluate the degree of tumor angiogenesis and capillary permeability, both of which are important biological markers related to malignancy, grading, and prognosis (particularly for gliomas) [17]. This chapter focuses on the three most widely used perfusion MR imaging methods to study and quantify brain tumor vasculature: dynamic susceptibility contrast (DSC), dynamic contrast enhancement (DCE), and arterial spin labeling (ASL).

Dynamic susceptibility contrast perfusion imaging

DSC perfusion MR imaging is increasingly becoming integrated into daily clinical practice as a diagnostic tool that provides maps of regional variations in the perfusion of the cerebral microvasculature, both in the normal and diseased brain [18–24]. As described in Chapter 2, DSC perfusion MR imaging utilizes the temporal changes of signal intensity following intravascular bolus administration of paramagnetic contrast agents, to calculate CBV, MTT, CBF, and other parameters.

While sophisticated algorithms for post-processing of DSC data are commonly used in the research environment, until recently there were almost no commercially available processing packages for clinical use. Therefore, in clinical practice, other simpler but perhaps less rigorous methods of data analysis have been used, such as peak height (PH), and percentage of signal intensity recovery (PSR). These latter two parameters have not been discussed previously, and are dependent on the parameters of the acquisition sequence; however, they can be easily calculated without complex modeling or utilization of sophisticated leakage correction algorithms, and may be of clinical value despite their rather unclear relationship to underlying physiological principles (Figure 11.1). The PH parameter is defined as:

$$PH = S_0 - S_{min} \qquad (11.1)$$

where S_{min} is the minimum signal intensity of the perfusion curve, and S_0 is the baseline signal intensity before contrast arrival. Note that the PH parameter

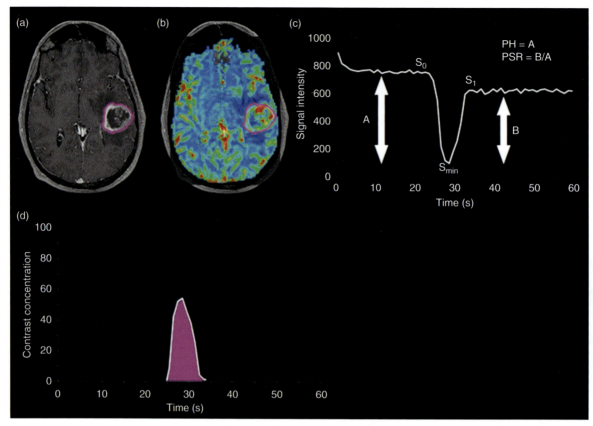

Figure 11.1 Calculation of DSC perfusion imaging parameters: CBV, peak height (PH), and percentage of signal intensity recovery (PSR). (a) Axial contrast-enhanced T_1-weighted image from a patient histologically diagnosed with glioblastoma multiforme (GBM) with (b) fused co-registered CBV map from the same location are used to calculate DSC parameters via placement of a region of interest (ROI) surrounding the contrast-enhancing component of the tumor (purple circle). (c) ROI placement allows for the generation of a signal intensity–time curve. PH is calculated as $S_0 - S_{min}$, where S_0 is the pre-contrast bolus baseline signal intensity and S_{min} is the minimum signal intensity obtained during the first pass of contrast. PSR is calculated as $(S_1 - S_{min}/S_0 - S_{min})$, where S_1 is the average post-bolus signal intensity. (d) Contrast concentration–time curve following baseline subtraction correction. CBV is proportional to the area under the concentration–time curve (purple shaded area).

can only be evaluated in a relative manner, by comparing with changes in a presumed normal region.

In tissues with a disrupted BBB, the interstitial pooling of contrast agent (that manifests as contrast enhancement on T_1-weighted images) may also result in the T_2^*-weighted signal in DSC not returning to baseline during the recirculation phase of the perfusion curve, depending on the DSC sequence parameters used and the relative amounts on T_1 and T_2^* weighting. The degree of residual T_2^* signal loss (PSR) may be estimated from

$$PSR = \frac{(S_1 - S_{min})}{(S_0 - S_{min})} \qquad (11.2)$$

where S_1 is the signal intensity during the recirculation phase of the perfusion curve (Figure 11.1).

Effects of contrast recirculation and leakage on DSC parameters

The estimation of DSC perfusion parameters has been described in Chapter 2. One common problem when analyzing DSC data is how to deal with contrast agent recirculation within the brain, and in the context of brain tumors, analysis is often more complicated due to contrast leakage into the tumor interstitium via a disrupted BBB. Given these issues, a number of modifications must be implemented to produce more physiologically accurate estimates of DSC perfusion parameters.

The idealized analysis of the contrast concentration–time curve assumes that following the passage of the contrast bolus the intravascular concentration becomes zero; however, in reality, residual intravascular contrast agent recirculates through the body. During the recirculation phase a second less prominent peak is measured (Figure 11.2). As the contrast material continues to recirculate through the body it becomes diluted through renal clearance and evenly distributed (mixed) in the bloodstream, resulting in broadening of the bolus in the second pass, and subsequently a slow decline of the signal in the brain as renal clearance occurs.

Several post-processing algorithms have been developed to calculate perfusion images in the presence of contrast agent recirculation. One of the most common ways is to utilize a curve-fitting technique, such as fitting a gamma-variate function to the first part of the concentration vs. time curve only. This allows for calculation of the area under the fitted contrast concentration–time curve instead of the original data, thereby approximating the curve that would have been obtained without the presence of contrast recirculation. However, in our experience the gamma-variate fit can be unstable. Small variations in the initial parameter estimates may yield wide variations in the end results. This instability occurs even with data averaged over multiple regions of interest (ROI) in areas of high perfusion and appears to be inherent to the technique. In practice, satisfactory fits can often be found only by repeating the procedure with multiple initial estimates until a set is found that causes the fitting algorithm to converge. This approach can be applied to fit concentration–time curves from multiple ROIs, since each fit takes very little time, but it is not suited for pixel-by-pixel calculations of CBV maps. To obtain CBV maps, alternative corrections for recirculation are preferable, which may be numerically more stable, such as the 'negative enhancement integral.'

The negative enhancement integral method is one of the simplest methods used clinically to calculate CBV, and is represented schematically in Figure 11.2C. The integral of $(S_0 - S_t)$ is calculated from the bolus arrival in the brain to either the end of the first pass, or (in some studies) to the end of the data acquisition, i.e., including both the initial and recirculation phases. It should be noted that calculation of CBV using the negative enhancement integral may result in either an underestimation or an overestimation of CBV in regions with disrupted BBB, due to competing T_1 and T_2 effects (discussed below).

Alternatively, the "baseline subtraction" method can be utilized to estimate CBV (Figure 11.2D). This method is similar to the negative enhancement integral but includes a simple linear correction estimation to account for a possible baseline shift during the passage of the contrast agent.

It should be noted that all of the parameters described above, i.e., PH, PSR, and CBV, determined either using the negative enhancement integral or baseline subtraction methods do not yield a linear or absolute measurement. As a result, it is always necessary to express the measurement relative to that in a reference region, which is usually chosen to be in contralateral, normal-appearing white matter.

Contrast leakage into tumor interstitium is a commonly encountered confounding factor that can adversely affect accurate CBV estimation. The leakage of contrast material into the tumoral interstitial space via the disrupted BBB can cause significantly increased signal, due to increased T_1 relaxation, both during the first pass and later phases of the signal intensity–time curve (Figure 11.3). This can significantly impact the CBV calculation. Several techniques have been utilized to reduce T_1 sensitivity. First, low flip angle gradient echo sequences can be used to reduce T_1 weighting, however, at the cost of reduced signal-to-noise ratio (SNR). Second, T_1 sensitivity can be largely eliminated through the use of dual-echo imaging techniques that first obtain a T_1-weighted echo to subsequently correct the predominantly T_2-weighted second echo [25, 26]. The use of dual-echo imaging is an effective way to remove the effects of changes in T_1; however, this technique necessitates a significant increase in sampling time (if parallel imaging is not used), which results in a decrease in the number of slices that can be covered within one TR time period. Finally, the interstitial space can be "pre-enhanced" (i.e., T_1-shortened) through the administration of a small contrast dose prior to the full bolus administration, thereby reducing the relaxivity-based signal intensity response to subsequent contrast doses [27, 28]. One problem with this technique is that its effectiveness is largely dependent upon the interstitial contrast concentration at the time of the bolus passage, which can significantly vary based on the rate of contrast material extravasation into the tumor interstitium, which cannot be predicted prior to contrast administration.

Techniques to reduce T_1 relaxation effects have specific advantages and disadvantages. The choice of

207

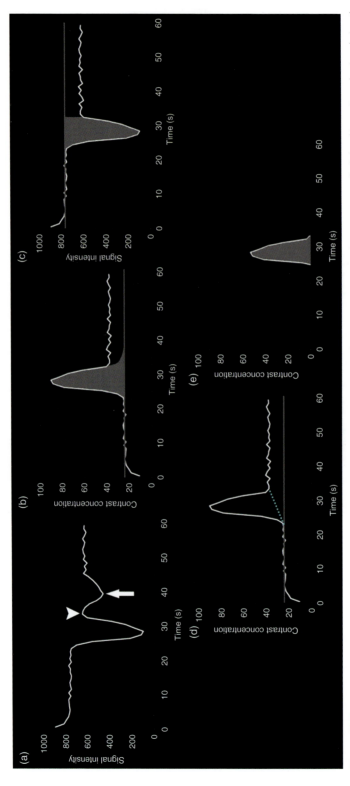

Figure 11.2 Idealized illustrations of effects of contrast recirculation on DSC parameters. (a) Signal intensity–time curve demonstrates marked signal intensity reduction during the first pass of intravascular contrast material followed by partial recovery (arrowhead). A second, less intense, signal decrease occurs as the contrast agent recirculates (arrow). (b) Curve-fitting the first-pass region of the graph to a gamma-variate function (the theoretical response of the heart-lung system to a contrast bolus) approximates the tissue ΔR_2^* curve that would have been obtained without the presence of contrast recirculation. Shaded area (integral) is proportional to relative CBV. (c) Estimating CBV (shaded area) from the original signal vs. time curve using the 'negative enhancement integral.' (d) Instead of using the pre-contrast baseline for integration, a shifted baseline formed by connecting the pre-contrast baseline signal intensity with the signal intensity at the end of the first pass of contrast can be used (blue dashed line, leading to (e) a recirculation corrected relative CBV measurement.

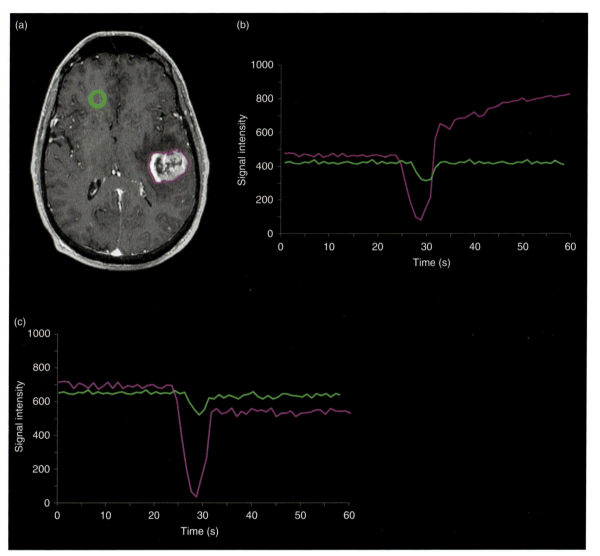

Figure 11.3 Effects of flip angle and contrast-agent leakage in DSC signal vs. time curve. (a) Contrast-enhanced T_1-weighted image demonstrates a left temporoparietal GBM with an ROI covering the entire contrast-enhancing region (purple ROI) and contralateral normal-appearing white matter (green circle). (b) Using a 90° flip angle, the signal intensity–time curve in the tumor ROI (purple) overshoots above the pre-contrast baseline due to T_1 relaxation effects as a result of contrast agent extravasation. The contralateral normal-appearing white matter curve (green) does not overshoot the pre-contrast baseline due to an intact BBB. (c) Use of a 35° flip angle minimizes T_1 relaxation effects.

which technique to implement in daily clinical practice will vary widely depending upon the tumor to be imaged and institutional policy. In general, at our institution, a combination of a repetition time (TR) (1250 ms) and a relatively low flip angle (35°) is used to minimize T_1 relaxation effects, and a gradient-echo technique with an echo time (TE) of 54 ms maximizes susceptibility contrast.

Clinical applications of dynamic susceptibility contrast tumor imaging

Vascular morphology and microvascular proliferation are important elements in the evaluation of tumor angiogenesis that can be utilized in characterizing tumor biological aggressiveness and histology. DSC perfusion imaging provides an in vivo CBV map that depicts overall tumor vascularity that permits the indirect assessment of tumor angiogenesis. CBV measurements have been shown to correlate with histological measurements of tumor angiogenesis [29, 30]. However, as demonstrated by meningioma and choroid plexus papilloma, elevated tumor angiogenesis is not synonymous with biological aggressiveness. With the recent interest in and development of anti-angiogenic cancer therapies, DSC perfusion imaging can be used as a non-invasive assessment of changes in tumor CBV during treatment, thereby, actively monitoring therapeutic efficacy. While conventional MR imaging is limited by its non-specificity to differentiate between tumor recurrence and therapy-related necrosis, DSC perfusion imaging has been shown to correlate better with clinical response in patients undergoing anti-angiogenic therapy [20].

CBV measurements may also be useful as an adjunct to conventional morphological MRI to facilitate assessment of tumor grade, differentiate tumor etiology, and identify tumor-mimicking lesions (such as radiation necrosis and tumefactive demyelinating lesion).

Preoperative grading of glioma

High-grade malignant gliomas (epitomized by glioblastoma multiforme [GBM], the most common primary brain tumor) are highly aggressive tumors that histologically demonstrate significant cellular invasion of surrounding neuropil structures and marked angiogenic features. The ability to recruit and synthesize vascular networks for further growth and proliferation is an important biological feature of GBM aggressiveness. The degree of vascular proliferation, a marker of angiogenesis, is a critical element in the determination of glioma grade. As the therapeutic approaches to low- and high-grade gliomas are drastically different, preoperative DSC assessment of glioma vascularity can provide information which may potentially alter therapeutic management.

Contrast-enhanced T_1-weighted imaging depicts tumor regions with a disrupted BBB; however, it is limited in its ability to accurately grade gliomas (Figure 11.4). DSC perfusion imaging, on the other hand, can quantify variations in regional CBV that reflect alterations in tumor angiogenesis and has shown promise in the preoperative grading of glioma. Catheter-based angiography has previously been the definitive imaging modality to depict tumor

vascularity, but this technique has largely been replaced by non-invasive techniques. CBV maps are particularly useful in glioma, an inherently heterogeneous tumor, by quantifying overall tumor microvascular proliferation and regional differential expression of angiogenic processes. Since CBV measurements have been shown to directly correlate with histological features of glioma angiogenesis, there is a growing consensus that CBV, in conjunction with conventional T_1- and T_2-weighted morphological MR sequences, may serve as a non-invasive surrogate marker of tumor aggressiveness that may be useful in the preoperative differentiation of low- and high-grade gliomas (Figure 11.4) [18, 19, 29, 30].

Low-grade gliomas exhibit significantly lower relative CBV (rCBV) when compared with higher grade gliomas (anaplastic astrocytomas and GBM), as initially described by Aronen et al. [18]. In general, low-grade gliomas tend to demonstrate little to no CBV elevation compared with the contralateral normal appearing brain (Figure 11.4A) [18, 19]. Among high-grade gliomas, anaplastic astrocytomas tend to demonstrate lower rCBV measurements when compared with GBM (Figure 11.4C). Oligodendrogliomas, regardless of grade, tend to demonstrate elevated CBV when compared with astrocytomas (Figure 11.4B). The finding that CBV measurements tend to increase with glioma grade and biological aggressiveness is consistent with histological studies demonstrating reduced microvascular proliferation and less deranged vascular morphology in low-grade gliomas compared to high-grade gliomas. While differentially higher CBV has been described with increasing glioma grade, it should be noted that this concept applies only to fibrillary astrocytomas [31].

Significant inter- and intra-tumoral CBV heterogeneity has been described in gliomas. This heterogeneity results in an overlap of CBV measurements between different glioma grades. This CBV heterogeneity is likely due to the observed inherent heterogeneity of angiogenic processes within gliomas. As a result of this overlap, CBV measurements should not be blindly utilized to preoperatively assign glioma grade. CBV maps should be interpreted concurrently with conventional contrast-enhanced T_1- and T_2-weighted images that provide additional morphological information, including BBB integrity and characteristics of tumor-related edema.

While great strides have been made to precisely characterize the biological significance of elevated

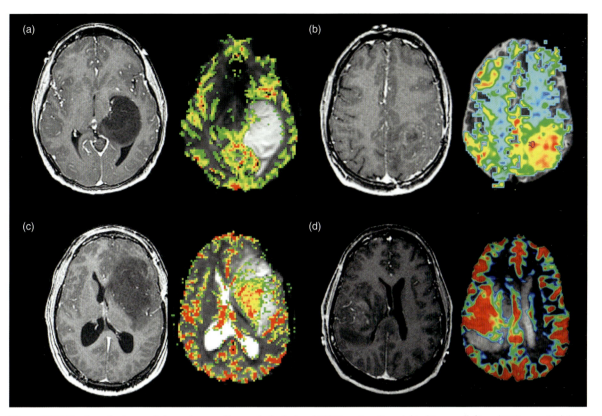

Figure 11.4 Grading of primary glial neoplasms with morphological and DSC imaging. T_1-weighted images (left) and CBV maps (right) in (a) grade II fibrillary astrocytoma, (b) grade II oligodendroglioma, (c) grade III anaplastic astrocytoma, and (d) grade IV GBM. Little to no contrast enhancement within the various tumors demonstrates the limited ability of T_1-weighted imaging to accurately grade primary glial neoplasms. CBV maps in conjunction with conventional imaging sequences are useful in the preoperative differentiation of low- and high-grade gliomas. Low-grade gliomas (a) exhibit significantly lower CBV when compared with higher-grade gliomas such as anaplastic astrocytomas (c) and GBMs (d). Among high-grade gliomas, anaplastic astrocytomas tend to demonstrate lower CBV measurements when compared with GBM. Oligodendroglioma (b), despite being a grade II tumor, can demonstrate elevated CBV, similar to GBM (d).

DSC perfusion parameters through direct correlation with histological features of cellular aggressiveness based on image-guided biopsy, there remain significant questions whether these perfusion parameters will be accepted clinically as "stand alone" biomarkers of tumor angiogenesis [29, 30], due in large part to the significant intra- and inter-tumoral biological heterogeneity of glioma and the non-specificity of CBV in distinguishing elevated microvascular density from dilated hyperplastic microvasculature. A prime example of the lack of specificity of CBV can be seen in the DSC perfusion evaluation of World Health Organization (WHO) grade I pilocytic astrocytoma. This common pediatric brain tumor often demonstrates vascular hyperplasia, composed primarily of dilated vessels of uniform morphology which is a relatively non-aggressive angiogenic feature (Figure 11.5). On the other hand, GBM (WHO grade IV)

frequently contains aggressive angiogenic features including elevated microvascular density and hyperplasia that can be morphologically quite heterogeneous, including classic glomeruloid vessels, simple endothelial hyperplasia, and delicate vasculature. Despite the markedly different expression of aggressive angiogenic features found between tumors there can be a great deal in overlap in individual tumor CBV values [32]. Due to the current limitations of DSC perfusion parameters, histological analysis of biopsy specimens remains the definitive method of determining tumor type and grade.

However, one important drawback of tissue biopsy when performed without MR imaging guidance is that it is subject to significant sampling error, resulting in under-grading in up to 30% of high-grade glioma cases [15, 16]. This is due to the extreme geographic heterogeneity of aggressive

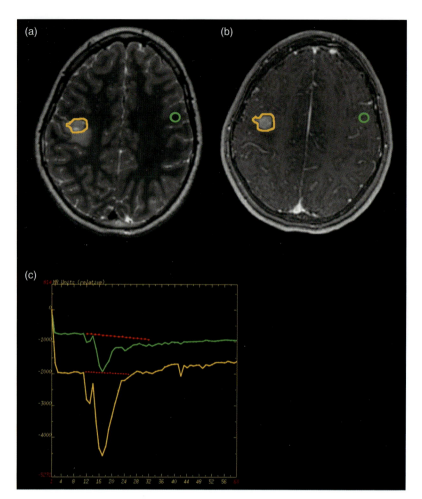

(a)

(b)

(c)

Figure 11.5 Elevated CBV within WHO grade I pilocytic astrocytoma. (a) Axial T_2-weighted, (b) T_1-weighted post-contrast images, and (c) signal intensity–time curve demonstrate elevated CBV within the contrast-enhancing region (gold ROI) when compared with contralateral normal-appearing gray matter (green ROI). Elevated CBV within this low-grade tumor is due to the presence of dilated vessels of uniform morphology, a relatively non-aggressive angiogenic feature.

cellular features within glioma. Ideally, grading should be based on histological evaluation of tissue obtained from the most biologically aggressive region; however, the intraoperative localization of these regions utilizing conventional morphological MR imaging features alone is quite challenging. At most institutions, the imaging modality used for intraoperative guidance is contrast-enhanced CT or T_1-weighted MRI, which are only capable of depicting regions of BBB breakdown. These regions of enhancement may or may not correspond to the tumor's most biologically aggressive region. CBV maps can depict regions of increased vascularity that may serve as additional targets for stereotactic biopsy. At our institution, such maps are routinely used to select biopsy sites for both enhancing and peritumoral non-enhancing regions. This methodology is thought to reduce sampling error and frequency of non-diagnostic biopsy sampling. The intraoperative use of CBV maps is particularly useful in patients with non-enhancing tumors, because they can be used to locate regions of increased tumor vascularity presumed to represent the region of highest biological malignancy (Figure 11.6) [30].

Differentiating low-grade gliomas

Up to 20% of all primary gliomas are low grade. The main preoperative differential diagnosis for a non-enhancing neoplastic mass lesion includes both diffuse astrocytoma and oligodendroglioma. The distinction has significant therapeutic and prognostic implications. As mentioned previously, pure and mixed oligodendrogliomas demonstrate high rCBV

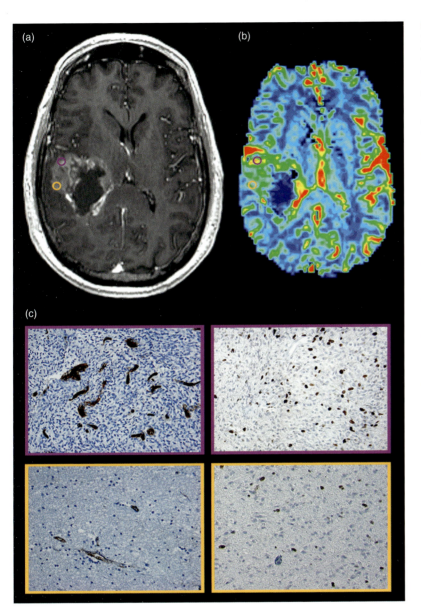

Figure 11.6 Ideally, tumor grading should be based on tissue obtained from the most biologically aggressive region of the lesion; however, identification of these regions based on conventional MRI alone can be challenging. (a) Axial T_1-weighted post-contrast and (b) co-registered CBV images of newly diagnosed GBM demonstrates variable CBV expression within similar appearing contrast-enhancing regions. (c) Enhancing region with elevated CBV (purple circle) demonstrates aggressive cellular characteristics including elevated microvascular density, simple and complex vascular morphology (top left) associated with elevated cellular proliferation (brown cells; top right) consistent with GBM. Conversely, sampling of enhancing region with relatively lower CBV (gold circle) demonstrates less aggressive cellular characteristics: delicate vascular morphology (bottom left) without associated elevated cellular proliferation (bottom right). Histological analysis of this biopsy region alone might have resulted in under-grading of the tumor due to sampling error. Histological slides courtesy of Joanna Phillips, UC San Francisco, USA.

measurements independent of tumor grade. Prior investigations have demonstrated that oligodendroglioma can manifest significantly elevated CBV values that, taken in isolation, can be confused with high-grade gliomas (Figure 11.4) [18, 19, 22, 29, 31, 33]. The increase in oligodendroglioma's relative CBV measurements may be due to the increased expression of morphologically delicate microvasculature. This is in contrast to WHO grade II astrocytomas that tend to demonstrate little or no CBV elevation [18, 19]. Additionally, oligodendrogliomas have characteristic morphological features on contrast-enhanced T_1- and T_2-weighted images, which include cortical involvement with frontal lobe predominance, intra-tumoral cysts, and susceptibility changes due to intra-tumoral calcification, that can also help pre-operatively to differentiate diffuse astrocytoma from oligodendroglioma.

Differentiating high-grade glioma from solitary metastatic intracerebral neoplasia

Intracranial metastases account for up to 50% of all brain tumors, and may be the first manifestation of systemic malignancy in approximately 30% of patients with cancer. The imaging diagnosis of intracranial metastases is usually straightforward, as metastatic lesions tend to be multiple, well circumscribed, and favor the gray–white matter junction. However, a diagnostic dilemma can ensue when a patient presents with a solitary lesion without a history of systemic cancer. It is clinically important to distinguish solitary intracranial metastasis from primary glioma, because medical staging, surgical planning, and therapeutic decisions are very different. Patients with primary glioma usually do not require systemic work up, because tumor spread outside of the central nervous system (CNS) is exceedingly rare. Patients with metastatic systemic malignancy are more likely to be treated with non-operative therapies and should undergo comprehensive systemic staging to determine the site of the primary malignancy. In this situation, conventional contrast-enhanced T_1- and T_2-weighted imaging characteristics of the solitary metastasis and primary high-grade glioma (enhancement associated with a variable degree of peritumoral edema) are non-specific, and therefore cannot be used with confidence to narrow the differential diagnosis.

Despite their similar morphological appearance, the ultrastructure of tumor capillaries is markedly different between primary glioma and brain metastasis. Histologically these two types of tumors widely vary in their extent of invasion and capillary morphology; these physiological features can be characterized utilizing DSC perfusion imaging. Metastatic tumors spread to the CNS via hematogenous routes, inducing intra-tumoral neovascularization as they expand. The newly formed capillaries resemble those of the primary systemic tumor, with gap junctions, fenestrated membranes, and open endothelial junctions, all of which are significantly different from normal brain capillaries. This unique intracerebral capillary morphology results in greatly increased capillary permeability uniformly throughout the tumor vasculature, causing peritumoral vasogenic edema. Conversely, the capillaries of primary glioma have various degrees of BBB disruption and a variety of morphological features, including glomeruloid capillaries, simple vascular hyperplasia, and delicate neocapillaries that simulate normal brain vessels. As a result, the degree of primary glioma capillary permeability can vary widely. Both types of tumors express varying degrees of peritumoral vasogenic edema; however, the peritumoral regions in patients with metastatic lesions demonstrate normal-appearing capillaries of intracerebral origin with no evidence of infiltrative metastatic cells beyond the macroscopic boundaries of the tumor. In contrast, high-grade astrocytomas demonstrate infiltrative peri-axonal tumor growth with morphologically deranged tumor capillaries.

The inherent differences in histological capillary features between primary glioma and metastatic lesions form the basis for tumor differentiation using DSC perfusion imaging. CBV measurements obtained from within the enhancing component of these tumors have not been shown to be useful in differentiating their histological origin [34]. However, CBV (and PH) measurements obtained from non-enhancing, peritumoral regions, and the tumor-wide PSR, have been shown to be helpful in differentiating GBM from solitary brain metastasis (Figure 11.7) [35]. CBV and PH are significantly elevated within primary glioma peritumoral regions when compared with metastatic lesions. Additionally, tumor-wide PSR values are significantly reduced within metastatic lesions when compared with primary gliomas. The observed differences in regional CBV, PH, and PSR can, in part, be explained by differences in histologically defined pathophysiology. In metastatic tumors, peritumoral edema represents pure vasogenic edema caused by increased interstitial water due to leaky capillaries without evidence of infiltrative tumor growth or elevated VEGF, and thereby microvascular expression; this manifests as reduced CBV and PH values when compared with primary glioma. Conversely, the significant reduction in PSR values within brain metastasis when compared with primary glioma is likely due to the differences in capillary permeability between the tumor types.

Differentiating recurrent high-grade glioma from radiation-induced necrosis

External beam radiation therapy (EBRT) has become an important therapeutic adjunct to surgical resection in patients with newly diagnosed high-grade glioma. However, a common complication of this therapy is delayed radiation necrosis. Conventional contrast-

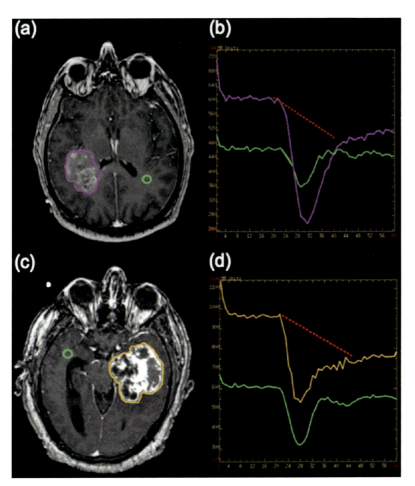

Figure 11.7 Differentiating high-grade glioma from solitary metastatic lesion with DSC perfusion imaging. (a) Post-contrast T_1-weighted image and (b) DSC signal intensity–time curves from GBM; (c) post-contrast T_1-weighted image and (d) DSC signal intensity–time curves from metastatic lung cancer. Post-contrast images demonstrate similar morphology with central regions of non-enhancement and minimal surrounding vasogenic edema. PSR values obtained from the entire enhancing region (purple and gold ROIs for GBM and metastasis, respectively) are significantly lower within the metastatic lesion (45% return to baseline) compared with GBM (75% return to baseline). Both enhancing lesions demonstrate similar relative CBV (area under the purple and gold curve bounded by red line) and relative PH (GBM = 2.3, metastasis = 1.8) measurements.

enhanced CT and MR imaging, in isolation, are not capable of distinguishing radiation necrosis from recurrent high-grade glioma. Both entities cause extensive vasogenic edema in white matter, either from diffuse neoplastic infiltration of recurrent tumor, or the demyelinating process of radiation necrosis and varying degrees of disruption in the BBB that result in mass effect and abnormal contrast enhancement. As a result, it is often difficult to determine whether a progressively enhancing lesion after EBRT is due to recurrent high-grade glioma or radiation necrosis.

The distinction between recurrent high-grade glioma and radiation-induced necrosis is not inconsequential. Both disease entities can manifest with progressive focal neurological deficits and signs of increased intracranial pressure. Therapeutically, recurrent tumor may benefit from surgical resection with adjuvant chemotherapy or additional targeted high-dose radiation therapy. Conversely, the surgical

manipulation of tissue expressing radiation necrosis can cause further damage to adjacent brain parenchyma. Therefore, radiation necrosis is generally treated conservatively with steroids.

Histological analysis is the only definitive clinically accepted means of differentiating between recurrent tumor and radiation necrosis. Pathologically, these two disease entities are markedly dissimilar. Radiation necrosis consistently demonstrates extensive microvascular injury manifested by endothelial damage associated with vascular dilation, and fibrinoid necrosis surrounded by relatively normal cerebral vasculature. In contrast, the hallmark of recurrent high-grade glioma is the presence of proliferative tumor associated with hyperplastic microvasculature. The inherent biological dissimilarities between these two disease processes can be exploited by DSC perfusion imaging.

Relative CBV and PH tend to be significantly elevated within contrast-enhancing tumor when compared with radiation necrosis. Additionally, diminished PSR has been found within regions of contrast-enhancing recurrent tumor when compared with similar-appearing regions of radiation necrosis (Figure 11.8) [36]. While CBV differences have been found between these two disease entities, it should be noted that a significant degree of measurement overlap has been described, making relative PH a more reliable predictor of recurrent tumor in two studies [36, 37]. DSC perfusion imaging measurements within contrast-enhancing recurrent tumor have been previously noted to be highly heterogeneous, with regions of both high and low CBV (Figure 11.9) [36, 37]. This CBV heterogeneity and overlap is likely caused by several factors: (1) regional tumor heterogeneity resulting from the coexistence of viable tumor vasculature with areas of radiation-induced dilated vasculature and fibrinoid tissue necrosis; (2) the inability of CBV measurements to differentiate elevated microvascular proliferation occurring within regions of residual tumor from radiation-induced hyperplastic dilated vasculature; and (3) the previously described inherent shortcomings associated with CBV measurements obtained from vasculature with a disrupted BBB.

PSR is an additional DSC perfusion imaging parameter that appears to be different in recurrent GBM and radiation necrosis. The observed reduced PSR within recurrent GBM is likely caused by the presence of a disrupted neoplastic BBB that is permeable to macromolecular contrast agents. In our experience, the degree of capillary leakiness, while quantifiably different, remains similar enough such that there is a large degree of PSR value overlap between the two disease entities, reducing the predictive ability of this parameter.

Differentiating recurrent metastatic intracerebral neoplasia from radiation necrosis following stereotactic radiosurgery

Following therapy with conformal stereotactic radiosurgery, the differentiation of recurrent metastatic tumor from radiation necrosis can be difficult when a progressively enhancing lesion is noted on follow-up MR imaging. A patient's clinical course, tissue sampling, and serial imaging have traditionally been used to distinguish tumor recurrence and radiation necrosis.

Despite their similar morphological MR imaging appearance, the microstructure of metastatic tumor is markedly different from that of irradiated non-tumor involved brain. Pathologically, these two processes demonstrate markedly different biological features. Enhancing, recurrent metastatic tumors histologically demonstrate elevated microvascular proliferation and elevated capillary permeability when compared with regions of irradiated brain. The capillaries of irradiated brain demonstrate some disruption of the BBB, which accounts for the presence of contrast enhancement. However, the BBB remains relatively intact when compared with the inherently leaky capillaries of recurrent metastatic tumor, which resemble those of the primary systemic tumor. The physiological differences in microvascular proliferation and capillary permeability between recurrent metastatic tumor and radiation necrosis form the basis for utilizing DSC perfusion imaging techniques to differentiate between these two disease processes.

PSR has been shown to be a reliable parameter that can accurately differentiate recurrent metastatic tumor from radiation necrosis (Figure 11.10) [38]. In a retrospective study involving patients suspected of having either recurrent metastatic tumor or radiation necrosis, it was observed that the PSR measurement obtained from contrast-enhancing regions was significantly reduced in patients with histologically proven recurrent tumor. A PSR threshold of 76.3% yielded a sensitivity and specificity of 96% and 100%, respectively. The utility of rCBV and PH in differentiating recurrent metastatic tumor and radiation necrosis has also been demonstrated in other studies [38, 39]. These parameters have been shown to be significantly elevated within recurrent metastatic tumor, though a large degree of overlap has been noted, suggesting that PSR may be a better prognostic indicator of metastatic tumor recurrence than either rCBV or PH.

Neoplastic-mimicking lesions: tumefactive demyelinating masses

Tumefactive demyelinating lesions (TDLs) are well known to mimic high-grade glial neoplasms when visualized with conventional MR sequences. A solitary TDL, at the time of clinical presentation, can pose a significant diagnostic dilemma. The gold standard for diagnosis and grading of glioma is

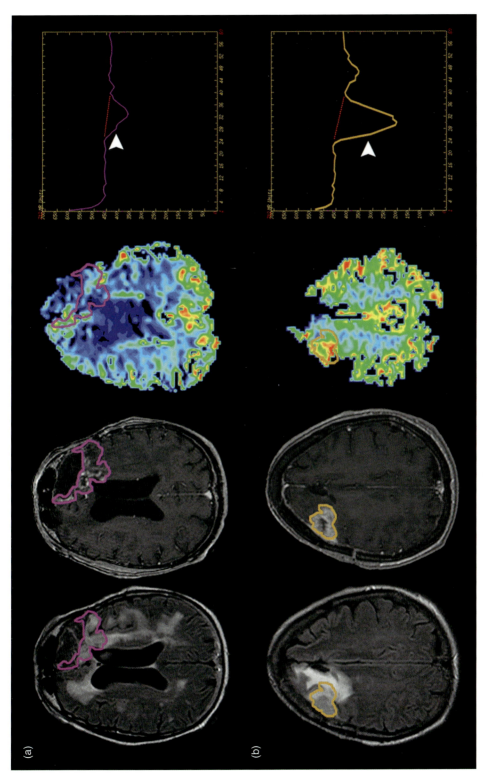

Figure 11.8 Differentiating recurrent high-grade glioma from radiation-induced necrosis utilizing DSC perfusion imaging. Axial FLAIR and T_1-weighted post-contrast images obtained from (a) a 62-year-old man with biopsy-proven radiation necrosis and (b) a 58-year-old man with biopsy-proven recurrent tumor demonstrate similar rim-enhancing lesions (purple and gold ROIs) with surrounding rim of vasogenic edema. Both patients received similar medical (temozolomide) and fractionated EBRT of 200 cGy per day for a total dose of 6000 cGy over approximately 6 weeks. The CBV map produced from the signal intensity–time curve of the enhancing ROIs (purple and gold) demonstrate significantly elevated CBV and PH (arrowhead) with reduced PSR in the recurrent tumor (b) when compared with radiation necrosis (a).

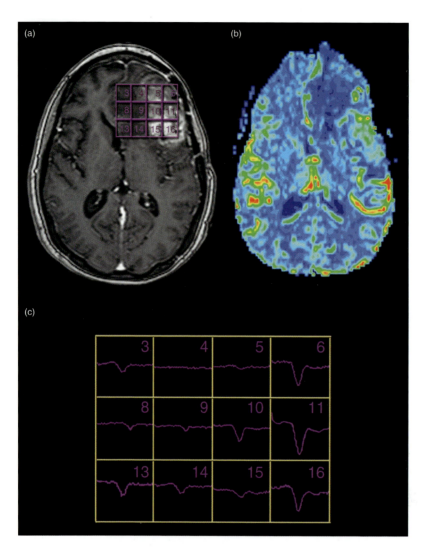

Figure 11.9 Regional heterogeneity of DSC parameters within GBM following medical and radiation therapy. (a) Post-contrast T_1-weighted image with overlying multi-voxel ROI (purple squares), (b) co-registered CBV map, and (c) corresponding signal intensity–time curves demonstrate a considerable degree of regional CBV and PH heterogeneity within similar-appearing contrast-enhancing tissues. Following surgery, this region was shown to contain a mixture of radiation necrosis and recurrent tumor. Contrast-enhancing regions within voxels 6, 11, and 16 demonstrate significantly elevated CBV and PH consistent with recurrent tumor when compared with voxels 4, 5, and 15, which are more consistent with radiation necrosis.

through surgical biopsy. TDLs, however, require no such intervention. Differentiating high-grade glioma from a solitary TDL is vital because an incorrect diagnosis of primary glioma can lead to unnecessary and potentially harmful surgical therapies. TDLs can appear very similar to high-grade gliomas on conventional contrast-enhanced T_1- and T_2-weighted images, demonstrating enhancement with varying degrees of peri-lesional vasogenic edema, mass effect, and central necrosis [40]. Histologically, TDLs typically demonstrate demyelination associated with perivascular inflammatory infiltration without microvascular proliferation. However, the presence of hypercellularity and atypical reactive astrocytes has been described, and this can confuse the clinical picture, sometimes

resulting in the misdiagnosis of tumor [41]. One of the key histopathological differences between TDLs and glioma is the absence of frank angiogenesis within TDLs. The blood vessels in areas of demyelination are intrinsically normal without evidence of neovascularization. TDLs demonstrate mild or no CBV elevation compared with normal white matter. One characteristic feature of TDLs is the presence of intra-lesional venous enhancement. Another is their propensity to occur close to periventricular tributary veins (Figure 11.11) [42]. These findings are in contrast to high-grade gliomas, which characteristically express markedly elevated CBV in both the tumor's enhancing and peritumoral non-enhancing regions.

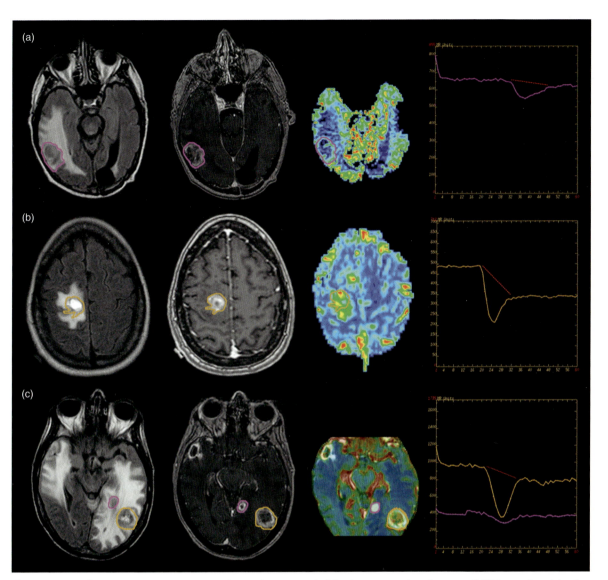

Figure 11.10 Differentiating recurrent metastases from radiation necrosis following stereotactic radiosurgery. FLAIR image, T$_1$-weighted post-contrast image, co-registered CBV map, and signal intensity–time curve are shown in three patients with histologically proven (a) radiation necrosis, (b) recurrent tumor, and (c) mixed radiation necrosis and recurrent tumor. CBV and PH in the contrast-enhancing regions are higher in recurrent metastasis (gold ROIs) compared with radiation necrosis (purple ROIs). Additionally, PSR is significantly reduced within recurrent tumor when compared with radiation necrosis. In (c), differences in perfusion imaging characteristics are helpful to differentiate between recurrent tumor and radiation necrosis in patients with multiple enhancing lesions.

Dynamic contrast-enhanced imaging

Unlike DSC techniques, which focus on characterizing CBV, DCE perfusion imaging is primarily utilized to quantify vascular permeability. Quantifying vascular permeability within the brain provides valuable physiological information about BBB integrity, vascular morphology, and microvascular pathophysiology. As described in Chapter 4, the degree of vascular permeability is usually expressed as the volume transfer constant (K^{trans}). Quantitative estimates of microvascular permeability obtained through DCE techniques have shown potential in preoperatively grading primary gliomas, differentiating recurrent high-grade gliomas from

219

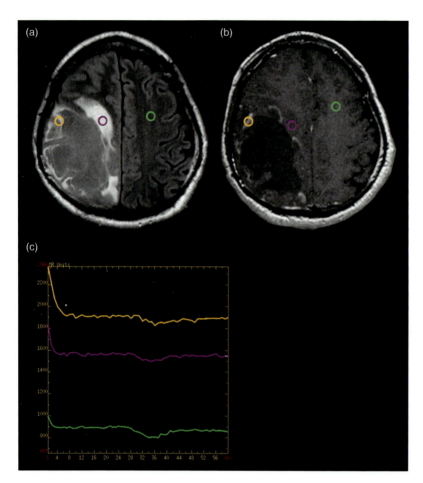

Figure 11.11 Characterization of a tumor-mimicking lesion with DSC perfusion imaging. (a) FLAIR image, (b) post-contrast T_1-weighted image, and (c) signal intensity–time curves from multiple ROIs within a rim-enhancing lesion associated with significant peritumoral edema, later proven to represent tumefactive demyelination. DSC perfusion measurements within enhancing (gold ROI) and non-enhancing (purple ROI) are similar to contralateral normal-appearing white matter (green ROI). The lack of elevated CBV within this lesion supports the diagnosis of TDL rather than a neoplastic process.

radiation-induced necrosis, and differentiating meningiomas from high-grade gliomas.

Pharmacokinetic modeling of intravascular paramagnetic contrast

The modeling of contrast agent uptake in enhancing intracerebral lesions is fully described in Chapter 4. In the setting of a disrupted BBB, contrast extravasates from the blood into the extravascular extracellular space (EES), manifesting as contrast enhancement on CT and MR imaging. The rate at which contrast agent permeates into the EES is governed by several factors: (1) the surface area of the disrupted BBB; (2) the degree of endothelial permeability; (3) the molecular size of the intravascular contrast agent; and (4) the contrast concentration gradient across the vascular wall. DCE perfusion imaging involves dynamic T_1-weighted images (often 3D spoiled gradient-recalled (SPGR) acquisition sequences) after intravenous (IV) contrast administration. The most widely applied technique to measure vascular permeability is based on a two-compartment pharmacokinetic model described by Tofts and Kermode [43–45], which fits the signal intensity–time curve to a three-parameter model. After determining the time course of the contrast agent concentration in blood plasma, referred to as the 'arterial input function' (AIF), measurement of the time course of contrast agent accumulation in tissue allows for the EES volume fraction and K^{trans} to be calculated.

It should be recognized, however, that this approach has two significant limitations in clinical practice: (1) the presence of intravascular signal within the tissue ROI; and (2) its dependence on the flow. Voxels containing cerebral vasculature will have a large signal change, giving rise to erroneously large K^{trans} values, sometimes referred to as a "pseudo-permeability effect." The pseudo-permeability effect is manifested as high permeability in areas of otherwise normal-appearing brain. Also, as described in Chapter 4, under certain conditions (particularly in the case of low CBF) the uptake of contrast agent in the tissue will be determined by the blood flow, rather than by the permeability. Due to these two shortcomings, modifications in the original compartmental pharmacokinetic modeling technique have been described [43].

Intuitively, it would seem that more complex models that more accurately estimate individual hemodynamic components would be more desirable than simpler analytical approaches; however, the addition of more variables into the curve-fitting process can lead to increased variability, resulting in increased uncertainty in the derived measurements. Therefore, the precise DCE perfusion MR imaging technique and post-processing strategy used is often dependent on the clinical question to be addressed.

In addition to pharmacokinetically based analytical modeling techniques, DCE data may also be analyzed to yield semi-quantitative-derived parameters that characterize a lesion's contrast enhancement dynamics. These measures include time to peak enhancement (TTP), peak enhancement level, maximum relative enhancement, maximum rate of signal change (maximal intensity change per unit time interval ratio; MITR), contrast enhancement washout rate, and initial area under the signal intensity–time curve (Figure 11.12). While easier to quantify, these non-pharmacokinetic parameters are subject to significant variability due to differences in patient cardiac physiology, MR scanner and sequences, and the non-linear relationship between contrast concentration and signal intensity. This non-linearity has a profound effect on the measurement accuracy, resulting in between-subjects variability. Despite these limitations, some investigators have demonstrated the clinical utility of some non-pharmacokinetic DCE perfusion parameters [19].

Clinical applications of dynamic contrast-enhanced perfusion imaging

Preoperative grading of glioma

K^{trans} represents a quantitative measure of contrast enhancement within the brain. Since it is well known that high-grade gliomas tend to demonstrate more enhancement than low-grade gliomas, it is to be expected that K^{trans} will correlate strongly with glioma grade [46, 47]. The presence of a disrupted BBB within glomeruloid vessels allows for the leakage of intravascular contrast material into the EES, which can be quantified utilizing K^{trans} measurements (Figure 11.13). Studies comparing tumor grade and estimates of K^{trans} show a close correlation in gliomas, with higher values seen in tumor grade III and IV than in low-grade, minimally enhancing masses. Additionally, studies have demonstrated a statistically significant correlation between K^{trans} and mitotic indices [47]. The characterization of DCE-derived K^{trans} in combination with DSC CBV provides additional physiological information about BBB integrity and elevated microvascular density which can further aid in the grading of primary glioma.

Differentiating meningioma from high-grade glioma

High-grade gliomas and meningiomas are the two most common primary brain tumors. The morphological and physiological vasculature properties of these two tumor types are markedly dissimilar. Meningiomas are highly vascular tumors with capillaries that completely lack a BBB due to their recruitment of the extra-axial blood supply. Conversely, the vasculature of high-grade gliomas expresses varying degrees of BBB disruption, depending on grade and histological subtype. As a result, the degree of capillary permeability in meningioma is generally higher than in primary high-grade gliomas. A study of five patients with glioma and five patients with meningioma, found that the EES was significantly larger within meningiomas ($34 \pm 7\%$) compared with gliomas ($22 \pm 4\%$) [48]. Additionally, K^{trans} was significantly lower within high-grade glioma ($0.15 \pm 0.03 \ \text{min}^{-1}$) when compared with meningioma ($0.28 \pm 0.20 \ \text{min}^{-1}$). While these perfusion parameters are very different, it is usually not a diagnostic challenge to differentiate a glioma from a meningioma on conventional MRI because of their different morphology.

Differentiating recurrent high-grade glioma from radiation-induced necrosis

Although both recurrent tumor and radiation necrosis typically exhibit contrast enhancement, some

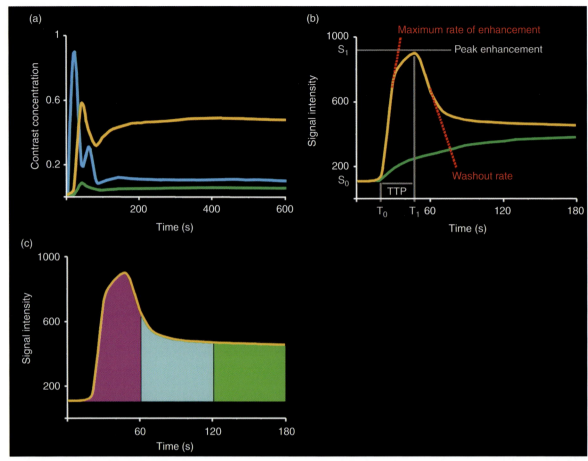

Figure 11.12 Quantitative pharmacokinetic and semi-quantitative parameters calculated with DCE imaging. (a) Contrast concentration–time curves obtained from the enhancing region of a GBM (gold), contralateral normal-appearing white matter (green), and AIF (blue) allows for the calculation of EES volume and bulk transfer coefficient (K^{trans}) as well as other quantitative pharmacokinetic measures. There are markedly elevated values of these parameters within the enhancing GBM tissue when compared with normal-appearing white matter. (b) Signal intensity–time curves obtained from another patient with GBM (gold) and contralateral normal-appearing white matter (green) demonstrate the calculation of semi-quantitative DCE parameters. Time-to-peak enhancement (TTP) is the period between the onset of enhancement (T_0) and peak enhancement (T_1). Peak enhancement is the absolute signal intensity value (S_1) during maximum enhancement. Maximum relative enhancement is the difference between the baseline signal intensity S_0 and S_1. Maximum rate of enhancement (MITR) and washout rates can also be measured. (c) Area under the signal intensity–time curve (AUC) from initial time point of contrast administration (T_0) can be measured by integrating over 60 sec (purple), 120 s (blue), or 180 s (green).

studies have indicated that DCE imaging may be useful to distinguish them. One study, using T_1-weighted fast spin-echo DCE, measured the maximum rate of signal change in 73 patients with either recurrent primary glial neoplasms or radiation necrosis [49]. Recurrent gliomas were found to demonstrate significantly elevated maximum rate of signal change ($5.85 \pm 1.78\,\mathrm{s}^{-1}$) when compared with histologically confirmed radiation necrosis ($1.90 \pm 0.78\,\mathrm{s}^{-1}$). This finding may reflect differences in blood flow rather than permeability, however.

Clinical trial endpoint: the utilization of DCE perfusion MR imaging

Over the last decade there has been significant progress in the development of anti-angiogenic therapies for primary brain tumors. With the increasing clinical implementation of these targeted therapeutics, there is a need for modalities that can non-invasively access their efficacy in vivo. DCE imaging has been proposed as a method to assess physiological treatment response of anti-angiogenic therapies. It has been

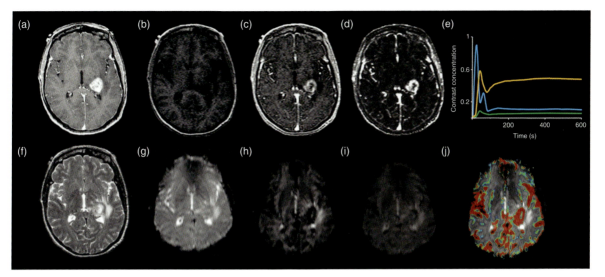

Figure 11.13 Combined analysis of DCE (b–e) and DSC (g–j) perfusion imaging in a 63-year-old man with a left dorsolateral thalamic GBM (grade IV). (a) T_1-weighted post-contrast and dynamic series of steady-state T_1-weighted 3D SPGR images (b) before and (c) after the administration of IV contrast demonstrate progressive enhancement consistent with increased permeability within the rim of the tumor. (e) Idealized illustration of contrast concentration–time curves in the enhancing portion of the GBM (gold), contralateral normal-appearing white matter (green), and AIF (blue). (f) T_2-weighted image and (g) series of T_2^*-weighted gradient-echo EPI (TR/TE 1250/54 ms) obtained before IV contrast, at the peak arrival time (h; 10 s after the bolus injection of contrast agent), and 50 s after injection (i) demonstrates marked signal intensity drop within the tumor and subsequent return of the signal intensity to baseline except in areas of disruption or lack of the BBB where leakage has occurred. (j) CBV map superimposed upon the SPGR image demonstrates elevated CBV in a similar location to the region of increased permeability.

recommended that K^{trans} and initial area under the signal intensity–time curve, obtained on a voxel-by-voxel basis, be used for the assessment of anti-angiogenic therapeutics. These two DCE imaging measures require calculation of instantaneous tumor contrast agent concentration, based on the change in T_1 relaxivity due to contrast uptake (ΔR_1). The ΔR_1 measurement requires (1) an estimate of contrast agent relaxivity in tumor vasculature and tissues; (2) measurement of tumor pre-contrast T_1 relaxation rate; (3) accurate T_1 measurement method; (4) AIF measurement; and (5) reproducible contrast injection, ideally with an MR-compatible power injector. These guidelines, initiated in 2002, are significant because they are the first to suggest that quantitative DCE imaging can be used as a primary endpoint for clinical trials in a standardized format.

Arterial spin labeling

The previous two sections have discussed techniques that utilize intravascular contrast agents to quantify tissue hemodynamics. DSC and DCE imaging techniques indirectly estimate tissue perfusion parameters through either the T_2^* or T_1 relaxation effects induced

by exogenous contrast material. While these methods have gained widespread clinical implementation, they have several limitations. A significant limitation is that patients with allergy to gadolinium (Gd) contrast agents and/or with impaired renal function cannot undergo such contrast-based methods. Additionally, repetitive measurements are difficult because multiple contrast injections would be required. In these situations, use of non-invasive MR perfusion techniques based on labeling of endogenous water in inflowing blood (ASL) may be preferable. Chapter 3 provides a full description of ASL acquisition and analysis methods. ASL has shown promise in the preoperative grading of glioma and in differentiating the etiology of solitary intracerebral enhancing lesions, and is also largely unaffected by the problems associated with confounding contrast enhancement which can occur with DSC. However, since ASL has only relatively recently become commercially available on most MR scanners, there are fewer ASL studies of brain neo-plasms compared to DSC/DCE, but the use of this technique is growing.

Most studies of ASL in brain tumors have also compared the findings with contrast-based DSC perfusion imaging. In general, similar findings are

223

present with both modalities, and it is generally concluded that ASL CBF and DSC-based rCBV are largely equivalent to identify regions of hyper- and hypoperfusion associated with tumors, particularly at 3 T [50–52]. One study [51] also showed that the use of a fast spin-echo ASL readout had significant advantages in reducing the susceptibility artifact seen in gradient-echo echo-planar imaging (EPI) DSC methods.

Clinical applications of arterial spin labeling

Differentiating intra-axial enhancing mass lesions

It can often be difficult to reliably distinguish between different malignant lesions (such as high-grade glioma, primary CNS lymphoma, and intra-axial metastasis) using conventional MR imaging. Additionally, it can also sometimes be difficult to differentiate these lesions from benign entities, such as meningioma and hemangioblastoma. ASL may add additional physiological information that can help with this diagnostic dilemma. As previously discussed, the biological microstructure of these three common malignant intra-axial lesions markedly differs, based on angiogenesis and tumor invasion beyond the contrast-enhancing regions. Histologically, high-grade gliomas demonstrate markedly increased infiltrative tumor and neovascularization within non-enhancing T_2 hyperintense regions. This increased angiogenesis within the peritumoral regions is histologically expressed as elevated microvascular density. Conversely, primary CNS lymphoma and metastatic tumors do not demonstrate infiltrative peri-axonal tumor spread or increased neovascularization beyond the region of enhancement. In the peritumoral regions, the T_2 hyperintensity is physiologically due to vasogenic edema resulting from the subtle BBB deficits. Therefore patterns of CBF increase as depicted on ASL may be helpful in distinguishing these lesion types.

Preoperative grading of gliomas

Similar to DSC, ASL estimates of CBF may provide a measure of angiogenesis and microvascular proliferation prior to a surgical tissue sampling. Additionally, given the heterogeneous biological expression patterns of primary glioma, ASL holds promise in

directing regional biopsy sampling to areas of elevated neovascularization, which may help to reduce undergrading of primary glial tumors due to sampling error. The first ASL study [53] to report elevated CBF in high-grade gliomas compared with either low-grade glioma or metastasis using a pulsed ASL method using multiple readout time points. This study also compared DSC and ASL results in the same patients, and concluded that both methods had equal sensitivity for making this distinction, though it was reported that CBF may have been underestimated at high flow rates with ASL, due to a reduced water extraction fraction at high CBF. In the same paper it was suggested that relative CBF (rCBF) may be more sensitive than absolute measurements, due to age dependence of normal CBF. Another study [54] used continuous ASL (CASL) at 3 T, also focusing on differentiating high-grade from low-grade glioma. It was also found that rCBF measures (defined as tumor CBF divided by the global CBF, excluding the tumor ROI) were better at separating the tumor groups than absolute CBF. Another study [55] assessed the benefit of adding flow-sensitive alternating inversion recovery (FAIR) ASL and diffusion-weighted imaging (DWI) to conventional imaging to distinguish between gliomas ranging from grade II to grade IV. While it is difficult to assess how much of the effect was due to ASL and how much due to DWI, it was found that observers diagnosed the correct glioma grade 70% of the time before evaluating the ASL and DWI sequences, and 88% of the time after evaluation, suggesting that such sequences add value to the workup of primary glioma. Specifically for distinguishing high-grade gliomas (grades III–IV) from low-grade (grade II), the use of a rCBF threshold of 1.24 (relative to the contralateral normal area) yielded sensitivity and specificity of 96% and 82%, respectively, with a high area under the curve (AUC) on the receiver-operating characteristic (ROC) plot (0.97).

In another study, two pulsed ASL (PASL) techniques (one based on FAIR, the other on a Q2TIPS approach) were used to quantify rCBF in patients with pathologically diagnosed primary gliomas of varying grades [56]. rCBF in this study was defined as the tumor CBF divided by the mean gray matter CBF. It was found that a moderate correlation existed between the two ASL sequences, and rCBF was found to be significantly elevated within GBM (rCBF 1.8) when compared with anaplastic astrocytoma (1.1) and low-grade gliomas (0.8) (Figure 11.14). The AUC of

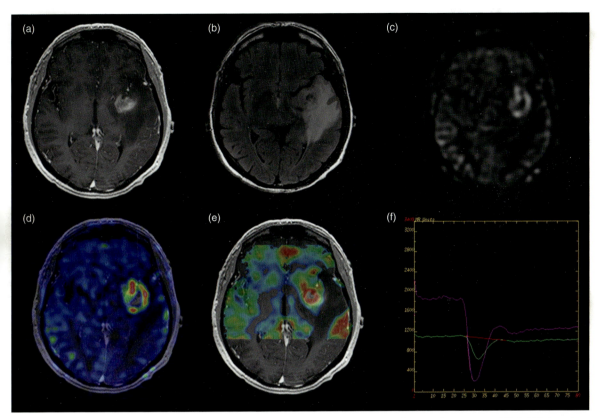

Figure 11.14 Example of ASL in a case of GBM: (a) Post-contrast T_1-weighted, (b) FLAIR, and (c) pseudo-continuous ASL (pCASL-based CBF images. Fused color (d) ASL CBF and (e) DSC-derived CBV maps demonstrate increased values within the contrast-enhancing regions of the tumor. (f) The signal intensity–time curve demonstrates elevated relative PH and greater than 60% return to baseline (PSR) in the lesion (purple), which in combination with elevated CBF and CBV suggests a high-grade glioma.

the ROC plot to distinguish GBM from anaplastic astrocytoma was 0.83, and using a rCBF threshold of 1.4, the sensitivity and specificity was 97% and 50%, respectively. For distinguishing GBM from low-grade glioma, the AUC was 0.94, and using a rCBF threshold of 1.6, the sensitivity and specificity were 94% and 78%, respectively. It was more difficult to distinguish between anaplastic astrocytoma and low-grade astrocytomas (AUC 0.76). While preoperative biopsy remains the gold standard for grading primary gliomas, the findings of this and other studies suggest that ASL shows promise for the assessment of new primary gliomas.

Distinguishing between GBM and other brain neoplasms

As with DSC, another potential application for ASL CBF imaging is to differentiate GBM from other brain neoplasms, the most common being either intracranial metastases or primary CNS lymphoma. In the previously discussed study [56], it was found

that GBM and intracranial metastases could be distinguished based on the CBF in the T_2-hyperintense regions surrounding the areas of enhancement. Using a rCBF threshold of 0.5 (relative to normal gray matter CBF), sensitivity and specificity values of 100% and 71%, respectively were found. Interestingly, neither rCBV (measured using DSC) nor rCBF (using either of two ASL sequences) within the enhancing region of the tumor itself could distinguish GBM from metastases. Comparing GBM and CNS lymphoma, it was found that an rCBF threshold of 1.2 yielded sensitivity and specificity of 97% and 80%, respectively. The results of this study demonstrate that ASL quantification of CBF is useful in distinguishing GBM from primary CNS lymphoma and intra-axial metastasis. More studies are needed to determine the relative sensitivity and specificity of ASL vs. DSC perfusion imaging for distinguishing primary glial neoplasms of all grades from other tumor types.

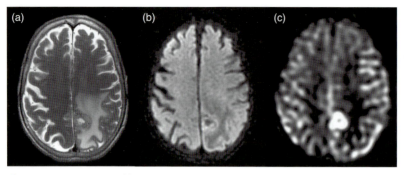

Figure 11.15 An 85-year-old women presenting with new seizure. (a) T$_2$-weighted image shows a small mass lesion in the left parietal lobe with extensive vasogenic edema. (b) There is no diffusion reduction to suggest an abscess or stroke. Contrast could not be given because of the patient's poor renal function and low creatinine clearance. (c) Non-contrast PCASL CBF imaging demonstrates that the lesion is hypervascular, suggesting a neoplasm. Biopsy revealed metastatic renal cell carcinoma, an entity known to be highly vascular. Case courtesy of Greg Zaharchuk, Stanford University, Stanford, USA.

Evaluating response to treatment

One advantage of ASL (compared to DSC) to evaluate response to treatment is its inherently quantitative nature, such that 'absolute CBF' may be compared over different time points in the same subject without the need for normalization. One ASL study [57] of intracranial metastases before and at several time points after stereotactic radiation found that pre-treatment rCBF (calculated as the ratio of the CBF in the tumor to the CBF of normal gray matter) was not predictive of local control. However, tumors that did not respond could be distinguished from those that either were stable or regressed as early as 6 weeks after treatment, with the rCBF decreasing significantly in the latter cases. This conclusion was the same regardless of whether ASL or DSC was used as the perfusion imaging method. An ASL case report [58] of a patient with GBM treated with an anti-angiogenic (bevacizumab) showed that while the enhancing region and FLAIR hyperintensity decreased during the first month after treatment, CBF (based on either ASL or DSC) continued to increase and predicted subsequent failure.

Special cases

Based on clinical experience, several investigators have determined that certain non-glial brain tumors appear especially prominent on ASL perfusion imaging. In particular, high CBF has been noted in hemangioblastoma and in renal cell carcinoma metastasis. Both of these lesions are known to be highly vascular. Hemangioblastoma is an uncommon tumor that primarily affects the posterior fossa and can be associated with

von Hippel–Lindau syndrome; one study [59] showed that the mean CBF from pathologically proven hemangioblastoma was significantly higher than that of a group of untreated solitary metastases. Using the PASL QUASAR method, a mean CBF of 437 ± 234 ml/100 g/min was found in four cases of hemangioblastoma, which was significantly higher than that from the group of metastases (125 ± 134 ml/100 g/min). It was also noted that the one outlier in terms of high CBF was a renal cell carcinoma metastasis, an entity known to have high vascularity (Figure 11.15).

Technical considerations, limitations, and pitfalls

Dynamic susceptibility contrast

The successful clinical implementation of DSC perfusion MR imaging techniques requires correct choice of data acquisition, a robust contrast agent bolus, and appropriate analysis software and visualization. For data acquisition, a fast MR imaging sequence, such as EPI, should be used to acquire multi-slice images with a temporal resolution of 1–2 s, usually with a gradient-echo EPI sequence. Sequence parameters depend on the field strength used, the desired coverage, and spatial and temporal resolution. At 1.5 T, TE values of 45–50 ms give excellent contrast with gradient-echo EPI and a single dose of Gd. At 3 T, shorter TE values between 30 and 45 ms may be used. Typical slice thicknesses are 3–5 mm with an in-plane resolution of ~2 mm. With these parameters it is usually possible to interleave about 20 slices within one TR time period, allowing more or less whole brain coverage. If higher spatial resolution is required for a lesion study, the number of slices and slice thickness can be reduced to only cover the lesion, but with higher temporal and spatial resolution. If a reduced flip angle excitation pulse (e.g., 35°) is used, effects of brain T_1 shortening due to BBB leakage may be somewhat reduced. Some investigators recommend use of a spin-echo EPI readout; however, contrast is much reduced in this case. Also, some investigators recommend 'pre-loading' with a low dose of contrast agent (e.g., 1–2 ml, ~1/10th of the DSC dose) a few min before the actual DSC experiment, in order to saturate the T_1 effect associated with BBB leakage. To cover the first pass through the brain and recirculation, a 60-second dynamic acquisition is probably sufficient; if permeability information is also desired, particularly for more slowly enhancing lesions, the scan can be extended for 2–3 min to capture slower BBB leakage effects.

Second, an MR-compatible power injector should be employed to administer a rapid, uniform, and well-defined contrast agent bolus. It is recommended that all patients undergo placement of an 18-gauge IV catheter prior to imaging, preferably in the right antecubital fossa. Using a right-arm injection site may reduce the occurrence of contrast agent reflux cephalad into the jugular vein. A single, weight-based dose of contrast (0.1 mmol/kg) should be administered at a rate of around 3–5 ml/s, so that the bolus duration is of the order of 3–5 s depending on the patient weight. Some institutions utilize a double dose of contrast agent to improve contrast, although this practice is declining with the increasing awareness of the risk of nephrogenic systemic fibrosis (NSF) for some Gd-based contrast agents. The injection should be followed by a saline flush of 20–30 ml delivered at the same rate, to ensure the entire bolus of contrast enters the circulation.

Third, a clinically assessable software program that allows for straightforward DSC imaging processing and rCBV measurements is required. Unfortunately, until recently, commercially available, US Food and Drug Administration (FDA)-approved DSC processing packages were not available, and processing tools provided by vendors of MRI scanners were limited in their capabilities. At most, some vendors would provide maps of TTP and rCBV. It is therefore preferable to perform offline reconstruction of DSC data. Processing steps may include motion correction, setting threshold values to remove

extraneous data from outside the head, and placing an ROI on an arterial branch in the hemisphere contralateral to the tumor to measure the AIF. Typically, the middle cerebral artery (MCA) or one of its proximal branches is used. The next step is to define the images corresponding to the baseline and first pass of the contrast agent, respectively. The pre-enhancement images are defined as the set of images just prior to the arrival of the bolus, and serve as a baseline for perfusion measurements. Typically the first few time points are excluded in order to allow the signal intensity to reach a steady state. The start of the first pass is defined by the point at which a signal change is first seen within the brain, and may extend either until the start of the second pass, or until the end of the data acquisition. There are relative advantages and disadvantages to each approach – by using the entire data acquisition the effects of slow flow are minimized (more of a problem in cerebrovascular disease than in tumors). However, if the passage of the bolus is rapid, using the whole data acquisition may lower SNR in the calculated perfusion images, and may also introduce motion artifact and increase sensitivity to both recirculation effects and the effects of BBB leakage.

Finally, the user must define the parameters of the CBV calculation method. As previously discussed, the CBV calculation methodology employed has significant implications in measured CBV values. The use of a gamma variate fitting curve technique can yield wide variations in CBV measurements with small changes to the initial measurement parameters. Negative enhancement integral techniques to calculate CBV are clinically very attractive because of their simple calculation methods; however, this image processing technique can result in systematic CBV errors in regions of BBB disruption. Once the methodology has been selected, CBV maps can be calculated on a voxel-by-voxel basis, as described in Chapter 2. PH and PSR parameters can be easily calculated as previously described, using the signal intensity–time curve for each ROI.

There are several important limitations associated with DSC perfusion imaging. First, because the technique is susceptibility-weighted, it is sensitive to structures or lesions that induce strong magnetic field inhomogeneity, such as blood products, calcium, melanin, metal, or lesions near a brain–bone–air interface, such as the anterior and middle cranial fossa or cerebellar hemisphere near the petrous apex. Macroscopic susceptibility may be somewhat decreased by increasing spatial resolution, but this can usually only be done at the expense of decreased coverage. Finally, the CBV calculation may be inaccurate in GBM or meningiomas in the setting of severe breakdown (or absence) of the BBB, unless appropriate acquisition or analysis techniques are used to correct for this. The use of rCBV measurements may lead to erroneous conclusions about absolute CBV changes if there are concomitant global CBV changes (for example, due to chemotherapy effects, or decreased cardiac function).

Dynamic contrast-enhanced imaging

Creating maps of the permeability parameter K^{trans} requires several steps. First, pre-contrast T_1 values must be measured. While several sequences can be used to estimate baseline T_1, a convenient method for this purpose is to use gradient echo sequences with variable flip angles. Then, the dynamic T_1-weighted contrast-enhanced sequence is performed, obtained through the tumor and the major vessels of the brain at a temporal resolution adequate to enable accurate AIF characterization. Again, a standardized contrast administration protocol is recommended, similar to that used for DSC perfusion imaging, although the rate of injection can be lower than that for DSC imaging (e.g., 2 ml/s) since rapid first-pass information is not required in DCE. Axial 3D T_1-weighted imaging with SPGR acquisition in the steady state is recommended for the dynamic T1-weighted acquisition with the following parameters: TR 6.5 ms, 1 excitation, flip angle 30°, in-plane resolution 2 mm, slice thickness 3 mm. A 30-s temporal resolution and a total scan time of around 6 min are recommended.

Following acquisition, generation of parametric maps may involve motion correction, the calculation of contrast concentration versus time, and the identification of the AIF. Measurement of the AIF can be affected by flow effects which can contribute to an apparent change in blood T_1; this can be minimized by using an inferior saturation slab to saturate inflowing spins. Once the AIF has been defined, K^{trans} values can be obtained on a voxel-by-voxel basis as described in Chapter 4 [43–45].

Arterial spin labeling

Quantifying CBF with ASL can be readily incorporated into routine clinical practice. Use of a 3 T scanner is recommended, since ASL has significantly higher SNR at 3 T compared with 1.5 T. PASL is a common

methodology and available commercially on several MRI scanners (Siemens and Philips) [60, 61]. Many investigators have utilized FAIR-based labeling PASL sequences to examine brain tumors. For this indication, using a FAIR approach for labeling has several advantages over EPI-based signal targeting by alternating radiofrequency pulses (EPISTAR), which labels a bolus of blood inferior to the acquired slices. On the other hand, FAIR allows for the non-selective application of an inversion pulse to intravascular water on either side of the imaged volume. Applying the inversion pulse in this manner allows for the intravascular water to contribute equally regardless of the direction from which the blood entered the imaged slices.

Another approach, with higher SNR than PASL, is pseudo-continuous ASL (pCASL), and at the time of writing, this is the standard product on GE scanners [62]. pCASL at 3 T is therefore recommended for tumor studies, with background-suppression, 3D fast spin-echo readout, and online reconstruction of quantitative CBF images. Other sequences currently commercially available are described in Chapter 3. Clinical requirements are multi-slice coverage in a reasonable scan time (4–6 min). Because ASL has relatively low SNR, typical voxel sizes and slice thickness are in the 4–5 mm range. pCASL labeling should be performed for at least 1200–1500 ms, followed by a similar post-labeling delay to allow the blood to transit to the brain. Since CBF images are calculated by subtraction, motion correction prior to subtraction is recommended.

ASL perfusion imaging in routine clinical practice has several limitations. First, ASL techniques allow for quantitative CBF estimation, but cannot monitor other parameters like CBV and K^{trans}. Second, one of the main drawbacks of ASL imaging is the lower SNR when compared with DSC and DCE imaging techniques. ASL methods with improved SNR have been developed [62, 63], and the technique itself is likely to continue to improve. Other drawbacks of ASL are more fully discussed in Chapter 3. Importantly, one of the largest problems with ASL for evaluating cerebrovascular pathologies, that of CBF underestimation in regions with long delay times, is less of a problem for brain tumor studies, since often CBF levels are higher, and arrival times are shorter, than in normal tissue. Finally, ASL techniques are sensitive to patient motion because they involve the subtraction of two images with signal intensities that differ by only a few percent. Single excitation imaging techniques such as EPI and the application of background suppression have helped to dramatically reduce motion-related error. Prospective motion correction approaches are also beginning to be applied to ASL imaging [64].

Conclusion

Perfusion imaging has been demonstrated to be a useful adjuvant to traditional morphological MR imaging, and is becoming increasingly useful in clinical practice for the diagnosis, prognostication, and prediction of response to therapy in patients with brain tumors. DSC, DCE, and ASL perfusion techniques provide quantitative estimates of tumor physiology that can be used to help in (a) the differentiation of tumor from non-neoplastic lesions, (b) evaluation of different tumor types, (c) prediction of tumor grade, (d) monitoring of tumor progression, and (e) monitoring the efficacy of anti-angiogenic therapy. Perfusion imaging techniques continue to develop, and with increasing integration into clinical practice, it is hoped that this will likely result in improved patient outcomes, by providing more accurate and timely diagnoses which can be used to select and guide optimal treatments.

References

1. Lund EL, Spang-Thomsen M, Skovgaard-Poulsen H, Kristjansen PE. Tumor angiogenesis–a new therapeutic target in gliomas. *Acta Neurol Scand* 1998;**97**:52–62.

2. Tate MC, Aghi MK. Biology of angiogenesis and invasion in glioma. *Neurotherapeutics* 2009;**6**:447–57.

3. Jensen RL. Brain tumor hypoxia: tumorigenesis, angiogenesis, imaging, pseudoprogression, and as a therapeutic target. *J Neurooncol* 2009;**92**:317–35.

4. Wong ML, Prawira A, Kaye AH, Hovens CM. Tumour angiogenesis: its mechanism and therapeutic implications in malignant gliomas. *J Clin Neurosci* 2009;**16**:1119–30.

5. Damert A, Machein M, Breier G, *et al.* Up-regulation of vascular endothelial growth factor expression in a rat glioma is conferred by two distinct hypoxia-driven mechanisms. *Cancer Res* 1997;**57**:3860–4.

6. Jouanneau E. Angiogenesis and gliomas: current issues and development of surrogate markers. *Neurosurgery* 2008;**62**:31–50; discussion 50–2.

7. Damert A, Ikeda E, Risau W. Activator-protein-1 binding potentiates the hypoxia-inducible factor-1-mediated hypoxia-induced transcriptional activation of vascular-endothelial growth factor expression in C6 glioma cells. *Biochem J* 1997;**327** (Pt 2):419–23.

8. Sage MR. Blood-brain barrier: phenomenon of increasing importance to the imaging clinician. *AJR Am J Roentgenol* 1982;**138**:887–98.

9. Pietsch T, Valter MM, Wolf HK, *et al.* Expression and distribution of vascular endothelial growth factor protein in human brain tumors. *Acta Neuropathol* 1997;**93**:109–17.

10. Provias J, Claffey K, delAguila L, *et al.* Meningiomas: role of vascular endothelial growth factor/vascular permeability factor in angiogenesis and peritumoral edema. *Neurosurgery* 1997;**40**:1016–26.

11. Dietzmann K, von Bossanyi P, Warich-Kirches M, *et al.* Immunohistochemical detection of vascular growth factors in angiomatous and atypical meningiomas, as well as hemangiopericytomas. *Pathol Res Pract* 1997;**193**:503–10.

12. Assimakopoulou M, Sotiropoulou-Bonikou G, Maraziotis T, Papadakis N, Varakis I. Microvessel density in brain tumors. *Anticancer Res* 1997;**17**:4747–53.

13. Rojiani AM, Dorovini-Zis K. Glomeruloid vascular structures in glioblastoma multiforme: an immunohistochemical and ultrastructural study. *J Neurosurg* 1996;**85**:1078–84.

14. Izycka-Swieszewska E. [Immunomorphological analysis of the vascular stroma in glioblastoma]. *Neurol Neurochir Pol* 2003;**37**:59–71.

15. Prayson RA, Agamanolis DP, Cohen ML, *et al.* Interobserver reproducibility among neuropathologists and surgical pathologists in fibrillary astrocytoma grading. *J Neurol Sci* 2000;**175**:33–9.

16. Coons SW, Johnson PC, Scheithauer BW, Yates AJ, Pearl DK. Improving diagnostic accuracy and interobserver concordance in the classification and grading of primary gliomas. *Cancer* 1997;**79**:1381–93.

17. Peters AM. Fundamentals of tracer kinetics for radiologists. *Br J Radiol* 1998;**71**:1116–29.

18. Aronen HJ, Gazit IE, Louis DN, *et al.* Cerebral blood volume maps of gliomas: comparisons with tumor grade and histological findings. *Radiology* 1994;**191**:41–51.

19. Knopp EA, Cha S, Johnson G, *et al.* Glial neoplasms: dynamic contrast-enhanced T2*-weighted

MR imaging. *Radiology* 1999;**211**:791–8.

20. Cha S, Knopp EA, Johnson G, *et al.* Dynamic contrast-enhanced T2-weighted MR imaging of recurrent malignant gliomas treated with thalidomide and carboplatin. *AJNR Am J Neuroradiol* 2000;**21**:881–90.

21. Sugahara T, Korogi Y, Shigematsu Y, *et al.* Perfusion-sensitive MRI of cerebral lymphomas: a preliminary report. *J Comput Assist Tomogr* 1999;**23**:232–7.

22. Sugahara T, Korogi Y, Shigematsu Y, *et al.* Value of dynamic susceptibility contrast magnetic resonance imaging in the evaluation of intracranial tumors. *Top Magn Reson Imaging* 1999;**10**:114–24.

23. Villringer A, Rosen BR, Belliveau JW, *et al.* Dynamic imaging with lanthanide chelates in normal brain: contrast due to magnetic susceptibility effects. *Magn Reson Med* 1988;**6**:164–74.

24. Rosen BR, Belliveau JW, Vevea JM, Brady TJ. Perfusion imaging with NMR contrast agents. *Magn Reson Med* 1990;**14**:249–65.

25. Vonken EJ, van Osch MJ, Bakker CJ, Viergever MA. Measurement of cerebral perfusion with dual-echo multi-slice quantitative dynamic susceptibility contrast MRI. *J Magn Reson Imaging* 1999;**10**:109–17.

26. Newbould RD, Skare ST, Jochimsen TH, *et al.* Perfusion mapping with multiecho multishot parallel imaging EPI. *Magn Reson Med* 2007;**58**:70–81.

27. Paulson ES, Schmainda KM. Comparison of dynamic susceptibility-weighted contrast-enhanced MR methods: recommendations for measuring relative cerebral blood volume in brain tumors. *Radiology* 2008;**249**:601–13.

28. Boxerman JL, Schmainda KM, Weisskoff RM. Relative cerebral blood volume maps corrected for contrast agent extravasation significantly correlate with glioma tumor grade, whereas uncorrected maps do not. *AJNR Am J Neuroradiol* 2006;**27**:859–67.

29. Sugahara T, Korogi Y, Kochi M, *et al.* Correlation of MR imaging-determined cerebral blood volume maps with histologic and angiographic determination of vascularity of gliomas. *AJR Am J Roentgenol* 1998;**171**:1479–86.

30. Barajas RF, Jr., Hodgson JG, Chang JS, *et al.* Glioblastoma multiforme regional genetic and cellular expression patterns: influence on anatomic and physiologic MR imaging. *Radiology* 2010;**254**:564–76.

31. Cha S, Tihan T, Crawford F, *et al.* Differentiation of low-grade oligodendrogliomas from low-grade astrocytomas by using quantitative blood-volume measurements derived from dynamic susceptibility contrast-enhanced MR imaging. *AJNR Am J Neuroradiol* 2005;**26**:266–73.

32. Senturk S, Oguz KK, Cila A. Dynamic contrast-enhanced susceptibility-weighted perfusion imaging of intracranial tumors: a study using a 3T MR scanner. *Diagn Interv Radiol* 2009;**15**:3–12.

33. Sugahara T, Korogi Y, Kochi M, Ushio Y, Takahashi M. Perfusion-sensitive MR imaging of gliomas: comparison between gradient-echo and spin-echo echo-planar imaging techniques. *AJNR Am J Neuroradiol* 2001;**22**:1306–15.

34. Law M, Cha S, Knopp EA, *et al.* High-grade gliomas and solitary metastases: differentiation by using perfusion and proton spectroscopic MR imaging. *Radiology* 2002;**222**:715–21.

35. Cha S, Lupo JM, Chen MH, *et al.* Differentiation of glioblastoma multiforme and single brain metastasis by peak height and percentage of signal intensity recovery derived from dynamic susceptibility-weighted contrast-enhanced perfusion MR imaging. *AJNR Am J Neuroradiol* 2007;**28**:1078–84.

36. Barajas RF, Jr., Chang JS, Segal MR, *et al.* Differentiation of recurrent glioblastoma multiforme from radiation necrosis after external beam radiation therapy with dynamic susceptibility-weighted contrast-enhanced perfusion MR imaging. *Radiology* 2009;**253**:486–96.

37. Sugahara T, Korogi Y, Tomiguchi S, *et al.* Posttherapeutic intraaxial brain tumor: the value of perfusion-sensitive contrast-enhanced MR imaging for differentiating tumor recurrence from nonneoplastic contrast-enhancing tissue. *AJNR Am J Neuroradiol* 2000;**21**:901–9.

38. Barajas RF, Chang JS, Sneed PK, *et al.* Distinguishing recurrent intra-axial metastatic tumor from radiation necrosis following gamma knife radiosurgery using dynamic susceptibility-weighted contrast-enhanced perfusion MR imaging. *AJNR Am J Neuroradiol* 2009;**30**:367–72.

39. Essig M, Waschkies M, Wenz F, *et al.* Assessment of brain metastases with dynamic susceptibility-weighted contrast-enhanced MR imaging: initial results. *Radiology* 2003;**228**:193–9.

40. Giang DW, Poduri KR, Eskin TA, *et al.* Multiple sclerosis masquerading as a mass lesion. *Neuroradiology* 1992;**34**:150–4.

41. Nesbit GM, Forbes GS, Scheithauer BW, Okazaki H, Rodriguez M. Multiple sclerosis: histopathologic and MR and/or CT correlation in 37 cases at biopsy and three cases at autopsy. *Radiology* 1991;**180**:467–74.

42. Cha S, Pierce S, Knopp EA, *et al.* Dynamic contrast-enhanced T2*-weighted MR imaging of tumefactive demyelinating lesions. *AJNR Am J Neuroradiol* 2001;**22**:1109–16.

43. Tofts PS, Brix G, Buckley DL, *et al.* Estimating kinetic parameters from dynamic contrast-enhanced T(1)-weighted MRI of a diffusable tracer: standardized quantities and symbols. *J Magn Reson Imaging* 1999;**10**:223–32.

44. Tofts PS, Kermode AG. Measurement of the blood-brain barrier permeability and leakage space using dynamic MR imaging. 1. Fundamental concepts. *Magn Reson Med* 1991;**17**:357–67.

45. Tofts PS. Modeling tracer kinetics in dynamic Gd-DTPA MR imaging. *J Magn Reson Imaging* 1997;**7**:91–101.

46. Patankar TF, Haroon HA, Mills SJ, *et al.* Is volume transfer coefficient (K(trans)) related to histologic grade in human gliomas? *AJNR Am J Neuroradiol* 2005;**26**:2455–65.

47. Roberts HC, Roberts TP, Bollen AW, *et al.* Correlation of microvascular permeability derived from dynamic contrast-enhanced MR imaging with histologic grade and tumor labeling index: a study in human brain tumors. *Acad Radiol* 2001;**8**:384–91.

48. Zhu XP, Li KL, Kamaly-Asl ID, *et al.* Quantification of endothelial permeability, leakage space, and blood volume in brain tumors using combined T1 and T2* contrast-enhanced dynamic MR imaging. *J Magn Reson Imaging* 2000;**11**:575–85.

49. Hazle JD, Jackson EF, Schomer DF, Leeds NE. Dynamic imaging of intracranial lesions using fast spin-echo imaging: differentiation of brain tumors and treatment effects. *J Magn Reson Imaging* 1997;**7**:1084–93.

50. Lehmann P, Monet P, de Marco G, *et al.* A comparative study of perfusion measurement in brain tumours at 3 Tesla MR: arterial spin labeling versus dynamic susceptibility contrast-enhanced MRI. *Eur Neurol* 2010;**64**:21–6.

51. Jarnum H, Steffensen EG, Knutsson L, *et al.* Perfusion MRI of brain tumours: a comparative study of pseudo-continuous arterial spin labelling and dynamic susceptibility contrast imaging. *Neuroradiology* 2010;**52**:307–17.

52. Tourdias T, Rodrigo S, Oppenheim C, *et al.* Pulsed arterial spin labeling applications in brain tumors: practical review. *J Neuroradiol* 2008;**35**:79–89.

53. Warmuth C, Gunther M, Zimmer C. Quantification of blood flow in brain tumors: comparison of arterial spin labeling and dynamic susceptibility-weighted contrast-enhanced MR imaging. *Radiology* 2003;**228**:523–32.

54. Wolf RL, Wang J, Wang S, *et al.* Grading of CNS neoplasms using continuous arterial spin labeled perfusion MR imaging at 3 Tesla. *J Magn Reson Imaging* 2005;**22**:475–82.

55. Kim HS, Kim SY. A prospective study on the added value of pulsed arterial spin-labeling and apparent diffusion coefficients in the grading of gliomas. *AJNR Am J Neuroradiol* 2007;**28**:1693–9.

56. Weber MA, Zoubaa S, Schlieter M, *et al.* Diagnostic performance of spectroscopic and perfusion MRI for distinction of brain tumors. *Neurology* 2006;**66**:1899–906.

57. Weber MA, Thilmann C, Lichy MP, *et al.* Assessment of irradiated brain metastases by means of arterial spin-labeling and dynamic susceptibility-weighted contrast-enhanced perfusion MRI: initial results. *Invest Radiol* 2004;**39**:277–87.

58. Fellah S, Girard N, Chinot O, Cozzone PJ, Callot V. Early evaluation of tumoral response to anti-angiogenic therapy by arterial spin labeling perfusion magnetic resonance imaging and susceptibility weighted imaging in a patient with recurrent glioblastoma receiving bevacizumab. *J Clin Oncol* 2011;**29**:e308–11.

59. Yamashita K, Yoshiura T, Hiwatashi A, *et al.* Arterial spin labeling of hemangioblastoma: differentiation from metastatic brain tumors based on quantitative blood flow measurement. *Neuroradiology* 2012;**54**:809–13.

60. Luh WM, Wong EC, Bandettini PA, Hyde JS. QUIPSS II with thin-slice TI1 periodic saturation: a method for improving accuracy of quantitative perfusion imaging using pulsed arterial spin labeling. *Magn Reson Med* 1999;**41**:1246–54.

61. Petersen ET, Lim T, Golay X. Model-free arterial spin labeling quantification approach for perfusion MRI. *Magn Reson Med* 2006;**55**:219–32.

62. Dai W, Garcia D, de Bazelaire C, Alsop DC. Continuous flow driven inversion for arterial spin labeling using pulsed radiofrequency and gradient fields. *Magn Reson Med* 2008;**60**:1488–97.

63. Guenther M, Oshio K, Feinberg DA. Single-shot 3D imaging techniques improve arterial spin labeling perfusion measurements. *Magn Reson Med* 2005;**54**:491–8.

64. Zhang J, Zaharchuk G, Moseley M, *et al.* Pulsed continuous arterial spin labeling (pcASL) with prospective motion correction (PROMO). *Proc Intl Soc Magn Reson Med*, Stockholm, Sweden, 2010;5034.

Differentiating oligodendroglioma from low-grade astrocytoma

History

(a) A 52-year-old man and (b) a 57-year-old woman present with new headache and onset of seizure activity.

Technique

Post-contrast T_1-weighted (left) and T_2^*-weighted gradient-echo EPI (right; TR/TE 1250/54 ms, flip angle 35°) with overlying CBV map calculated utilizing the baseline subtraction method.

Imaging findings

See Figure 11.16.

Discussion

Contrast enhancement is a non-specific imaging finding which reflects the presence of a disrupted BBB. However, in patient (a), the combination of enhancement, cortical expansion, and markedly elevated CBV is suggestive of low-grade oligodendroglioma or GBM. The lack of elevated CBV within the region of contrast enhancement in patient (b) suggests the presence of a

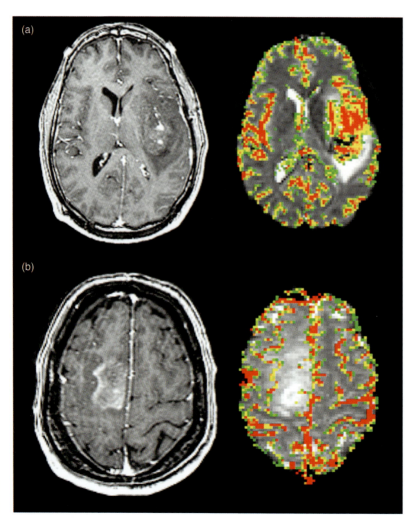

(a)

(b)

Figure 11.16 Both patients demonstrate regions of abnormal contrast enhancement associated with surrounding decreased T_1 signal and mass effect suggestive of vasogenic edema in the setting of a primary glial neoplasm. Additionally, patient (a) demonstrates significant cortical expansion with the tumor centered in the left frontal lobe. Markedly elevated CBV is observed within patient (a). In contrast, the lesion of patient (b) does not have elevated CBV. Image-guided biopsy analysis of regions with elevated CBV in patient (a) resulted in a diagnosis of WHO grade II oligodendroglioma. Tissue obtained from patient (b) was consistent with a diagnosis of WHO grade II astrocytoma.

low-grade glial neoplasm, such as a fibrillary astrocytoma. In this case, a tumefactive demyelinating lesion cannot be entirely excluded given these findings, and histological analysis is required for definitive clinical diagnosis.

Key points

- Oligodendroglioma should be included in the differential diagnosis of an enhancing glial neoplasm with elevated CBV.
- Low-grade fibrillary astrocytomas may have a variable degree of contrast enhancement, but generally do not demonstrate elevated CBV.

Bibliography

Aronen HJ, Gazit IE, Louis DN, *et al*. Cerebral blood volume maps of gliomas: comparison with tumor grade and histologic findings. *Radiology* 1994;**191**:41–51.

Knopp EA, Cha S, Johnson G, *et al*. Glial neoplasms: dynamic contrast-enhanced T2*-weighted MR imaging. *Radiology* 1999;**211**:791–8.

History

(a) A 55-year-old man and (b) a 62-year-old woman without a pertinent past medical history present with severe progressive headache.

Technique

Post-contrast T_1-weighted (left) and T_2*-weighted signal intensity–time curve obtained from gradient-echo EPI (right; TR/TE 1250/54 ms, flip angle 35°) with ROIs placed on the enhancing lesion (green) and normal-appearing white matter (purple) (Figure 11.17).

Imaging findings

See Figure 11.17.

Discussion

The inherent differences in capillary permeability due to the differential expression of the BBB between high-grade primary glioma and metastases form the basis for tumor differentiation using DSC perfusion imaging. Quantification of tumor-wide PSR measurements based on the signal intensity–time curves can be helpful in differentiating GBM from solitary brain metastasis. Treatment-naïve GBM typically demonstrate greater than 65% recovery to baseline. Conversely, intracerebral

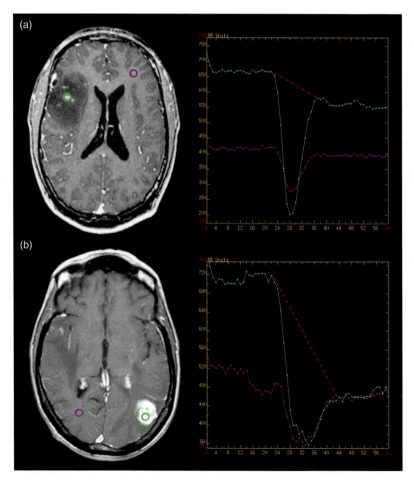

Figure 11.17 Both patients demonstrate abnormal but non-specific solitary foci of contrast enhancement. Interrogation of the signal intensity–time curve demonstrates greater than 75% return of signal intensity to baseline during the post-bolus phase in patient (a) (green curve). Conversely, patient (b) demonstrates significantly reduced signal intensity following the bolus phase of contrast administration (green curve). Both patients demonstrate similar relative PH and CBV. Image-guided biopsy analysis of the enhancing regions demonstrated GBM within patient (a), while patient (b) was histologically diagnosed with metastatic breast cancer.

metastases typically demonstrate less than 50% of signal intensity recovery. Enhancement and CBV measurements are typically not as useful in differentiating between these two entities.

Key points

- PSR is markedly diminished within enhancing metastatic foci when compared with treatment-naïve high-grade glial neoplasms.
- CBV and PH measurements obtained from enhancing regions are less useful for this distinction.

Bibliography

Law M, Cha S, Knopp EA, *et al.* High-grade gliomas and solitary metastases: differentiation by using perfusion and proton spectroscopic MR imaging. *Radiology* 2002;**222**(3):715–21.

Cha S, Lupo JM, Chen MH, *et al.* Differentiation of glioblastoma multiforme and single brain metastasis by peak height and percentage of signal intensity recovery derived from dynamic susceptibility-weighted contrast-enhanced perfusion MR imaging. *AJNR Am J Neuroradiol* 2007;**28**(6): 1078–84.

History

A 60-year-old woman with loss of consciousness.

Technique

(a) Non-contrast CT was the initial study. Based on this, MRI was performed 2 days later, including (b) FLAIR, (c) post-contrast T_1-weighted imaging, (d) PCASL, and (e) bolus DSC perfusion-weighted imaging (PWI)-based rCBV. (f) Six days later, biopsy was performed at the lateral aspect of the lesion. (g) One month later, post-contrast T_1-weighted imaging was repeated (Figure 11.18).

Imaging findings

See Figure 11.18.

Discussion

This case demonstrates the problems of sampling error in clinical biopsies and the use of perfusion imaging to guide the best site to biopsy. Initially, in this case, there was enhancement surrounding the hematoma, and biopsy was performed at the most clinically accessible site, the lateral aspect; however, this region was not enhancing because of neoplasm, but rather due to reactive changes following hematoma. Lesion growth and subsequent biopsy of the medial aspect of this mass confirmed the presence of GBM.

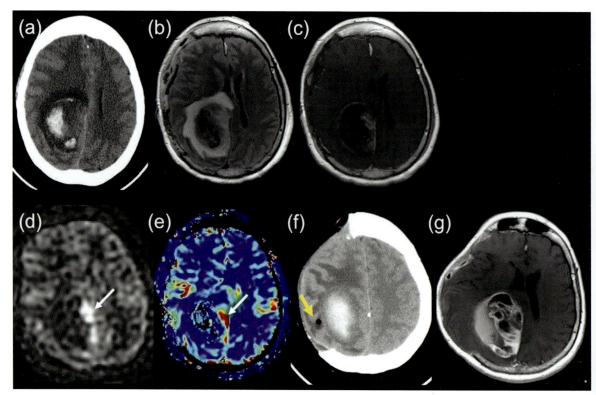

Figure 11.18 (a) Initial non-contrast CT showed an intraparenchymal hematoma in the right frontal lobe. (b) Subsequent MRI showed a (c) ring-enhancing lesion with significant edema. (d) ASL demonstrated increased CBF, while (e) DSC showed elevated rCBV limited to the medial aspect of the hematoma (arrows). Unfortunately, the neurosurgeons performed the biopsy at the lateral aspect of the lesion, which returned 'no neoplasm.' (f) Post-operative CT demonstrates site of tissue sampling denoted by foci of air (yellow arrow). The patient returned one month later, at which point, (g) a repeat MRI was performed and demonstrated marked increase in size and enhancement of the mass, primarily in the medial region where the perfusion imaging was abnormal. Repeat biopsy of the medial aspect of the mass was performed, and pathology demonstrated glioblastoma multiforme (GBM).

- Perfusion imaging can help guide the biopsy toward the highest-grade part of an enhancing mass.
- Both ASL CBF and DSC rCBV can be used for this purpose.

Bibliography

Maia AC, Jr., Malheiros SM, da Rocha AJ, *et al.* Stereotactic biopsy guidance in adults with supratentorial nonenhancing gliomas: role of perfusion-weighted magnetic resonance imaging. *J Neurosurg* 2004; **101**(6):970–6.

Chapter

12

MR perfusion imaging in oncology: applications outside the brain

James P. B. O'Connor and Geoff J. M. Parker

Key points

- Among non-neurological applications, perfusion MRI is mainly used in breast, liver, and prostate cancer.
- The most common application is the use of enhancement pattern to characterize lesions as malignant or benign.
- Other applications include targeting of biopsy and monitoring of treatment response.
- DSC is less frequently used outside the brain, but may be included as part of a multi-parametric response.
- DCE-MRI is being increasingly used as an indicator of treatment response in vascular-based (anti-VEGF) tumor therapies.
- Perfusion MRI in organ systems outside the CNS for oncological applications remains an active area of research.

Introduction

The MRI-based methods for measuring perfusion and related vascular characteristics that are described in this book have multiple research and clinical applications in oncology. The oncological applications specific to the brain are detailed in Chapter 11. This current chapter provides an overview of oncology applications outside the brain, covering both current clinical practice and research techniques. The technical aspects of image acquisition and analysis are only alluded to briefly, except where these details form a critical component of understanding the study data and their interpretation.

Various perfusion MRI techniques are performed in oncology imaging. Outside the brain, the majority of applications are based on T_1-weighted dynamic contrast-enhanced (DCE)-MRI, although dynamic susceptibility contrast (DSC) and arterial spin labeling (ASL) are now used increasingly often in research studies. In this section, all 'MR perfusion imaging' refers to T_1-weighted DCE-based techniques unless explicitly stated otherwise. It is important to appreciate that T_1-weighted DCE-MRI is an umbrella term that covers many similar acquisition and analysis approaches, which may have important differences in their practical application and for comparison between studies.

In most clinical applications, DCE-MRI is performed in non-specialist centers and analysis is tailored towards describing simple qualitative metrics such as curve shape or rapidity of enhancement and washout, although in some instances pharmacokinetic modeling may be performed. In most scenarios, the technique is used to characterize lesions as malignant or not, and is used as part of a wider MRI examination, including anatomical and other advanced techniques such as diffusion-weighted imaging (DWI). Here, interpretation is largely qualitative and reliant on clinical interpretation by a radiologist on a per patient basis. In distinction, many research applications involve the derivation of quantitative metrics that estimate values of blood flow, volume, or vessel permeability. These methods require highly refined acquisition and analysis protocols, and interpretation is largely quantitative and based on statistical analysis of data across a group of patients.

Conventional clinical practice

The most commonly accepted use for DCE in oncology outside of the brain is for the diagnosis and/or characterization of lesions. In addition, in some circumstances, the technique is also used for screening,

Clinical Perfusion MRI: Techniques and Applications, ed. Peter B. Barker, Xavier Golay, and Greg Zaharchuk. Published by Cambridge University Press. © Peter B. Barker, Xavier Golay, and Greg Zaharchuk 2013.

improving lesion detection, and monitoring for evidence of lesion progression. Other applications have been investigated, such as using enhancement curves to distinguish between tumor recurrence and response to therapy, for example in bladder cancer [1], but as yet are not routinely used in clinical practice. In this section, three common clinical examples are discussed, to illustrate current use of perfusion MRI in clinical practice.

Imaging primary breast tumors

MR perfusion imaging in breast cancer is covered in detail in Chapter 13. A brief overview of the topic is presented here because of its importance in oncological imaging in the body. Breast cancer is the most frequently diagnosed cancer worldwide. It accounts for nearly one-quarter of all new cancer cases and 14% of all cancer deaths in 2008 [2]. Most patients with breast cancer undergo triple assessment (clinical, ultrasound, and X-ray mammography) without need for MRI. However, indications for using MRI in general and DCE in particular have increased over the last decade.

Breast MRI is performed with a dedicated coil, with the patient prone and the breasts lying centrally within the receiver apparatus, which is designed to minimize patient movement and provide support for the breasts. Typically, 3D DCE sequences are acquired with a temporal resolution of around 20–30 s, near isotropic resolution in the mm range, and with fat suppression. At 1.5 T, some compromise must be made between requirements for acceptable temporal resolution, high spatial resolution, and signal-to-noise ratio (SNR), but at 3 T these difficulties are largely overcome, and it is now routine to acquire high-quality volumetric images through both breasts simultaneously at a rate of around one volume every 15 s [3], with the option of performing advanced analysis (pharmacokinetic modeling) as well as routine curve analysis. The technical issues surrounding image acquisition at 1.5 and 3 T are reviewed in detail in reference [4] and in Chapter 13.

Analysis techniques used in breast DCE MRI

A variety of techniques are used clinically in the analysis of breast tumor DCE data (reviewed in [4]). At one end of the spectrum, simple visual inspection of signal intensity (SI) curves can be performed with data acquired every 30–60 s or so, to define enhancement rate and SI curve shape. This work,

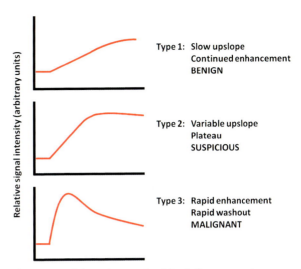

Figure 12.1 Schematic example of simple SI curves used to characterize breast lesions: most (but not all) malignant lesions are characterized by rapid arterial enhancement and rapid washout. In clinical practice, these features are important but are always used in conjunction with other morphological MRI features to determine the index of suspicion for a tumor being malignant. More examples are shown in Chapter 13.

for example as reported by Kuhl *et al.* [5], is simple to perform with a region of interest (ROI) drawn on a series of images with or without correction for motion. This method has proved useful in distinguishing benign from malignant lesions (Figure 12.1) and is routinely used by radiologists for the clinical evaluation of breast lesions.

Several techniques of increasing complexity can be performed on conventional clinical workstations as well as in centers with dedicated specialist analysis support. These range from deriving parameters based on the SI curve (such as the time to peak; TTP) through to pharmacokinetic analysis using one of various available models to describe the passage of contrast agent through tissue, all of which are variants of the kinetic model described by Kety [6] and presented in Chapters 1 and 4. These more advanced analyses typically utilize data registration to reduce artifacts from motion, and require calculation or estimation of tissue T_1 and an arterial input function (AIF). A formal ROI must be defined either by the radiologist or by the use of an automated software package [7].

Malignant breast lesion detection with DCE

DCE has been used since the 1990s to characterize malignant breast lesions. In general terms, malignant lesions were found to have washout of contrast agent after initial rapid enhancement, the latter feature relating in part to greater microvessel density [8] and higher microvascular permeability [9]. This information can be combined with other features available from contrast-enhanced MRI, such as the presence or absence of rim enhancement and lesion speculation. Such features have been incorporated into scoring systems such as the American College of Radiology "BIRADS" lexicon, which provides a consistent method for reporting the likelihood of malignancy in a breast lesion [10].

While there has been considerable variation in the spatial coverage, spatial resolution, and temporal resolution of analysis used in studies, DCE has a sensitivity of over 95% [11, 12]. The cited specificity is highly variable (between 40% and 95%], depending in part on acquisition and analysis methodology [12]. Multiple studies suggest that the area under the curve for receiver operator characteristic (ROC) curve analysis is typically 0.8 to 0.9 depending on study analysis [13]. In practice, most patients still undergo ultrasound or X-ray mammographic assessment and DCE is reserved for problem solving of cases that remain equivocal. Therefore, the true positive predictive value for the technique as used in clinical practice may be less than the above figures imply, and DCE may not obviate the need to perform a biopsy to determine the lesion pathology.

Screening in high-risk populations with DCE

Several gene mutations have been identified that predispose women to higher risk of developing breast cancer. Mutations in the *BRCA1* and *BRCA2* genes result in a cumulative risk of breast cancer by the age of 70 of 39–87% for *BRCA1* and 26–91% for *BRCA2* [14], and in many cases women with these mutations develop cancer at an early age. Some rarer gene mutations such as *TP53* also confer high risks, and evidence is growing of further mutations in a range of genes that individually cause a small increase in risk, but may significantly increase breast cancer risk in some women who carry multiple mutations [15]. These women with an elevated risk of breast cancer can be identified by performing genetic testing, and/ or by evaluating family history. Since many of these patients are young, there is a need for appropriate screening methods [16].

While X-ray mammography is an effective screening method in the normal population, particularly in those over 50 years of age, it is less effective in

younger, high-risk women, where the higher proportion of breast parenchyma to fat often results in dense mammograms that are difficult to interpret. Several large multicenter studies have evaluated the role of DCE in screening for cancers in women with a high genetic risk of breast cancer [17, 18]. While there are between-study differences in the age range of patients, and in the percentage risk for developing breast cancer relative to the normal population required for entry into each study, these studies have shown consistently that DCE is the most sensitive method of detecting cancer in women with a strong familial risk of breast cancer. For example, in the Magnetic Resonance Imaging in Breast Cancer Screening (MARIBS) study [18], a standardized acquisition and analysis approach was used in 22 centers, following training to ensure compliance. Prescriptive analyses were followed, using both morphology (well or poorly defined, spiculation), enhancement pattern (homogeneous, heterogeneous, rim-like), simple quantification of enhancement upslope, and washout pattern (based on the grading system of Kuhl *et al.* [5]). This system allowed lesions to be graded as malignant, suspicious, or benign.

Across these eight studies, the sensitivity of DCE was approximately twice that of X-ray mammography (75–90% vs. 40%). Combined with mammography, DCE had a sensitivity of over 90%. The additional benefit due to DCE was largely from detection of small, node-negative tumors. The strength of these results has enabled guidelines to be issued regarding the high-risk groups who may benefit from annual breast screening using DCE [19].

Staging loco-regional disease with DCE

There is emerging evidence that DCE increases the sensitivity of detecting intra-ductal carcinoma and can better delineate extensive multi-focal disease when compared to ultrasound and X-ray mammography [4]. However, the technique is not particularly specific, which results in a relatively high false positive rate (manifested as overcalling of disease extent) in around 20% of patients. The value of adding DCE to standard triple assessment has recently been evaluated in a 45-center-wide study of patients scheduled for wide local excision [20]. A total of 1623 patients were randomized for triple assessment with or without additional DCE. While MRI improved ability to localize disease pre-operatively, this additional imaging did not alter re-operation rates. Furthermore, it was not shown to improve quality of life or to be economically viable.

DCE-based early assessment of response to chemotherapy

Around 5% of patients with breast cancer receive cytotoxic neo-adjuvant chemotherapy (NAC). Since approximately one-third respond poorly to this therapy, there is interest in using advanced imaging techniques to identify those patients who are responding to NAC as soon as possible, rather than wait to the end of a course of chemotherapy after many months. Multiple independent studies have reported a statistically significant reduction in either the initial area under curve taken up to 60 s post injection ($IAUC_{60}$) or K^{trans} in breast cancer at or around two completed cycles of therapy in patients treated with a variety of different cytotoxic regimens. These small studies suggest that larger reductions in K^{trans} appear to indicate a subsequent favorable response [21–23]. This finding is consistent with preliminary evidence from 120 patients which suggests that those with persistent higher K^{trans} values after around two cycles of treatment with NAC have a significantly worse overall survival compared to those with a lower/reduced K^{trans} value, using multivariate analysis that included other imaging and non-imaging indicators of prognosis [24]. Further studies are required to test if these findings are reproducible, robust, and whether they can be translated into altering treatment selection and improving outcome for those patients who show early indicators of poor response to NAC.

Imaging liver metastases

Primary liver tumors are relatively rare, accounting for approximately 2% of all cancers in the USA in 2010 [2], although incidence is higher in Asia and sub-Saharan Africa [25]. In distinction, the liver is a frequent site of metastatic disease in many common and uncommon cancers. Precise rates depend on underlying tumor stage, grade, histology, genetic profile, treatment exposure, and other factors. For example, approximately 20% of patients with early stage HER2-positive breast cancer will develop liver metastases within 10 years [26], but nearer to 50% of patients with advanced breast, colorectal, and lung cancer develop liver metastases [27].

For most patients, conventional contrast-enhanced CT allows detection of metastases and adequate evaluation of the number of lesions, as well as their distribution and relationship to vital anatomical structures. Comparison with previous CT imaging allows radiologists to be confident that any 'new' lesions are malignant. Conventional CT is also ideal for the assessment of response to chemotherapy and localized therapies (such as embolization or ablation) in most tumor types [28]. T_1- and T_2-weighted anatomical MRI and DWI outperform CT in accurate detection and delineation of both primary and some secondary lesions, such as breast cancer metastases [29].

Lesion characterization with liver DCE

The main clinical application for perfusion MRI in the liver is to characterize lesions in patients with a known primary cancer, where the tumor and nodal stage [30] is known, but there is doubt over whether a liver lesion represents a distant metastasis. This is a common clinical scenario, and in many cases, lesions are shown to be benign pathologies such as hemangioma, focal nodular hyperplasia, or cysts. Correct diagnosis may make a significant difference to patient management, for instance by avoiding unnecessary treatment for benign lesions and for determining suitability for surgical resection of the primary cancer.

In most centers, initial T_1- and T_2-weighted sequences are performed along with in/out of phase imaging and DWI, followed by the perfusion sequence. This is typically a T_1-weighted 3D FLASH (fast low angle shot), FFE (fast field echo), or equivalent sequence acquired during gentle free breathing, although a breath-hold technique may be used in first-pass studies. Depending on local preferences and contrast agent choice, images are acquired up to every few seconds, but must include pre-contrast, arterial phase, portal venous phase, and delayed phase images (at around 10 min after initial gadolinium administration). Signal intensity differences are examined between the different phases of contrast agent uptake (Figure 12.2). Features of malignancy include a peripheral vascular rim, rapid arterial enhancement, and early washout of contrast agent [31].

It should be emphasized that in this scenario, perfusion MRI is one of many sequences performed in an examination of the liver and it is the overall signal characteristics on all the sequences that influence whether a lesion is designated as malignant or benign. It is also important to note that in many cases, malignant lesions do not behave 'typically' and can be difficult to characterize confidently, particularly in cases where lesions have been pre-treated, such as in metastatic breast cancer [32].

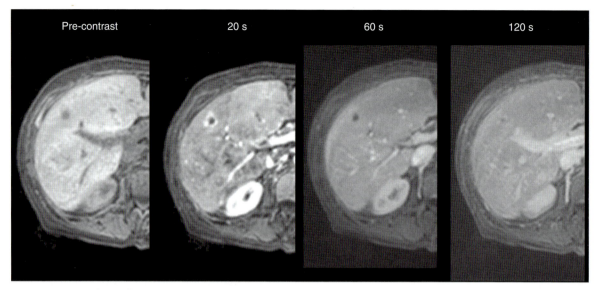

| Pre-contrast | 20 s | 60 s | 120 s |

Figure 12.2 Clinical DCE of the liver. In this 57-year-old woman with biopsy-proven rectal cancer, multiple T_1-weighted images show a solitary lesion with low signal intensity, exhibiting peripheral rim enhancement in the arterial phase (at 20 s) and then gradual washout as the remainder of the liver enhances. These features are highly suggestive of malignancy in the appropriate clinical context.

Other applications of perfusion MRI in the liver

Some studies have attempted to determine the tumor histology or grade using perfusion imaging (both DCE-MRI and perfusion CT methods) [33], akin to techniques performed in neuroimaging. As yet there are no convincing reproducible data to support this application in liver imaging [29]. There may be potential for perfusion MRI to detect early changes in the perfusion patterns of livers at risk of developing liver metastases. Based on early studies in CT [34], it was shown that a composite, non-model-based hepatic perfusion index (HPI) parameter was increased in patients with overt metastases compared with patients without metastases, reflecting subtle changes in the arterial perfusion in the liver [35]. Finally, physiological imaging including perfusion MRI may have a role in detecting response to embolization and anti-vascular therapies where change in size may be minimal following therapy. This indication is yet to translate to routine practice, but is discussed in detail below (in the section "Research applications").

Imaging tumors within the prostate

Prostate cancer is a major health concern with a nearly 8% cumulative risk of men developing the disease by 75 years of age, making it the second most frequently diagnosed cancer worldwide, and accounting for 14% of all cancer deaths [2]. Diagnosis is made

by ultrasound-guided biopsies, following prostate-specific antigen (PSA) measurement and digital rectal examination. Nearly all patients then undergo MRI for staging assessment. There is considerable variation in MRI technique in examining the prostate, particularly in field strength and in use of body or endorectal coils. Few studies have examined these issues in detail, and at present the value of high field strength and use of an endorectal coil are not proven [36].

Considerable variation is present in the acquisition and analysis of DCE in prostate cancer and its role in multi-parametric imaging. This has prompted the development of expert consensus recommendations concerning the use of guidelines on the use of imaging in prostate cancer [37]. However, several commentators have questioned whether these guidelines are based on sound scientific criteria or are ready for routine clinical use, and have pointed out a lack of consensus on over one-third of issues surrounding data acquisition and analysis [38]. Thus, the value of DCE in the assessment of prostate cancer is yet to be fully determined despite the considerable promise shown to date.

Lesion detection and localization with DCE

Primary tumors are notoriously difficult to identify accurately within the prostate gland using conventional T_1- and T_2-weighted MRI. DCE measurements of blood flow have been shown to be elevated in

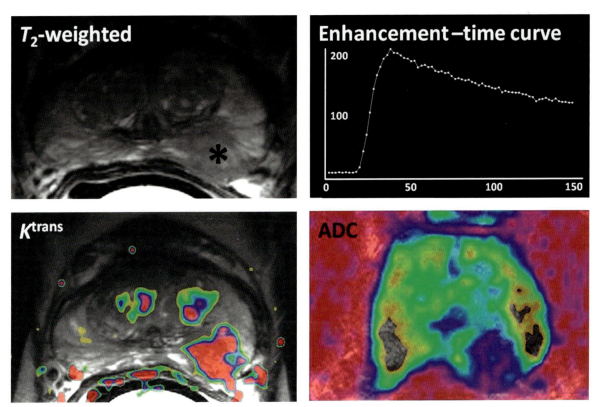

Figure 12.3 Clinical DCE-MRI of the prostate. Multi-parametric images in a 62-year-old man with T3a Gleason 4 + 3 prostatic carcinoma. The T_2-weighted image shows an ill-defined low signal nodule in the left peripheral zone (denoted by *). The DCE enhancement–time curve over the nodule shows rapid enhancement followed by washout, suggesting malignancy. K^{trans} and apparent diffusion coefficient (ADC) maps show the tumor extent, with early extra-capsular infiltration into surrounding peri-prostatic fat. Images are courtesy of Dr. Thomas Hambrock, Department of Radiology, University Medical Center Nijmegen, Nijmegen, the Netherlands.

prostate cancer relative to the normal glandular tissue [39]. This has prompted interest in how DCE, DWI, and other techniques might be used to aid prostate cancer diagnosis and monitoring [36]. At present, DCE along with DWI and magnetic resonance spectroscopy (MRS) are widely but inconsistently used across specialist cancer centers for these purposes [38] (Figure 12.3).

Initial work suggests that DCE may increase detection accuracy in prostate cancer, but this benefit is likely to be as part of a multi-parametric approach [36]. It is well documented that significant spatial heterogeneity can exist across the tumor in functional image parameters such as K^{trans}, making definition of tumor margins difficult [40]. Although parameters derived from DSC can be measured in the prostate [41], their role (if any) is yet to be determined. Consequently, the ability of functional techniques to define accurately tumor margins is poor. With ROC curve

analysis, the area under the curve (AUC) is approximately 0.65 for perfusion-based parameters (similar to DWI) [42]. However, combination of DCE, DWI, and anatomical T_1- and T_2-weighted sequences improves sensitivity of cancer detection in the peripheral zone, from around 63% to 80% [43]. In addition, combination of DCE with DWI best improves localization accuracy, with a sensitivity of approximately 80% (compared with 70% for anatomical sequences alone) [44], helping to improve local staging.

Targeting biopsy with functional imaging

Gleason score (a histopathological grading system) is a key prognostic determinant in prostate cancer, but has a high sampling error when performed on tissue obtained using ultrasound-guided biopsy [36]. This can lead to both under- and over-treatment of lesions assigned an incorrect Gleason score. Initial studies with physiological MRI have shown correlations with image parameters and Gleason grade at prostatectomy [45]. This work requires further evaluation in large prospective studies to determine specificity, but such methods show promise in targeting tumor biopsy, akin to the use of relative cerebral blood flow (rCBV) for targeting biopsy in brain tumors (Chapter 11).

Research applications: current practice and unmet needs

The MRI methods described in this book are inherently quantitative and thus enable measurement of characteristics such as blood flow, blood volume, and vessel permeability. An extensive, but by no means exhaustive, list of features that can be measured by DSC, DCE, and ASL are provided in Table 12.1. These MRI-derived estimates of microvascular features are examples of biological markers (termed biomarkers) that are objectively measured and evaluated as indicator(s) of normal biological processes, pathogenic processes, or therapeutic responses to a pharmacological or other intervention [46]. Biomarkers have multiple uses, including being used to monitor response once a therapy has begun (therapeutic biomarkers) and to predict response either regardless of the specific therapy used (prognostic biomarkers) or for a specific given therapy (predictive biomarkers). These applications are discussed below.

Therapeutic biomarkers: early indicators of response

In most conventional imaging, the first image-based assessment of response is at several cycles (usually weeks to months) post therapy to evaluate whether tumors have responded. Size-based response criteria, such as RECIST (Response Evaluation Criteria in Solid Tumors) are used, where the percentage change in size is measured in one [47] or two dimensions [48]. Tumor- or therapy-specific criteria are essentially modifications of this approach, for example, with the addition of density measurement in the Choi criteria [49] and glucose metabolism assessment in the Cheson criteria [50].

However, there is interest in using physiological imaging methods (including perfusion) as indicators of therapeutic effect. Two main indications are to evaluate targeted therapies that induce minimal change in tumor size but improve patient survival [51]; and to provide early indication of anti-tumoral efficacy before significant changes in tumor size are detected [52].

Evidence for anti-vascular effects with MRI

Over 100 studies have used MRI-based measurement of tumor perfusion to evaluate drugs with proposed anti-vascular mechanisms of action [53]. These compounds include anti-vascular endothelial growth

Table 12.1. Microvascular features measured by DSC, DCE, and ASL

Parameter	Definition	Unit
T_1-weighted DCE		
K^{trans}	Volume transfer constant between plasma and the EES	min^{-1}
$IAUC_{60}$	Initial area under gadolinium concentration agent–time curve at 60 s	mM min
F	Blood flow	ml/min/ml
PS	Permeability surface area product per unit mass of tissue	ml/min/ml
k_{ep}	Rate constant between EES and plasma	min^{-1}
v_p	Blood plasma volume	ml/ml
$T_2{*}$-weighted DSC		
rBF	Relative blood flow	ml/min/ml
rBV	Relative blood volume	ml/ml
Arterial spin labeling		
F	Blood flow	ml/min/ml

EES, extravascular extracellular space.

factor (VEGF) antibodies, tyrosine kinase receptor inhibitors (of VEGF and other growth factors that mediate tumor angiogenesis), and vascular disrupting agents. Despite the now common use of MRI in many trials, it should be noted that the overwhelming majority of such studies still do not use functional imaging of any kind.

Most studies have used T_1-weighted DCE and have calculated either $IAUC_{60}$ or K^{trans}. There is compelling evidence that $IAUC_{60}$, K^{trans}, and related parameters (k_{ep} and PS) are consistently reduced following administration of several anti-vascular compounds with a proven anti-vascular mechanism of action. For example, statistically significant reductions in K^{trans} have been reported in nine published DCE studies of bevacizumab monotherapy with pooled data from 162 patients [54–62] (example parameter maps are shown in Figure 12.4). This finding is consistent across multiple patient populations, at various time points between 4 hrs and 28 days, and is congruent with data from CT perfusion studies of bevacizumab-treated patients [63]. These findings support the notion that VEGF blockade causes rapid and sustained anti-vascular effects that occur during a single cycle of anti-VEGF therapy [56].

Comparable results have been reported in studies of patients with solid tumors treated with clinically effective tyrosine kinase inhibitors. These include multiple studies of cediranib [64–66], sorafenib [67, 68], sunitinib [69, 70], and pazopanib [71]. Consistent reduction in $IAUC_{60}$ or K^{trans} between 4 hrs and 5 days has also been reported with the anti-tubulin agent fosbretabulin [72–74]. Similar results have also been seen in studies that incorporate DSC-or ASL-derived biomarkers [75, 76].

The relationship between an image biomarker and anti-tumor efficacy must also be accompanied by a change in plasma or tumor pharmacokinetics if the biomarker is to be regarded as a true pharmacological indicator of drug efficacy. Clear dose-dependent relationships (reduction in $IAUC_{60}$ or K^{trans} from baseline) have been identified in trials of cediranib [64], vatalanib [77], sorafenib [67], and pazopanib [78], where linear relationships between drug dose and vascular response were modeled over the dose range examined. In many of these and other phase I studies, pharmacokinetics data demonstrate that active drug concentrations are reached within individual patients' plasma. The area under the plasma concentration–time curve at a steady state (AUC_{ss}), or the maximum drug concentration in the plasma (C_{max}) have correlated significantly with change in $IAUC_{60}$ or K^{trans} following cediranib [64], vatalanib [77, 79, 80], pazopanib [78], and brivanib [81].

Two further examples of how DCE measurement of perfusion can benefit drug development are in selecting optimum drug dose and schedule for future studies. In four unrelated studies of the anti-tubulin agent fosbretabulin, vascular response was observed at 45 mg/m^2 or greater, defining a therapeutic window between the biologically active dose and the clinical maximum tolerated dose of 68 mg/m^2 [72–74, 82]. A study of brivanib [81] evaluated different dose schedules in multiple cohorts with 12–15 patients per cohort, to determine the optimum schedule for phase II studies. Statistically significant reductions in $IAUC_{60}$ and K^{trans} were seen with brivanib either 400 mg twice daily, or 800 mg once daily, in continuous daily dosing, but not with 800 mg intermittent dosing or at lower dose levels.

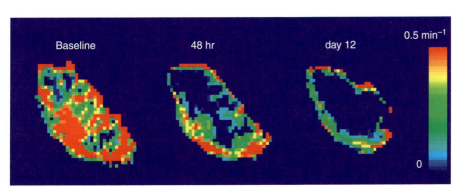

Figure 12.4 K^{trans} parameter maps in a 73-year-old man with a colorectal liver metastasis before and after bevacizumab treatment: the distribution of K^{trans} is spatially heterogeneous with high values in the periphery and low values in the core. K^{trans} was reduced after 2 days and further reduced after 12 days of treatment compared with baseline.

Importantly, drugs that have been found to demonstrate limited clinical benefits show little or no significant reduction in $IAUC_{60}$ or K^{trans}, for example in studies of semaxanib [83] and vandetanib in tumors that show little clinical response to the drug [84]. Unfortunately, this clarity – significant reduction in biomarkers with active compounds and lack of change in biomarkers with ineffectual compounds – is not seen in all studies. Reductions in K^{trans} seen in studies of vatalanib [77, 79, 80] were comparable to those seen with bevacizumab, cediranib, sorafenib, and fosbretabulin, yet vatalanib has failed to demonstrate a survival benefit at phase III testing in colorectal cancer when used in combination therapy with cytotoxic agents [85]. Thus, anti-vascular activity does not guarantee phase III success [86]; it appears that a statistically significant change in MRI-based perfusion biomarkers is a necessary but not necessarily sufficient evidence of clinically significant efficacy of therapies secondary to anti-vascular mechanisms. As such, DCE might be used as a gatekeeper to avoid pushing potentially inefficient new therapies to phase III clinical trials.

There are still many unresolved issues surrounding the use of perfusion MRI in early phase clinical trials of anti-vascular agents. These include: choice of biomarker (e.g., established primary endpoints such as $IAUC_{60}$ or K^{trans}, versus alternative parameters such as enhancing tumor volume or fractional plasma volume); timing of image measurements; how T_1 is calculated or estimated; how an AIF is calculated or estimated; and whether the ROI is limited to a few slices or includes the whole tumor [87]. These discrepancies are present in the existing literature and limit direct comparison between study data. Despite these factors, there is now considerable evidence for using DCE in phase I/II studies to help indicate biological efficacy, elucidate the mechanism of action, and to determine the biologically active dose and schedule.

Prognostic and predictive biomarkers: indicators of outcome

One rapidly developing research area is how imaging biomarkers may be used to inform clinical outcome irrespective of the treatment prescribed (a prognostic indicator) or directly relating to the therapy given (a predictive indicator). Both baseline parameters and early pharmacokinetic changes in a parameter have been investigated for this end, for example as reviewed in the section on breast cancer above. Elsewhere, there is emerging evidence that image biomarkers relate to survival in several phase I and phase II clinical trials of novel therapies.

An illustrative example is found in studies of anti-VEGF monotherapy in patients with metastatic renal clear cell cancer (RCC), with multiple studies evaluating image biomarkers of tumor vascularity measured both before treatment and 3–12 weeks following therapy. Two independent studies of patients with metastatic RCC treated with sorafenib have reported that high baseline values of K^{trans} were associated with longer progression-free survival (PFS) [67, 68]. In one of these studies, higher baseline plasma volume was also related to a longer PFS [67]. An equivalent relationship between K^{trans} and PFS has been shown in a study of sunitinib in metastatic RCC [88]. Since K^{trans} is a composite parameter reflecting flow and permeability it is not possible to determine exactly which biological entity relates to outcome.

There is also evidence that early reduction in perfusion parameters may relate to outcome. K^{trans} reduction following sorafenib therapy has shown a statistically significant relationship to progression in one small study [68], but not in another larger study with more tightly controlled imaging protocols [67]. Comparable studies of vatalanib assessed by ASL (where flow was measured) [75] and thalidomide assessed by dynamic CT (where flow and permeability were measured) [89] do however suggest that this approach may be useful. Overall, there is evidence that high baseline perfusion and rapid early reduction in perfusion may relate to beneficial outcome following anti-VEGF therapy.

Comparable findings have been found in studies of other solid tumors [77, 90] and hematological malignancies [76, 91] using both DCE and ASL. Since all of these studies are small and many are retrospective, conclusions from such data must be interpreted with caution, but overall, these studies suggest that perfusion MRI may provide clinically important information regarding patient response to therapy.

Advanced image analysis techniques

Most of the quantitative MR perfusion imaging parameters described in this chapter are simple average values of K^{trans}, flow, or equivalent metrics. There is considerable recent interest in exploring how more advanced analysis methods may be applied to these basic signals (DCE, DSC, and ASL) and used to calculate alternative biomarkers, including parameters that measure overall spatial complexity and parameters that relate to specific tumor sub-regions [92]. These methods are still in their infancy and their precise value is at present unclear. Nonetheless, it seems increasingly likely that some of these advanced analysis methods will find clinical utility in years to come.

Tumors are biologically complex structures. There is a substantial literature that has looked at how tumor spatial complexity can be quantified using texture, fractal, and other related metrics. For example, in breast cancer, texture analysis-derived biomarkers have shown a higher ROC curve value for discriminating malignant tumors from benign lesions compared to traditional enhancement parameters, suggesting that incorporation of these more complex measurements could improve computer-aided diagnosis systems [93]. Fractal analysis has been used to quantify tumor spatial complexity in many studies. In one example of liver metastases from colorectal cancer, fractal parameters derived from DCE measured prior to chemotherapy explained over 80% of the variation in tumor shrinkage after 10 weeks of therapy, where simple baseline measurements such as tumor size and average K^{trans} failed to do so [94] (Figure 12.5).

Other areas of interest include how perfusion MRI may be used to identify those regions within a tumor that are biologically important in driving response to therapy, resistance, and subsequent tumor progression. Early work some 10 years ago showed that different tumor sub-regions respond variously to therapy, for example greater reduction in K^{trans} in the tumor center compared with the tumor periphery when PC-3 tumors were challenged with the VEGF-related tyrosine kinase inhibitor vandetanib [95]. Similar results to these data based on a-priori approaches have been seen in other studies of VEGF inhibitors where significant reductions in K^{trans} were seen in tumor deemed 'viable' by its T_2-weighted and ADC signal, but not in tissue deemed 'necrotic' by its T_2-weighted and ADC signal [96]. Formal image segmentation without a-priori assumptions has shown that similar differential changes occur in tumor sub-regions following challenge with bevacizumab in human tumors [97], but further work is required before such techniques can be shown to have clear clinical application.

Conclusions

Clinically available perfusion MRI techniques have begun to find several applications in both routine oncological practice and in research applications. In clinical practice, DCE is typically used in combination

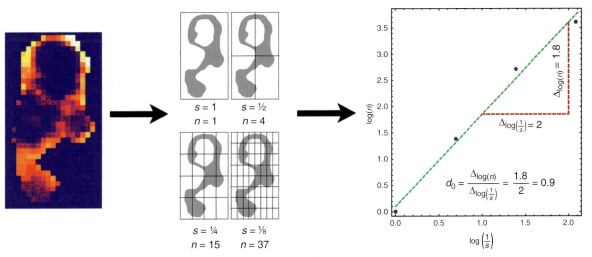

Figure 12.5 Schematic representation of fractal parameter derivation: a K^{trans} map from a single slice through a tumor shows marked spatial heterogeneity. A criterion is applied to the contrast agent concentration time series to identify enhancing voxels and a box surrounding the object defined by the enhancing voxels is successively divided, defining a range of scales (s) at which the number of boxes containing a part of the object is counted (n). The fractal parameter d_0 is the slope of the line of best fit through the points (log n, log 1/s) and quantifies the space-filling properties of the parameter map.

with morphological imaging and DWI. In this context, perfusion MRI has already found a role as a component of a multi-parametric approach to lesion characterization, delineation, and identification of aggressive tumor foci. Research applications, focused on the evaluation of anti-vascular therapies, have driven a desire for parameter quantification using pharmacokinetic modeling, and by doing so enable other applications – such as whether baseline values of perfusion are prognostic of outcome – to be applied to clinical datasets, as in breast cancer.

However, the role of perfusion MRI in prediction of treatment response and prognosis is as yet unclear.

The next few decades will see continued development of novel therapies, an increase in the complexity and capacity of novel MRI methods, and continued desire to personalize therapeutic monitoring (as well as the therapy itself). This can only result in an increased application of advanced MRI techniques, including DCE, DSC, and ASL, in the management of cancer patients both in routine clinical practice and in drug development.

References

1. Dobson MJ, Carrington BM, Collins CD, *et al*. The assessment of irradiated bladder carcinoma using dynamic contrast-enhanced MR imaging. *Clin Radiol* 2001;**56**:94–8.

2. Jemal A, Bray F, Center MM, *et al*. Global cancer statistics. *CA Cancer J Clin* 2011;**61**:69–90.

3. Henderson E, Rutt BK, Lee TY. Temporal sampling requirements for the tracer kinetics modeling of breast disease. *Magn Reson Imaging* 1998;**16**:1057–73.

4. Turnbull LW. Dynamic contrast-enhanced MRI in the diagnosis and management of breast cancer. *NMR Biomed* 2009;**22**:28–39.

5. Kuhl CK, Mielcareck P, Klaschik S, *et al*. Dynamic breast MR imaging: are signal intensity time course data useful for differential diagnosis of enhancing lesions? *Radiology* 1999;**211**: 101–10.

6. Kety SS. The theory and applications of the exchange of inert gas at the lungs and tissues. *Pharmacol Rev* 1951;**3**: 1–41.

7. Szabo BK, Aspelin P, Wiberg MK. Neural network approach to the segmentation and classification of dynamic magnetic resonance images of the breast: comparison with empiric and quantitative kinetic parameters. *Acad Radiol* 2004;**11**:1344–54.

8. Buckley DL, Drew PJ, Mussurakis S, Monson JR, Horsman A. Microvessel density of invasive breast cancer assessed by dynamic Gd-DTPA enhanced MRI. *J Magn Reson Imaging* 1997;**7**: 461–4.

9. Knopp MV, Weiss E, Sinn HP, *et al*. Pathophysiologic basis of contrast enhancement in breast tumors. *J Magn Reson Imaging* 1999;**10**:260–6.

10. Erguvan-Dogan B, Whitman GJ, Kushwaha AC, Phelps MJ, Dempsey PJ. BI-RADS-MRI: a primer. *AJR Am J Roentgenol* 2006;**187**:W152–60.

11. Shimauchi A, Jansen SA, Abe H, *et al*. Breast cancers not detected at MRI: review of false-negative lesions. *AJR Am J Roentgenol* 2010;**194**:1674–9.

12. Benndorf M, Baltzer PA, Vag T, *et al*. Breast MRI as an adjunct to mammography: Does it really suffer from low specificity? A retrospective analysis stratified by mammographic BI-RADS classes. *Acta Radiol* 2010;**51**: 715–21.

13. El Khouli RH, Macura KJ, Jacobs MA, *et al*. Dynamic contrast-enhanced MRI of the breast: quantitative method for kinetic curve type assessment. *AJR Am J Roentgenol* 2009;**193**: W295–300.

14. Robson M, Offit K. Clinical practice. Management of an inherited predisposition to breast cancer. *N Engl J Med* 2007;**357**:154–62.

15. Easton DF, Pooley KA, Dunning AM, *et al*. Genome-wide association study identifies novel breast cancer susceptibility loci. *Nature* 2007;**447**:1087–93.

16. Leach MO. Breast cancer screening in women at high risk using MRI. *NMR Biomed* 2009;**22**:17–27.

17. Kriege M, Brekelmans CT, Boetes C, *et al*. Efficacy of MRI and mammography for breast-cancer screening in women with a familial or genetic predisposition. *N Engl J Med* 2004;**351**:427–37.

18. Leach MO, Boggis CR, Dixon AK, *et al*. Screening with magnetic resonance imaging and mammography of a UK population at high familial risk of breast cancer: a prospective multicentre cohort study (MARIBS). *Lancet* 2005;**365**: 1769–78.

19. NICE. *Familial Breast cancer: The Classification and Care of Women at Risk of Familial Breast Cancer in Primary, Secondary and Tertiary Care – Update*. London: National Institute for Clinical Excellence, 2006. Available from: http://www.nice.org.uk/guidance/cg41 (accessed January 9, 2013).

20. Turnbull LW, Brown SR, Olivier C, *et al*. Multicentre randomised controlled trial examining the cost-effectiveness of contrast-enhanced high field

magnetic resonance imaging in women with primary breast cancer scheduled for wide local excision (COMICE). *Health Technol Assess* 2010;**14**:1–182.

21. Hayes C, Padhani AR, Leach MO. Assessing changes in tumour vascular function using dynamic contrast-enhanced magnetic resonance imaging. *NMR Biomed* 2002;**15**:154–63.

22. Martincich L, Montemurro F, De Rosa G, *et al.* Monitoring response to primary chemotherapy in breast cancer using dynamic contrast-enhanced magnetic resonance imaging. *Breast Cancer Res Treat* 2004;**83**:67–76.

23. Baar J, Silverman P, Lyons J, *et al.* A vasculature-targeting regimen of preoperative docetaxel with or without bevacizumab for locally advanced breast cancer: impact on angiogenic biomarkers. *Clin Cancer Res* 2009;**15**:3583–90.

24. Li SP, Makris A, Beresford MJ, *et al.* Use of dynamic contrast-enhanced MR imaging to predict survival in patients with primary breast cancer undergoing neoadjuvant chemotherapy. *Radiology* 2011;**260**:68–78.

25. Yu MC, Yuan JM. Environmental factors and risk for hepatocellular carcinoma. *Gastroenterology* 2004;**127**:S72–8.

26. Kennecke H, Yerushalmi R, Woods R, *et al.* Metastatic behavior of breast cancer subtypes. *J Clin Oncol* 2010;**28**:3271–7.

27. Husband JE, Reznek RH. *Imaging in Oncology*. London: Taylor & Francis, 2004.

28. Eisenhauer EA, Therasse P, Bogaerts J, *et al.* New response evaluation criteria in solid tumours: revised RECIST guideline (version 1.1). *Eur J Cancer* 2009;**45**:228–47.

29. Koh DM, Padhani AR. Functional magnetic resonance imaging of the liver: parametric assessments beyond morphology. *Magn Reson Imaging Clin N Am* 2010;**18**:565–85, xii.

30. Edge SB, Byrd DR, Compton CC, *et al. AJCC Cancer Staging Handbook*, 5th edn. New York: Springer, 2010.

31. Silva AC, Evans JM, McCullough AE, *et al.* MR imaging of hypervascular liver masses: a review of current techniques. *Radiographics* 2009;**29**:385–402.

32. Semelka RC, Worawattanakul S, Noone TC, *et al.* Chemotherapy-treated liver metastases mimicking hemangiomas on MR images. *Abdom Imaging* 1999;**24**:378–82.

33. Abdullah SS, Pialat JB, Wiart M, *et al.* Characterization of hepatocellular carcinoma and colorectal liver metastasis by means of perfusion MRI. *J Magn Reson Imaging* 2008;**28**:390–5.

34. Miles KA, Hayball MP, Dixon AK. Functional images of hepatic perfusion obtained with dynamic CT. *Radiology* 1993;**188**:405–11.

35. Totman JJ, O'Gorman RL, Kane PA, Karani JB. Comparison of the hepatic perfusion index measured with gadolinium-enhanced volumetric MRI in controls and in patients with colorectal cancer. *Br J Radiol* 2005;**78**:105–9.

36. Hoeks CM, Barentsz JO, Hambrock T, *et al.* Prostate cancer: multiparametric MR imaging for detection, localization, and staging. *Radiology* 2011;**261**:46–66.

37. Dickinson L, Ahmed HU, Allen C, *et al.* Magnetic resonance imaging for the detection, localisation, and characterisation of prostate cancer: recommendations from a European consensus meeting. *Eur Urol* 2011;**59**:477–94.

38. deSouza NM, Sala E. Imaging: standardizing the use of functional MRI in prostate cancer. *Nat Rev Urol* 2011;**8**:127–9.

39. Buckley DL, Roberts C, Parker GJ, Logue JP, Hutchinson CE. Prostate cancer: evaluation of vascular characteristics with dynamic contrast-enhanced T1-weighted MR imaging–initial experience. *Radiology* 2004;**233**:709–15.

40. Riches SF, Payne GS, Morgan VA, *et al.* MRI in the detection of prostate cancer: combined apparent diffusion coefficient, metabolite ratio, and vascular parameters. *AJR Am J Roentgenol* 2009;**193**:1583–91.

41. Alonzi R, Taylor NJ, Stirling JJ, *et al.* Reproducibility and correlation between quantitative and semiquantitative dynamic and intrinsic susceptibility-weighted MRI parameters in the benign and malignant human prostate. *J Magn Reson Imaging* 2010;**32**:155–64.

42. Langer DL, van der Kwast TH, Evans AJ, *et al.* Prostate cancer detection with multi-parametric MRI: logistic regression analysis of quantitative T2, diffusion-weighted imaging, and dynamic contrast-enhanced MRI. *J Magn Reson Imaging* 2009;**30**: 327–34.

43. Delongchamps NB, Rouanne M, Flam T, *et al.* Multiparametric magnetic resonance imaging for the detection and localization of prostate cancer: combination of T2-weighted, dynamic contrast-enhanced and diffusion-weighted imaging. *BJU Int* 2011;**107**: 1411–18.

44. Futterer JJ, Heijmink SW, Scheenen TW, *et al.* Prostate cancer localization with dynamic contrast-enhanced MR imaging and proton MR spectroscopic imaging. *Radiology* 2006;**241**: 449–58.

45. Hambrock T, Somford DM, Huisman HJ, *et al.* Relationship between apparent diffusion coefficients at 3.0-T MR imaging and Gleason grade in peripheral

249

zone prostate cancer. *Radiology* 2011;**259**:453–61.

46. NIH BDWG. Biomarkers and surrogate endpoints: preferred definitions and conceptual framework. *Clin Pharmacol Ther* 2001;**69**:89–95.

47. Therasse P, Arbuck SG, Eisenhauer EA, *et al.* New guidelines to evaluate the response to treatment in solid tumors. European Organization for Research and Treatment of Cancer, National Cancer Institute of the United States, National Cancer Institute of Canada. *J Natl Cancer Inst* 2000;**92**:205–16.

48. World Health Organization. *WHO Handbook for Reporting Results of Cancer Treatment.* Geneva: World Health Organization, 1979.

49. Choi H, Charnsangavej C, Faria SC, *et al.* Correlation of computed tomography and positron emission tomography in patients with metastatic gastrointestinal stromal tumor treated at a single institution with imatinib mesylate: proposal of new computed tomography response criteria. *J Clin Oncol* 2007;**25**:1753–9.

50. Cheson BD, Pfistner B, Juweid ME, *et al.* Revised response criteria for malignant lymphoma. *J Clin Oncol* 2007;**25**:579–86.

51. O'Connor JP, Jackson A, Asselin MC, *et al.* Quantitative imaging biomarkers in the clinical development of targeted therapeutics: current and future perspectives. *Lancet Oncol* 2008;**9**:766–76.

52. Michaelis LC, Ratain MJ. Measuring response in a post-RECIST world: from black and white to shades of grey. *Nat Rev Cancer* 2006;**6**:409–14.

53. O'Connor JPB, Jackson A, Parker GJM, Roberts C, Jayson GC. Dynamic contrast-enhanced MRI in clinical trials of antivascular therapies. *Nat Rev Clin Oncol* 2012;**9**:167–77.

54. Wedam SB, Low JA, Yang SX, *et al.* Antiangiogenic and antitumor effects of bevacizumab in patients with inflammatory and locally advanced breast cancer. *J Clin Oncol* 2006;**24**:769–77.

55. Li SP, Taylor NJ, Mehta S, *et al.* Evaluating the early effects of anti-angiogenic treatment in human breast cancer with intrinsic susceptibility-weighted and diffusion-weighted MRI: initial observations. *Proc Intl Soc Magn Reson Med*, Montreal, Canada, 2011;342.

56. O'Connor JP, Carano RA, Clamp AR, *et al.* Quantifying antivascular effects of monoclonal antibodies to vascular endothelial growth factor: insights from imaging. *Clin Cancer Res* 2009;**15**:6674–82.

57. Barboriak DP, DesJardins A, Rich J, *et al.* Treatment of recurrent glioblastoma multiforme with bevacizumab and irinotecan leads to rapid decreases in tumor plasma volume and Ktrans. *RSNA* 2007;**93**: SST09–05.

58. Gutin PH, Iwamoto FM, Beal K, *et al.* Safety and efficacy of bevacizumab with hypofractionated stereotactic irradiation for recurrent malignant gliomas. *Int J Radiat Oncol Biol Phys* 2009;**75**: 156–63.

59. Zhang W, Kreisl TN, Solomon J, *et al.* Acute effects of bevacizumab on glioblastoma vascularity assessed with DCE-MRI and relation to patient survival. *Proc Intl Soc Magn Reson Med*, Montreal, Canada, 2009;282.

60. Gururangan S, Chi SN, Young Poussaint T, *et al.* Lack of efficacy of bevacizumab plus irinotecan in children with recurrent malignant glioma and diffuse brainstem glioma: a Pediatric Brain Tumor Consortium study. *J Clin Oncol* 2010;**28**:3069–75.

61. Kreisl TN, Zhang W, Odia Y, *et al.* A phase II trial of single-agent bevacizumab in patients with recurrent anaplastic glioma. *Neuro Oncol* 2011;**13**: 1143–50.

62. Siegel AB, Cohen EI, Ocean A, *et al.* Phase II trial evaluating the clinical and biologic effects of bevacizumab in unresectable hepatocellular carcinoma. *J Clin Oncol* 2008;**26**:2992–8.

63. Willett CG, Duda DG, di Tomaso E, *et al.* Efficacy, safety, and biomarkers of neoadjuvant bevacizumab, radiation therapy, and fluorouracil in rectal cancer: a multidisciplinary phase II study. *J Clin Oncol* 2009;**27**:3020–6.

64. Drevs J, Siegert P, Medinger M, *et al.* Phase I clinical study of AZD2171, an oral vascular endothelial growth factor signaling inhibitor, in patients with advanced solid tumors. *J Clin Oncol* 2007;**25**:3045–54.

65. Batchelor TT, Sorensen AG, di Tomaso E, *et al.* AZD2171, a pan-VEGF receptor tyrosine kinase inhibitor, normalizes tumor vasculature and alleviates edema in glioblastoma patients. *Cancer Cell* 2007;**11**:83–95.

66. Mitchell CL, O'Connor JP, Roberts C, *et al.* A two-part phase II study of cediranib in patients with advanced solid tumours: the effect of food on single-dose pharmacokinetics and an evaluation of safety, efficacy and imaging pharmacodynamics. *Cancer Chemother Pharmacol* 2011;**68**:631–41.

67. Hahn OM, Yang C, Medved M, *et al.* Dynamic contrast-enhanced magnetic resonance imaging pharmacodynamic biomarker study of sorafenib in metastatic renal carcinoma. *J Clin Oncol* 2008;**26**:4572–8.

68. Flaherty KT, Rosen MA, Heitjan DF, *et al.* Pilot study of DCE-MRI to predict progression-free survival with sorafenib therapy in

renal cell carcinoma. *Cancer Biol Ther* 2008;7:496–501.

69. Zhu AX, Sahani DV, Duda DG, *et al.* Efficacy, safety, and potential biomarkers of sunitinib monotherapy in advanced hepatocellular carcinoma: a phase II study. *J Clin Oncol* 2009;27:3027–35.

70. Machiels JP, Henry S, Zanetta S, *et al.* Phase II study of sunitinib in recurrent or metastatic squamous cell carcinoma of the head and neck: GORTEC 2006–01. *J Clin Oncol* 2010;28:21–8.

71. Hurwitz HI, Dowlati A, Saini S, *et al.* Phase I trial of pazopanib in patients with advanced cancer. *Clin Cancer Res* 2009;15:4220–7.

72. Galbraith SM, Maxwell RJ, Lodge MA, *et al.* Combretastatin A4 phosphate has tumor antivascular activity in rat and man as demonstrated by dynamic magnetic resonance imaging. *J Clin Oncol* 2003;21:2831–42.

73. Stevenson JP, Rosen M, Sun W, *et al.* Phase I trial of the antivascular agent combretastatin A4 phosphate on a 5-day schedule to patients with cancer: magnetic resonance imaging evidence for altered tumor blood flow. *J Clin Oncol* 2003;21:4428–38.

74. Nathan P, Zwifel M, Padhani AR, *et al.* Phase 1 trial of combretastatin A4 phosphate (CA4P) in combination with bevacizumab in patients with advanced cancer. *Clin Cancer Res* 2012;18:3428–39.

75. de Bazelaire C, Alsop DC, George D, *et al.* Magnetic resonance imaging-measured blood flow change after antiangiogenic therapy with PTK787/ZK 222584 correlates with clinical outcome in metastatic renal cell carcinoma. *Clin Cancer Res* 2008;14:5548–54.

76. Fenchel M, Konaktchieva M, Weisel K, *et al.* Early response assessment in patients with

multiple myeloma during anti-angiogenic therapy using arterial spin labelling: first clinical results. *Eur Radiol* 2010;20:2899–906.

77. Morgan B, Thomas AL, Drevs J, *et al.* Dynamic contrast-enhanced magnetic resonance imaging as a biomarker for the pharmacological response of PTK787/ZK 222584, an inhibitor of the vascular endothelial growth factor receptor tyrosine kinases, in patients with advanced colorectal cancer and liver metastases: results from two phase I studies. *J Clin Oncol* 2003;21:3955–64.

78. Murphy PS, Roberts C, Whitcher B, *et al.* Vascular response of hepatocellular carcinoma to pazopanib measured by dynamic contrast-enhanced MRI: pharmacokinetic and clinical activity correlations. *Proc Intl Soc Magn Reson Med,* Stockholm, Sweden 2010;2720.

79. Mross K, Drevs J, Muller M, *et al.* Phase I clinical and pharmacokinetic study of PTK/ZK, a multiple VEGF receptor inhibitor, in patients with liver metastases from solid tumours. *Eur J Cancer* 2005;41:1291–9.

80. Thomas AL, Morgan B, Horsfield MA, *et al.* Phase I study of the safety, tolerability, pharmacokinetics, and pharmacodynamics of PTK787/ZK 222584 administered twice daily in patients with advanced cancer. *J Clin Oncol* 2005;23:4162–71.

81. Jonker DJ, Rosen LS, Sawyer MB, *et al.* A phase I study to determine the safety, pharmacokinetics and pharmacodynamics of a dual VEGFR and FGFR inhibitor, brivanib, in patients with advanced or metastatic solid tumors. *Ann Oncol* 2011;22:1413–19.

82. Akerley WL, Schabel M, Morrell G, *et al.* A randomized phase 2 trial of combretastatin A4 phosphate (CA4P) in

combination with paclitaxel and carboplatin to evaluate safety and efficacy in subjects with advanced imageable malignancies. *J Clin Oncol (Meetings Abstracts)* 2007;25 (18S):14060.

83. O'Donnell A, Padhani A, Hayes C, *et al.* A phase I study of the angiogenesis inhibitor SU5416 (semaxanib) in solid tumours, incorporating dynamic contrast MR pharmacodynamic end points. *Br J Cancer* 2005;93: 876–83.

84. Miller KD, Trigo JM, Wheeler C, *et al.* A multicenter phase II trial of ZD6474, a vascular endothelial growth factor receptor-2 and epidermal growth factor receptor tyrosine kinase inhibitor, in patients with previously treated metastatic breast cancer. *Clin Cancer Res* 2005;11:3369–76.

85. Hecht JR, Trarbach T, Hainsworth JD, *et al.* Randomized, placebo-controlled, phase III study of first-line oxaliplatin-based chemotherapy plus PTK787/ZK 222584, an oral vascular endothelial growth factor receptor inhibitor, in patients with metastatic colorectal adenocarcinoma. *J Clin Oncol* 2011;29:1997–2003.

86. Ellis LM. Antiangiogenic therapy: more promise and, yet again, more questions. *J Clin Oncol* 2003;21:3897–9.

87. O'Connor JP, Jackson A, Parker GJ, Jayson GC. DCE-MRI biomarkers in the clinical evaluation of antiangiogenic and vascular disrupting agents. *Br J Cancer* 2007;96:189–95.

88. Bjarnason GA, Williams R, Hudson JM, *et al.* Microbubble ultrasound (DCE-US) compared to DCE-MRI and DCE-CT for the assessment of vascular response to sunitinib in renal cell carcinoma (RCC). *J Clin Oncol (Meetings Abstracts)* 2011;29(S):4627.

251

89. Faria SC, Ng CS, Hess KR, *et al.* CT quantification of effects of thalidomide in patients with metastatic renal cell carcinoma. *AJR Am J Roentgenol* 2007;**189**:378–85.

90. Yopp AC, Schwartz LH, Kemeny N, *et al.* Antiangiogenic therapy for primary liver cancer: correlation of changes in dynamic contrast-enhanced magnetic resonance imaging with tissue hypoxia markers and clinical response. *Ann Surg Oncol* 2011;**18**:2192–9.

91. Hillengass J, Wasser K, Delorme S, *et al.* Lumbar bone marrow microcirculation measurements from dynamic contrast-enhanced magnetic resonance imaging is a predictor of event-free survival in progressive multiple myeloma. *Clin Cancer Res* 2007;**13**:475–81.

92. Jackson A, O'Connor JP, Parker GJ, Jayson GC. Imaging tumor vascular heterogeneity and angiogenesis using dynamic contrast-enhanced magnetic resonance imaging. *Clin Cancer Res* 2007;**13**:3449–59.

93. Karahaliou A, Vassiou K, Arikidis NS, *et al.* Assessing heterogeneity of lesion enhancement kinetics in dynamic contrast-enhanced MRI for breast cancer diagnosis. *Br J Radiol* 2010; **83**:296–309.

94. O'Connor JP, Rose CJ, Jackson A, *et al.* DCE-MRI biomarkers of tumour heterogeneity predict CRC liver metastasis shrinkage following bevacizumab and FOLFOX-6. *Br J Cancer* 2011;**105**:139–45.

95. Checkley D, Tessier JJ, Kendrew J, Waterton JC, Wedge SR. Use of dynamic contrast-enhanced MRI to evaluate acute treatment with ZD6474, a VEGF signalling inhibitor, in PC-3 prostate tumours. *Br J Cancer* 2003;**89**:1889–95.

96. Berry LR, Barck KH, Go MA, *et al.* Quantification of viable tumor microvascular characteristics by multispectral analysis. *Magn Reson Med* 2008;**60**:64–72.

97. Buonaccorsi GA, Rose CJ, O'Connor JP, *et al.* Cross-visit tumor sub-segmentation and registration with outlier rejection for dynamic contrast-enhanced MRI time series data. *Lect Notes Comp Sci* 2010;**6363**:121–8.

Liver metastasis from colorectal cancer

History

A 57-year-old woman with locally advanced T3 rectal cancer and nodal metastasis (circled in Figure 12.6) became unwell with tiredness, abdominal pain, and weight loss, 3 years after initial chemo-radiotherapy. Computed tomography showed ill-defined low attenuation in liver segments VIII and IVa (arrow in CT image, Figure 12.6).

Technique

T_1- and T_2-weighted axial images of the liver and DCE-MRI (baseline, arterial and portal venous, and delayed 10 min phases).

Imaging findings

See Figure 12.6.

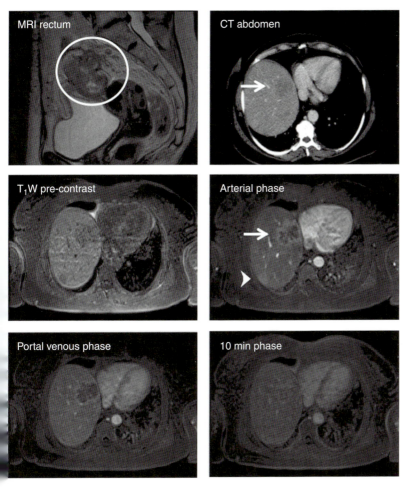

Figure 12.6 A 7 × 5 cm ring enhancing lesion was demonstrated in segment VIII/IVa with rapid arterial enhancement and subsequent washout, consistent with metastasis (arrow). Additional lesions not visible on the CT images were also demonstrated (arrowhead), confirming disease progression.

Discussion

DCE liver MRI confirmed the presence of metastatic disease and also demonstrated an additional lesion not visualized on CT. The perfusion pattern (rapid enhancement/washout) suggested a malignant rather than benign lesion.

Key points

- Liver MRI has increased sensitivity over CT for detecting liver lesions.

- DCE sequences help to characterize lesion morphology, distinguishing malignant and benign tumors from one another.

Bibliography

Koh DM, Padhani AR. Functional magnetic resonance imaging of the liver: parametric assessments beyond morphology. *Magn Reson Imaging Clin N Am* 2010;**18**:565–85.

MR perfusion imaging in breast cancer

Riham H. El Khouli, Katarzyna J. Macura, and David A. Bluemke

Key points

- Breast cancer is the most commonly diagnosed cancer in women, and is a major cause of morbidity and mortality.
- Clinical perfusion MRI in the breast is based on T_1-weighted DCE measurements following bolus injection of gadolinium-based contrast agent.
- Malignant breast tumors are typically associated with increased blood flow, vascular permeability, and cell density (leading to decreased extravascular extracellular space).
- Various methods of analysis of DCE data are available, including measurements of signal enhancement, wash-in/washout pattern, model-based analyses, and computer-aided diagnosis (CAD).
- The temporal enhancement patterns seen on DCE (types I, II, or III) are classified into 'persistent,' 'plateau,' and 'washout,' respectively. There is increasing risk of malignancy going from type I to type III.
- CAD-based analysis of DCE data is increasingly used to generate voxel-by-voxel color-coded maps that rate the likelihood of malignancy. However, diagnostic accuracy is not 100% so MRI does not obviate the need for breast biopsy in many patients.
- DCE is being increasingly used as a screening tool for select patient groups carrying one or several genetic mutations who are at higher risk for breast cancer.
- DCE may also be useful for predicting or monitoring tumor response to neoadjuvant chemotherapy.

Introduction

Breast cancer is the most common cancer diagnosed in women in the United States, with about 200 000 new cases diagnosed in the USA in 2010, and it is the second most common cause of death among females, after lung cancer [1]. Pathophysiology of breast cancer is related to vascular and perfusion anomalies. Living cells require oxygen and nutrients to survive; for that reason they need to develop new blood vessels, since the largest distance compatible with simple oxygen diffusion is 200 µm. When small malignant lesions develop in the breast, they can satisfy oxygen and nutrient demands through simple diffusion; however, as malignant tumors enlarge, they are no longer capable of relying on diffusion. Demands for oxygen and nutrients exceed supply, leading to an ischemic and hypoglycemic state (metabolic stressors). These metabolic stressors along with many other identified stressors, such as mechanical (pressure generated by proliferating cells in the tumor space), immune/inflammatory cells, or genetic mutations (activation of oncogenes or deletion of suppressor genes), stimulate the release of many biochemical factors, among which is the vascular endothelial growth factor (VEGF). VEGF promotes the formation of new branching and feeding vessels from pre-existing peritumoral capillaries [2]. Circulating endothelial cells that were shed from the vascular wall and bone marrow may contribute to the angiogenesis as well [3, 4].

Tumor vessels are structurally and functionally abnormal. Grossly, they are tortuous and unevenly dilated, with excessive branching and arteriovenous shunting. This results in uneven and variable flow in different areas within the tumor, and can create low oxygen tension (hypoxic) regions. Microscopically, tumor vascular walls are fenestrated, due to numerous endothelial defects and transcellular holes, wide intra-endothelial junctions, and absent basement membrane [5–8]. VEGF plays a role in maintaining the high fraction of immature vessels within the tumor. Immature vessels do not have investing pericytes and/or smooth muscle cells; therefore, they are the most permeable vessels. All the above factors lead to increase in permeability of vascular walls within tumors, which leads to the fast leakage of contrast material into the extravascular extracellular space (EES) and the early contrast washout from the tumor that characterizes malignant lesions on dynamic contrast-enhanced (DCE)-MRI studies (as described in detail in Chapter 4). Another characteristic of malignant lesions of the breast is the high replication and turnover rates of tumor cells within a small space, which leads to increased cellular density of the tumor when compared with that of normal glandular breast tissue. The increase in cellular density results in decreased EES volume in tumor regions. On the other hand, in benign breast tissues there is usually no alteration of the vascular bed or extracellular spaces.

For these reasons, DCE has been of considerable interest over the last three decades for the detection and characterization of breast lesions. The initial emphasis was on the assessment of tumor morphology with high spatial resolution scans at a single time point after contrast administration. Contrast-enhanced MRI was shown to have a very high sensitivity with a moderate specificity for identifying malignancy. During the late 1990s, two large multi-center trials took place to evaluate the role of DCE, where multiple scans acquired at high temporal resolution were obtained after intravenous (IV) contrast administration. These trials were conducted by the American College of Radiology Imaging Network (ACRIN), and the International Breast MR Consortium. The investigators highlighted the importance of DCE in improving the specificity to distinguish benign from malignant breast lesions [9–14]. Since the publication of the results of these studies, DCE has been accepted as a part of the routine breast MRI exam. Using DCE, several tissue perfusion parameters can be assessed, including contrast enhancement rate, intensity, and pattern of contrast uptake. Pharmacokinetic modeling can also be performed to derive quantitative markers to complement the assessment of lesion morphology.

DCE parameters: semi-quantitative and qualitative

The peak percentage enhancement and early wash-in rate

Peak percentage enhancement is very important in differentiating benign from malignant lesions. The initial (or wash-in) part of the kinetic curve is categorized into three categories; *slow* (initial enhancement <60% of peak), *intermediate* (initial enhancement 60–80% of peak), or *fast* (initial enhancement >80% of peak) [15]. Lesions that show early intense enhancement are highly suspicious for malignancy. The peak percentage enhancement and its timing (within the first 2 min) are both important; if the peak percentage enhancement is greater than 80% in the first 2 min, the suspicion for breast cancer increases. Categorizing enhancement in this manner resulted in a positive predictive value (PPV) of 47% and a negative predictive value (NPV) of 87% [15].

Time–intensity curve (kinetic curve)

The most popular method to interpret DCE is the kinetic curve (or time–intensity curve), a plot of the change in signal intensity (on the y-axis) versus time (on the x-axis) (Figure 13.1). The kinetic curve can be created using two methods; the first is by simply plotting the absolute signal intensity on the y-axis, and the other is by plotting the percentage enhancement. Percentage enhancement is calculated according to the equation [16, 17]:

$$\frac{S_{post} - S_{pre}}{S_{pre}} \times 100$$

where S_{pre} is the signal intensity in the pre-contrast image and S_{post} is the signal intensity in the post-contrast image. Plotting the percentage enhancement instead of the absolute signal intensity has several advantages; it is a normalized value that relates the post-contrast signal intensity to the pre-contrast one, which eliminates the confounding effect of the many factors, including scanning parameters, that may influence the signal intensity in the patient. It also simplifies the interpretation of the kinetic curve, as the peak percentage enhancement is the initial parameter of interest during the interpretation.

The most commonly used method for assessment of the kinetic curve shape is a qualitative assessment

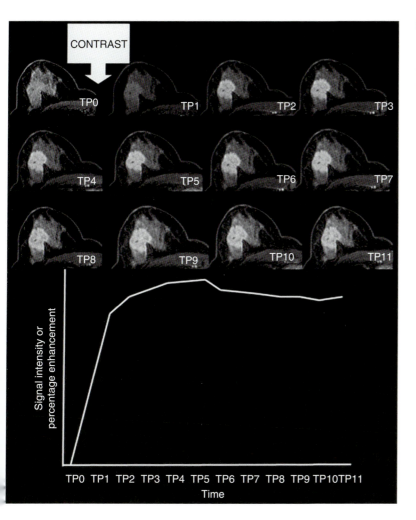

Figure 13.1 The kinetic curve (time–intensity curve) constructed by plotting the signal intensity (% enhancement) changes in different DCE phases on the Y-axis versus time on the X-axis. TP, time point.

which was reported to have a variable inter-observer agreement, ranging from a kappa of 0.27 [18, 19] to 0.8 [9]. The qualitative method depends on subjectively categorizing the shape of the washout curve into three types (Figure 13.2) [9, 15, 18, 20]:

Type I (persistently enhancing): a gradual slow and continuous enhancement over the scanning period. This type is further categorized into type IA and type IB according to the enhancement pattern in the first 2 min. In type IA the enhancement is slowly progressing, while in type IB there is an early marked enhancement sometimes exceeding 80% enhancement followed by a slower continuous enhancement (Figure 13.2). Both types IA and IB are considered good predictors of a benign lesion, with an NPV of 94% [15], unless architectural features indicate otherwise.

Type II (plateau): intense early enhancement within the first 2 min equal to or exceeding 80% peak enhancement followed by persistence of the same percentage enhancement over the scanning period. This type of curve carries intermediate probability as both benign and malignant lesions can show this perfusion behavior. It is considered somewhat suspicious, and correlation with morphological features is critical. If both are indeterminate, further workup is usually recommended.

Type III (washout): intense early enhancement equal to or exceeding 80% of peak enhancement followed by a decrease in the percentage enhancement (washout). This type of curve reflects the expected dynamics of malignant tumors and is considered a strong indicator of malignancy, with a PPV of 87% [15].

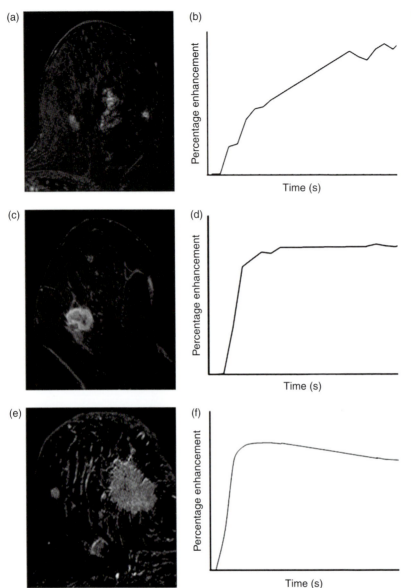

Figure 13.2 Breast lesions and different types (shapes) of the time–intensity curve. (a–b) Type I is a persistently enhancing curve, indicative of benign etiology. (c–d) Type II (plateau) curve has an intermediate probability for malignancy (in this case, the lobulated lesion was proven at pathology to be invasive ductal carcinoma) (e–f) Type III (washout) curve is indicative of malignancy (infiltrating ductal carcinoma).

The assessment of the kinetic curve shape can also be performed with a quantitative approach that is independent of subjective interpretation by individual observers [21]. In the study by El Khouli et al. [21], two parameters were calculated from the kinetic curves: the average washout slope and the absolute washout percentage-enhancement difference. Average washout slope was calculated as the mean slope of the line from the peak enhancement (defined as peak enhancement within the first 2 min) until the last time point (including all intermediate time points). The washout percentage-

enhancement difference was calculated by subtracting the percentage enhancement from the last time point from the peak (beginning and ending time points only).

The quantitative results were categorized into three categories analogous to the qualitative results. Both parameters were categorized as persistently enhancing, plateau, or washout, based on their values relative to thresholds placed symmetrically above and below zero. The percentage-enhancement threshold was 5%, while the washout slope cutoff point was 0.03%/s. An example of the quantitative categorization using one

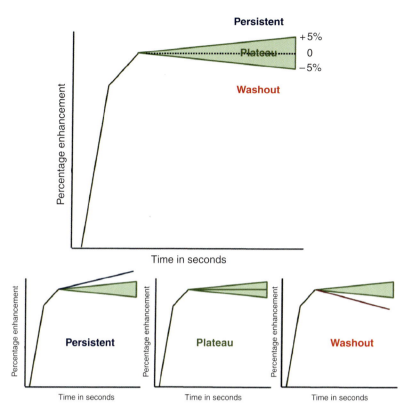

Figure 13.3 Illustration of a quantitative method for kinetic curve type assessment by categorizing the washout parameters (percentage-enhancement difference). If the change in percentage enhancement between the peak and subsequent time points is less than ±5% the pattern is considered as "plateau" (shaded area), more than 5% change is considered "persistent," and more than −5% is considered "washout."

of these thresholds (±5% cutoff range) is shown in Figure 13.3.

Washout rate

This is a quantitative assessment of the washout part of the kinetic curve. As we mentioned above, washout curves (with negative washout rate) are considered a high predictor for malignancy while the persistently enhancing (positive washout rate) is considered a good predictor of benignity.

Enhancement pattern

Another feature of DCE studies is the enhancement pattern [16, 22]. The pattern of enhancement can be divided into centrifugal and centripetal (Figure 13.4).

In the centrifugal pattern, the lesion starts enhancing from the center and progresses to the periphery, and that pattern is considered as a benign feature.

In the centripetal pattern the lesion starts enhancing from the periphery and progresses to the central portion, and that pattern is considered as a malignant feature.

Using these enhancement pattern features resulted in 95% sensitivity, 86% specificity, and 93% accuracy in one study [22].

Unilateral increased vascularity

This feature, first described in 2001, is based on the changes in breast vascularity that are thought to be associated with malignancy [23, 24]. Maximum intensity projection (MIP) images are generated from the dynamic post-contrast MR images and vascularity of both breasts is compared. A breast vascularity score may then be derived [24] depending on the number of vessels per breast that are ≥ 3 cm in length and ≥ 2 mm in maximum transverse diameter (Table 13.1). When the difference in the number of vessels between the two breasts is ≥ 2, the breast with higher vascularity is considered to have unilateral increased vascularity. It was hypothesized that this is a good predictor of ipsilateral invasive breast cancer (Figure 13.5). The reported sensitivity was 88%, specificity 82%, and overall accuracy 87%. The PPV was 94% and NPV 70%.

259

Pharmacokinetic modeling

Computer-assisted diagnosis (CAD) [25] was initially applied in mammography and then later to breast MRI. In mammography, CAD detects calcifications and masses associated with malignancy based on automated image feature analysis. In MRI, CAD is based on analysis of tissue perfusion using pharmacokinetic modeling of enhancement kinetics. Pharmacokinetic modeling offers many advantages over the qualitative assessment of the DCE studies; it provides quantitative parameters that reflect physiological and

Table 13.1. Vascularity map Scoring

Score 0:   Absent or very low vascularity (no vessels*)

Score 1:   Low vascularity (only one vessel*)

Score 2:   Moderate vascularity (2–4 vessels*)

Score 3:   High vascularity (≥ 5 vessels*)

* Vessels ≥ 3 cm long and ≥ 2 mm diameter

anatomical information about the lesion. It has been shown that breast MRI CAD allows characterization of *de novo* breast lesions as well as treatment response in neoadjuvant chemotherapy [26, 27].

The baseline T_1 mapping sequence

Pharmacokinetic modeling relies on accurate calculation of contrast concentration within the tissue of interest in each dynamic phase. The simplest way to measure the change in contrast concentration is to assume that the change in signal intensity is directly proportional to the tissue contrast concentration. However, this assumption is not correct, as the relationship between the contrast concentration and signal intensity is not linear. However, the change in relaxivity ($R_1 = 1/T_1$) has a more linear relationship with contrast concentration. Therefore, for an accurate measurement of contrast concentration, the baseline mapping of T_1 and equilibrium magnetization should be the first step in DCE pharmacokinetic

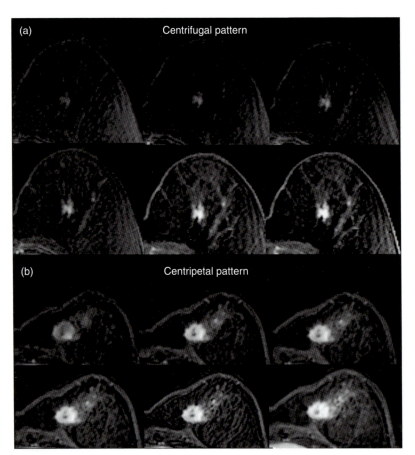

(a) Centrifugal pattern

(b) Centripetal pattern

Figure 13.4 Focal lesion enhancement displaying (a) centrifugal and (b) centripetal patterns. (a) Benign lesion, proven histologically to be sclerosing adenosis, that was morphologically highly suspicious for malignancy due to the spiculated margin. The enhancement started at the center of the lesion and progressed to the periphery (centrifugal). (b) Infiltrating ductal carcinoma showing enhancement starting at the periphery and progressing to the center of the mass (centripetal).

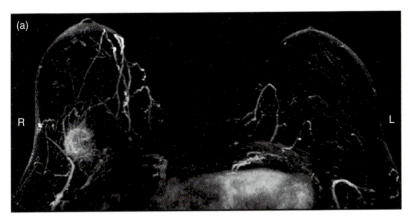

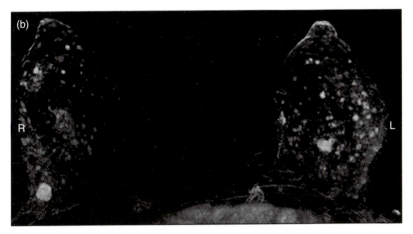

Figure 13.5 The application of 'unilateral increased vascularity index' in assessing a breast lesion. Maximum intensity projections (MIPs) of high spatial resolution subtraction images were constructed, showing (a) a case with unilateral increased vascularity according to the breast vascularity scoring system, with the right breast showing five vessels (each longer than 3 cm and thicker than 2 mm), while the left breast showing only one such vessel. The difference between the right and left breast vascularity is four. The lesion was proven histopathologically to be infiltrating ductal carcinoma. (b) A case with multiple enhancing lesions bilaterally. The unilateral increased vascularity sign is absent. Biopsy of the most suspicious lesion demonstrated fibroadenoma.

analysis. This T_1 mapping corrects for the non-linearity between the signal intensity changes and the underlying contrast material concentration changes [28–31]. Multiple methods have been described to acquire the T_1 map, among which the variable flip angle technique is the most widely used due to its short acquisition time and reasonable accuracy [32–35]. However, T_1 mapping is rarely performed in routine clinical breast MRI, as qualitative assessment is more common than quantitative assessment.

The dynamic series

The images acquired in the dynamic series should include in the field of view both the tissue of interest and a large blood vessel. The contrast versus time profile in the blood vessel allows measurement of the plasma contrast concentration over time, which is known as the vascular or arterial input function (VIF or AIF). The contrast material concentration within the breast tissue over time is measured as well.

The VIF/AIF is used to calculate the contrast concentration gradient between the blood and lesion. The combined information about contrast concentration changes over time in both the lesion and the AIF is required to perform pharmacokinetic modeling [36, 37].

Pharmacokinetic parameters

As described in Chapter 4, there are various quantitative parameters that can be extracted from the DCE data:

1. K^{trans} *(transfer constant):* the rate of contrast agent transfer from plasma compartment to extravascular extracellular spaces (wash-in rate).
2. k_{ep} *(washout rate constant):* the rate of escape of contrast agent from the extracellular spaces to the plasma compartment (washout rate). k_{ep} is the ratio of the transfer constant to the extravascular extracellular space fractional volume (v_e).

3. v_e *(Extravascular extracellular space (EES) fractional volume, or EVF):* volume of the interstitial space.
4. *Peak enhancement:* maximum tissue enhancement.

Other quantitative parametric interpretation of DCE includes the measurement of the initial area under the curve (IAUC) of the contrast agent concentration within the initial 2 min. It was reported to be reproducible and correlates well with tissue permeability, especially when normalized to the surrounding normal tissue [38].

CAD principles in DCE

There are several commercially available CAD software packages, which are based on one of two different principles for dynamic MRI data analysis. The first one relies on the *three time points (3TP)* analysis in which the color coding of breast tissue depends on acquiring three series of images; the pre-contrast or baseline series (TP0); the 2 min post-contrast series (TP1), and the 6 min post-contrast series (TP2). The resulting 3TP kinetic curve is then divided into two parts: TP0–TP1 corresponding to wash-in, and TP1–TP2 corresponding to washout. Subsequently, the color encoding has two components. The first is to determine the color hue depending on the washout part (TP1–TP2) of the kinetic curve, with the blue for persistently enhancing (progressively increasing signal intensity), green for plateau, and red for washout (decreasing signal intensity). The second part determines the intensity of the color and depends on the wash-in part of the curve (TP0–TP1), with dark color for slow wash-in rate, bright with the fast wash-in rate, and intermediate color for intermediate wash-in rate [39]. Looking at the overall color map gives a good idea of the kinetic pattern of any part of the tissue, to facilitate the placement of a region of interest (ROI) in the most suspicious part of the lesion for further evaluation.

The second principle aims to extract more detailed functional quantitative data, by analyzing the contrast distribution in relation to the vascularity of focal breast lesions [28, 31, 40–47]. Since the 1990s, many studies have been conducted to investigate compartmental modeling theories. These models are based on assessing the exchange of contrast between different body compartments. The simplest model describes two compartments: one compartment being the tissue

of interest and the second compartment being the plasma. The greater the number of compartments in the model, the more accurate it is expected to be [31, 48, 49]. The four compartmental modeling theoretically divides the body into four units; plasma, normal extracellular space, tumoral leakage spaces, and the kidneys. Three main kinetic coefficients (K^{trans}, k_{ep}, and v_e) can be extracted from the data by analyzing the wash-in and washout slopes and appropriate fitting of the dynamic curves [31, 48–50].

Color map

Pharmacokinetic models characterize breast lesions in terms of multiple parameters that describe contrast delivery, accumulation, and washout, rather than using a single observational parameter such as percentage of contrast washout (Figure 13.6). Unfortunately, multiple complex parameters are often difficult to interpret in a clinical setting. Therefore, typically, CAD software packages combine multiple parameters into a color-coded display that enables the radiologist to rapidly determine whether the DCE data are suggestive of malignancy or not. In this manner, the color map produced represents the result of analysis of DCE and calculations of both permeability and EES volume fraction values on a voxel-by-voxel basis. The CAD software implements categorization of lesions by mapping these parameters into one of the three colors representing a probability range from benign, through indeterminate, to malignant. The color code combines values of the permeability and EES volume fraction based on several studies that have determined appropriate cutoff points. Blue represents normal contrast kinetics, green represents indeterminate to suspicious, and red represents highly suspicious. Once an ROI is drawn on the most suspicious part of the lesion identified by CAD, the results of the quantitative analysis, including the lesion kinetic curve, may be displayed (Figures 13.7, 13.8, and 13.9).

However, within a single lesion, voxels with both malignant and benign parameters may be present. The percentage distribution of each color can be calculated. Typically, the best test performance for identifying a malignant lesion occurs if the lesion is composed of more than approximately 16% of red "malignant" voxels. Likewise, the best test performance to identify benign lesions occurs if the lesion is composed of 20% or more blue "benign" voxels [42–46, 51, 52].

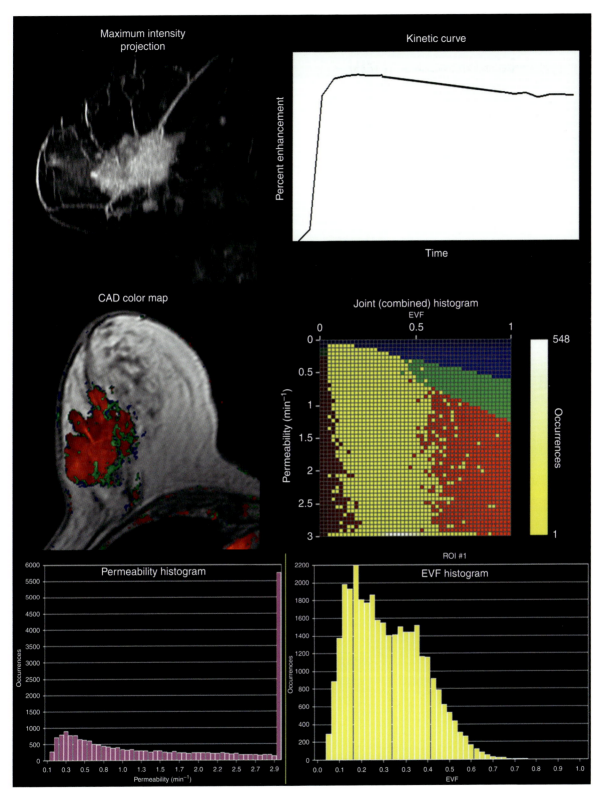

Figure 13.6 Post-processing of DCE images of the breast with CAD software (iCAD View, iCad, Inc.). Sagittal MIP (top left) shows a spiculated mass that on histology was found to be an infiltrating ductal carcinoma. The contrast enhancement kinetic curve for the whole lesion (top right) indicates a type III (washout) pattern. The CAD color map (middle left) shows that the mass was assigned red (high association with malignancy) and green (moderate association with malignancy) based on each voxel's permeability and extracellular volume fraction (EVF). The distribution of lesion voxels is overlaid (in yellow) on the joint histogram (middle right, indicating standardized likelihood of malignancy color coding, based on permeability and EVF values), showing that most of the lesion pixels are suggestive of malignancy (red). Bottom left and right panels show the histograms of lesion permeability and EVF, respectively.

263

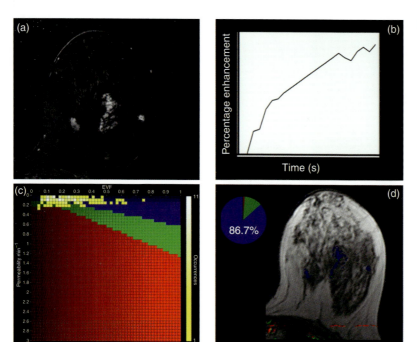

Figure 13.7 Suspicious breast lesion on mammography referred for breast MRI. (a) An axial high spatial resolution subtracted image shows areas of clumped, non-mass-like enhancement in the upper left breast. (b) The corresponding kinetic curve shows a Type I (persistently enhancing) curve that is indicative of a benign lesion. (c) The joint histogram showing the distribution of the lesion pixels (yellow) within the blue and green color-coded regions, again consistent with a low level of suspicion for a malignant lesion. (d) The color map shows that 87% of the lesion exhibits blue color (benign perfusion pattern). Histopathological examination revealed benign fibrocystic changes.

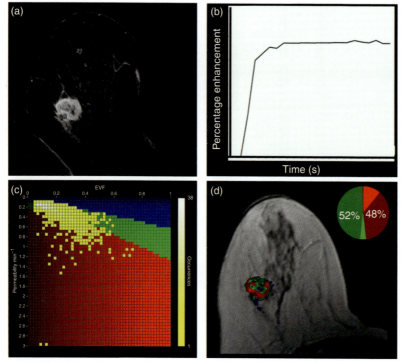

Figure 13.8 Patient recently diagnosed with right breast cancer. (a) An axial high spatial resolution subtracted image shows a spiculated enhancing mass at the upper outer quadrant of the right breast. (b) The corresponding kinetic curve shows a Type II (plateau) pattern that is indeterminate but which might be considered suspicious for a malignant lesion. (c) The joint histogram shows the distribution of the lesion voxels within the red and green color-coded regions, suggesting a high level of suspicion. (d) The color map shows that 48% of the lesion exhibits red color, which is highly suggestive of a malignant lesion.

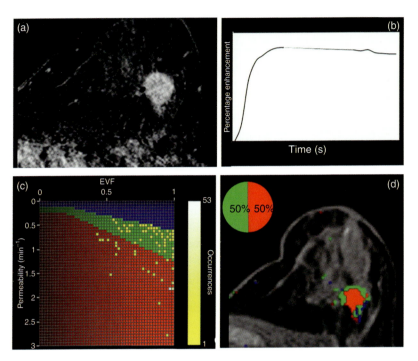

Figure 13.9 A case of a patient with a strong family history of breast cancer that was referred for screening. (a) An axial high spatial resolution subtracted image shows a spiculated, enhancing mass at the 3 o'clock position of the left breast. (b) The corresponding kinetic curve shows a Type III (washout) curve that is indicative of malignant enhancement pattern. (c) The joint histogram showing the distribution of the lesion voxels within the red and green color-coded regions suggests a high level of suspicion for a malignant lesion. (d) The color map shows that 50% of the lesion exhibits red color, which is highly suggestive of malignancy.

Role of CAD in improving breast MRI diagnostic performance

Applying pharmacokinetic parameters to characterize breast lesions as benign or malignant capitalizes on the principle that high vascular permeability and low EES volume fraction is a signature of malignancy [39, 53–56]. Using the intensity-modulated color-coded display method in CAD based on the kinetic curve shape, detection and characterization of breast lesions is quick and easy to interpret. Improved diagnostic performance (i.e., confidence for both detection and characterization of lesions) compared to conventional display techniques was achieved using this type of automated CAD software, with 93% sensitivity, 86% specificity, and 91% accuracy in one study [53]. It was also documented that CAD significantly reduced the false positive rates compared to qualitative interpretation by 33% when using 80% threshold for enhancement, and by 50% when using 100% threshold [57]. By using quantitative pharmacokinetic modeling, a significant difference in distribution of color hue and depth between benign and malignant lesions was achieved [39] and resulted in preserving high sensitivity (93%) while significantly reducing the false positive rate by 23% when using 100% enhancement threshold as compared to the initial interpretation without CAD software [54].

Pharmacokinetic modeling approaches should be used as an adjunct to the information from high spatial resolution 3D MRI, and is an area of continuing research. In one study, analysis of lesion morphology coupled with low temporal resolution (86 s per acquisition) kinetic images resulted in an AUC value of 0.84 for distinguishing malignant from benign lesions [58], while a more recent study showed that both the kinetic curve type classification and pharmacokinetic modeling are likely to produce similar overall performance, both of which are improved compared to morphological analysis of imaging features on high spatial resolution scans alone [59]. A very recent study showed that K^{trans} correlated with the final diagnosis with an AUC of 0.96, while v_e did not, showing an AUC of only 0.58 [60]. Clearly, this is an area of much ongoing research.

Treatment response assessment following neoadjuvant therapy

Since the early 1970s, there has been increasing interest in the non-radical treatment of early breast cancer. Many studies reported the absence of any significant difference in the outcome between conservative breast surgery and classic mastectomy [61, 62]. Neoadjuvant chemotherapy is often used before surgery to shrink the size of large cancers (locally advanced breast cancer), either to allow inoperable cases to become operable or to perform a localized resection in a patient who would otherwise require a mastectomy. Neoadjuvant chemotherapy also may treat possible undetected micro-metastases. The assessment of tumor response to neoadjuvant therapy is important for clinical decision-making, for instance to distinguish patients who benefit from the treatment from those who do not, and who therefore require a change of management as early as possible. Large clinical trials have investigated the degree of tumor response and patient survival in patients receiving neoadjuvant chemotherapy [63, 64]. Although both mammography and ultrasound are routinely used to monitor response to neoadjuvant chemotherapy, DCE has proven to be more accurate in assessing tumor response [65, 66].

Tumor size

Tumor size is the basic criterion upon which tumor response to treatment is determined. In the early 1980s, the World Health Organization (WHO) developed guidelines for assessment of tumor response to treatment in an attempt to standardize criteria for both clinical and research evaluations. Since then, WHO criteria have been used widely as the standard method. WHO criteria are based on the *bi-dimensional measurement*, where tumor size is determined by measuring the longest diameter of the tumor and then its perpendicular diameter and subsequently calculating the sum of both diameters. Many studies were done to compare the accuracy of uni-dimensional and bi-dimensional measurements in the assessment of tumor treatment response; the

biggest was a study by James *et al.* [67] in which the authors retrospectively studied over 4000 patients from 14 different centers and concluded that there was no change in the measured response rate to treatment when using uni- or bi-dimensional lesion measurements. At the same time, the change in the maximal tumor diameter correlated more with the fixed proportion of killed tumor cells by the effect of chemotherapy than did the bi-dimensional measurement [68]. At the end of the last century, three research groups; the European Organization for Research and Treatment of Cancer (EORTC), the National Cancer Institute of the United States, and the National Cancer Institute of Canada Clinical Trials Group developed new guidelines modifying the WHO criteria with the acronym RECIST (Response Evaluation Criteria In Solid Tumors). Both WHO and RECIST classified response to treatment into four categories (Table 13.2). There are many differences between the WHO and RECIST criteria but the main difference is that RECIST uses the *uni-dimensional measurement* (the longest diameter of the tumor) as its main indicator for treatment response. Due to the complexity of the WHO guidelines, many investigators prefer the RECIST criteria due to their simplicity, especially since many studies have confirmed its accuracy and usefulness, and the high concordance between the uni-dimensional and bi-dimensional criteria [69].

Recently, *3D volume* change in tumor size was suggested to be more predictive of recurrence-free survival in patients undergoing neoadjuvant chemotherapy (Figure 13.10) [70]. The 3D tumor volume is usually calculated according to the following equation:

$$\text{Tumor volume} = (\pi/6) \times d_1 \times d_2 \times d_3 \qquad (13.1)$$

where d_i = diameter in each of the three dimensions.

Table 13.2. Objective treatment response categories

		WHO	RECIST
1. **Complete response CR:**	Disappearance of all lesions confirmed at 4 weeks	–	–
2. **Partial response PR:**	Partial decrease in tumor size confirmed at 4 weeks	50% decrease	30% decrease
3. **Progressive disease PD:**	Increase in tumor size without a previous CR or PR	25% increase	20% increase
	New lesion	–	–
4. **Stable disease SD:**	If criteria do not meet either PR or PD		

(a)　　　　　　　　　　　　　　(b)

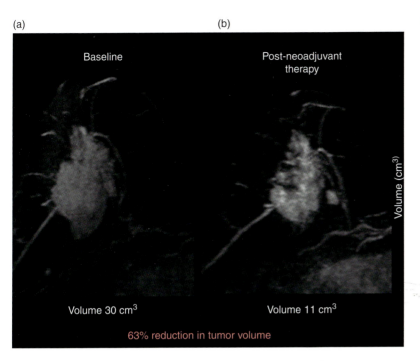

Baseline

Post-neoadjuvant therapy

Volume 30 cm^3　　　　　　　Volume 11 cm^3

63% reduction in tumor volume

Volume (cm^3)

Figure 13.10 Response to chemotherapy demonstrated by breast MRI. (a) Baseline pre-treatment mass (dimensions $6.5 \times 5.0 \times 1.8$ cm, volume 30 cm^3) was diagnosed as infiltrating ductal carcinoma. (b) The same lesion post-neoadjuvant chemotherapy (dimensions $4.5 \times 3.1 \times 1.5$ cm, volume 11 cm^3). According to the RECIST (uni-dimensional measurement) there was a 30% decrease in the size of the mass, which classifies the patient in the partial response category. According to the WHO classification (bi-dimensional measurement), there was a 34% decrease in the tumor size, which classifies the patient in the non-responder category (stable disease). According to the recently introduced volume criteria, there was a 63% reduction in tumor volume, which classifies the patient into the partial response category. In such ambiguous cases, perfusion imaging may provide helpful information.

DCE parameter analysis in clinical trials

Many studies have been performed to evaluate the role of DCE in assessing response to neoadjuvant chemotherapy. Generally, most of these studies have concluded that while a change in tumor size may be observed only after the third cycle of chemotherapy, dynamic pharmacokinetic changes may already be detected after the first cycle. Vascular density, permeability, and perfusion have been suggested to be the factors that best differentiated responders from non-responders (see Table 13.3, Figure 13.11). Changes in the transport constant (K^{trans}), washout constant (k_{ep}) and extravascular extracellular volume (v_e) are discussed below:

1. K^{trans}: two important factors were reported concerning K^{trans} value:

    a. A significant reduction in K^{trans} compared with baseline was observed in many studies from the early post-chemotherapy period, and this reduction became more evident during the course of treatment in clinico-pathologically proven responders [71–73]. In the same study, proven non-responders showed either an increase or no change in K^{trans} with a right shift of the histogram (towards high K^{trans} values). These changes in K^{trans} are thought to be caused by changes in both microvascular density and permeability. It is hypothesized that chemotherapeutic agents cause reduction of angiogenic factors such as VEGF, which is a strong stimulus for neo-angiogenesis and a promoter of permeability. VEGF reduction would cause reversal of these processes, which would explain the decrease in K^{trans} in the responder group. On the other hand, tumors in non-responders may keep producing VEGF, which will result in stable or increased K^{trans} values.

    b. The change in K^{trans} is correlated with its pre-treatment value, which suggests that the pre-treatment K^{trans} value may predict both the tumor pathological response, and also the length of disease-free survival. One possible explanation of this observation is that chemotherapy agents will be delivered at higher concentrations to tumors with greater permeability (K^{trans}), leading to better response [71].

2. k_{ep} showed the same correlation as K^{trans}; significant reductions of k_{ep} values from baseline at early post-treatment periods were found in responders, while k_{ep} was constant or even increased in non-responders [71–73].

267

Table 13.3. How DCE-MRI pharmacokinetic parameters change in response to treatment

K^{trans} **Pre-treatment** → The higher the K^{trans} in pre-treatment study, the more probable the lesion will respond to treatment
Post-treatment → Responders → significant reduction from the baseline
→ Non-responders → no changes or slight increase

k_{ep} **Post-treatment** → Responders → significant reduction from the baseline
→ Non-responders → no changes or slight increase

v_e **Pre-treatment** → Significantly higher for responders compared with non-responders
Post-treatment → Responders → no changes or slight decreased
→ Non-responders → significant rise from the baseline

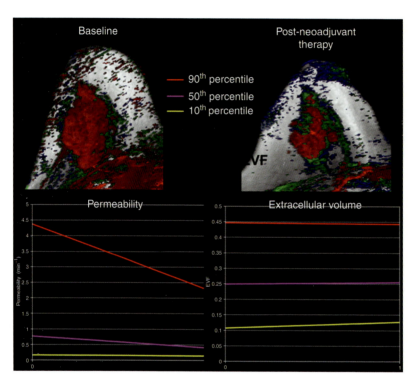

Figure 13.11 Response to chemotherapy demonstrated by perfusion MRI. Although the reduction in tumor size did not meet the WHO or RECIST criteria for partial response, there was a marked reduction in the permeability of the tumor after administration of neoadjuvant chemotherapy with stable EES volume fraction (EVF). A significant change in the color codes of the lesion can be seen after therapy.

3. v_e: the initial v_e value was shown to be high for responders and significantly lower for non-responders. During treatment, there was a significant rise in v_e in non-responders, unlike non-responders where v_e remained static or even decreased [73].

Hardware, software and scanning considerations for breast MRI

Field strength

Until recently, 1.5 T was the magnetic field strength most widely used in breast MRI in clinical practice. However, many recent research trials have been performed using 3 T magnets, given the expected linear increase in signal-to-noise ratio (SNR) with magnetic field strength [74–76]. These benefits come with some challenges when shifting from 1.5 T to 3 T. With increased field strength, *susceptibility artifacts* (variation of local magnetic field at the boundaries between different types of tissues) are increased, and transmit radiofrequency (RF) coil homogeneity is also worse, which may lead to worse fat suppression if care is not taken to set up the acquisition properly.

Unilateral versus bilateral acquisition

Bilateral image acquisition for breast MRI is preferred over unilateral acquisition for several reasons. First, it is useful for comparison of symmetry, a very important concept in breast diagnosis in general, to include physical exam, mammography, and MRI. Second, a large study, part of the International Breast MRI Consortium (IBMC) trial, reported that in women with recent breast cancer, about 4% will have a contralateral invasive breast cancer detected on MRI that is otherwise occult on other breast imaging modalities [10], which underlines the absolute importance of bilateral coverage in clinical breast MRI.

Sagittal versus axial

The sagittal plane was routinely used in the past for breast MRI, both because it has several advantages over other orientations, and also because of its similarity to conventional mammographic views (Table 13.4). Recently, bilateral simultaneous acquisition of sagittal images has been implemented; however, this requires a relatively long imaging time, making it difficult to acquire high temporal resolution dynamic series in this plane. Currently, bilateral axial protocols are widely used in clinical practice, capitalizing on advantages of scanning both breasts simultaneously and in a short time. Also, the axillary tail of the breast and the axillae are well visualized in the axial view.

2D versus 3D acquisitions

In breast MRI, scans can be acquired either in a multi-slice 2D mode or with 3D sequences where signal from the whole breast is detected on every shot.

Table 13.4. Advantages and disadvantages of imaging in the sagittal plane

ADVANTAGES OF SAGITTAL PLANE:
1. Correlates very well anatomically and easier for surgeons
2. Needs small FOV → Improves spatial resolution at a given matrix
   → Relatively homogeneous field across the breast
   ↓
   Better fat-suppression results

DISADVANTAGES OF SAGITTAL PLANE:
1. Increased number of slices to cover both breasts
2. Breasts are often scanned sequentially (not simultaneously) → not suitable for bilateral DCE-MRI of breast

FOV, Field of view.

There are advantages and disadvantages to each approach; however, when high spatial resolution, good SNR, and extended coverage are required, 3D sequences are more efficient. For this reason, most high-resolution breast MRI is performed using 3D encoding.

Fat suppression versus subtraction

The breast is composed of glandular (water) and adipose (fat) tissue. Fat tissue is bright on T_1-weighted images because of its short T_1 relaxation time. After contrast injection, a breast lesion may enhance and become isointense to fat, which explains the importance of fat suppression. However, the use of fat-suppression pulses within the pulse sequence lengthens the minimum repetition time (TR) that can be used, and therefore increases the scan time, which is unfavorable for dynamic imaging. Another problem with fat suppression, especially when scanning both breasts simultaneously in the axial plane, is the inhomogeneity of the magnetic field. However, with recent advances in scanner hardware, shimming techniques, and the development of more sophisticated fat-suppression approaches, it is possible to use fat suppression in high temporal resolution dynamic bilateral scans.

Another option to improve the contrast between enhancing breast lesions and breast fat is the image subtraction technique in which post-contrast images are subtracted from pre-contrast images, resulting in a new image highlighting only enhancing tissues. There are many reasons to examine both fat-suppressed and subtraction images. On high-resolution fat-suppressed images, lesions may be detected, even if they show no enhancement, and some of these lesions may be malignant. A small percentage of malignant lesions do not enhance, thus showing that morphological features must also be considered. Lesions that show suspicious architectural features but do not enhance must be detectable, and the problem with looking only at subtraction images is that these lesions will not be visible. Also, subtraction images are sensitive to misregistration problems due to breathing or other motion between acquisitions, which are aggravated with increasing spatial resolution (and smaller voxel size). An example of a fat-suppressed and a subtraction image, which has some loss in detail, is shown in Figure 13.12.

269

(a)

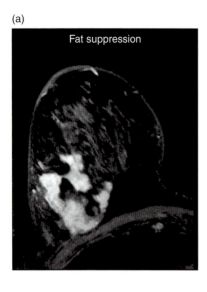

Fat suppression

(b)

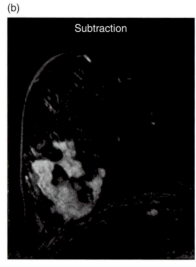

Subtraction

Figure 13.12 Fat suppression versus image subtraction. (a) Fat-suppressed high spatial resolution image (0.5 mm voxel size). (b) Subtraction image (post-contrast – pre-contrast). While the subtraction image offers more accurate assessment of degree and pattern of enhancement, the post-contrast image offers more details of glandular tissue, which may be critical to the assessment of morphology, e.g., lesion margins.

Breast MRI artifacts

Some of the common artifacts in breast MRI and the suggested methods to correct them are listed in Table 13.5 [77].

Temporal resolution versus spatial resolution

DCE breast protocols vary widely between institutions, with most significant differences in spatial and temporal resolutions. Current MRI scanners and pulse sequences can rapidly image the entire breast in 15 s or less. However, this high temporal resolution (important for kinetic analysis) comes at the expense of reduced spatial resolution (Figure 13.13), which is crucial for the morphological assessment of a suspicious breast lesion. Three common approaches are generally employed. The first places a higher value on the diagnostic value of the morphological information compared with the information obtained from the dynamic scan. This approach focuses on acquiring a high spatial resolution sequence with a low temporal resolution (usually around 120 s per image). In a typical protocol, one pre- and at least three post-contrast phases are acquired and used to create the kinetic curve with four or more time points. The second approach strives to achieve a balance between spatial and temporal resolution [14, 20, 78] considering the importance of morphological features [78–80]. With this approach, a sequence with a modest spatial and temporal resolution (usually around 60 s per image) is acquired [20]. The third approach uses a hybrid protocol with both high spatial and high temporal resolution sequences. In such a protocol, pre-contrast high temporal and high spatial resolution series are obtained, after which a set of early post-contrast dynamic (high temporal resolution) series are acquired over the first 2 min (to record the wash-in phase of the contrast agent) followed by a single post-contrast high spatial resolution sequence (to obtain the morphological information at peak enhancement), and at the end another set of dynamic series is performed to capture the washout phase (Figure 13.14).

The introduction of pharmacokinetic modeling techniques and the subsequent development of CAD software has led to a rapid rise in the clinical application of breast DCE [48]. Note, however, that all studies that have investigated the accuracy, applicability, and significance of pharmacokinetic modeling have acquired dynamic scans with a temporal resolution of 20 s or less [31, 48, 49, 81, 82].

Parallel imaging

As explained earlier, high temporal resolution is an important requirement for accurate dynamic DCE analysis, whether using a qualitative approach, semi-quantitative approach, or pharmacokinetic modeling. Reducing scan time is possible in various ways, and recently fast imaging techniques based on parallel imaging with multiple receiver coils have become popular. Sensitivity encoding (SENSE) is one of these techniques, and has found recent and wide acceptance

Table 13.5. MRI artifacts

Artifact	How to detect it?	How to correct it?
Improper positioning	Areas of high signal intensity where breast tissue is adjacent to coil elements	Breast should be centered within the coil
Motion	Misregistration errors in subtraction images	1. Explaining the importance of staying still to the patient 2. Ensuring that the position is comfortable for the patient 3. Applying mild compression to the breast 4. Sedation for claustrophobic patients
Susceptibility artifact (metallic artifact)	Local signal intensity void and distortion	1. Removing any metallic objects if possible 2. Using titanium (MR compatible) biopsy clips instead of the ferromagnetic ones
Wraparound artifact	Tissues outside the FOV become superimposed on structures within the FOV	Increase FOV
Zebra artifact	Black and white bands within the image	1. Increase FOV 2. Apply phase over-sampling
Chemical shift artifact	Bright or dark band perpendicular to frequency-encoding direction where fat and water are adjacent to each other	Increase bandwidth per pixel of the imaging sequence

(a)

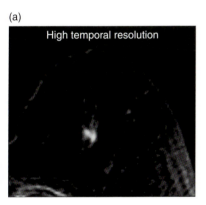

High temporal resolution

(b)

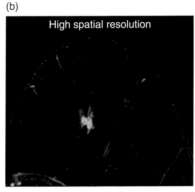

High spatial resolution

Figure 13.13 High temporal versus high spatial resolution images. (a) High temporal resolution (5 mm slice thickness and 15 s scan duration) versus (b) high spatial resolution (with 2.5 mm slice thickness and 2.5 min scan duration). While the high temporal resolution image (a) offers short acquisition time (15 s), which is critical for DCE, it is associated with architectural detail loss compared with the high spatial resolution image (b).

for breast DCE. Parallel imaging takes advantage of the spatial information that the phased-array RF coils encode to shorten the acquisition time by decreasing the number of k-space lines sampled, thus increasing temporal resolution. The reduction in the number of phased encoding steps is referred to as the reduction factor (R) (parallel imaging scan time = full scan time/R), which is typically 2 or more [83, 84]. The SENSE technique requires the acquisition of a reliable sensitivity mapping of each coil element, called the 'reference scan,' prior to the dynamic acquisition. Other parallel imaging techniques such as GRAPPA also work in a similar manner, albeit without the need for a reference scan.

Parallel imaging may also be used to improve spatial resolution with similar scan times as conventional acquisitions, and can be used to trade off between the temporal and spatial resolution. An important limitation of parallel imaging is a reduction in the SNR due to the shorter scan time and possible noise enhancement through suboptimal receiver coil arrangement, which leads to the potential to introduce image artifacts. Other parallel imaging artifacts are caused by the mismatch between the reference scan and the data acquisition. These mismatches can be caused by motion (respiration or gross patient motion), local susceptibility, strong fat signals, or inappropriately small field of view [83, 84].

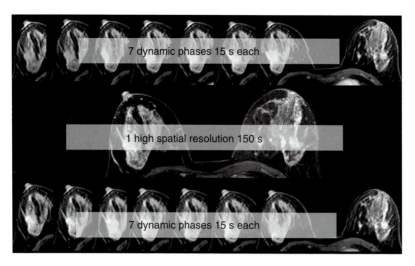

7 dynamic phases 15 s each

1 high spatial resolution 150 s

7 dynamic phases 15 s each

Figure 13.14 Illustration of a hybrid scanning protocol that interleaves both high temporal and high spatial resolution imaging. After contrast injection, seven dynamic phases, each at 15 s temporal resolution, are obtained to characterize the wash-in phase of contrast enhancement, followed by a high spatial resolution scan (2.5 min after contrast injection) for morphological assessment, followed by another seven dynamic phases to characterize the washout phase.

Gadolinium contrast agent

No systematic study has been performed to document differences between the various gadolinium-based MRI contrast agents that are available for breast imaging. The relaxivity of most of these agents is quite similar (range $4.3–4.8\,\mathrm{mM^{-1}\,s^{-1}}$), with the exception being gadobenate dimeglumine (Gd-BOPTA, MultiHance) (relaxivity $9.7\,\mathrm{mM^{-1}s^{-1}}$). Gd-BOPTA has weak protein interactions, and the impact of this on detection of malignancy is unknown. Due to this higher relaxivity, thresholds for enhancement of malignant lesions using Gd-BOPTA may be different compared with these other contrast agents and this must be taken into account in the pharmacokinetic modeling process [85]. It should also be noted that contrast agent effects on tissue relaxation times may be different between 1.5 T and 3 T.

Conclusion

MRI of the breast has proven to be a valuable diagnostic tool in detecting, characterizing, and assessing the extent of breast cancer and its response to treatment. DCE provides not only morphological information about breast tissue but also functional information about tissue perfusion and vascular permeability that permits the evaluation of breast lesions with improved diagnostic accuracy compared to anatomical imaging alone. Enhancement kinetics based on DCE provide objective information on cancer detection and characterization, as well as treatment planning and post-treatment evaluation. However, sensitivity and specificity of DCE are still generally considered not high enough to eliminate the need to perform biopsies in most patients. Breast DCE is currently favored for the screening evaluation of patients who are considered high risk for breast cancer, for instance those with known genetic mutation *BRCA*, or with a greater than 20% lifetime risk based on family history, dense breasts, and those with a prior history/recent diagnosis of breast cancer. Breast DCE may also be useful to monitor treatment response after neoadjuvant chemotherapy and to identify a primary lesion in patients diagnosed with metastatic axillary adenocarcinoma of unknown origin.

References

1. American Cancer Society. *Cancer Facts & Figures 2010*. Atlanta: American Cancer Society, Inc., 2010.

2. Pham CD, Roberts TP, van Bruggen N, *et al.* Magnetic resonance imaging detects suppression of tumor vascular permeability after administration of antibody to vascular endothelial growth factor. *Cancer Invest* 1998;**16**:225–30.

3. Kerbel RS. Tumor angiogenesis: past, present and the near future. *Carcinogenesis* 2000;**21**: 505–15.

4. Patan S, Munn LL, Jain RK. Intussusceptive microvascular growth in a human colon adenocarcinoma xenograft: a novel mechanism of tumor angiogenesis. *Microvasc Res* 1996;**51**:260–72.

5. Knopp MV, Giesel FL, Marcos H, von Tengg-Kobligk H, Choyke P.

Dynamic contrast-enhanced magnetic resonance imaging in oncology. *Top Magn Reson Imaging* 2001;**12**:301–8.

6. Dadiani M, Seger D, Kreizman T, *et al.* Estrogen regulation of vascular endothelial growth factor in breast cancer *in vitro* and *in vivo*: the role of estrogen receptor alpha and c-Myc. *Endocr Relat Cancer* 2009;**16**:819–34.

7. Kadambi A, Mouta Carreira C, Yun CO, *et al.* Vascular endothelial growth factor (VEGF)-C differentially affects tumor vascular function and leukocyte recruitment: role of VEGF-receptor 2 and host VEGF-A. *Cancer Res* 2001;**61**:2404–8.

8. Carmeliet P, Jain RK. Angiogenesis in cancer and other diseases. *Nature* 2000;**407**:249–57.

9. Bluemke DA, Gatsonis CA, Chen MH, *et al.* Magnetic resonance imaging of the breast prior to biopsy. *JAMA* 2004;**292**:2735–42.

10. Lehman CD, Blume JD, Thickman D, *et al.* Added cancer yield of MRI in screening the contralateral breast of women recently diagnosed with breast cancer: results from the International Breast Magnetic Resonance Consortium (IBMC) trial. *J Surg Oncol* 2005;**92**:9–15; discussion 15–16.

11. Lehman CD, Gatsonis C, Kuhl CK, *et al.* MRI evaluation of the contralateral breast in women with recently diagnosed breast cancer. *N Engl J Med* 2007;**356**:1295–303.

12. Lehman CD, Isaacs C, Schnall MD, *et al.* Cancer yield of mammography, MR, and US in high-risk women: prospective multi-institution breast cancer screening study. *Radiology* 2007;**244**:381–8.

13. Schnall MD, Blume J, Bluemke DA, *et al.* Diagnostic architectural and dynamic features at breast MR imaging: multicenter study. *Radiology* 2006;**238**:42–53.

14. Schnall MD, Rosten S, Englander S, Orel SG, Nunes LW. A combined architectural and kinetic interpretation model for breast MR images. *Acad Radiol* 2001;**8**:591–7.

15. Kuhl CK, Mielcareck P, Klaschik S, *et al.* Dynamic breast MR imaging: are signal intensity time course data useful for differential diagnosis of enhancing lesions? *Radiology* 1999;**211**:101–10.

16. Kaiser WA, Deimling M. [A new multislice measurement sequence for the complete dynamic MR examination of the larger organs: application to the breast]. *Rofo* 1990;**152**:577–82.

17. Kaiser WA, Zeitler E. MR imaging of the breast: fast imaging sequences with and without Gd-DTPA. Preliminary observations. *Radiology* 1989;**170**:681–6.

18. Kinkel K, Helbich TH, Esserman LJ, *et al.* Dynamic high-spatial-resolution MR imaging of suspicious breast lesions: diagnostic criteria and interobserver variability. *AJR Am J Roentgenol* 2000;**175**:35–43.

19. Stoutjesdijk MJ, Futterer JJ, Boetes C, *et al.* Variability in the description of morphologic and contrast enhancement characteristics of breast lesions on magnetic resonance imaging. *Invest Radiol* 2005;**40**:355–62.

20. Kuhl CK, Schild HH, Morakkabati N. Dynamic bilateral contrast-enhanced MR imaging of the breast: trade-off between spatial and temporal resolution. *Radiology* 2005;**236**:789–800.

21. El Khouli RH, Macura KJ, Jacobs MA, *et al.* Dynamic contrast-enhanced MRI of the breast: quantitative method for kinetic curve type assessment. *AJR Am J Roentgenol* 2009;**193**:W295–300.

22. Boetes C, Barentsz JO, Mus RD, *et al.* MR characterization of suspicious breast lesions with a gadolinium-enhanced TurboFLASH subtraction technique. *Radiology* 1994;**193**:777–81.

23. Mahfouz AE, Sherif H, Saad A, *et al.* Gadolinium-enhanced MR angiography of the breast: is breast cancer associated with ipsilateral higher vascularity? *Eur Radiol* 2001;**11**:965–9.

24. Sardanelli F, Iozzelli A, Fausto A, Carriero A, Kirchin MA. Gadobenate dimeglumine-enhanced MR imaging breast vascular maps: association between invasive cancer and ipsilateral increased vascularity. *Radiology* 2005;**235**:791–7.

25. D'Orsi CJ. Computer-aided detection: there is no free lunch. *Radiology* 2001;**221**:585–6.

26. Jackson A, O'Connor JP, Parker GJ, Jayson GC. Imaging tumor vascular heterogeneity and angiogenesis using dynamic contrast-enhanced magnetic resonance imaging. *Clin Cancer Res* 2007;**13**:3449–59.

27. O'Connor JP, Jackson A, Parker GJ, Jayson GC. DCE biomarkers in the clinical evaluation of antiangiogenic and vascular disrupting agents. *Br J Cancer* 2007;**96**:189–95.

28. Brix G, Semmler W, Port R, *et al.* Pharmacokinetic parameters in CNS Gd-DTPA enhanced MR imaging. *J Comput Assist Tomogr* 1991;**15**:621–8.

29. Taylor JS, Tofts PS, Port R, *et al.* MR imaging of tumor microcirculation: promise for the new millennium. *J Magn Reson Imaging* 1999;**10**:903–7.

30. Evelhoch JL. Key factors in the acquisition of contrast kinetic data for oncology. *J Magn Reson Imaging* 1999;**10**:254–9.

31. Tofts PS, Brix G, Buckley DL, *et al.* Estimating kinetic parameters from dynamic contrast-enhanced T(1)-weighted MRI of a diffusable tracer: standardized quantities and symbols. *J Magn Reson Imaging* 1999;**10**:223–32.

273

32. Wang HZ, Riederer SJ, Lee JN. Optimizing the precision in T1 relaxation estimation using limited flip angles. *Magn Reson Med* 1987;**5**:399–416.

33. Deoni SC, Rutt BK, Peters TM. Rapid combined T1 and T2 mapping using gradient recalled acquisition in the steady state. *Magn Reson Med* 2003;**49**:515–26.

34. Deoni SC, Peters TM, Rutt BK. High-resolution T1 and T2 mapping of the brain in a clinically acceptable time with DESPOT1 and DESPOT2. *Magn Reson Med* 2005;**53**:237–41.

35. Deoni SC, Peters TM, Rutt BK. Determination of optimal angles for variable nutation proton magnetic spin-lattice, T1, and spin-spin, T2, relaxation times measurement. *Magn Reson Med* 2004;**51**:194–9.

36. Parker GJ, Roberts C, Macdonald A, *et al.* Experimentally-derived functional form for a population-averaged high-temporal-resolution arterial input function for dynamic contrast-enhanced MRI. *Magn Reson Med* 2006;**56**:993–1000.

37. Buonaccorsi GA, Roberts C, Cheung S, *et al.* Comparison of the performance of tracer kinetic model-driven registration for dynamic contrast enhanced MRI using different models of contrast enhancement. *Acad Radiol* 2006;**13**:1112–23.

38. Roberts C, Issa B, Stone A, *et al.* Comparative study into the robustness of compartmental modeling and model-free analysis in DCE studies. *J Magn Reson Imaging* 2006;**23**:554–63.

39. Hauth EA, Jaeger H, Maderwald S, *et al.* Evaluation of quantitative parametric analysis for characterization of breast lesions in contrast-enhanced MR mammography. *Eur Radiol* 2006;**16**:2834–41.

40. Boxerman JL, Bandettini PA, Kwong KK, *et al.* The intravascular contribution to fMRI signal change: Monte Carlo modeling and diffusion-weighted studies *in vivo*. *Magn Reson Med* 1995;**34**:4–10.

41. Buckley DL, Drew PJ, Mussurakis S, Monson JR, Horsman A. Microvessel density of invasive breast cancer assessed by dynamic Gd-DTPA enhanced MRI. *J Magn Reson Imaging* 1997;**7**:461–4.

42. Bhujwalla ZM, Artemov D, Glockner J. Tumor angiogenesis, vascularization, and contrast-enhanced magnetic resonance imaging. *Top Magn Reson Imaging* 1999;**10**:92–103.

43. Jackson A, Jayson GC, Li KL, *et al.* Reproducibility of quantitative dynamic contrast-enhanced MRI in newly presenting glioma. *Br J Radiol* 2003;**76**:153–62.

44. Mussurakis S, Buckley DL, Horsman A. Dynamic MRI of invasive breast cancer: assessment of three region-of-interest analysis methods. *J Comput Assist Tomogr* 1997;**21**:431–8.

45. Yankeelov TE, Luci JJ, Lepage M, *et al.* Quantitative pharmacokinetic analysis of DCE data without an arterial input function: a reference region model. *Magn Reson Imaging* 2005;**23**:519–29.

46. Yankeelov TE, Rooney WD, Huang W, *et al.* Evidence for shutter-speed variation in CR bolus-tracking studies of human pathology. *NMR Biomed* 2005;**18**:173–85.

47. Radjenovic A, Dall BJ, Ridgway JP, Smith MA. Measurement of pharmacokinetic parameters in histologically graded invasive breast tumours using dynamic contrast-enhanced MRI. *Br J Radiol* 2008;**81**:120–8.

48. Tofts PS. Modeling tracer kinetics in dynamic Gd-DTPA MR imaging. *J Magn Reson Imaging* 1997;**7**:91–101.

49. Tofts PS, Berkowitz B, Schnall MD. Quantitative analysis of dynamic Gd-DTPA enhancement in breast tumors using a permeability model. *Magn Reson Med* 1995;**33**:564–8.

50. El Khouli RH, Jacobs MA, Bluemke DA. Magnetic resonance imaging of the breast. *Semin Roentgenol* 2008;**43**:265–81.

51. Huang W, Li X, Morris EA, *et al.* The magnetic resonance shutter speed discriminates vascular properties of malignant and benign breast tumors *in vivo*. *Proc Natl Acad Sci U S A* 2008;**105**:17943–8.

52. Haris M, Husain N, Singh A, *et al.* Dynamic contrast-enhanced (DCE) derived transfer coefficient (ktrans) is a surrogate marker of matrix metalloproteinase 9 (MMP-9) expression in brain tuberculomas. *J Magn Reson Imaging* 2008;**28**:588–97.

53. Pediconi F, Catalano C, Venditti F, *et al.* Color-coded automated signal intensity curves for detection and characterization of breast lesions: preliminary evaluation of a new software package for integrated magnetic resonance-based breast imaging. *Invest Radiol* 2005;**40**: 448–57.

54. Williams TC, DeMartini WB, Partridge SC, Peacock S, Lehman CD. Breast MR imaging: computer-aided evaluation program for discriminating benign from malignant lesions. *Radiology* 2007;**244**:94–103.

55. Hauth EA, Jaeger H, Maderwald S, *et al.* [Quantitative parametric analysis of contrast-enhanced lesions in dynamic MR mammography]. *Radiologe* 2008;**48**:593–600.

56. Hauth EA, Jaeger HJ, Maderwald S, *et al.* Quantitative 2- and 3-dimensional analysis of pharmacokinetic model-derived variables for breast lesions in dynamic, contrast-enhanced MR mammography. *Eur J Radiol* 2008;**66**:300–8.

57. Lehman CD, Peacock S, DeMartini WB, Chen X. A new automated software system to evaluate breast MR examinations: improved specificity without decreased sensitivity. *AJR Am J Roentgenol* 2006;**187**:51–6.

58. Veltman J, Stoutjesdijk M, Mann R, *et al.* Contrast-enhanced magnetic resonance imaging of the breast: the value of pharmacokinetic parameters derived from fast dynamic imaging during initial enhancement in classifying lesions. *Eur Radiol* 2008;**18**: 1123–33.

59. El Khouli RH, Macura KJ, Kamel IR, Jacobs MA, Bluemke DA. 3-T dynamic contrast enhanced magnetic resonance imaging of the breast: pharmacokinetic parameters versus conventional kinetic curve analysis, *AJR Am J Roentgenol* 2011;**197**:1498–505.

60. Huang W, Tudorica LA, Li X, *et al.* Discrimination of benign and malignant breast lesions by using shutter-speed dynamic contrast-enhanced MR imaging. *Radiology* 2011;**261**:394–403.

61. Sarrazin D, Le MG, Arriagada R, *et al.* Ten-year results of a randomized trial comparing a conservative treatment to mastectomy in early breast cancer. *Radiother Oncol* 1989;**14**:177–84.

62. Fisher B, Bauer M, Margolese R, *et al.* Five-year results of a randomized clinical trial comparing total mastectomy and segmental mastectomy with or without radiation in the treatment of breast cancer. *N Engl J Med* 1985;**312**:665–73.

63. Fisher B, Bryant J, Wolmark N, *et al.* Effect of preoperative chemotherapy on the outcome of women with operable breast cancer. *J Clin Oncol* 1998;**16**:2672–85.

64. Buchholz TA, Hill BS, Tucker SL, *et al.* Factors predictive of outcome in patients with breast cancer refractory to neoadjuvant chemotherapy. *Cancer J* 2001;**7**:413–20.

65. Rosen EL, Blackwell KL, Baker JA, *et al.* Accuracy of MRI in the detection of residual breast cancer after neoadjuvant chemotherapy. *AJR Am J Roentgenol* 2003;**181**:1275–82.

66. Cheung YC, Chen SC, Su MY, *et al.* Monitoring the size and response of locally advanced breast cancers to neoadjuvant chemotherapy (weekly paclitaxel and epirubicin) with serial enhanced MRI. *Breast Cancer Res Treat* 2003;**78**:51–8.

67. James K, Eisenhauer E, Christian M, *et al.* Measuring response in solid tumors: unidimensional versus bidimensional measurement. *J Natl Cancer Inst* 1999;**91**:523–8.

68. Therasse P. Measuring the clinical response. What does it mean? *Eur J Cancer* 2002;**38**:1817–23.

69. Park JO, Lee SI, Song SY, *et al.* Measuring response in solid tumors: comparison of RECIST and WHO response criteria. *Jpn J Clin Oncol* 2003;**33**:533–7.

70. Partridge SC, Gibbs JE, Lu Y, *et al.* MRI measurements of breast tumor volume predict response to neoadjuvant chemotherapy and recurrence-free survival. *AJR Am J Roentgenol* 2005;**184**:1774–81.

71. Padhani AR, Hayes C, Assersohn L, *et al.* Prediction of clinicopathologic response of breast cancer to primary chemotherapy at contrast-enhanced MR imaging: initial clinical results. *Radiology* 2006;**239**:361–74.

72. Wasser K, Klein SK, Fink C, *et al.* Evaluation of neoadjuvant chemotherapeutic response of breast cancer using dynamic MRI with high temporal resolution. *Eur Radiol* 2003;**13**:80–7.

73. Pickles MD, Lowry M, Manton DJ, Gibbs P, Turnbull LW. Role of dynamic contrast enhanced MRI in monitoring early response of locally advanced breast cancer to neoadjuvant chemotherapy. *Breast Cancer Res Treat* 2005;**91**:1–10.

74. Kuhl CK, Jost P, Morakkabati N, *et al.* Contrast-enhanced MR imaging of the breast at 3.0 and 1.5 T in the same patients: initial experience. *Radiology* 2006;**239**:666–76.

75. Rakow-Penner R, Daniel B, Yu H, Sawyer-Glover A, Glover GH. Relaxation times of breast tissue at 1.5T and 3T measured using IDEAL. *J Magn Reson Imaging* 2006;**23**:87–91.

76. Rausch DR, Hendrick RE. How to optimize clinical breast MR imaging practices and techniques on Your 1.5-T system. *Radiographics* 2006;**26**:1469–84.

77. Harvey JA, Hendrick RE, Coll JM, *et al.* Breast MR imaging artifacts: how to recognize and fix them. *Radiographics* 2007;**27** Suppl 1: S131–45.

78. Nunes LW, Schnall MD, Orel SG. Update of breast MR imaging architectural interpretation model. *Radiology* 2001;**219**: 484–94.

79. Nunes LW, Schnall MD, Orel SG, *et al.* Breast MR imaging: interpretation model. *Radiology* 1997;**202**:833–41.

80. Nunes LW, Schnall MD, Siegelman ES, *et al.* Diagnostic performance characteristics of architectural features revealed by high spatial-resolution MR imaging of the breast. *AJR Am J Roentgenol* 1997;**169**:409–15.

81. Collins DJ, Padhani AR. Dynamic magnetic resonance imaging of tumor perfusion. Approaches and biomedical challenges. *IEEE Eng Med Biol Mag* 2004;**23**:65–83.

82. Dale BM, Jesberger JA, Lewin JS, Hillenbrand CM, Duerk JL. Determining and optimizing the precision of quantitative

measurements of perfusion from dynamic contrast enhanced MRI. *J Magn Reson Imaging* 2003;**18**:575–84.

83. Kurihara Y, Yakushiji YK, Tani I, Nakajima Y, Van Cauteren M. Coil sensitivity encoding in MR imaging: advantages and disadvantages in clinical practice. *AJR Am J Roentgenol* 2002;**178**:1087–91.

84. Glockner JF, Hu HH, Stanley DW, Angelos L, King K. Parallel MR imaging: a user's guide. *Radiographics* 2005;**25**: 1279–97.

85. Sardanelli F, Fausto A, Esseridou A, Di Leo G, Kirchin MA. Gadobenate dimeglumine as a contrast agent for dynamic breast magnetic resonance imaging: effect of higher initial enhancement thresholds on diagnostic performance. *Invest Radiol* 2008;**43**:236–42.

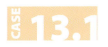

CASE 13.1 DCE-MRI in infiltrating ductal carcinoma

History

A 54-year-old woman presenting with a palpable mass in the right breast. The mass was not detected with mammography or ultrasound. MR imaging, including perfusion DCE imaging, was performed.

Technique

Two series of T_1-weighted images were acquired pre- and post-administration of 0.1 mmol/kg gadolinium contrast; one series was performed with high spatial resolution, and the other with high temporal resolution. Subtraction images were calculated, and the dynamic series were analyzed with iCAD software, using a four-compartmental pharmacokinetic model.

Imaging findings

See Figure 13.15.

Discussion

The patient underwent surgical biopsy that revealed an infiltrating ductal carcinoma of type luminal A (low grade, estrogen receptor positive).

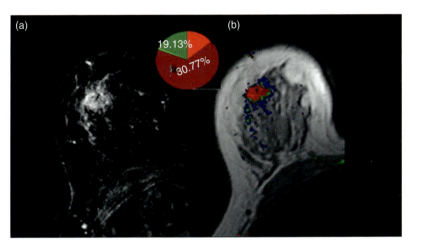

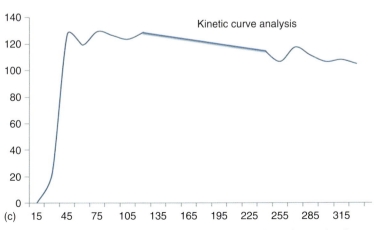

Figure 13.15 The high spatial resolution subtraction image (a) showed a spiculated mass measuring 2.2 × 2.2 × 1.9 cm in the upper outer quadrant of the right breast. CAD color map (b) and joint histogram (d) demonstrated that 80.77% of the lesion exhibits perfusion suspicious for malignancy (red). The kinetic curve (c) demonstrated a type III (washout) pattern characteristic of malignancy. Individual lesion histograms for permeability (e), extracellular volume fraction (EVF) (f), and k_{ep} (g) show that the majority of voxels in the mass lie in the high permeability, low EVF, and high k_{ep} regions. This pattern of perfusion is consistent with malignancy.

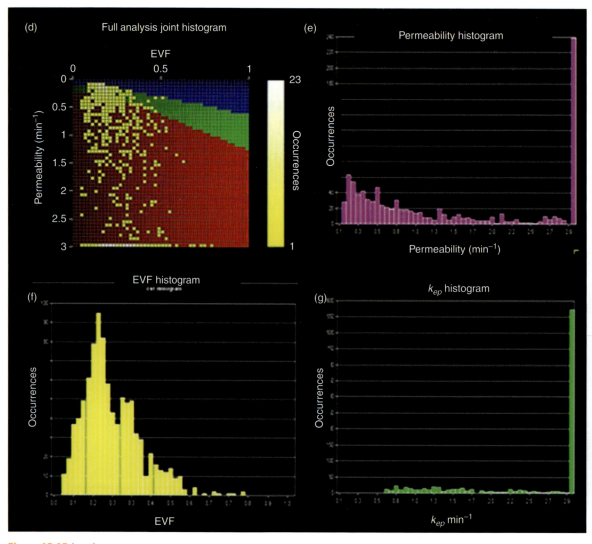

Figure 13.15 (cont.)

Contrast-enhanced MRI of the breast has a very high sensitivity for detecting breast cancer. Adding DCE perfusion imaging to the conventional breast MR exam helps improve specificity. Spiculated margins along with washout kinetic curve are strong predictors of breast cancer. Breast cancers demonstrate distorted tumoral vascularity along with increased cellularity, leading to increased permeability along with decreased extracellular space volume. Pharmacokinetic modeling offers additional insight into these two physiological parameters.

Key points

- Contrast-enhanced MRI can detect malignant lesions that may not be detected with mammography or ultrasound.
- Spiculated tumor margins and washout kinetic curve pattern are strong predictors of malignancy.
- Pharmacokinetic modeling offers quantitative assessment of perfusion in breast lesions. Breast cancer demonstrates high permeability and low EES values.

DCE-MRI in fibroadenoma

History

A 42-year-old woman presenting for a workup of micro-calcifications that revealed ductal carcinoma *in situ* (DCIS), a pre-malignant lesion. She was subsequently referred to MRI for the evaluation of extent of disease. MR imaging showed a well-circumscribed lobulated mass in the upper inner quadrant of the right breast.

Technique

Two series of T_1-weighted images were acquired pre- and post-administration of 0.1 mmol/kg gadolinium contrast; one series was performed with high spatial resolution, and the other with high temporal resolution. Subtraction images were calculated, and the dynamic series were analyzed with iCAD software, using a four-compartmental pharmacokinetic model.

Imaging findings

See Figure 13.16.

Discussion

This lesion was proven to be a fibroadenoma on biopsy. Fibroadenoma is the most common benign tumor of the breast and the most common breast tumor in

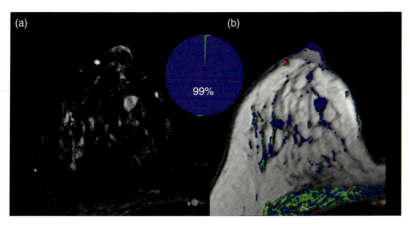

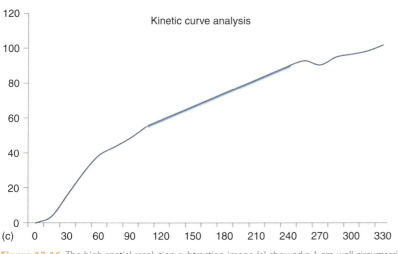

Figure 13.16 The high spatial resolution subtraction image (a) showed a 1-cm well-circumscribed, lobulated enhancing mass in the upper inner quadrant of the right breast. CAD color map (b) and joint histogram (d) demonstrated that 99% of the lesion exhibits a benign perfusion pattern (blue color). The kinetic curve (c) also demonstrated a type I (persistently enhancing) pattern suggestive of benign nature. Individual histograms for permeability (e), extracellular volume fraction (EVF) (f), and k_{ep} (g) show that most voxels in the mass are located in the low permeability, intermediate EVF, and low k_{ep} regions. This pattern of perfusion is consistent with a benign lesion.

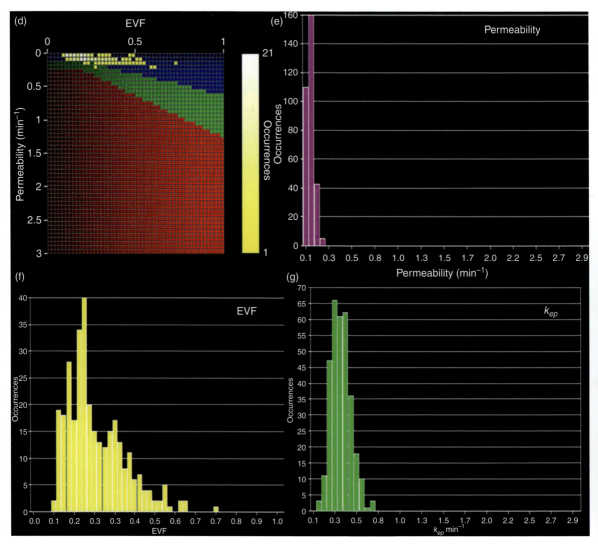

Figure 13.16 (cont.)

women under age 30. Differentiating fibroadenoma from breast cancer is sometimes challenging. Perfusion studies when added to morphological assessment demonstrated significant improvement in specificity. Lobulated margin along with a persistently enhancing (type I) kinetic curve suggest benign process.

Key points

- DCE perfusion studies improve the specificity of contrast-enhanced MRI of the breast.

- Lobulated tumor margins along with a persistently enhancing kinetic curve pattern suggest a benign diagnosis.
- Pharmacokinetic modeling offers quantitative assessment of perfusion in breast lesions. Normal glandular tissue and typically presenting benign breast lesions demonstrate low permeability and intermediate to high EES values.

MR perfusion imaging in the body: kidney, liver, and lung

Pottumarthi V. Prasad and Robert R. Edelman

Key points

- Perfusion methods that have been initially demonstrated in neuroimaging are now becoming more commonly used for body imaging applications, but must be adapted to account for the increased motion and unique physiology of these organ systems.
- These methods enable functional and physiological organ assessment, and are not reserved to oncological applications.
- ASL and blood oxygenation level-dependent (BOLD) imaging methods may be uniquely suited for renal and liver applications, since they do not require the use of exogenous agents, which are frequently contraindicated in patients with renal or liver dysfunction.
- Body perfusion techniques are most advanced in the kidneys, due to the great clinical need for physiological imaging and their inherently high blood flow.
- While compelling preliminary studies have been performed in the liver and lung, these applications are currently less frequently applied in clinical studies.
- Consensus on protocols and post-processing methodology is an essential next step, which will enable more widespread clinical use of these techniques.

Introduction

This chapter will discuss body perfusion MRI applications, specifically related to three organs: kidneys, liver, and lungs. Each section begins with a short description of the scientific and/or clinical rationale for perfusion imaging and then describes what is known to date regarding the feasibility and/or status of performing these measurements, along with their potential significance. Unlike neurological and oncological applications described in Chapters 8–13, perfusion MRI in the body is still evolving, and so no specific, standardized methods of data acquisition and analysis have yet emerged. However, a brief description of all methods available to date and relevant references are provided. The perfusion MRI techniques discussed fall under two primary categories, either those based on exogenous contrast agent administration, or those based on endogenous contrast mechanisms.

Kidney

Scientific/clinical rationale

In 1938, Goldblatt [1, 2] demonstrated a relationship between hypertension and renal ischemia. He was able to consistently produce elevations in systolic blood pressure by producing renal ischemia with a constricting clamp in an animal model. Removal of the clamp restored blood pressure to the reference range. Based on this finding, Burkland et al. performed nephrectomy of a unilateral ischemic kidney as a cure for hypertension [3]. This remained the method of surgical treatment until 1960 when Lambeth et al. reported resolving hypertension by correction of renal artery stenosis (RAS) [4]. In the 1960s, the delineation of the renin–angiotensin system and its relation to hypertension [5] also had a large impact on the medical therapy and diagnostic studies used in renovascular hypertension.

Hypertension is a common occurrence with almost 65 million cases diagnosed in the USA, based on a report from the National Health and Nutrition

Clinical Perfusion MRI: Techniques and Applications, ed. Peter B. Barker, Xavier Golay, and Greg Zaharchuk. Published by Cambridge University Press. © Peter B. Barker, Xavier Golay, and Greg Zaharchuk 2013.

Examination Survey (NHANES) in 2005–2006 and coincident US population estimates. Of these, an estimated 1 to 5% have renovascular disease (RVD) as the underlying cause [6]. As one of the few potentially curable causes of hypertension, RVD remains an important yet challenging diagnosis. Not all patients with RAS have RVD; in fact, those with essential hypertension tend to develop accelerated atherosclerosis, which can lead to RAS. These diagnostic limitations have generated controversies surrounding treatment. Most anatomical tests, such as conventional angiography, MR angiography (MRA) and CT angiography (CTA), are limited in their ability to diagnose RVD because they rely on RAS as the sole criterion. Most of the randomized prospective trials have not shown benefit of revascularization over medical management [7]. It is suspected that this is related to the fact that large vessel occlusive disease leads to changes in microvascular environment in the kidney, which may remain unchanged upon revascularization of the large vessel. Therefore, it appears that there is a need to carefully identify those subjects who may benefit from revascularization.

Renal vascular imaging

Catheter angiography remains the gold standard for anatomical depiction of renal vasculature owing to its exquisite spatial and temporal resolution [8]. Additionally, it allows for a functional assessment of hemodynamic significance in terms of pressure drop across the stenosis [9, 10]. As an invasive test, however, catheter angiography has the highest associated risk, including those associated with conscious sedation, iodinated contrast, ionizing radiation, atheroembolic disease, bleeding, dissection, thrombosis, and arterial injury sometimes requiring surgical repair. Catheter angiography is also the most expensive, both in the financial cost and in the amount of time, effort, and inconvenience for the patient. Because RAS is responsible for only a small fraction of hypertension and renal failure cases, catheter angiography is not suitable as a screening technique [11]. Ultrasound would be an ideal modality to serve as a screening procedure based on widespread availability, low cost, ease of use, and lack of ionizing radiation [11]. However, the spatial resolution is limited to the main renal arteries, except in the case of transplants where the superficial nature of the location allows for higher frequency transducers to be used. In addition

to anatomy, ultrasound also allows for functional assessment in terms of Doppler flow within the vessels. Pitfalls of ultrasound include limited accuracy (only ∼60%), operator dependence, and susceptibility to technical issues in the presence of abdominal fat and gas. Also, ultrasound is not good for evaluating accessory renal arteries. In addition, Doppler techniques cannot evaluate the entire length of the artery. CTA provides exquisite vascular depiction without the risks involved with invasive catheter angiography. While CTA has sufficiently high sensitivity and specificity compared to catheter angiography [11], it still has risks associated with radiation and also nephrotoxicity of iodinated contrast agents.

It is now well appreciated that the presence of RAS is only part of the diagnosis of renovascular hypertension, because revascularization does not cure hypertension in the majority of cases [12]. Measuring perfusion and glomerular filtration rate (GFR) can be used to evaluate the functional significance of RAS. Today, these are measured using nuclear medicine approaches that do not provide evaluation of renal arteries. Since MRI and CT are primarily utilized for angiography and have the ability to provide additional functional information, they are ideal techniques to provide comprehensive studies. There is preliminary evidence that combined MR perfusion and angiography can improve sensitivity and specificity compared to MRA alone in differentiating renovascular from other renal parenchymal diseases [13].

Renal perfusion imaging

Given that the primary function of the kidneys is to remove waste products from the blood, they receive almost a fourth of the cardiac output. However, most of the blood flow is directed towards the renal cortex (400–500 ml/100 g/min) [14] and only a small fraction supplies the medulla. The medulla is subdivided in to the inner and outer medulla, each with differences in their level of perfusion. Most available data regarding renal perfusion have been obtained from rodent models with microprobes [15] or microspheres [16], which have limited spatial resolution. This makes the kidneys very interesting in terms of perfusion imaging techniques that can depict the spatial differences, especially in humans.

Most quantitative perfusion imaging has been performed using radionuclides, where the tissue concentration of a radioactive tracer is measured over time and, using suitable tracer kinetic models (e.g., see Chapter 1), several physiological parameters related to blood flow are estimated [17, 18]. However, these techniques suffer from modest spatial resolution and do not depict the heterogeneity in the distribution of blood flow within the kidneys. The tracer kinetic principles can be readily extended to other modalities, as long as the tracer concentration can be estimated. The availability of micro-bubbles that can be used as an ultrasound contrast agent has led to perfusion imaging based on contrast-enhanced ultrasound (CEUS) [12]. There are several advantages of this approach, including being inexpensive, portable, widely available; and enabling serial examinations at short time intervals without exposure to radiation or nuclear tracers. While relative regional blood flow estimates are feasible, absolute quantitation is still limited by issues of linearity in response, inadequate compensation for micro-bubble attenuation, and other factors. Overall, ultrasound techniques are limited by operator dependence and limited spatial resolution. Contrast-enhanced CT is another viable option [12]. With the availability of electron beam CT (EBCT) and multi-detector CT (MDCT), high spatial and temporal resolutions with large spatial coverage are possible. These techniques also afford a linear response with concentration of the contrast agent. While feasibility in humans has been shown [13], the technique is limited by radiation dose and by nephrotoxicity concerns, especially in subjects with compromised renal function [12]. MRI offers a variety of approaches to study perfusion based on both exogenous and endogenous contrast mechanisms.

Perfusion MRI

Techniques based on exogenous contrast administration

With the evolution of ultra-fast MRI techniques [19, 20], the possibility of monitoring exogenous tracer kinetics in vivo using MRI has become a reality, not only in the brain but in most organs in the body. Several gadolinium (Gd) chelates are approved for routine use as contrast agents in MRI and can serve as tracers for blood flow measurements (see Chapter 2 for more details). Since signal changes can be related to changes in local Gd concentration, tracer kinetic principles can be applied to relate the measured concentration–time curves to different physiological parameters. As described in detail in Chapter 1, from the measurements of the tissue and arterial

concentration curves ($c_{tissue}(t)$ and $c_{arterial}(t)$) the volume of distribution (V) of the agent can be calculated directly as:

$$V = \frac{\int_0^\infty c_{tissue}(t)\,dt}{\int_0^\infty c_{arterial}(t)\,dt} \qquad (14.1)$$

If the contrast material is restricted to the intravascular space (as is the case in the brain), the volume of distribution reflects the blood volume V_b within the tissue. The arterial concentration–time curve can be measured using additional simultaneously acquired images that include the feeding artery [21]. However, even in the absence of arterial sampling, relative blood volumes can be inferred, assuming all the voxels within the image are fed by a single arterial source. It has been shown that with intravascular agents accurate blood volume measurements can be obtained, but measurement of perfusion is more difficult [22]. The central volume principle, introduced by Stewart more than a century ago, relates the blood flow and blood volume to the mean transit time (MTT) [23]:

$$MTT = \frac{Regional\ blood\ volume\ (V)}{Regional\ blood\ flow\ (F)} \qquad (14.2)$$

MTT is usually estimated by calculating the first moment of the measured concentration–time curve as shown below:

$$\frac{V}{F} = \frac{\int_0^\infty t\,c_{out}(t)\,dt}{\int_0^\infty c_{out}(t)\,dt} \qquad (14.3)$$

where $c_{out}(t)$ is the concentration of the indicator measured at the outlet. This formulation, however, cannot be applied to imaging measurements because MR and other imaging measurements estimate the concentration within the tissue rather than at the outlet [24]. Flow measurements made using the above formulation may yield a semi-quantitative index that can be clinically useful [24]. Equation 14.3 also assumes that $c_{out}(t)$ is measured in response to an instantaneous bolus of the tracer (mathematically described as a delta function). Since this is not achievable in practice, it is necessary to obtain an independent measure of the arterial concentration–time curve, and deconvolve its distribution from the measured tissue concentration–time data.

While commonly used Gd chelates behave as intravascular tracers in the brain owing to the blood–brain barrier, in most other organs they behave as extracellular agents. However, with the recent introduction of ultrasmall superparamagnetic iron oxide (USPIO) particles as intravascular MR contrast agents, it is possible to perform first-pass contrast-enhanced perfusion measurements. Morell et al. [25] have recently shown the feasibility of obtaining quantitative cortical blood flow measurements in human kidneys. Their estimate of 339 ± 60 ml/100 g/min is in reasonable agreement with the literature values of 350 to 460 ml/100 g/min [14, 26, 27].

Alternately, first-pass data with Gd chelates can be used to obtain semi-quantitative (and model-free) estimates of renal blood flow. While lacking absolute quantitation, these methods could still provide a means to perform relative measurements. It was shown that this method can be used to document redistribution of flow in regions directly affected by extracorporeal shock wave lithotripsy compared to the contralateral kidney [28]. Clinical feasibility of using contrast-enhanced perfusion MRI has been demonstrated in the evaluation of RAS [29]. It was found that the MTT showed significant differences between severe RAS and the normal contralateral kidney. Reduced perfusion in regions supplied by stenotic segmental renal arteries was also observed (Figure 14.1).

DCE-MRI methods

Perfusion MRI techniques based on exogenous contrast agents typically acquire data during the first pass of the agent through the tissue. Since Gd chelates are excreted through the kidneys, extended acquisition allows for estimation of excretory function. There are a number of different approaches proposed for evaluating renal function, and it is beyond the scope of this chapter to provide detailed discussion. However, a recent report compared different analysis models using the same data set and found most of them provided good estimates of GFR [30]. While

some models only estimate GFR, there are others that also estimate renal plasma flow (RPF) [31].

Angiotensin-converting enzyme inhibitor (ACE-I) renal scintigraphy is thought to be a predictor of response to therapy because it is a functional test of renal ischemia [12]. It does not, however, supply anatomical information that is needed for therapeutic planning. Decreased renal perfusion pressure in patients with RAS activates the renin–angiotensin system and increases production of angiotensin II. Angiotensin II causes vasoconstriction of the efferent glomerular arteriole and restores renal perfusion pressure and glomerular filtration to normal or near-normal levels. This compensated RAS may not manifest any perfusion or filtration abnormalities on renal scintigraphy or MR renography.

Administering ACE-I lowers GFR in the setting of RVD because it blocks the production of angiotensin II, decreasing efferent glomerular arteriolar vasoconstriction and reducing perfusion pressure. Figure 14.2 shows an example of MR renography with administration of the ACE-I captopril in a swine model of induced unilateral RAS. While this example illustrates the efficacy of the method, for practical routine clinical use other factors need to be considered. Since the objective is to combine such functional information with anatomical depiction of the RAS, the protocol should also include MRA. Since contrast-enhanced MRA is now standard clinical practice for renal MRA, the total dose of contrast agent administered is a key issue. One approach [32] is to implement a protocol which utilizes a small dose of contrast for MR renography (2 ml or 0.013 mmol/kg of Gd-DTPA) in combination with a larger dose for MRA. The higher spatial resolution available with MRI (compared to scintigraphy) allows the differentiation of the signal intensity versus time curves independently for the cortex and medulla. Among patients with normal serum creatinine levels, administration of ACE-I unmasked decreased GFR by depressing medullary enhancement in patients with RAS.

Overall, several papers support the feasibility of MR-based GFR measurements [30, 31, 33–39]. Unfortunately, however, there is no consensus yet for these to be translated to the clinic. A significant concern is the risk of developing nephrogenic systemic fibrosis (NSF) [40] in subjects with compromised renal function when using Gd-based contrast agents. Clearly, patients with potentially

(a)

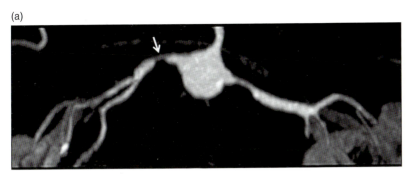

(b)

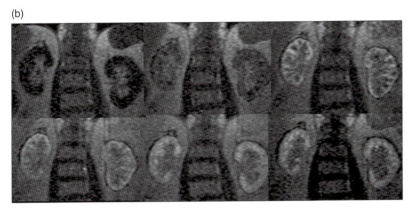

(c)

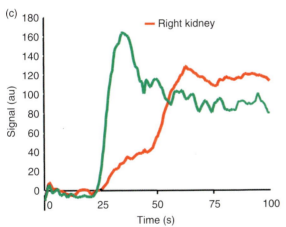

Time (s)

Figure 14.1 (a) Maximum intensity projection of renal arteries obtained from contrast-enhanced 3D MRA in a 60-year-old male with hypertension. Note the stenosis on the right renal artery (arrow). (b) Images taken at representative time points from the contrast-enhanced first-pass perfusion series. Note the qualitative difference in the uptake kinetics between the two kidneys. The right kidney has patchy and delayed enhancement compared to the contralateral kidney. (c) Signal intensity vs. time curves for each kidney (green – left and red – right). Note the clearly delayed uptake in the kidney supplied by the stenosed renal artery. Data provided by Dr. Henrik Michaely, University Medical Centre Mannheim, Mannheim, Germany.

compromised renal function would be a target population for the use of MRI-based GFR measurements. There is evidence that the use of macrocyclic agents (such as ProHance, Gadovist, and Dotarem) minimizes the risk of NSF in this population [41, 42]. However, with incomplete understanding of the pathophysiology of NSF, regulatory authorities continue to have concern about the entire class of Gd-based agents in patients with poor renal function [42].

Endogenous contrast mechanisms for perfusion MRI
Arterial spin labeling (ASL)
ASL uses magnetically labeled water as a tracer [43]. A number of approaches based on this idea have been proposed, and are described in detail in Chapter 3. All are based on manipulating the magnetization of inflowing arterial blood and involve acquiring a *flow-insensitive* image and a *flow-sensitive* image, and subtracting the former from the latter to remove the

285

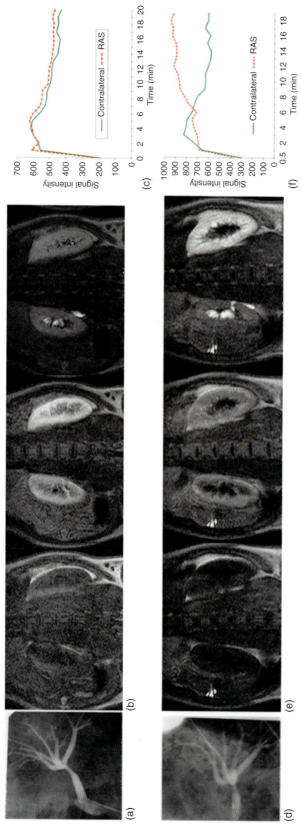

Figure 14.2 (a) Antero-posterior angiogram obtained 3 weeks after surgical placement of a constrictor in a swine shows a moderately stenotic vessel. (b) Coronal T$_1$-weighted images obtained using 3D fast imaging with steady-state precession (FISP) (TR/TE, 3.5/1.4 ms; flip angle, 20°) to acquire 10 partitions within a single breath-hold of about 5 s. Images of a single, representative slice at three representative time points after captopril administration are shown. Prior to administration of gadopentetate dimeglumine (Gd-DTPA) (left), the kidneys have little signal intensity. The middle image obtained 30 s after Gd-DTPA administration shows perfusion or an uptake phase. At 16 min after Gd-DTPA administration (right), both kidneys show a decrease in signal intensity, which signifies symmetric washout or excretion. (c) Signal intensity vs. time curves illustrate symmetric uptake and washout phases in both kidneys, indicating that even when captopril is administered, no substantial left-to-right differences are apparent and that the level of stenosis was not hemodynamically significant. (d, e, f) Similar images obtained in the same animal 3 weeks later when the stenosis has progressed to be significant (d). (e) Coronal MR renograms show again symmetric perfusion on the uptake phase (middle); however, at 16 min after Gd-DTPA administration (right) there is substantial accumulation of contrast material in the kidney supplied by the stenosed vessel. (f) Signal intensity vs. time curves illustrate the asymmetry in the washout phase, demonstrating the presence of hemodynamically significant stenosis. Adapted from Prasad *et al.* [108].

TI = 600 ms   TI = 700 ms   TI = 800 ms   TI = 900 ms

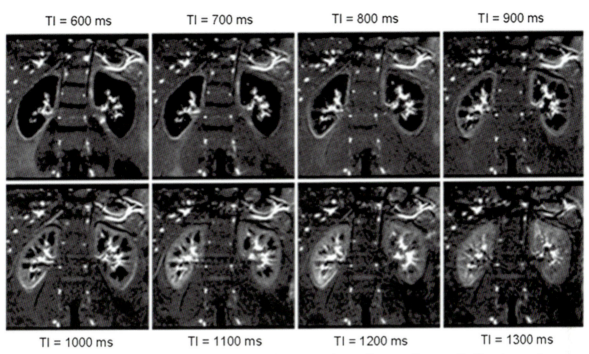

TI = 1000 ms   TI = 1100 ms   TI = 1200 ms   TI = 1300 ms

Figure 14.3 ASL data acquired using true-FISP readout in a healthy young volunteer. Two sets of images with different preparation pulses, one with a non-selective inversion pulse (flow-insensitive) and the other with a selective pulse (flow-sensitive) were acquired. Acquisition parameters included TR/TE/TI/BW/slice thickness/acquisition matrix = 10 s/2.8 ms/600–1300 ms/965 Hz/pixel/5 mm/192 × 72 and 36 cm field of view, resulting in a pixel size of 1.9 × 5 mm^2. The longer TI delay allows for more of the labeled spins to reach the renal parenchyma.

background tissue signals. For each image there is a delay period (inversion time [TI] for pulsed ASL and post-label delay [PLD] for continuous or pseudo-continuous ASL) during which the arterial blood enters the voxel in proportion to the perfusion rate f. There are various implementations of this method in practice, but all of them can be analyzed in similar ways [44]. The technique is limited by the blood T_1 relaxation time, and the magnitude of the signal change between the labeled and unlabeled images is small. Nevertheless, sufficiently high signal-to-noise ratio (SNR) can be achieved with appropriate experimental design, so that these small changes can be reliably measured. In addition, the observed signal changes can be modeled directly in terms of f, thus providing the potential for obtaining quantitative measurement of perfusion.

Recent progress in acquisition techniques, and the introduction of higher field scanners, have given rise to an implementation that shows promise for routine clinical application in the kidneys. Figure 14.3 shows images acquired in a healthy subject that illustrate the sensitivity of the measurement to changes in blood flow. Images were obtained with different delay (i.e., inflow) times following the application of the labeling pulse. At short

delays the blood flow does not reach the renal parenchyma. At TI = 900 ms, enhancement begins to be visible in the outer cortex of the parenchyma. This is consistent with the known vascular architecture within the kidney. At longer delay times the enhancement extends into the medulla. The flow-related signal change is also influenced by the T_1 of tissue and blood, since the delay times are comparable to the T_1 values.

The images in Figure 14.3 are ΔM maps, i.e., differences in signal intensity between the flow-sensitive and flow-insensitive images at different delay times. With additional information about M_0 and T_1, it is possible to estimate blood flow in quantitative units. Perfusion rates in healthy renal cortex and medulla have been estimated to be 220–280 ml/ 100 g/min and 50–120 ml/100 g/min, respectively [45]. This compares well with clearance techniques or positron emission tomography (PET) measurements considered as gold standard for correct physiological values (300–550 ml/100 g/min) for the renal cortex [14, 46]. More recently, using the same approach as in [45], ASL measurements were directly compared to renal plasma flow as estimated by para-aminohippurate (PAH) plasma clearance method in hypertensive subjects before and after treatment with an ACE-I [47]. A fairly good correlation between the MRI-derived measures and those estimated by PAH clearance technique was observed, as shown Figure 14.4. However, the MRI measurements in this study were from a single slice, and therefore not necessarily reflective of kidney perfusion as a whole. This may in part explain the relatively moderate level of correlation observed between the two measurements. However, compared to the logistical complexity of the PAH measurements, ASL estimates are relatively straightforward to perform. Figure 14.5 shows an example of a patient with a stenosis of the renal artery, in which ASL is used to demonstrate improved kidney blood flow after correction of the vascular lesion with a stent.

Blood oxygenation level-dependent (BOLD) MRI

Although perfusion MR measures the amount of blood per unit volume of tissue, ultimately the physiologically most significant parameter is how much nutrient, especially oxygen, is received. In most organs, tissue oxygenation often parallels blood flow status. However, strictly speaking, tissue oxygenation is a reflection of the net effect of oxygen supply *via* blood flow and regional oxygen consumption. Since oxygen consumption at rest in most tissue remains constant (i.e., independent of oxygen supply), tissue oxygenation tracks with the regional blood flow. However, this is not true in certain regions of the kidney. This makes oxygenation measurements especially relevant in renal physiology and pathophysiology, where active tubular reabsorption demands more oxygen consumption, resulting in filtration and blood flow rising together [48]. Over a wide range of normal blood flows, the renal arteriovenous oxygen difference is remarkably constant. For the purposes of function and oxygen supply, the mammalian kidney can be considered to be made of two separate systems, the cortex and medulla [48]. The flow of blood to the renal cortex normally supplies oxygen far in excess of its metabolic needs. By contrast, blood flow to the renal medulla is parsimonious. In addition, oxygen diffuses from the arterial to venous *vasa recta*,

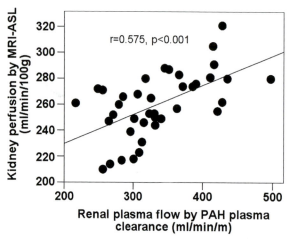

Figure 14.4 Correlation between kidney perfusion assessed by MRI–ASL (ml/min/100 g) and renal plasma flow assessed by PAH plasma clearance (ml/min/m) [47]. Reproduced with kind permission from Oxford University Press.

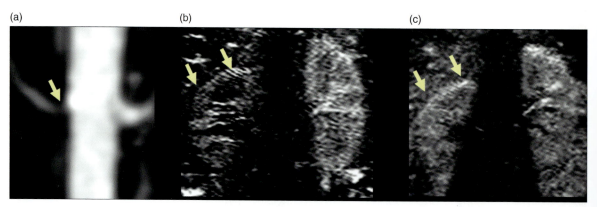

Figure 14.5 Example of the combined morphological and functional MR kidney examination. (a) MRA of a 52-year-old female patient with right renal artery stenosis of 60%. (b) ASL perfusion-weighted image shows reduced signal intensity of the right kidney. The SNR of the affected kidney is 4.8 vs. 8.6 in the healthy left kidney. (c) The same kidney after stenting of the affected artery. Both kidneys now appear equally intense with a SNR of 7.0 (formerly affected kidney) vs. 7.5 (healthy kidney). Figure provided by Dr. Henrik Michaely, University Medical Centre Mannheim, Mannheim, Germany, adapted from Michaely *et al.* [109].

and the process of generating an osmotic difference by active reabsorption of sodium requires a large amount of oxygen. All of these combined results in a poorly oxygenated medulla. This medullary hypoxia has consequences to renal physiology and pathophysiology [49] and hence evaluation of in vivo renal oxygenation is important.

Most widely applied methods to study renal medullary hypoxia in animal models use invasive microelectrodes [50–52]. Recently a novel laser-based probe for oxygen tension (pO2) has become available [53]. With the probe size in the order of a couple of hundred microns, as opposed to tens of microns with conventional microelectrodes, there are some fundamental differences in the data obtained. However, considering the extremely fragile microelectrodes, the laser probes may have practical advantages. There are histological methods, e.g., pimonidazole, that have been used to map hypoxic regions [54]. Pimonidazole mapping is not a quantitative technique and is typically sensitive only at pO2 levels of less than 10 mmHg. Recently, use of an endogenous hypoxia marker such as upregulation of hypoxia inducible factor-α (HIF-α) has been demonstrated [55–58]. Electron paramagnetic resonance (EPR) has been shown to be useful in measuring changes related to tissue oxygenation [57, 58]. It necessitates introducing lithium phthalocyanine (LiPc) crystals whose EPR signals can then be monitored. The line width of the LiPc signals is then directly related to surrounding tissue pO2. More recently, EPR imaging has also been shown possible in concert with suitable spin probes [59]. However, because of their invasive nature, none of these methods is currently applicable to studies in humans.

BOLD MRI has been used extensively in organs such as the brain [60–62]. The BOLD technique exploits the variation of the magnetic properties of hemoglobin, depending on whether it is in the oxygenated or deoxygenated form. This affects the T_2^* relaxation time of the neighboring water molecules, and in turn influences the MRI signal on T_2^*-weighted images. The rate of spin dephasing R_2^* ($= 1/T_2^*$) is closely related to the tissue microvasculature content of deoxyhemoglobin. Since the pO2 of venous blood is thought to be in equilibrium with the surrounding tissue, changes estimated by BOLD MRI can be interpreted as changes in tissue pO2 [63–65]. Good agreement has been demonstrated between renal BOLD measurements in humans [64, 65] and rodents [66] with earlier animal data obtained using invasive microelectrodes [52]. This was done by demonstrating changes in R_2^* images following administration of furosemide, and comparing them with those following acetazolamide. Furosemide, a loop diuretic, reduces the reabsorptive work in the thick ascending limbs situated in the medulla, and hence improves medullary oxygenation (Figure 14.6). Conversely, while

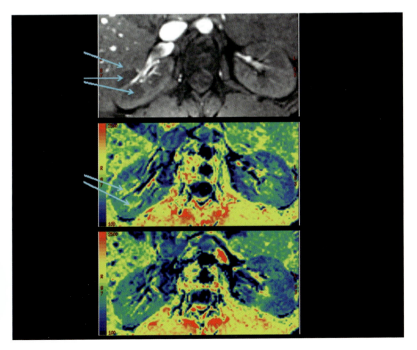

Figure 14.6 (Top) Anatomic MRI of the kidneys; (middle) R_2^* map at baseline; (bottom) R_2^* map after administration of furosemide (20 mg IV). R_2^* maps are shown in pseudo-color along with a color bar showing the range of R_2^* values (2–50 s^{-1}). Higher R_2^* values imply lower tissue oxygenation (i.e., more deoxyhemoglobin), due to higher levels of hypoxia and/or lower blood flow [65]. Note that the medulla turns bluer in the post-furosemide R_2^* map, implying an improved oxygenation level approaching that of the cortex.

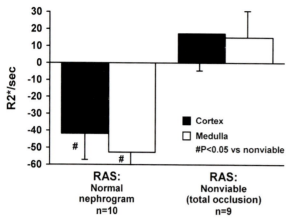

Figure 14.7 Changes in BOLD MR measurements (ΔR_2^* (s^{-1})) before and after furosemide infusion in patients undergoing evaluation for RAS. Kidneys were classified as either "normal" or "non-viable" (with total occlusion) based on conventional renography. Non-functioning kidneys demonstrated no R_2^* response after intravenous furosemide, whereas normal kidneys had consistent reduction in R_2^* after furosemide, particularly in medullary regions [67]. Reproduced with the kind permission from American Society of Nephrology.

acetazolamide results in a similar diuretic effect, it acts on the cortical portion of the nephron, and therefore shows minimal change in the medullary oxygenation.

One study [67] has reported on R_2^* measurements in human subjects with RAS. In normal-sized kidneys downstream of high-grade renal arterial stenoses, R_2^* was elevated at baseline (suggesting enhanced hypoxia) and fell after administration of furosemide (Figure 14.6). This was true even when the GFR was significantly reduced. These results are supported by previous reports of preserved cortical tissue volume in post-stenotic kidneys, despite reduced function as measured by isotope renography [68]. These in turn may suggest that GFR might be recoverable for such cases and that non-filtering kidney tissue represents a form of "hibernation" in the kidney with the potential for restoring kidney function after restoring blood flow [68]. On the other hand, atrophic kidneys beyond totally occluded renal arteries demonstrated low levels of R_2^* (improved oxygenation) that did not change after furosemide [67] (Figure 14.7). This suggests non-functioning kidney with limited or no oxygen consumption.

There are a few examples of applications of perfusion MRI to kidneys in clinical settings. These include evaluation of renal transplants where diagnosis of acute rejection versus acute tubular necrosis (ATN)

is important, which currently requires a biopsy to be performed. BOLD has been shown to facilitate distinction of acute rejection versus ATN by three different groups [69–71]. ASL has also been shown to be useful in evaluating anti-angiogenic therapy in renal cell carcinoma [72, 73].

Liver

Scientific/clinical rationale

Liver, unlike any other organ, has a dual blood supply with the majority (75%) from the portal venous circulation and 25% from the hepatic artery [74]. This distribution is known to change in disease conditions such as cirrhosis [75, 76]. There are multiple other situations where perfusion changes in the liver could be anticipated, including portal vein obstruction, hepatic neoplasms, hepatic trauma, hereditary hemorrhagic telangiectasia (HHT), hepatic vein obstruction, steal phenomenon by hypervascular tumors, inflammatory changes, aberrant blood supply, hepatic parenchymal compression, and others. The dual supply requires a modified dual-input single/multi-compartment model to describe the concentration–time relationship.

Cirrhosis is a consequence of chronic liver disease characterized by replacement of liver tissue by fibrosis, scar tissue, and regenerative nodules resulting in a loss of liver function. It is caused most commonly by alcoholism, hepatitis B and C, and fatty liver disease, and includes some unknown causes. Early imaging studies using radioisotopes showed differences in contribution from the hepatic artery and portal vein [77]. With the availability of MDCT, contrast-enhanced dynamic CT has been used to perform liver perfusion imaging. Using such dynamic information with sufficient temporal resolution, arterial and venous contributions can be separated [78]. These methods also demonstrated changes in hepatic artery versus portal venous contributions in cirrhosis [79].

Currently, the use of MRI for liver perfusion imaging is rather limited. One study [80] applied a 2D single-slice technique to acquire dynamic image acquisition with 2 s temporal resolution in a swine model of portal venous occlusion. More recently a similar acquisition with three slices acquired every 5.5 s was applied to evaluate liver transplants [81]. Another study [82] used a 3D dynamic acquisition with about 4 s temporal resolution to evaluate

(a)

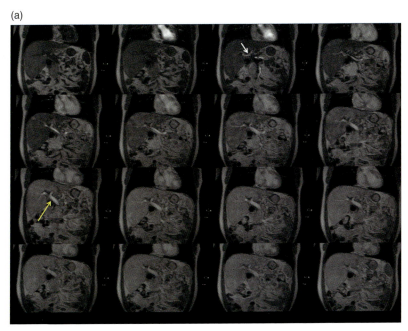

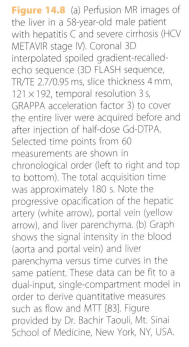

Figure 14.8 (a) Perfusion MR images of the liver in a 58-year-old male patient with hepatitis C and severe cirrhosis (HCV METAVIR stage IV). Coronal 3D interpolated spoiled gradient-recalled-echo sequence (3D FLASH sequence, TR/TE 2.7/0.95 ms, slice thickness 4 mm, 121 × 192, temporal resolution 3 s, GRAPPA acceleration factor 3) to cover the entire liver were acquired before and after injection of half-dose Gd-DTPA. Selected time points from 60 measurements are shown in chronological order (left to right and top to bottom). The total acquisition time was approximately 180 s. Note the progressive opacification of the hepatic artery (white arrow), portal vein (yellow arrow), and liver parenchyma. (b) Graph shows the signal intensity in the blood (aorta and portal vein) and liver parenchyma versus time curves in the same patient. These data can be fit to a dual-input, single-compartment model in order to derive quantitative measures such as flow and MTT [83]. Figure provided by Dr. Bachir Taouli, Mt. Sinai School of Medicine, New York, NY, USA.

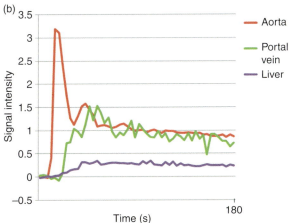

lesion-specific permeability, while another applied a similar 3D dynamic MRI data acquisition to study perfusion using a dual-input single-compartment model [83]. Figure 14.8 shows an example of data obtained using this technique. In a small group of patients with established cirrhosis, three model-derived parameters (arterial flow, MTT and Gd-distribution volume) were able to predict advanced fibrosis with high sensitivity (84.6%) and specificity (100%) [84]. A more recent study addressed the significance of accurate timing of the arterial phase for liver perfusion imaging [85]. A bolus tracking approach commonly used for contrast-enhanced

MRA (CE-MRA) showed significant benefit over fixed time acquisitions in terms of optimal timing for capturing perfusion images during the arterial phase.

The application of MRI perfusion to the liver is still evolving, and a recent review article summarizes the current status and future directions [86]. Currently, there is more experience with CT perfusion imaging, and there are several issues still in need of consensus. In terms of analysis of MR perfusion data, both single- and multiple-compartment models with dual inputs have been proposed, as well as model-free methods [87]. The latter ones have the advantage of relative simplicity, and hence more widespread availability. Since patients with advanced, chronic liver disease usually also have compromised renal function, the risk of NSF is also relevant to this population, which limits the use of Gd-based contrast agents as discussed above. Thus, there is increased interest in the non-contrast agent-based approaches for MR measurements of liver perfusion. Currently, there are no reports of ASL applied to liver; however, BOLD methods have been applied, usually in concert with a physiological or pharmacological challenge, to monitor oxygenation changes [88–90].

Lungs

Scientific/clinical rationale

Since the lungs receive the entire cardiac output, there is not much of a need for perfusion measurements in healthy lungs. However, the ability to image blood flow has advanced the understanding of lung physiology significantly. Again, early imaging studies of perfusion were performed using nuclear medicine methods [91]. MRI perfusion and ventilation imaging have provided great avenues for studying lung physiology [92].

Pulmonary embolism (PE) is the third most common cardiovascular disease, after myocardial infarction and stroke, and results in thousands of deaths each year [93]. Early and accurate diagnosis is highly desirable because PE is not suspected in 70% of those who die of the disease. Approximately 65% of the subjects die within 1 hr of presentation of PE and above 90% die within 2.5 hrs [94]. Pulmonary angiography is the reference standard for the diagnosis and exclusion of PE. However, with the current availability of techniques with much less risk, it is no longer the first line of testing for PE. Ventilation perfusion (V/Q) scans (usually performed with a gamma camera, using inhaled and intravenous injection of radioactive technetium compounds, respectively) have high positive and negative predictive values, and are associated with minimal risks and radiation burden [95]. The major limitation of this method is the lack of direct visualization of the clot. Also, if the clot is not fully occlusive, the mismatch of V/Q may not be observed. CT pulmonary angiography has gained acceptance to diagnose or exclude PE [81, 96]. However, pulmonary CTA is associated with significant

radiation dosage, and may be contraindicated in pregnancy and in those with compromised renal function. Therefore, there is a need for alternate technology, and MRI offers potential in this regard.

CE-MRA and perfusion MRI

Interest in pulmonary MRA has been around for over two decades. Owing to the enormous tissue–air interface in the lungs, MRI of the lungs remained inaccessible until the early 1990s. However, with the availability of very short echo times in gradient echo sequences, pulmonary angiography was shown to be feasible as early as 1992 [97]. However, the acquisition time was in the order of 10 min, making it non-viable for routine clinical use. With the introduction of CE-MRA, shorter acquisition times are possible, making the technique a viable option for the diagnosis of PE [98]. The recently published report [99] based on PIOPED III (Prospective Investigation of Pulmonary Embolism Diagnosis III) concluded that when technically adequate data were available, the sensitivity and specificity of MR arteriography for detection of PE were 78% and 99% respectively. When combined with MR venography (MRV), the sensitivity improved to 92%; however 52% of the subjects had technically inadequate studies. Contrast-enhanced first-pass perfusion MRI has also been shown to be feasible [100], in a study which detected PE in an embolic swine model based on absence of enhancement in the region distal to the occluded vessel (Figure 14.9) [101]. However, there have been few subsequent studies after these initial reports. It is conceivable that a combination of MR perfusion with MRA may have a better diagnostic efficacy than either alone, and that MR perfusion imaging may not be as prone to technical failures as MRV, although this remains to be determined.

With the extremely high blood volume in the lungs, ASL is extremely efficacious for lung perfusion imaging [102–104] (Figure 14.10) and has been shown to detect PE [105]. Without the need for exogenous contrast administration, the acquisition can be repeated, for instance in the case of technical failures or other issues. However, again, there have been few studies evaluating this technique in the clinic. This is probably related to the fact that these measurements should be performed in conjunction with MRA to localize the clot, and until viable non-contrast MRA methods that are effective are available for routine clinical use, ASL perfusion may play very

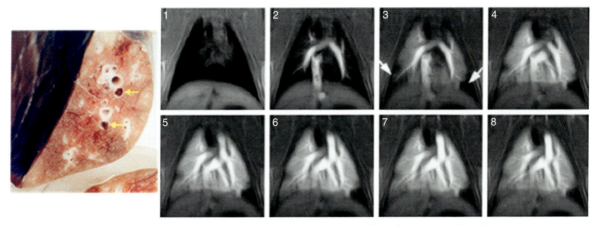

Figure 14.9 Contrast-enhanced time-resolved MR perfusion images from a pig model of pulmonary embolism. Multiple perfusion defects (arrows) are observed corresponding to regions distal to the emboli (verified at necropsy, yellow arrows). Adapted from Chen *et al.* [101].

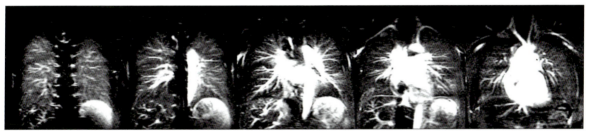

Figure 14.10 ASL-FAIR (flow-sensitive alternating inversion recovery) images of the lungs obtained in a healthy human subject. Note the pulmonary vessels appear bright, many of which are seen to bifurcate to successively smaller vessels. A diffuse blush throughout the lungs is seen from flow within the microvasculature. Later images show the label transit into the systemic arterial circulation.

little role in the evaluation of PE. Note that ASL cannot be performed after contrast administration, since blood T_1 becomes very short. There are other conditions where perfusion MRI may be useful, such as early detection of changes associated with cystic fibrosis [106], pulmonary hypertension [107], and other conditions. Also, the study of the physiology of both healthy and diseased lungs is still an active area of research amongst pulmonologists, and arguably MRI may be best suited for those applications, particularly with the development of hyperpolarized gases for imaging of lung ventilation.

Conclusions

Since the applications to kidney, liver, and lungs are still evolving, it is premature to discuss or recommend specific protocols and analysis techniques for clinical use at the current time. In terms of analysis methods, when considering conventional Gd chelates as MRI

contrast agents for perfusion imaging, either single- or multiple-compartment models can be used, based on the level of sophistication desired. While the multiple-compartment models are potentially more accurate, they are not always easy to prove in practice, because not all the fit parameters can be compared with a physical measurement. For most routine clinical applications, it could be argued that precision is more important than accuracy, because the clinical interest is mostly to differentiate disease from healthy conditions. Further, the simpler the technique, the more likely it will be adopted for widespread use, so semi-quantitative or model-free approaches are often reported in the literature. With the availability of USPIO and other blood pool agents, the question regarding the best contrast agent also remains open. With the use of blood pool agents, analysis tools already developed for use in neurological applications may be used, and are readily available. However, approaches still need to be developed to deal with

293

other problems specifically associated with body imaging, such as cardiac and respiratory motion. While both ASL and contrast-based perfusion measurements in the body have been available for some time, the utility of these techniques is still limited to a few academic sites, predominantly for research purposes. While these methods can be performed on most commercial MR scanners, analysis is usually done offline, and as stated above, there is currently no consensus on optimal analysis techniques. ASL is less widely available on scanners, and also there is no consensus on the implementation and analysis for body applications. In principle, contrast-enhanced MRI measurements are believed to be more sensitive especially at low-flow situations, because of the greater signal changes they elicit.

Even though feasibility of perfusion MRI has been established in kidney, liver, and lungs (to variable degrees for each application), translation to routine use in the clinic will take a concerted effort from investigators, the respective clinical and radiology departments, and the various equipment vendors. An initiative similar to Quantitative Imaging Biomarkers Alliance (QIBA) under the Radiological Society of North America (RSNA) may be necessary to collectively translate these physiological MRI methods into common practice, and establish their superiority to alternative diagnostic procedures. Such efforts are critical to enable these promising methodologies to go beyond the feasibility stage and enter routine clinical practice.

References

1. Goldblatt H. Experimental hypertension induced by renal ischemia: Harvey Lecture, May 19, 1938. *Bull N Y Acad Med* 1938;**14**(9):523–53. Epub 1938/09/01.

2. Goldblatt H. Studies on experimental hypertension: VII. The production of the malignant phase of hypertension. *J Exp Med* 1938;**67**(5):809–26. Epub 1938/04/30.

3. Burkland CE, Goodwin WE, Leadbetter WF. The cure of hypertension by nephrectomy; a ten-year follow-up of a case. *Surgery* 1950;**28**(1):67–70. Epub 1950/07/01.

4. Lambeth CB, Derrick JR, Hansen AE. Stenosis of a branch of the renal artery causing hypertension in a child, including a complication of translumbar renal arteriography. *Pediatrics* 1960;**26**:822–7. Epub 1960/11/01.

5. Taquini AC, Jr., Taquini AC. The renin-angiotensin system in hypertension. *Am Heart J* 1961;**62**:558–64. Epub 1961/10/01.

6. Pickering TG, Mann SJ. Is there a role for non-invasive screening tests in diagnosing renal artery stenosis? *J Hypertens* 1996;**14**(11):1265–6. Epub 1996/11/01.

7. Textor SC, Lerman L. Renovascular hypertension and ischemic nephropathy. *Am J Hypertens* 2010;**23**(11):1159–69. Epub 2010/09/25.

8. Kim D, Porter DH, Brown R, *et al.* Renal artery imaging: a prospective comparison of intra-arterial digital subtraction angiography with conventional angiography. *Angiology* 1991;**42**(5):345–57. Epub 1991/05/01.

9. Nahman NS, Jr., Maniam P, Hernandez RA, Jr., *et al.* Renal artery pressure gradients in patients with angiographic evidence of atherosclerotic renal artery stenosis. *Am J Kidney Dis* 1994;**24**(4):695–9. Epub 1994/10/01.

10. Delin NA, Ekestrom S, Hoglund NO. Arteriographic appearance of renal artery stenosis compared to resistance measured at operation. Effect of artery reconstruction on flow, pressure gradient and resistance. *Acta Chir Scand Suppl.* 1966;**356B**:150–62. Epub 1966/01/01.

11. Zhang HL, Sos TA, Winchester PA, Gao J, Prince MR. Renal artery stenosis: imaging options, pitfalls, and concerns. *Prog Cardiovasc Dis* 2009;**52**(3):209–19. Epub 2009/11/18.

12. Safian RD, Textor SC. Renal-artery stenosis. *N Engl J Med* 2001;**344**(6):431–42. Epub 2001/02/15.

13. Attenberger UI, Sourbron SP, Schoenberg SO, *et al.* Comprehensive MR evaluation of renal disease: added clinical value of quantified renal perfusion values over single MR angiography. *J Magn Reson Imaging* 2010;**31**(1):125–33. Epub 2009/12/23.

14. Dworkin LD, Brenner BM. The renal circulation. In: Brenner BM, Rector FC, editors, *The Kidney.* Philadelphia: Saunders, 1981.

15. Badzynska B, Sadowski J. Opposed effects of prostaglandin E2 on perfusion of rat renal cortex and medulla: interactions with the renin-angiotensin system. *Exp Physiol* 2008;**93**(12):1292–302. Epub 2008/07/01.

16. Young LS, Regan MC, Barry MK, Geraghty JG, Fitzpatrick JM. Methods of renal blood flow measurement. *Urol Res* 1996;**24**(3):149–60. Epub 1996/01/01.

17. Lassen NA, Perl W. *Tracer Kinetic Methods in Medical Physiology.* New York: Raven, 1979.

18. Zierler KL. Equations for measuring blood flow by external monitoring of radioisotopes. *Circ*

Res 1965;**16**:309–21. Epub 1965/04/01.

19. Davis CP, McKinnon GC, Debatin JF, von Schulthess GK. Ultra-high-speed MR imaging. *Eur Radiol* 1996;**6**(3):297–311. Epub 1996/01/01.

20. Nitz WR. Fast and ultrafast non-echo-planar MR imaging techniques. *Eur Radiol* 2002;**12**(12):2866–82. Epub 2002/11/20.

21. Perman WH, Gado MH, Larson KB, Perlmutter JS. Simultaneous MR acquisition of arterial and brain signal-time curves. *Magn Reson Med* 1992;**28**(1):74–83. Epub 1992/11/01.

22. Lassen NA. Cerebral transit of an intravascular tracer may allow measurement of regional blood volume but not regional blood flow. *J Cereb Blood Flow Metab* 1984;**4**(4):633–4. Epub 1984/12/01.

23. Stewart GN. Researches on the circulation time in organs and on the influences which affect it: Parts I.-III. *J Physiol* 1893; **15**(1–2):1–89. Epub 1893/07/01.

24. Weisskoff RM, Chesler D, Boxerman JL, Rosen BR. Pitfalls in MR measurement of tissue blood flow with intravascular tracers: which mean transit time? *Magn Reson Med* 1993;**29**(4):553–8. Epub 1993/04/01.

25. Morell A, Ahlstrom H, Schoenberg SO, *et al.* Quantitative renal cortical perfusion in human subjects with magnetic resonance imaging using iron-oxide nanoparticles: influence of T1 shortening. *Acta Radiol* 2008; **49**(8):955–62. Epub 2008/07/11.

26. Giebisch G, Windhager E. Glomerular filtration and renal blood flow. In: Boron WF, Boulpaep EL, editors. *Medical physiology: A Cellular and molecular approach*. Philadelphia: Saunders, 2003;757–73.

27. Greger R. Introduction to renal function, renal blood flow and the formation of filtrate. In: Greger R, Windhorst U, editors, *Comprehensive Human Physiology: From Cellular Mechanisms to Integration*. Berlin: Springer, 1996;1469–87.

28. Mostafavi MR, Chavez DR, Cannillo J, Saltzman B, Prasad PV. Redistribution of renal blood flow after SWL evaluated by Gd-DTPA-enhanced magnetic resonance imaging. *J Endourol* 1998;**12**(1):9–12. Epub 1998/04/08.

29. Michaely HJ, Schoenberg SO, Oesingmann N, *et al.* Renal artery stenosis: functional assessment with dynamic MR perfusion measurements–feasibility study. *Radiology* 2006;**238**(2):586–96. Epub 2006/01/27.

30. Bokacheva L, Rusinek H, Zhang JL, Chen Q, Lee VS. Estimates of glomerular filtration rate from MR renography and tracer kinetic models. *J Magn Reson Imaging* 2009;**29**(2):371–82. Epub 2009/01/24.

31. Jones RA, Votaw JR, Salman K, *et al.* Magnetic resonance imaging evaluation of renal structure and function related to disease: technical review of image acquisition, postprocessing, and mathematical modeling steps. *J Magn Reson Imaging* 2011;**33**(6):1270–83. Epub 2011/05/19.

32. Lee VS, Rusinek H, Johnson G, *et al.* MR renography with low-dose gadopentetate dimeglumine: feasibility. *Radiology* 2001;**221**(2):371–9.

33. Annet L, Hermoye L, Peeters F, *et al.* Glomerular filtration rate: assessment with dynamic contrast-enhanced MRI and a cortical-compartment model in the rabbit kidney. *J Magn Reson Imaging* 2004;**20**(5):843–9. Epub 2004/10/27.

34. Baumann D, Rudin M. Quantitative assessment of rat kidney function by measuring the clearance of the contrast agent Gd (DOTA) using dynamic MRI. *Magn Reson Imaging* 2000;**18**(5):587–95. Epub 2000/07/29.

35. Buckley DL, Shurrab AE, Cheung CM, *et al.* Measurement of single kidney function using dynamic contrast-enhanced MRI: comparison of two models in human subjects. *J Magn Reson Imaging* 2006;**24**(5):1117–23. Epub 2006/08/31.

36. Hackstein N, Heckrodt J, Rau WS. Measurement of single-kidney glomerular filtration rate using a contrast-enhanced dynamic gradient-echo sequence and the Rutland-Patlak plot technique. *J Magn Reson Imaging* 2003;**18**(6):714–25. Epub 2003/11/25.

37. Katzberg RW, Buonocore MH, Low R, *et al.* MR determination of glomerular filtration rate in subjects with solitary kidneys in comparison to clinical standards of renal function: feasibility and preliminary report. *Contrast Media Mol Imaging* 2009;**4**(2):51–65. Epub 2009/03/11.

38. Lee VS, Rusinek H, Bokacheva L, *et al.* Renal function measurements from MR renography and a simplified multicompartmental model. *Am J Physiol Renal Physiol* 2007;**292**(5):F1548–59. Epub 2007/01/11.

39. Niendorf ER, Grist TM, Lee FT, Jr., Brazy PC, Santyr GE. Rapid in vivo measurement of single-kidney extraction fraction and glomerular filtration rate with MR imaging. *Radiology* 1998;**206**(3):791–8. Epub 1998/03/12.

40. Agarwal R, Brunelli SM, Williams K, *et al.* Gadolinium-based contrast agents and nephrogenic systemic fibrosis: a systematic review and meta-analysis. *Nephrol Dial Transplant* 2009;**24**(3):856–63. Epub 2008/10/28.

41. Chrysochou C, Buckley DL, Dark P, Cowie A, Kalra PA.

Gadolinium-enhanced magnetic resonance imaging for renovascular disease and nephrogenic systemic fibrosis: critical review of the literature and UK experience. *J Magn Reson Imaging* 2009;**29**(4):887–94. Epub 2009/03/24.

42. Kuo PH. Gadolinium-containing MRI contrast agents: important variations on a theme for NSF. *J Am Coll Radiol* 2008;**5**(1):29–35. Epub 2008/01/09.

43. Williams DS. Quantitative perfusion imaging using arterial spin labeling. *Methods Mol Med* 2006;**124**:151–73. Epub 2006/03/02.

44. Buxton RB, Frank LR, Wong EC, *et al.* A general kinetic model for quantitative perfusion imaging with arterial spin labeling. *Magn Reson Med* 1998;**40**(3):383–96. Epub 1998/09/04.

45. Martirosian P, Klose U, Mader I, Schick F. FAIR true-FISP perfusion imaging of the kidneys. *Magn Reson Med* 2004;**51**(2):353–61. Epub 2004/02/03.

46. Lorenz CH, Powers TA, Partain CL. Quantitative imaging of renal blood flow and function. *Invest Radiol* 1992;**27** Suppl 2:S109–14. Epub 1992/12/01.

47. Ritt M, Janka R, Schneider MP, *et al.* Measurement of kidney perfusion by magnetic resonance imaging: comparison of MRI with arterial spin labeling to para-aminohippuric acid plasma clearance in male subjects with metabolic syndrome. *Nephrol Dial Transplant* 2010;**25**(4):1126–33. Epub 2009/11/24.

48. Epstein FH, Agmon Y, Brezis M. Physiology of renal hypoxia. *Ann N Y Acad Sci* 1994;**718**:72–81; discussion 81–2. Epub 1994/04/15.

49. Brezis M, Rosen S. Hypoxia of the renal medulla–its implications for disease. *N Engl J Med* 1995;**332**(10):647–55. Epub 1995/03/09.

50. Brezis M, Agmon Y, Epstein FH. Determinants of intrarenal oxygenation. I. Effects of diuretics. *Am J Physiol* 1994;**267**(6 Pt 2):F1059–62. Epub 1994/12/01.

51. Liss AG, Liss P. Use of a modified oxygen microelectrode and laser-Doppler flowmetry to monitor changes in oxygen tension and microcirculation in a flap. *Plast Reconstr Surg* 2000;**105**(6):2072–8. Epub 2000/06/06.

52. Palm F, Cederberg J, Hansell P, Liss P, Carlsson PO. Reactive oxygen species cause diabetes-induced decrease in renal oxygen tension. *Diabetologia* 2003;**46**(8):1153–60. Epub 2003/07/25.

53. Braun RD, Lanzen JL, Snyder SA, Dewhirst MW. Comparison of tumor and normal tissue oxygen tension measurements using OxyLite or microelectrodes in rodents. *Am J Physiol Heart Circ Physiol* 2001;**280**(6):H2533–44.

54. Zhong Z, Arteel GE, Connor HD, *et al.* Cyclosporin A increases hypoxia and free radical production in rat kidneys: prevention by dietary glycine. *Am J Physiol* 1998;**275**(4 Pt 2):F595–604. Epub 1998/10/01.

55. Rosenberger C, Goldfarb M, Shina A, *et al.* Evidence for sustained renal hypoxia and transient hypoxia adaptation in experimental rhabdomyolysis-induced acute kidney injury. *Nephrol Dial Transplant* 2008;**23**(4):1135–43. Epub 2007/12/01.

56. Rosenberger C, Khamaisi M, Abassi Z, *et al.* Adaptation to hypoxia in the diabetic rat kidney. *Kidney Int* 2008;**73**(1):34–42. Epub 2007/10/05.

57. Hirayama A, Nagase S, Ueda A, *et al.* In vivo imaging of oxidative stress in ischemia-reperfusion renal injury using electron paramagnetic resonance. *Am J Physiol Renal Physiol* 2005;**288**(3):F597–603. Epub 2004/11/13.

58. Subramanian S, Yamada K, Irie A, *et al.* Noninvasive in vivo oximetric imaging by radiofrequency FT EPR. *Magn Reson Med* 2002;**47**(5):1001–8. Epub 2002/04/30.

59. Kempe S, Metz H, Mader K. Application of electron paramagnetic resonance (EPR) spectroscopy and imaging in drug delivery research – chances and challenges. *Eur J Pharm Biopharm* 2010;**74**(1):55–66. Epub 2009/09/03.

60. Matthews PM, Jezzard P. Functional magnetic resonance imaging. *J Neurol Neurosurg Psychiatry* 2004;**75**(1):6–12. Epub 2004/01/07.

61. Rajagopalan P, Krishnan KR, Passe TJ, Macfall JR. Magnetic resonance imaging using deoxyhemoglobin contrast versus positron emission tomography in the assessment of brain function. *Prog Neuropsychopharmacol Biol Psychiatry.* 1995;**19**(3):351–66. Epub 1995/05/01.

62. Ugurbil K, Hu X, Chen W, *et al.* Functional mapping in the human brain using high magnetic fields. *Philos Trans R Soc Lond B Biol Sci* 1999;**354**(1387):1195–213. Epub 1999/08/31.

63. Dunn JF, Swartz HM. Blood oxygenation. Heterogeneity of hypoxic tissues monitored using bold MR imaging. *Adv Exp Med Biol* 1997;**428**:645–50. Epub 1997/01/01.

64. Prasad PV, Chen Q, Goldfarb JW, Epstein FH, Edelman RR. Breath-hold R2* mapping with a multiple gradient-recalled echo sequence: application to the evaluation of intrarenal oxygenation. *J Magn Reson Imaging* 1997;**7**(6):1163–5. Epub 1997/12/24.

65. Prasad PV, Edelman RR, Epstein FH. Noninvasive evaluation of intrarenal oxygenation with BOLD MRI. *Circulation* 1996;**94**(12):3271–5. Epub 1996/12/15.

66. Priatna A, Epstein FH, Spokes K, Prasad PV. Evaluation of changes in intrarenal oxygenation in rats using multiple gradient-recalled echo (mGRE) sequence. *J Magn Reson Imaging* 1999;**9**(6):842–6. Epub 1999/06/18.

67. Textor SC, Glockner JF, Lerman LO, *et al*. The use of magnetic resonance to evaluate tissue oxygenation in renal artery stenosis. *J Am Soc Nephrol* 2008;**19**(4):780–8. Epub 2008/02/22.

68. Cheung CM, Shurrab AE, Buckley DL, *et al*. MR-derived renal morphology and renal function in patients with atherosclerotic renovascular disease. *Kidney Int* 2006;**69**(4):715–22. Epub 2006/01/06.

69. Han F, Xiao W, Xu Y, *et al*. The significance of BOLD MRI in differentiation between renal transplant rejection and acute tubular necrosis. *Nephrol Dial Transplant* 2008;**23**(8):2666–72. Epub 2008/03/01.

70. Djamali A, Sadowski EA, Samaniego-Picota M, *et al*. Noninvasive assessment of early kidney allograft dysfunction by blood oxygen level-dependent magnetic resonance imaging. *Transplantation* 2006;**82**(5):621–8. Epub 2006/09/14.

71. Sadowski EA, Fain SB, Alford SK, *et al*. Assessment of acute renal transplant rejection with blood oxygen level-dependent MR imaging: initial experience. *Radiology* 2005;**236**(3):911–19. Epub 2005/08/25.

72. de Bazelaire C, Alsop DC, George D, *et al*. Magnetic resonance imaging-measured blood flow change after antiangiogenic therapy with PTK787/ZK 222584 correlates with clinical outcome in metastatic renal cell carcinoma. *Clin Cancer Res* 2008;**14**(17):5548–54. Epub 2008/09/04.

73. De Bazelaire C, Rofsky NM, Duhamel G, *et al*. Arterial spin labeling blood flow magnetic resonance imaging for the characterization of metastatic renal cell carcinoma(1). *Acad Radiol* 2005;**12**(3):347–57. Epub 2005/03/16.

74. Chiandussi L, Greco F, Sardi G, *et al*. Estimation of hepatic arterial and portal venous blood flow by direct catheterization of the vena porta through the umbilical cord in man. Preliminary results. *Acta Hepatosplenol* 1968;**15**(3):166–71.

75. Gulberg V, Haag K, Rossie M, Gerbes AL. Hepatic arterial buffer response in patients with advanced cirrhosis. *Hepatology* 2002;**35**(3):630–4.

76. Richter S, Mucke I, Menger MD, Vollmar B. Impact of intrinsic blood flow regulation in cirrhosis: maintenance of hepatic arterial buffer response. *Am J Physiol Gastrointest Liver Physiol* 2000;**279**(2):G454–62.

77. Sarper R, Fajman WA, Rypins EB, *et al*. A noninvasive method for measuring portal venous/total hepatic blood flow by hepatosplenic radionuclide angiography. *Radiology* 1981;**141**(1):179–84.

78. Miles KA, Hayball MP, Dixon AK. Functional images of hepatic perfusion obtained with dynamic CT. *Radiology* 1993;**188**(2):405–11.

79. Bolton RP, Mairiang EO, Parkin A, *et al*. Dynamic liver scanning in cirrhosis. *Nucl Med Commun* 1988;**9**(3):235–47.

80. Zapletal C, Mehrabi A, Scharf J, *et al*. Experimental evaluation of dynamic MRI for quantification of liver perfusion. *Transplant Proc* 1999;**31**(1–2):421–2. Epub 1999/03/20.

81. Scharf J, Kemmling A, Hess T, *et al*. Assessment of hepatic perfusion in transplanted livers by pharmacokinetic analysis of dynamic magnetic resonance measurements. *Invest Radiol* 2007;**42**(4):224–9. Epub 2007/03/14.

82. Jackson A, Haroon H, Zhu XP, *et al*. Breath hold perfusion and permeability mapping of hepatic malignancies using magnetic resonance imaging and a first-pass leakage profile model. *NMR Biomed* 2002;**15**(2):164–73. Epub 2002/03/01.

83. Hagiwara M, Rusinek H, Lee VS, *et al*. Advanced liver fibrosis: diagnosis with 3D whole-liver perfusion MR imaging–initial experience. *Radiology* 2008;**246**(3):926–34. Epub 2008/01/16.

84. Patel J, Sigmund EE, Rusinek H, *et al*. Diagnosis of cirrhosis with intravoxel incoherent motion diffusion MRI and dynamic contrast-enhanced MRI alone and in combination: preliminary experience. *J Magn Reson Imaging* 2010;**31**(3):589–600. Epub 2010/02/27.

85. Sharma P, Kalb B, Kitajima HD, *et al*. Optimization of single injection liver arterial phase gadolinium enhanced MRI using bolus track real-time imaging. *J Magn Reson Imaging* 2011;**33**(1):110–18. Epub 2010/12/25.

86. Do RK, Rusinek H, Taouli B. Dynamic contrast-enhanced MR imaging of the liver: current status and future directions. *Magn Reson Imaging Clin N Am* 2009;**17**(2):339–49. Epub 2009/05/02.

87. Thng CH, Koh TS, Collins DJ, Koh DM. Perfusion magnetic resonance imaging of the liver. *World J Gastroenterol* 2010;**16**(13):1598–609. Epub 2010/04/01.

88. Haque M, Koktzoglou I, Li W, Carbray J, Prasad P. Functional MRI of liver using BOLD MRI: effect of glucose. *J Magn Reson Imaging* 2010;**32**(4):988–91. Epub 2010/10/01.

89. Fan Z, Elzibak A, Boylan C, Noseworthy MD. Blood oxygen level-dependent magnetic

resonance imaging of the human liver: preliminary results. *J Comput Assist Tomogr* 2010;**34**(4):523–31. Epub 2010/07/27.

90. Jin N, Deng J, Chadashvili T, *et al.* Carbogen gas-challenge BOLD MR imaging in a rat model of diethylnitrosamine-induced liver fibrosis. *Radiology* 2010;**254**(1):129–37. Epub 2009/12/25.

91. Worsley DF, Alavi A. Radionuclide imaging of acute pulmonary embolism. *Semin Nucl Med* 2003;**33**(4):259–78. Epub 2003/11/20.

92. Hopkins SR, Prisk GK. Lung perfusion measured using magnetic resonance imaging: new tools for physiological insights into the pulmonary circulation. *J Magn Reson Imaging* 2010;**32**(6):1287–301. Epub 2010/11/26.

93. Stein PD, Hull RD, Ghali WA, *et al.* Tracking the uptake of evidence: two decades of hospital practice trends for diagnosing deep vein thrombosis and pulmonary embolism. *Arch Intern Med* 2003;**163**(10):1213–19. Epub 2003/05/28.

94. Stein PD, Henry JW. Prevalence of acute pulmonary embolism among patients in a general hospital and at autopsy. *Chest* 1995;**108**(4):978–81. Epub 1995/10/01.

95. Leblanc M, Paul N. V/Q SPECT and computed tomographic pulmonary angiography. *Semin Nucl Med* 2010;**40**(6):426–41. Epub 2010/10/06.

96. Rubins JB. The current approach to the diagnosis of pulmonary embolism: lessons from PIOPED II. *Postgrad Med* 2008;**120**(1):1–7. Epub 2008/05/10.

97. Wielopolski PA, Haacke EM, Adler LP. Three-dimensional MR imaging of the pulmonary vasculature: preliminary experience. *Radiology* 1992;**183**(2):465–72. Epub 1992/05/01.

98. Meaney JF, Weg JG, Chenevert TL, *et al.* Diagnosis of pulmonary embolism with magnetic resonance angiography. *N Engl J Med* 1997;**336**(20):1422–7. Epub 1997/05/15.

99. Stein PD, Chenevert TL, Fowler SE, *et al.* Gadolinium-enhanced magnetic resonance angiography for pulmonary embolism: a multicenter prospective study (PIOPED III). *Ann Intern Med* 2010;**152**(7):434–43, W142–3. Epub 2010/04/07.

100. Hatabu H, Gaa J, Kim D, *et al.* Pulmonary perfusion: qualitative assessment with dynamic contrast-enhanced MRI using ultra-short TE and inversion recovery turbo FLASH. *Magn Reson Med* 1996;**36**(4):503–8. Epub 1996/10/01.

101. Chen Q, Levin DL, Kim D, *et al.* Pulmonary disorders: ventilation-perfusion MR imaging with animal models. *Radiology* 1999;**213**(3):871–9. Epub 1999/12/02.

102. Hatabu H, Tadamura E, Prasad PV, *et al.* Noninvasive pulmonary perfusion imaging by STAR-HASTE sequence. *Magn Reson Med* 2000;**44**(5):808–12. Epub 2000/11/07.

103. Hatabu H, Wielopolski PA, Tadamura E. An attempt of pulmonary perfusion imaging utilizing ultrashort echo time turbo FLASH sequence with signal targeting and alternating radio-frequency (STAR).

Eur J Radiol 1999;**29**(2):160–3. Epub 1999/06/22.

104. Mai VM, Berr SS. MR perfusion imaging of pulmonary parenchyma using pulsed arterial spin labeling techniques: FAIRER and FAIR. *J Magn Reson Imaging* 1999;**9**(3):483–7. Epub 1999/04/09.

105. Keilholz SD, Mai VM, Berr SS, Fujiwara N, Hagspiel KD. Comparison of first-pass Gd-DOTA and FAIRER MR perfusion imaging in a rabbit model of pulmonary embolism. *J Magn Reson Imaging* 2002;**16**(2):168–71. Epub 2002/08/31.

106. Eichinger M, Heussel CP, Kauczor HU, Tiddens H, Puderbach M. Computed tomography and magnetic resonance imaging in cystic fibrosis lung disease. *J Magn Reson Imaging* 2010;**32**(6):1370–8. Epub 2010/11/26.

107. Ley S, Grunig E, Kiely DG, van Beek E, Wild J. Computed tomography and magnetic resonance imaging of pulmonary hypertension: pulmonary vessels and right ventricle. *J Magn Reson Imaging* 2010;**32**(6):1313–24. Epub 2010/11/26.

108. Prasad PV, Goldfarb J, Sundaram C, *et al.* Captopril MR renography in a swine model: toward a comprehensive evaluation of renal arterial stenosis. *Radiology* 2000;**217**(3):813–18.

109. Michaely HJ, Schoenberg SO, Ittrich C, *et al.* Renal disease: value of functional magnetic resonance imaging with flow and perfusion measurements. *Invest Radiol* 2004;**39**(11):698–705. Epub 2004/10/16.

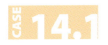

Chronic kidney disease

Huan Tan and Pottumarthi V. Prasad

History

A 57-year-old female patient with stage 3 chronic kidney disease (CKD) with estimated GFR = 43 ml/min.

Technique

Single-slice ASL with a 2D navigator-gated FAIR perfusion preparation and true-FISP readout.

Imaging findings

See Figure 14.11.

Discussion

Decreased renal perfusion values have been found in CKD patients compared with healthy controls. Hypoxia is known to play a major role in both initiation and progression of CKD [1, 2] and since vascular changes are partly responsible for the hypoxia [2], quantitative perfusion MRI could be a useful biomarker.

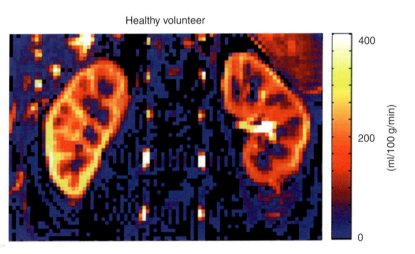

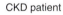

Figure 14.11 The mean perfusion in the CKD patient was 150 and 35 ml/100 g/min for the renal cortex and medulla, respectively, compared with 235 and 52 ml/100 g/min obtained in a healthy volunteer (male, 21 years old).

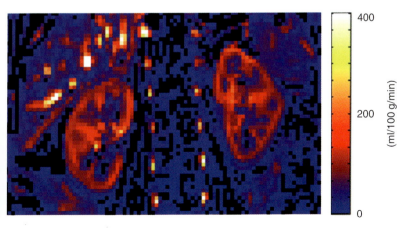

- Subjects with CKD are contraindicated for the use of contrast agents (MRI and X-ray based), and hence ASL-based perfusion MRI is attractive.
- Combination of ASL perfusion along with BOLD MRI (for assessing hypoxia) and diffusion MRI (for assessing fibrosis) could provide for a comprehensive, non-invasive, and potentially early detection of subjects with CKD at risk of progression.

References

1. Fine LG, Orphanides C, Norman JT. Progressive renal disease: the chronic hypoxia hypothesis. *Kidney Int Suppl* 1998;**65**:S74–8. Epub 1998/04/29.

2. Nangaku M. Chronic hypoxia and tubulointerstitial injury: a final common pathway to end-stage renal failure. *J Am Soc Nephrol* 2006;**17**(1):17–25. Epub 2005/11/18.

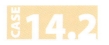

ASL in renal transplantation

Isky Gordon

History

An 18-year-old boy underwent a renal transplant after being on dialysis for 4 years. ASL MRI was undertaken shortly post transplantation and approximately 6 months later.

Technique

Oblique-coronal ASL data volumes were acquired on a 1.5 T Siemens Avanto scanner (Siemens Healthcare, Erlangen, Germany) with a dedicated abdominal TIM 32-channel body phased array coil. ASL was performed using a multi-TI FAIR labeling scheme and 3D GRASE imaging module. Background suppression and respiratory triggering were used to maximize measurement precision. Images were acquired following selective and non-selective inversion at 14 TI values spaced every 200 ms from 100 ms to 2700 ms. Repetition time (TR) was set to 3000 ms and echo time (TE) to 28.25 ms. The voxel size was $3.1 \times 3.1 \times 5.0 \, \text{mm}^3$ with a matrix size of 128×104. Total scan time for the ASL acquisition was approximately 5 min. T_1 maps of the kidney were acquired using the same sequence with background suppression disabled.

Imaging findings

See Figure 14.12.

Discussion

Kidneys with good function (estimated glomerular filtration rate (eGFR) $> 60 \, \text{ml/min per } 1.73 \, \text{m}^2$) have been shown to have higher perfusion than those with eGFR < 60 [1]; also native kidneys typically have higher perfusion than transplants, in which the mean eGFR is usually lower than in native kidneys as well [1]. Renal cortical perfusion has also been shown to correlate with eGFR, both in native and transplanted kidneys. Finally, a drop in perfusion might be an early indicator of acute rejection, which is not the case in this patient.

Key points

- Quantitative ASL of the kidneys is feasible in the clinical environment.
- ASL may be useful for monitoring kidney function post-transplant.

Reference

1. Artz NS, Sadowski EA, Wentland AL, *et al.* Arterial spin labeling MRI for assessment of perfusion in native and transplanted kidneys. *Magn Reson Imaging* 2011;**29**(1):74–82.

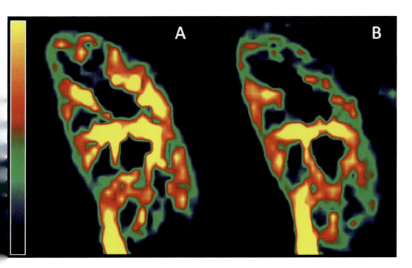

Figure 14.12 Eight days following the transplant ASL showed mean renal cortical perfusion of 155 ml/100 g/min and a median perfusion of 129 ml/100 g/min (a). Twenty-eight weeks following the transplant repeat ASL showed renal cortical perfusion of mean 114 ml/100 g/min and a median perfusion of 105 ml/100 g/min (b).

MR perfusion imaging in cardiac diseases

Jürg Schwitter

Key points

- Perfusion MRI detects myocardial ischemia with high diagnostic performance.
- Perfusion MRI using bolus contrast agent injection is a technique with excellent spatial resolution which allows the detection of small subendocardial perfusion deficits.
- Perfusion MRI is free of attenuation problems and delivers high-quality perfusion information in most patients.
- Perfusion MRI can detect coronary artery disease (CAD) and has been shown to be superior to SPECT in several large multicenter trials. It is an ideal test to confirm or exclude the presence of CAD, particularly in women and young adults, subjects who may be relatively more susceptible to radiation exposure. It is also an ideal method

for repetitive studies, i.e., to monitor CAD progression or treatment response.
- Perfusion MRI aids in the characterization of cardiac masses, specifically to differentiate tumors from thrombi.

Introduction: clinical Background

Coronary artery disease (CAD) is the leading cause of death in the industrialized world [1]. As shown in Figure 15.1, CAD can manifest in different ways, including both chest pain during exercise (stable angina pectoris) and as acute ST-segment (on the ECG) elevation myocardial infarction (STEMI), which requires immediate revascularization. The diagnosis of STEMI is relatively simple and straightforward, with typical chest pain, ST-segment elevation in the resting ECG, and positive serum troponins. However, the non-ST-segment elevation

Clinical presentations of CAD and its progression towards HF

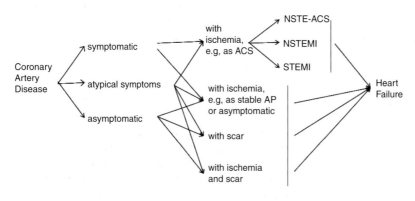

Figure 15.1 Clinical presentations and progression of CAD into heart failure (HF). CAD can present with typical or atypical symptoms or may develop without symptoms. The time course of CAD is also variable, with acute manifestions (ACS – acute coronary syndrome) or with stable progression. With further progression of the disease, particularly if infarcts develop with scar formation, CAD finally ends with heart failure. AP, angina pectoris; MI, myocardial infarction; NSTE, non-ST-segment elevation.

MI (NSTEMI) or its precursor, the non-ST-segment elevation acute coronary syndrome (NSTE-ACS) without relevant necrosis, are more difficult to diagnose. In these patients ischemia should be detected by non-invasive imaging tests or by visualization of coronary stenoses by invasive coronary angiography. Despite substantial progress in the treatment of STEMI by percutaneous coronary interventions (PCI), these patients still suffer from a higher in-hospital mortality rate than those with NSTE-ACS (7% vs. 5%, respectively), but the mortality rates become similar at 6 months of approximately 12% [2, 3].

It is generally accepted that symptomatic patients should undergo further diagnostic workup to establish the diagnosis of CAD, to assess the extent and severy of ischemia, and to plan treatment. In patients with a low probability for CAD of <10–20%, it is recommended to treat risk factors, but not to procede to ischemia testing (e.g., by a treadmill exercise test or non-invasive imaging tests). In patients with an intermediate pre-test probability for CAD, it is generally recommended to perform a treadmill exercise test (= stress ECG) and/or to perform ischemia testing by non-invasive imaging utilizing stress echocardiography, single-photon emission computed tomography (SPECT), dobutamine stress MRI, or perfusion MRI. At a high pre-test probability (higher than 80–90%), it is generally accepted to proceed directly to invasive coronary X-ray angiography (CXA).

Drug treatment and revascularizations by PCI or by surgery are well established as efficacious options in symptomatic patients to reduce angina and/or dyspnea as ischemic equivalent. However, the therapeutic efforts should not focus exclusively on symptoms reduction, but should also aim to reduce the risk for an acute myocardial infarction (AMI). In the United States, larger registries document that about 50% of men and approximately 67% of women do not exhibit chest pain before the first heart attack [1], indicating that an AMI is often the first manifestation of CAD. In a large cohort of 13 969 patients published recently, patients presenting with angina had a better all-case mortality over 5 years compared with asymptomatic patients [4]. In the asymptomatic population with silent ischemia, 47% of deaths occurred in patients with diabetes mellitus and/or dyspnea. Thus, ischemia detection and workup of suspected CAD should not exclusively be targeted on symptomatic patients as this strategy would miss between 50% and 67% of

patients with CAD before their first heart attack [5]. The precise profile of asymptomatic patients that should undergo further ischemic testing is not yet well defined, however, and prospective trials addressing this issue are needed. While ischemia burden is known as a prognostic factor, scar tissue in asymptomatic patients is less well established as a risk factor. With the advent of precise and reliable detection of scar tissue by MRI, this patient population was investigated recently. Kwong and coworkers followed patients without a history of MI, but with documented scar tissue by MRI, over approximately 1.5 years. Small amounts of scar tissue of 1–2% of the left ventricular (LV) mass increased the risk for major adverse cardiac events (MACE) 7-fold [6]. In that study, detection of scar tissue by the presence of late gadolinium enhancement on MRI was also a stronger predictor for MACE than regional wall motion abnormalities [6].

In patients with reduced LV function and a history of MI, a workup of ischemia including a viability assessment is crucial for decision-making with respect to revascularization versus drug treatment alone. In patients with a substantial amount of dysfunctional but viable myocardium, revascularization significantly improves outcome, as was demonstrated in a large meta-analysis [7]. In a prospective randomized trial, positron emission tomography (PET) was useful for clinical decision-making in the patients where revascularizations were technically feasible [8]. In the recent Simplified Treatment Intervention to Control Hypertension (STICH) substudy in which SPECT was used to assess viability, outcome did not improve when using this nuclear medicine-based approach, suggesting that this technique is probably not reliable enough to guide patient management [9]. In this context, it should be noted that the spatial resolution of gadolinium-enhanced MRI for viability imaging is superior in comparison to nuclear medicine techniques. Subendocardial scars are often missed by nuclear medicine techniques, whereas late gadolinium enhancement detects fibrotic regions as small as 0.5 ml with high reproducibility [10].

Ischemic burden is one of the most powerful prognostic factors in patients with CAD [11], so it is important not only to detect and quantify ischemia in these patients, but also to exclude ischemia to identify patients that can safely avoid further testing. In symptomatic patients, Jahnke and coworkers assessed ischemia by perfusion MRI and outcome was excellent with event

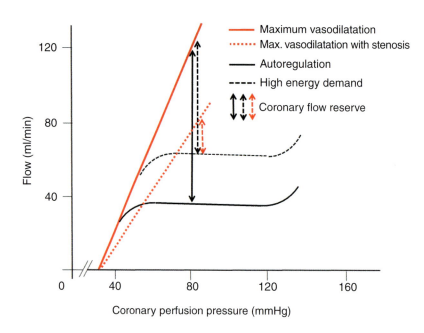

Figure 15.2 Concept of pathophysiology of coronary circulation. The black lines correspond to the condition of autoregulation, while the red lines correspond to the situation of maximum hyperemia.

Pathophysiology of coronary perfusion: "stress-only" versus "stress-rest" tests

The heart has an enormous need for oxygen as it beats about 100 000 times and pumps about 10 tons of blood through the body per day. To meet these oxygen needs, the heart muscle has a high blood flow and oxygen extraction. This makes further extraction of oxygen an inefficient strategy to match increased demand. Thus, variable demand by the heart is met primarily by adjusting coronary blood flow to the prevailing metabolic conditions. Over a range of perfusion pressures of approximately 60 to 120–140 mmHg coronary blood flow remains constant, representing the zone of "autoregulation" of coronary circulation [15, 16]. Within this pressure range, coronary resistance is varied within the different layers of the myocardial wall to maintain stable coronary blood flow. The fall in flow at low perfusion pressures indicates that vasodilatation can no longer compensate for a decrease in perfusion pressure. Once the microvasculature is maximally dilated (and vascular

rates of 0.3–0.5%/year in those without ischemia [12, 13]. Similar results were obtained with dobutamine stress MRI [14]. Thus, MRI is able to exclude CAD and to identify patients with a good prognosis, despite a positive history of CAD and MI.

resistance is minimal), flow becomes pressure dependent. This is the case for the relationship represented by the red lines in Figure 15.2. These lines represent the maximum coronary flow achievable during maximum vasodilatation, for example during reactive hyperemia (after transient coronary vessel occlusion) or during an adenosine infusion. Within the range of perfusion pressures with preserved autoregulation (the horizontal black lines in Figure 15.2), the relationship between coronary flow and perfusion pressure is governed by the microvascular resistance of the vessels of the coronary vascular bed. During conditions of elevated cardiac work or elevated coronary flow, such as in patients suffering from anemia, the level of autoregulation is elevated (the horizontal line is shifted upwards).

Some of the factors that affect the level of autoregulation are baseline metabolic needs, heart rate, contractility, and loading conditions [17]. Thus, the coronary flow reserve (CFR), defined as the maximum hyperemic flow divided by the resting flow, strongly depends on factors that regulate resting oxygen demand. Maximum myocardial blood flow depends on several factors as well. During conditions of increased extravascular compressive forces such as tissue edema, increased contractility, or increased blood viscosity, maximum blood flow is reduced (dotted red line in Figure 15.2). Also, thickening of coronary vessels or microvascular disease can reduce this maximum coronary flow [18]. Finally, a hemodynamically relevant coronary stenosis will also reduce the maximum hyperemic flow. Flow during autoregulation (resting flow) is not a constant but can be modified by various factors, which explains why the degree of stenosis of a coronary artery is not always tightly linked to a reduced CFR. This has been observed in many studies using PET to assess significance of coronary stenoses, where the correlation between percent stenosis and hyperemic flow was tighter than that for CFR [19–22].

Based on these considerations, it appears reasonable to assess myocardial blood flow by perfusion MRI methods during hyperemic conditions only. Several studies utilized this "stress-only" protocol and yielded excellent results in the detection of CAD in comparison with PET [23], or by utilizing the criterion of ≥50% diameter stenoses on invasive coronary angiography (CXA) as the standard of reference [23–27].

Perfusion studies in CAD and other diseases

Ischemia testing in stable CAD

Perfusion MRI is mainly utilized in the setting of known or suspected CAD [28, 29]. In the European registry on cardiovascular MR, about one-third of all MRI exams are performed to exclude or confirm ischemia in known or suspected CAD [30]. In that registry, perfusion MRI was used in two-thirds and dobutamine stress MRI in one-third for the detection of ischemia [30]. In multicenter studies of patients with known or suspected CAD, perfusion MRI yielded sensitivities and specificities for the detection of CAD (≥50% diameter stenosis on CXA in vessels of ≥ 2 mm diameter) of 91% and 78% [25]; and 85% and 67% [26], respectively, corresponding to areas under the receiver operator characteristic (ROC) curves (AUC) of 0.91[25] and 0.86 (see Figure 15.3) [26]. These studies relied on stress-only analyses where a quantitative upslope analysis was used in one study [25] and a visual assessment in the other [26]. The upslope approach quantifies the signal increase in the myocardium during the first pass of the contrast agent and compares it with values from a normal database. This approach also clearly demonstrated the importance of an adequate contrast agent dose to achieve an

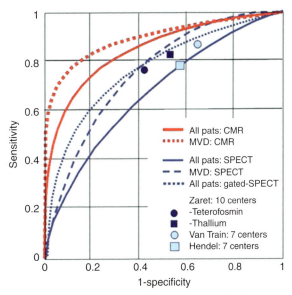

Figure 15.3 Diagnostic performance (ROC curve) of perfusion MRI (cardiac MR – CMR) to detect CAD (defined as ≥50% stenosis by invasive coronary angiography) in comparison to SPECT and gated-SPECT. Performance of SPECT in the MR-IMPACT trial is comparable to those of previous multicenter SPECT trials (given as squares and circles) reported by Zaret et al. [69], Van Train et al. [70], and Hendel et al. [71]. Better performance is obtained with perfusion MRI vs. SPECT (p = 0.013), particularly when patients had multivessel disease (MVD) (p = 0.006). Modified from Schwitter et al. [26, 29] with permission from Oxford University Press.

appropriate diagnostic performance. The high sensitivies and specificities mentioned above were obtained with a dose of 0.1 mmol/kg of a conventional (extravascular) gadolinium-based contrast agent. When a dose of 0.05 mmol/kg of the same contrast agent was used in one of these multicenter trials at 1.5 T, the AUC for CAD detection was as low as 0.53, yielding a specificity of only 25% at a sensitivity level of 94%, which is clinically not useful [25]. This high diagnostic performance was recently confirmed in the largest multicenter perfusion MRI trial performed so far, which included 33 participating centers [31].

Despite these positive results, several studies also used a "stress-rest" perfusion protocol to calculate a myocardial perfusion reserve index using MRI. At a threshold for a pathological myocardial perfusion reserve index of 1.1, this approach yielded a sensitivity of 88% and specificity of 90% for detecting CAD in patients with suspected CAD [32]. Other perfusion MRI studies based on a stress-rest protocol yielded sensitivities and specificities of 88% and 82%, respectively (AUC of 0.91) [33], and 91% and 62%, respectively [34].

305

Perfusion MRI is well established at a field strength of 1.5 T, and all multicenter studies performed so far used 1.5 T systems [25, 26]. A few smaller studies have explored the technique at 3 T and similar results were obtained as for 1.5 T [27]. Yet, cardiovascular imaging in general is more challenging at 3 T, due to increased artifacts from B_0 and B_1 inhomogeneities in most sequences. Thus, there is currently no evidence that demonstrates better perfusion MRI performance at 3 T compared with 1.5 T.

Ischemia testing in acute coronary syndrome (ACS)

While the resting ECG with ST-segment elevation and positive troponins are the cornerstone for the diagnosis of STEMI, NSTE-ACS remains a diagnostic challenge, as typically no or minimal necrosis is present, but there is an ischemic burden that typically requires treatment, such as revascularization. Since transient ischemia causes stunning, functional assessment and detection of regional hypokinesia is a practical approach to detect CAD and critical stenosis in acute chest pain patients [35]. However, in these patients with at least 30 min of chest pain but without ST-segment elevation on ECG, perfusion MRI detected MI with a sensitivity and specificity of 100% and 79%, respectively. The combined primary endpoint of NSTEMI and unstable angina was detected by MRI with a sensitivity of 84% and a specificity of 85% [35]. In patients with acute chest pain and AMI excluded by serial resting ECGs and negative troponins, perfusion MRI performed within 72 hrs of presentation yielded a sensitivity and specificity of 100% and 93%, respectively, for the detection of ACS [36]. In addition, no patients with a negative MRI scan had any cardiovascular outcomes during the 1-year follow-up [36]. Similarly, Plein and coworkers studied NSTE-ACS patients and significant coronary stenoses were detected by adenosine perfusion MRI (performed within 72 hrs of presentation) with a sensitivity and specificity of 88% and 83%, respectively, which increased to 96% and 83%, respectively, when using images of diagnostic quality only [37].

Perfusion testing for the differentiation of cardiac masses

Recent studies also focused on the value of perfusion MRI in the evaluation of cardiac masses. Here, differentiation of cardiac tumors versus thrombi is of particular clinical importance. Localization of masses and their relation to hypo- or akinetic regions are the important criteria for differentiation [38]. However, such a distinction is not always straightforward. Similarly, a pericardial effusion can occur in the setting of an infiltrative tumor process or can be associated with an acute infarction that can also provoke thrombus formation at the endocardial surface. Also, T_1- and T_2-weighted acquisitions do not allow reliable differentiation between benign and malignant masses. However, tissue perfusion as assessed with MRI has been shown to be useful to distinguish thrombi from tumor masses [39, 40]. The differentiation between lipomas and other tumors and thrombi is readily achievable by applying fat saturation techniques [40].

To detect thrombi, late gadolinium enhancement on MRI is a robust and sensitive observation. This application is relevant, as thrombi in the LV cavity occur in up to 20–30% of patients with AMI. In a study of 361 patients with intracardiac thrombi (confirmed by surgery or pathology), three different imaging techniques, (MRI, transesophageal [TEE], and transthoracic echocardiography [TTE]) all showed high specificity for the detection of thrombi of 99%, 96%, and 96%, respectively. However, MRI was much more sensitive, with a sensitivity of 88%, while sensitivities were 27% and 40% for TEE and TTE, respectively [41]. Detection rate was particularly high by MRI for small apical and parietal thrombi that might be missed by echocardiography.

Comparison with other modalities, limitations, and pitfalls

Principles of ischemia assessment by MRI versus nuclear medicine techniques

As discussed above, a perfusion MRI protocol for the assessment of CAD can consist of a stress-only acquisition or of a combined stress-rest strategy. In this context, it should be recognized, that the stress-rest MRI protocol does not mimic the stress and rest injections of a SPECT examination (Table 15.1). With SPECT imaging the stress injection detects ischemia during hyperemia (i.e., it detects a reduced maximum flow during pharmacological vasodilatation), while the rest injection exploits the uptake of the radioactive tracer into viable myocytes, thus probing viability rather than resting perfusion. Conversely, the rest injection in perfusion MRI measures resting

Table 15.1. Imaging methods in cardiology

	Ischemia		Viability	
	CM/Tracer	Technique	CM/Tracer	Technique
CMR	Gd chelate	First-pass stress injection or CFR with rest and stress	Gd chelate	LGE rest injection
SPECT	^{99m}Tc-tracer	Perfusion stress injection	^{99m}Tc-Tracer	Re-distribution rest injection
PET	^{13}N-ammonia ^{15}O-water	CFR with rest and stress injection	^{18}F-fluorodeoxy-glucose	Rest injection

CM, contrast medium; CMR, cardiovascular magnetic resonance; LGE, late gadolinium enhancement.

perfusion in order to calculate CFR when combined with the hyperemic flow measurement. The "MRI analog" of the SPECT rest injection is late gadolinium enhancement that depicts the uptake of contrast agent into fibrotic tissue, allowing the differentiation between scar and viable tissue. The PET analogs for the stress-rest MRI protocol to calculate CFR are flow-based tracers such as ^{13}N-ammonia or ^{15}O-water, performed both at rest and during hyperemia. The PET technique to determine viability (i.e., the comparable test to presence or absence of late gadolinium enhancement on MRI) uses ^{18}F-fluorodeoxyglucose (FDG), which probes the active uptake of the glucose analog FDG into the myocyte [42].

The CFR concept based on the considerations given in Figure 15.2 requires a quantitative measurement of tissue perfusion. Therefore, the PET approach to calculate CFR appears reasonable since PET is a quantitative technique, and several studies have demonstrated the relationship between CFR measured by PET and the degree of coronary stenoses [19, 20]. For the first-pass perfusion MRI technique, the upslope of the signal change during this first pass is often used as a quantitative measure of perfusion [23–25]. This approach is robust for the detection of a severe reduction of perfusion, e.g., in the setting of major coronary stenoses. However, for quantitative assessment of blood flow, a full analysis with measurement of an arterial input function (AIF) is required, which is often necessary when evaluating patients with reduced LV function. Therefore, several investigators have proposed to measure the signal within the LV blood pool as an estimate of the AIF. This approach may improve the overall performance

of the upslope analyses, although no comparative studies between quantitative and qualitative approaches are available so far. In addition, this type of AIF estimate tends to underestimate flow since the signal in the LV blood pool may be "clipped" at the high contrast agent concentrations that occur during the first pass [23]. Two techniques have been proposed to mitigate this problem. The first one utilizes two contrast agent boluses to measure hyperemic flow by perfusion MRI; one bolus is injected at a very low contrast agent concentration to measure the AIF, thereby avoiding "clipping" of the blood pool signal, and then a higher concentration contrast agent bolus is injected in order to achieve an adequate signal response in the myocardial tissue [43]. The second approach requires one single contrast agent injection during hyperemia only, which is an advantage [44]. With this latter technique, the signal in the LV blood pool is measured a very short time interval after a saturation pulse is applied that prevents the magnetization from achieving full relaxation prior to readout. As a result the signal in the LV blood pool is accurately determined even when relatively high contrast agent doses are administered.

When measuring the AIF, in order to save time, the acquisition of blood pool information from the LV can be acquired at a lower spatial resolution. The blood pool acquisition is immediately followed by additional saturation preparations and readouts at high spatial resolution with longer preparation times and readout intervals to obtain the first pass of the bolus passage through the tissue with higher sensitivity (the tissue contrast concentration being lower than in the blood pool). It should be noted that a precise AIF is only one prerequisite for accurate quantification of perfusion. Other factors to consider in the calculation of flow are extravasation of the conventional gadolinium-based contrast agent during the first pass, and proton exchange between the intra- and extravascular compartments, similar to methods employed in DCE elsewhere in the body. These factors are discussed in more detail in Chapters 1 and 4.

Comparison of diagnostic performance of perfusion MRI with nuclear medicine techniques

Using ^{13}N-ammonia PET as a reference standard, first-pass perfusion MRI detected regions of ischemia (i.e., regions with reduced stress perfusion) with a sensitivity and specificity of 91% and 94%, respectively [26]. In the same study, perfusion MRI detected coronary artery stenoses with a diameter reduction of >50% in vessels with a minimal diameter of > 2 mm with a sensitivity and specificity of 87% and 85%, respectively [26]. In an international multicenter perfusion MRI dose-finding study, MRI with a gadolinium dose of 0.1 mmol/kg (n = 41) performed better in a comparison with SPECT (n = 227) [25]. Perfusion MRI with a gadolinium dose of 0.1 mmol/kg also detected >50% diameter stenoses with an AUC of 0.86, versus 0.67 for SPECT (p = 0.013) [26]. This multicenter study ("MR-IMPACT"), performed in 18 centers in Europe and the USA, was not designed to compare perfusion MRI with gated-SPECT, however. Therefore, the "MR-IMPACT II" was conducted in 33 US and European sites to compare perfusion MRI versus gated-SPECT. CXA was used as the reference standard to define CAD (i.e., presence of >50% diameter stenosis). In 425 patients, all three modalities (CXA, perfusion MRI, and SPECT) were performed and entered into the analysis. For MRI and SPECT the dropout rate was 5.6% and 3.7%, respectively (not significantly different), due to inadequate quality as determined by three expert readers. The ROC analysis yielded a higher AUC for the detection of CAD for perfusion MRI than for SPECT (whether gated or ungated) [31].

The better performance of perfusion MRI than SPECT is most likely due to: (1) the higher spatial resolution of perfusion MRI and (2) the lack of attenuation artifacts that may be present on SPECT scans. Perfusion MRI yielded 10–20 times higher volume resolution. The lower spatial resolution of SPECT is further deteriorated by respiratory motion that may be largely avoided with perfusion MRI, as MRI can be performed during a single breath-hold. The high spatial resolution of perfusion MRI particularly increases its sensitivity to detect small subendocardial perfusion deficits. Note that the requirement for breath-hold might in certain cases reduce the performance of perfusion MRI with respect to SPECT, in cases where the patients do not or cannot cooperate. In several studies, the analysis of the subendocardial layer of the myocardium yielded better results for detecting coronary artery stenoses than analysis of the full myocardial wall thickness [23, 24]. The lack of attenuation artifacts in perfusion MRI improves its performance particularly in the inferior wall (e.g., in patients with large abdominal fat mass) or in the anterior wall (e.g., in women). In the MR-IMPACT II study, perfusion MRI performed better than SPECT in both genders [31]. This identifies perfusion MRI as an ideal test for CAD detection, particularly in women. This is important, as CAD appears to be underdiagnosed in women, and the outcome of an MI in women < 50 years is worse than for men. In addition to these considerations, there is evidence that women are more susceptible to ionizing radiation than men [45]. This fact was also corroborated by another study that followed approximately 82 000 patients for 5 years after the first AMI, and examined the occurrence of cancer in relationship to the doses of radiation exposure [46]. Radiation exposure was mainly due to catheterization (with or without PCI of the infarct-related artery), but about one-third of the radiation dose originated from SPECT scans. It was found that there was an increased risk of cancer incidence of 3% over 5 years per incremental exposure of 10 mSv. Hence, it is important in CAD patients to balance the benefit of a diagnostic test with its risks. These results of Eisenberg *et al.* are in close agreement with previous studies, e.g., that of Cardis *et al.*, who followed approximately 500 000 individuals for 10 years [47]. General recommendations about the effects of radiation on biological tissue can be found in reference [45]. Since the sensitivity to radiation is higher at a younger age, minimizing radiation exposure in young adults and particularly in children is important. In a recent study, the first-pass perfusion MRI technique was applied in children and a sensitivity of 87% and a specificity of 95% was achieved for the detection of

>50% diameter stenoses on CXA, indicating it to be a sensitive and specific alternative to CXA without involving any radiation [48].

Other approaches to probe coronary perfusion, CAD, and CFR by MRI

In routine clinical practice, the perfusion techniques mentioned above are generally applied to detect hemodynamically significant coronary artery stenoses. However, atherosclerosis actually begins in young adulthood and develops over many years, or decades, before it causes severe flow-limiting stenoses. Coronary atherosclerosis is thought to progress through repetitive plaque ruptures [49], with one of the first manifestations of CAD being impaired endothelial function. In the intact coronary vessel, increasing flow causes elevated shear stresses that act on the healthy endothelium to stimulate nitric oxide (NO) production, which dilates the vessel in order to adapt to increased flow demand. In a diseased vessel, such as in patients with early atherosclerosis, or even in patients with morphologically intact vessels but several cardiovascular risk factors, the ability of the vessel to react to increased shear stress is reduced and adequate NO production is lacking. This is speculated to trigger further atherosclerosis. For the peripheral vasculature of patients with risk factors, a phase-contrast (PC)-MRA method was developed to measure the reactive hyperemic response (change in blood flow) in the superficial femoral artery after a 4-min occlusion of the lower leg vascular bed [50]. This reactive hyperemic flow is based on a flow-mediated NO production, and this vascular responsiveness was progressively impaired with an increasing number of risk factors. Thus, such a test could be used as a bio-assay in patients to detect and quantify endothelial dysfunction in vivo as an early indicator of atherogenesis. In addition to the conventional risk factors, a negative correlation of the endothelial function with the visceral fat mass was also found. The PC-MRA acquisition technique for this approach was based on spatially selective pulses which restricted signal excitation to a small region, allowing high spatial resolution images to be recorded while still maintaining high temporal resolution [50].

As the influence of risk factors on the coronary circulation is of major clinical interest, endothelial function of the coronary vasculature has also been evaluated by MRI phase-contrast flow measurements.

In order to increase the sensitivity of these flow measurements to detect subtle changes in vascular reactivity, flow to or from a large mass of myocardial tissue should be assessed, which can be achieved by measuring flow in the coronary sinus (CS). The CS drains approximately two-thirds of the entire LV myocardial mass and lies in the atrioventricular groove, draining into the right atrium at the inferior surface of the heart. Also, its dimension of approximately 4–8 mm in diameter makes it an ideal vessel for such measurements. To localize the CS precisely, and to yield adequate temporal and spatial resolution, a navigator-based free-breathing approach is usually applied for these measurements. For accurate flow measurements in this vessel, a high temporal resolution is mandatory as the flow pattern in this vessel is highly pulsatile, as illustrated in Figure 15.4. To increase the navigator efficiency, dedicated algorithms were developed that collect central k-space lines multiple times when the vessel (i.e., the dome of the right hemidiaphragm) is in the central position of the acceptance window (see Figure 15.4). This technique measures CFR with high reproducibility, with differences of $-1.1 \pm 4.9\%$ (absolute differences of -0.21 ± 0.13) at a mean CFR of 2.55 as determined in healthy post-menopausal women [51]. As an example of the use of this technique, a study was designed to investigate whether hormone replacement therapy (HRT, using natural 17β-estradiol) in post-menopausal women can reverse the endothelial dysfunction which typically develops in women after menopause [51]. Previous large observational studies have yielded support for a positive effect of HRT in post-menopausal women to reduce CAD and its complications. However, the phase-contrast MRI study, performed with a double-blind randomized placebo-controlled cross-over design, yielded no evidence that 17β-estradiol substitution could improve or restore CFR (Figure 15.5) [51]. More recent, large prospective randomized HRT trials using clinical endpoints are in line with these MRI results, and currently HRT is not recommended as a treatment to prevent or mitigate CAD in post-menopausal women. As for the peripheral vasculature, CFR measurements in the CS also confirmed the presence of endothelial dysfunction in patients with cardiovascular risk factors and CAD [52]. Another reason for impaired CFR in elderly subjects is the reduction of the vascular density in the coronary circulation of hypertrophied myocardium (Figure 15.1), which reduces the

Motion adapted gating (MAG) and interactive window control "on the fly"

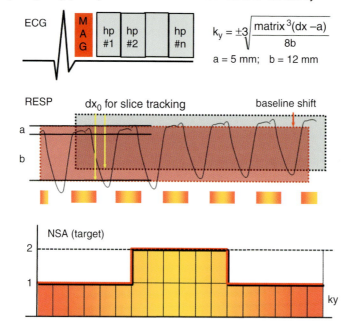

$$k_y = \pm 3 \sqrt{\frac{\text{matrix}^3(dx - a)}{8b}}$$

$a = 5\,\text{mm}; \quad b = 12\,\text{mm}$

Figure 15.4 Schematic illustration of the navigated, cardiac-gated PC-MRA acquisition technique for CS blood flow measurements. Immediately after the R-wave trigger, motion adapted gating (MAG) is applied. Variable phase-encoding gradients are applied according to the displacement (dx) of the diaphragm determined by MAG. Displacements $\leq 5\,\text{mm}$ led to acquisitions for profile $k_y = 0$, while displacements $\leq 12\,\text{mm}$ corresponded to higher k_y values. A target function defined the minimum number of signal averages (NSA (target)) required per k_y value. The acquisition is repeated until the target function is fulfilled.

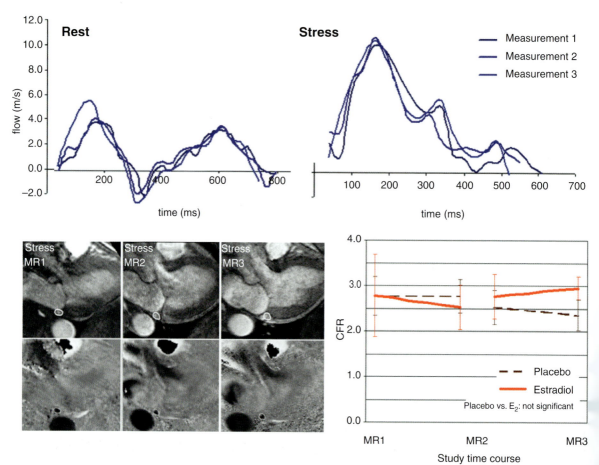

Figure 15.5 Time-resolved CS blood flow profiles at rest and during hyperemic stress are shown on the top row for three different sessions in the same patients, indicating high reproducibility. Image examples for these flow curves are given in the bottom row; the white circles indicate the CS regions used for the flow measurement. In post-menopausal women during placebo and 17β-estradiol treatment, no effect of the hormonal substitution on coronary endothelial function was observed as evidenced by a stable CFR in all patients. Adapted from Schwitter et al. [51]

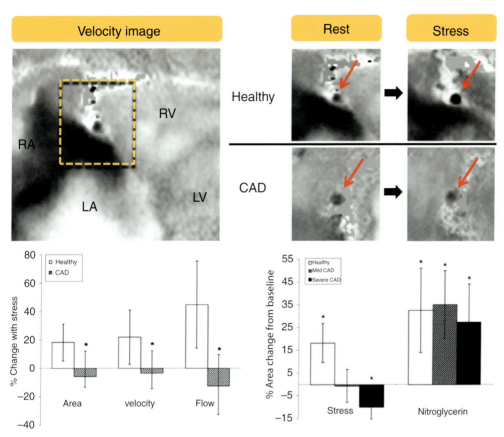

Figure 15.6 Measurements of coronary artery area, flow, and velocity in healthy volunteers and patients with CAD, showing both endothelial-dependent and -independent coronary vasomotion. Velocity images are shown in a healthy volunteer as well as in a patient with known CAD on the top row. During isometric handgrip stress, the vessel diameter in the healthy volunteer increases compared with baseline and maximum velocity also increases, whereas in the CAD patient, vessel diameter decreases slightly, and flow increase is blunted. Group mean results of changes in area, flow, and velocity with isometric handgrip stress for healthy subjects and CAD patients are shown bottom left. In contrast, the panel on the bottom right shows the results of administration of nitroglycerin, an endothelium-independent vasodilator, to healthy volunteers and patients with both mild and severe CAD. With nitroglycerin administration, coronary vessels dilate in both patients and controls, unlike in isometric stress. LA, left atrium; RA, right atrium; RV, right ventricle; LV, left ventricle.

maximum hyperemic flow. Maladaptation of the coronary circulation has been demonstrated by CS flow measurements in patients with LV hypertrophy in the setting of orthotopic heart transplantation[17], as well as in hypertrophic cardiomyopathy [53].

While the phase-contrast MRI approach can evaluate hyperemic flow in the CS that reflects the vasoreactivity of the microvasculature, MRI can also indirectly assess the local ability to produce NO in the conduit vessels. For example, the ability of the superficial femoral artery to dilate in response to a reactive hyperemic stimulus is already largely absent in individuals above 40 years of age with vascular risk factors [51]. However, in the coronary vasculature, vasoreactivity appears to be better preserved. One study used a high-resolution spiral breath-hold acquisition

$(0.89 \times 0.89$ mm in-plane resolution) to measure the coronary artery cross-sectional area at rest as well as during moderate isometric exercise (4 min of handgrip exercise) [54]. Impaired local vasodilatation of the right coronary artery was found in patients with known stenoses in the left anterior descending coronary artery compared with healthy subjects who did not have any stenoses in the coronary vascular tree (Figure 15.6).

Other MRI-based approaches to assess myocardial perfusion: research studies

The techniques discussed in this section are still under development and are not yet considered mature enough to be used for clinical decision-making in patients.

Blood oxygenation level-dependent (BOLD) imaging

While oxygenated hemoglobin is slightly diamagnetic, deoxygenated hemoglobin is paramagnetic and therefore shortens the T_2 and $T_2{}^*$ relaxation times of both blood and tissue containing deoxyhemoglobin within its microvasculature. Consequently, differences in the tissue content of oxygenated blood can be estimated from T_2- or $T_2{}^*$-weighted pulse sequences. During hyperemic conditions induced by pharmacological vasodilators, oxygen extraction will be lower in these hyperemic territories, while extraction will be higher (and the content of oxygenated blood lower) in tissue supplied by stenotic vessels. Initial work demonstrated that changes could be seen in the signal intensity of the myocardium following dipyridamole infusion using $T_2{}^*$-weighted imaging [55]. While in an experimental setting flow may increase during vasodilatation up to 4-fold, signal differences in normally perfused regions versus hyperemic regions were reported to be as low as 32% [56]. Similarly, in another study, a 100% increase in flow yielded a signal increase of only 5% (equal to a change in myocardial relaxation rate [R_2] of $0.94 \, \mathrm{s}^{-1}$ per unit change in flow) [57]. This limitation in signal difference is a significant limitation, since first-pass contrast agent-based studies suggested several hundred percent signal change is required for reliable stenosis detection [24]. Another limitation is that the BOLD approach is also sensitive to magnetic field inhomogeneities, which typically occur in the posterior wall close to the CS, which drains deoxygenated blood.

Arterial spin labeling (ASL)

Various approaches to ASL are described in detail in Chapter 3. In the heart, ASL is often performed based on the apparent shortening of the tissue T_1 relaxation times as unsaturated water spins enter the heart [58]. ECG-triggered T_1 measurements are performed after both global and slice-selective spin preparation, and absolute tissue perfusion is then calculated by assuming a two-compartment model [59]. This technique relies on accurate local registration of both acquisitions, which is difficult to achieve in the beating heart, so there have been comparatively few cardiac ASL studies reported in humans to date [60], in spite of the larger perfusion present in the cardiac muscle compared with the brain.

Hyperpolarized contrast agent techniques

While BOLD imaging is somewhat limited by the very small changes in signal that relate to changes in flow, recently it has been shown that hyperpolarization of nuclei other than protons boosts the perfusion signal dramatically [61]. In particular, carbon-13 (^{13}C) in various molecules can be hyperpolarized by dynamic nuclear polarization (DNP), and during a relatively short period of time of 1–2 min (depending on the T_1 of the hyperpolarized compound), a signal up to 10 000 times higher than in conventional ^{1}H MRI can be obtained [61]. Recently, hyperpolarized ^{13}C perfusion MRI was demonstrated to be feasible in the pig heart [62]. In addition, this technique theoretically allows for absolute quantification of perfusion, as the signal received is proportional to the amount of ^{13}C-compound as long as the calculation accounts for the T_1 decay of the hyperpolarized magnetization. The hyperpolarized signal is also strong enough even to allow for near real-time spectroscopic measurements of the heart muscle, and this technology will most likely represent the key application for metabolic heart studies in the future [63].

Safety aspects and contraindications for perfusion MRI examinations

In addition to the general contraindications that apply to MR examinations, some additional safety issues must be considered in order to perform cardiac MRI perfusion safely. Stress-test MRI involves the creation of hyperemia by administration of pharmacological vasodilators such as adenosine, regadenoson, ATP, or dipyridamole. These typically do not induce ischemia, since a steal effect is only provoked by these vasodilators in myocardium supplied by severely stenosed coronary arteries (in the order of 80–90% or higher). However, atrioventricular (AV)-block 2 and 3 or bronchospasm can occur during vasodilatory infusion. Therefore, a prior AV-block 1 or higher, as well as a history of asthma or pulmonary arterial hypertension, are contraindications for vasodilators. During stress MRI, i.e., during drug infusion and during the recovery period, continuous monitoring of heart rate, respiration, blood pressure, and heart rhythm is required. Also, adequate equipment must be available at the MRI site to perform emergency treatment if needed. Finally, during stress MRI examinations experienced personnel trained in basic and advanced life support should be present, who can manage cardiac and/or respiratory arrest. When these precautions are observed, this type of MR examination is very safe, as has been demonstrated in several multicenter perfusion trials [25, 26]. An excellent safety profile of perfusion MRI was also documented in the European MRI registry [30].

Unlike perfusion MRI with vasodilator infusions, perfusion MRI using dobutamine as the stressor may induce ischemia in patients with CAD, which results in regional hypokinesia that can be detected by functional cine MRI. Thus, dobutamine stress MRI frequently causes angina and/or dyspnea in patients with CAD. There is also a certain risk for tachyarrhythmia or even ventricular fibrillation during inotropic stimulation using dobutamine. Therefore, the frequency of side effects and complications is somewhat higher for dobutamine stress MRI [64, 65].

As for any MR examination, electronic devices are contraindicated. Here, a special note should be added as an increasing number of cardiac patients are also implanted with pacemakers (PMs) or implanted cardioverter-defibrillators (ICDs). During the past years, large efforts have been put into the development of MR-compatible devices, and a few MR-compatible PMs and leads are now available on the market. These devices were tested in large trials that resulted in the European Medicines Agency (EMEA) and US Food and Drug Administration (FDA) approval [66]. For ICDs, MR-compatible devices with regulatory approval are not yet available.

Data on the safety of coronary stents are rather scarce. In one study, no adverse effects were noted when MRI was performed within 1 week of stent implantation [67]. In general, coronary stents are considered safe in the MR environment at least for 1.5 T, although official FDA or EMEA approval is lacking. Similarly, most heart valves are considered safe for MR examinations. For valves and other devices, information is often available from the manufacturers, or from the literature [28].

Recommended protocols/analysis techniques for specific indications

A prerequisite for a successful diagnostic perfusion MRI study is adequate quality of the MRI data. Several parameters have been tested regarding their influence on image quality, such as saturation recovery time, readout flip angle, cardiac coverage [24], and

the contrast agent dose [25, 26]. Protocols and parameter settings are given in the literature [28, 29] as well as in Table 15.2. Powerful acceleration strategies-based parallel MRI acquisition techniques have been developed in recent years (exploiting coil sensitivities and spatio-temporal correlations) which allow for excellent spatial resolution (on the order of 1×1 mm in plane) [27, 68]. These techniques have not yet been tested in larger cohorts, however, and comparative studies versus "conventional" acquisition techniques are relatively scarce. Nevertheless, as long as parameters are achieved as given in Table 15.2, these novel techniques are likely to yield similar diagnostic results and good image quality.

Analyses of perfusion data can be either visual or quantitative, where the quantitative approach can be either "absolute" or relative, i.e., quantification based on perfusion-related parameters such as signal upslope during first pass, contrast agent arrival time, time-to-peak signal, mean transit time, area under the signal intensity–time curve, and others. The "upslope" technique has been applied in many single center studies [23, 24] and also proved high diagnostic performance for the detection of CAD in a multicenter trial as well [25]. The visual approach also proved diagnostically useful in CAD detection, and was superior to the diagnostic performance of SPECT performed in the same patients [26]. Conversely, a fully quantitative analysis yielding perfusion estimates in ml/100 g tissue/min has been applied in several single center studies [43, 44], but its diagnostic performance in a multicenter setting has not yet been evaluated.

How to perform perfusion MRI: recommendations

In order to minimize artifacts in perfusion MRI data and to ensure sufficient signal sensitivity to contrast agent concentration, i.e., to provide a large dynamic range of signal response in the myocardium during first pass, several aspects of the acquisition are crucial. In order to reduce motion-associated artifacts, the readout acquisition window should be < 150 ms per slice, the pulse sequence ECG-triggered, and acquisitions should occur in mid-late systole and mid-diastole (so as to avoid cardiac phases with rapid motion, e.g., early systole, early diastole, or late diastole during atrial contraction). One acquisition (i.e., a stack of 3–5 short-axis slices) every 1–2 heart beats

Table 15.2. Cardiac MR applications

MR Modality	Types of diagnoses possible	Parameters	Time
Localizer images	Aortic dissection Aortic aneurysm Pleural effusion Large pneumonia Intrathoracic masses Congenital heart diseases ARVC	fGRE sequences or SSFP sequences fGRE with and without fat saturation (to detect or exclude fatty infiltration in ARVC)	1–2 min
Cine MRI	Global LV or RV function abnormalities Regional wall motion abnormalities Hypertrophic cardiomyopathy LV aneurysms Pericardial effusion Valve abnormalities (valve orifice) Congenital heart diseases	Spatial resolution: 1–2 mm × 1–2 mm Temporal resolution: 40–60 ms Preferred sequence type: SSFP Slice thickness: 6–10 mm, gap 0–2 mm	5–10 min
Stress perfusion MRI Hyperemia: – Adenosine: 0.14 mg/kg/min for 3 min – Dipyridamole: 0.56 mg/kg for 4 min CM: 0.075–0.10 mmol/kg injected at 5 ml/s into antecubital vein	Ischemia detection: – Stress-induced perfusion deficit (adenosine, dipyridamole) – Stress-induced segmental dysfunction (cine MRI with dobutamine) Detection of CAD Workup of patients with known CAD for treatment decisions Workup of patients after CABG Risk stratification in CAD	Spatial resolution: at least 2–3 mm × 2–3 mm to minimize susceptibility artifacts along the blood pool–myocardial interface Temporal resolution: 1 short-axis stack/1–2 beats Acquisition window/slice: < 100 ms to minimize cardiac motion artifacts Signal increase during first pass: >250–300% 90°-preparation delay time: 100–150 ms/slice Coverage: ≥3 short-axis slices Slice thickness of 8–10 mm	10 min
Dobutamine stress MRI Dobutamine doses of 10/20/30/40 µg/kg (for 3 min each). Atropine up to 2 mg is added, if target heart rate (220 – age) is not reached.		Sequence: see cine MRI 3 short-axis and 3 long-axis acquisitions per dose of dobutamine	10–20 min
Rest perfusion	Rest myocardial ischemia/abnormal perfusion Microvascular obstruction Tumor (differentiation vs. thrombus)	Sequence: see stress perfusion MRI	1 min
Late gadolinium enhancement (LGE)	MI Myocardial fibrosis Myocarditis Various non-ischemic cardiomyopathies Thrombus Amyloidosis	Spatial resolution: 1.5–2.0 mm × 1.5–2.0 mm Preferred sequence type: segmented inversion recovery (IR) fGRE Slice thickness: 5–8 mm, gap 0–4 mm CM: 0.15–0.2 mmol/kg IV Start of imaging: 10–20 min after CM injection	5–15 min

MRI provides a multi-modal integrated assessment of patients with suspected CAD, possible or definite ACS, and CHF. Selection of different imaging modalities should be customized to the likely diagnoses and individualized to a given patient. Time estimates are rough estimates. ACS, acute, coronary syndrome; ARVC arrhythmogenic right ventricular cardiomyopathy; CABG, coronary artery bypass grafting; CHF, congestive heart failure; CM, contrast medium; fGRE, fast gradient echo; SSFP, steady-state free precession.

is sufficient with respect to temporal resolution [25, 26, 28, 31]. The patient should be instructed to hold his/her breath during the first pass to avoid any breathing-related artifacts. A high-quality ECG is key to guarantee correct triggering during first pass. To minimize susceptibility artifacts (e.g., in the subendocardium), a high spatial resolution of 1.5–2.5 mm in-plane (slice thickness 8–10 mm) is needed. Finally, a bolus of 0.075–0.1 mmol/kg IV of a conventional gadolinium-based contrast agent is recommended [26] to achieve a signal increase in the myocardium of 250–300% above the baseline pre-contrast myocardial signal [24–26]. More details on perfusion MRI protocols are available elsewhere [28]. These protocol recommendations are derived from large multicenter trials and their implementation should yield results comparable to the large trials (e.g., MR-IMPACT I and II) [25, 26, 28].

Conclusions

Perfusion MRI exploits the first-pass dynamics of conventional gadolinium-based contrast agents to detect myocardial ischemia. As coronary autoregulation tends to match myocardial perfusion (oxygen demand) over a wide range of perfusion pressures, detection of ischemic myocardial territories requires the administration of pharmacological vasodilators.

This test has been demonstrated to be safe in large studies performed at experienced sites that are properly equipped to perform the procedures.

Perfusion MRI has been shown to have high diagnostic accuracy. Its excellent spatial resolution allows the detection of small subendocardial perfusion deficits. As perfusion MRI is free of any attenuation artifacts, it delivers high-quality perfusion information in most patients, even in the posterior wall. There is also increasing evidence that patients without ischemic findings on perfusion MRI generally have an excellent prognosis.

Large multicenter trials have also proven perfusion MRI to be superior to SPECT. Therefore, it is an ideal test to confirm or exclude the presence of CAD, particularly in women and young adults, as these patient groups are particularly susceptible to radiation exposure. Due to its lack of radiation exposure, perfusion MRI can be applied repeatedly in the same patient, which is ideal to monitor CAD activity e.g., before and after revascularization procedures, or in patients with progressive disease.

Finally, perfusion MRI aids in the characterization of cardiac masses, specifically to differentiate tumors from thrombi, and advanced MRI applications can also assess coronary vasomotion and endothelial function in the coronary vascular bed.

References

1. Lloyd-Jones D, Adams R, Carnethon M, et al. American Heart Association Statistics Committee and Stroke Statistics Subcommittee. Heart disease and stroke statistics – 2009 update: report from the American Heart Association Statistics Committee and Stroke Statistics Subcommittee. *Circulation* 2009;**119**.

2. Volmink J, Newton J, Hicks N, et al. Coronary event and case fatality rates in an English population: results of the Oxford myocardial infarction incidence study. The Oxford Myocardial Infarction Incidence Study Group. *Heart* 1998;**80**:40–4.

3. Savonitto S, Ardissino D, Granger C, et al. Prognostic value of the admission electrocardiogram in acute coronary syndromes. *JAMA* 1999;**281**: 707–13.

4. Hachamovitch R, Rozanski A, Shaw L, et al. Impact of ischaemia and scar on the therapeutic benefit derived from myocardial revascularization vs. medical therapy among patients undergoing stress-rest myocardial perfusion scintigraphy. *Eur Heart J* 2011;**32**:1012–24.

5. Schwitter J. Future strategies in the management of coronary artery disease. *Fut Cardiol* 2006;**2**(5):555–65.

6. Kwong RY, Chan AK, Brown KA, et al. Impact of unrecognized myocardial scar detected by cardiac magnetic resonance imaging on event-free survival in patients presenting with signs or symptoms of coronary artery disease. *Circulation* 2006; **113**(23):2733–43.

7. Allman K, Shaw L, Hachamovitch R, Udelson J. Myocardial viability testing and impact of revascularization on prognosis in patients with coronary artery disease and left ventricular dysfunction: a meta-analysis. *J Am Coll Cardiol* 2002;**39**:1151–8.

8. Beanlands RS, Ruddy TD, deKemp RA, et al. Positron emission tomography and recovery following

revascularization (PARR-1): the importance of scar and the development of a prediction rule for the degree of recovery of left ventricular function. *J Am Coll Cardiol* 2002;**40**(10):1735–43.

9. Bonow RO, Maurer G, Lee KL, *et al.* Myocardial viability and survival in ischemic left ventricular dysfunction. *N Engl J Med* 2011;**364**(17):1617–25.

10. Wagner A, Mahrholdt H, Holly TA, *et al.* Contrast-enhanced MRI and routine single photon emission computed tomography (SPECT) perfusion imaging for detection of subendocardial myocardial infarcts: an imaging study. *Lancet* 2003;**361** (9355):374–9.

11. Iskander S, Iskandrian AE. Risk assessment using single-photon emission computed tomographic technetium-99m sestamibi imaging. *J Am Coll Cardiol* 1998;**32**(1):57–62.

12. Jahnke C, Nagel E, Gebker R, *et al.* Prognostic value of cardiac magnetic resonance stress tests: adenosine stress perfusion and dobutamine stress wall motion imaging. *Circulation* 2007;**115**:1769–76.

13. Steel K, Broderick R, Gandla V, *et al.* Complementary prognostic values of stress myocardial perfusion and late gadolinium enhancement imaging by cardiac magnetic resonance in patients with known or suspected coronary artery disease. *Circulation* 2009;**120**:1390–400.

14. Hundley WG, Morgan TM, Neagle CM, *et al.* Magnetic resonance imaging determination of cardiac prognosis. *Circulation* 2002;**106**(18):2328–33.

15. Hoffman JIE, Spaan JAE. Pressure-flow relations in coronary circulation. *Physiol Rev* 1990;**70**:331–90.

16. Mosher P, Ross JJ, McFate P, Shaw R. Control of coronary blood flow by an autoregulatory mechanism. *Circ Res* 1964;**14**:250–9.

17. Schwitter J, DeMarco T, Kneifel S, *et al.* Magnetic resonance-based assessment of global coronary flow and flow reserve and its relation to left ventricular functional parameters: a comparison with positron emission tomography. *Circulation* 2000;**101**(23):2696–702.

18. Tomanek R, Palmer P, Pfeiffer G, *et al.* Morphometry of canine coronary arteries, arterioles and capillaries during hypertension and left ventricular hypertrophy. *Circ Res* 1986;**58**:38–46.

19. Uren N, Melin J, De Bruyne B, *et al.* Relation between myocardial blood flow and the severity of coronary artery stenosis. *N Engl J Med* 1994;**330**:1782–8.

20. Picano E, Parodi O, Lattanzi F, *et al.* Assessment of anatomic and physiological severity of single-vessel coronary artery lesions by dipyridamole echocardiography. Comparison with positron emission tomography and quantitative arteriography. *Circulation* 1994;**89**:753–61.

21. Di Carli MF, Czernin J, Hoh C, *et al.* Relation among stenosis severity, myocardial blood flow, and flow reserve in patients with coronary artery disease. *Circulation* 1995;**91**:1944–51.

22. Sambuceti G, Parodi O, Marcassa C, *et al.* Alterations in regulation of myocardial blood flow in one-vessel coronary artery disease determined by positron emission tomography. *Am J Cardiol* 1993;**72**:538–43.

23. Schwitter J, Nanz D, Kneifel S, *et al.* Assessment of myocardial perfusion in coronary artery disease by magnetic resonance: a comparison with positron emission tomography and coronary angiography. *Circulation* 2001;**103**(18):2230–5.

24. Bertschinger KM, Nanz D, Buechi M, *et al.* Magnetic resonance myocardial first-pass perfusion imaging: parameter optimization for signal response and cardiac coverage. *J Magn Reson Imaging* 2001;**14**(5):556–62.

25. Giang T, Nanz D, Coulden R, *et al.* Detection of coronary artery disease by magnetic resonance myocardial perfusion imaging with various contrast medium doses: first European multicenter experience. *Eur Heart J* 2004;**25**:1657–65.

26. Schwitter J, Wacker C, van Rossum A, *et al.* MR-IMPACT: comparison of perfusion-cardiac magnetic resonance with single-photon emission computed tomography for the detection of coronary artery disease in a multicentre, multivendor, randomized trial. *Eur Heart J* 2008;**29**:480–9.

27. Plein S, Kozerke S, Suerder D, *et al.* High spatial resolution myocardial perfusion cardiac magnetic resonance for the detection of coronary artery disease. *Eur Heart J* 2008; **29**:2148–55.

28. Schwitter J. *CMR Update*, 2nd edn. Lausanne: Schwitter, J. 2012; Available from www.herz-mri.ch (accessed November 19, 2012).

29. Schwitter J, Arai A. Imaging: assessment of cardiac ischaemia and viability: role of cardiovascular magnetic resonance. *Eur Heart J* 2011;**32**:799–809.

30. Bruder O, Schneider S, Nothnagel D, *et al.* EuroCMR (European Cardiovascular Magnetic Resonance) Registry. *J Am Coll Cardiol* 2009;**54**:1457–66.

31. Schwitter J, Wacker CM, Wilke N, *et al.* Superior diagnostic performance of perfusion-cardiovascular magnetic resonance versus SPECT to detect coronary artery disease: the

secondary endpoints of the multicenter multivendor MR-IMPACT II (Magnetic Resonance Imaging for Myocardial Perfusion Assessment in Coronary Artery Disease Trial). *J. Cardiovasc Magn Reson* 2012;**14**:61–71.

32. Nagel E, Klein C, Paetsch I, *et al.* Magnetic resonance perfusion measurements for the noninvasive detection of coronary artery disease. *Circulation* 2003; **108**(4):432–7.

33. Plein S, Radjenovic A, Ridgway JP, *et al.* Coronary artery disease: myocardial perfusion MR imaging with sensitivity encoding versus conventional angiography. *Radiology* 2005;**235**(2):423–30.

34. Paetsch I, Jahnke C, Wahl A, *et al.* Comparison of dobutamine stress magnetic resonance, adenosine stress magnetic resonance, and adenosine stress magnetic resonance perfusion. *Circulation* 2004;**110**(7):835–42.

35. Kwong R, Schussheim A, Rekhraj S, *et al.* Detecting acute coronary syndrome in the emergency department with cardiac magnetic resonance imaging. *Circulation* 2003;**107**:531–7.

36. Ingkanisorn WP, Kwong RY, Bohme NS, *et al.* Prognosis of negative adenosine stress magnetic resonance in patients presenting to an emergency department with chest pain. *J Am Coll Cardiol* 2006;**47**(7):1427–32.

37. Plein S, Greenwood J, Ridgeway J, *et al.* Assessment of non-ST-segment elevation acute coronary syndromes with cardiac magnetic resonance imaging. *J Am Coll Cardiol* 2004;**44**:2173–81.

38. Hoffmann U, Globits S, Schima W, *et al.* Usefulness of magnetic resonance imaging of cardiac and paracardiac masses. *Am J Cardiol* 2003;**92**(7):890–5.

39. Schuler P, Weber A, Bode P, *et al.* MRI of intimal sarcoma of the

pulmonary arteries. *Circ Cardiovasc Imaging* 2009;**2**:e37–9.

40. Fussen S, De Boeck BWL, Zellweger MJ, *et al.* Cardiovascular magnetic resonance imaging for diagnosis and clinical management of suspected cardiac masses and tumours. *Eur Heart J* 2011; **32**(12):1551–60.

41. Srichai MB, Junor C, Rodriguez LL, *et al.* Clinical, imaging, and pathological characteristics of left ventricular thrombus: a comparison of contrast-enhanced magnetic resonance imaging, transthoracic echocardiography, and transesophageal echocardiography with surgical or pathological validation. *Am Heart J* 2006;**152**(1):75–84.

42. Knuesel PR, Nanz D, Wyss C, *et al.* Characterization of dysfunctional myocardium by positron emission tomography and magnetic resonance: relation to functional outcome after revascularization. *Circulation* 2003;**108**(9):1095–100.

43. Christian TF, Rettmann DW, Aletras AH, *et al.* Absolute myocardial perfusion in canines measured by using dual-bolus first-pass MR imaging. *Radiology* 2004;**232**(3):677–84.

44. Gatehouse PD, Elkington AG, Ablitt NA, *et al.* Accurate assessment of the arterial input function during high-dose myocardial perfusion cardiovascular magnetic resonance. *J Magn Reson Imaging* 2004;**20**(1):39–45.

45. Biological effects of ionizing radiation (BEIR) reports VII-Phase 2. National Research Council. Available from: www.nap.edu/catalog/11340.html (accessed November 19, 2012).

46. Eisenberg M, Afilalo J, Lawler P, *et al.* Cancer risk related to low-dose ionizing radiation from cardiac imaging in patients after acute myocardial

infarction. *CMAJ* 2011; **183**:430–6.

47. Cardis E, Vrijheid M, Blettner M, *et al.* Risk of cancer after low doses of ionising radiation: retrospective cohort study in 15 countries. *Br Med J* 2005;**331**:77–82.

48. Buechel ER, Balmer C, Bauersfeld U, Kellenberger CJ, Schwitter J. Feasibility of perfusion cardiovascular magnetic resonance in paediatric patients. *J Cardiovasc Magn Reson* 2009;**11**:51.

49. Burke A, Kolodgie F, Farb A, *et al.* Healed plaque ruptures and sudden coronary death: evidence that subclinical rupture has a role in plaque progression. *Circulation* 2001;**103**:934–40.

50. Schwitter J, Oelhafen M, Wyss BM, *et al.* 2D-spatially-selective real-time magnetic resonance imaging for the assessment of microvascular function and its relation to the cardiovascular risk profile. *J Cardiovasc Magn Reson* 2006;**8**(5):759–69.

51. Schwitter J, Kozerke S, Bremerich J, *et al.* Oral administration of 17beta-estradiol over 3 months without progestin co-administration does not improve coronary flow reserve in post-menopausal women: a randomized placebo-controlled cross-over CMR study. *J Cardiovasc Magn Reson* 2007;**9**:665–72.

52. Koskenvuo J, Hartiala J, Knuuti J, *et al.* Assessing coronary sinus blood flow in patients with coronary artery disease *AJR Am J Roentgenol* 2001;**177**:1161–6.

53. Kawada N, Sakuma H, Yamakado T, *et al.* Hypertrophic cardiomyopathy: MR measurement of coronary blood flow and vasodilator flow reserve in patients and healthy subjects. *Radiology* 1999;**211**:129–35.

54. Hays A, Hirsch G, Kelle S, *et al.* Noninvasive visualization of

317

coronary artery endothelial function in healthy subjects and in patients with coronary artery disease. *J Am Coll Cardiol* 2010;**56**:1657–65.

55. Niemi P, Poncelet BP, Kwong KK, *et al.* Myocardial intensity changes associated with flow stimulation in blood oxygenation sensitive magnetic resonance imaging. *Magn Reson Med* 1996;**36**:78–82.

56. Fieno DS, Shea SM, Li Y, *et al.* Myocardial perfusion imaging based on the blood oxygen level-dependent effect using T2-prepared steady-state free-precession magnetic resonance imaging. *Circulation* 2004;**110**:1284–90.

57. Wright K, Klocke F, Deshpande V, *et al.* Assessment of regional differences in myocardial blood flow using T2-weighted 3D BOLD imaging. *Magn Reson Med* 2001;**46**:573–8.

58. Reeder S, Atalay M, McVeigh E, Zerhouni E, Forder J. Quantitative cardiac perfusion: a noninvasive spin-labeling method that exploits coronary vessel geometry. *Radiology* 1996;**200**:177–84.

59. Belle V, Kahler E, Waller C, *et al.* In vivo quantitative mapping of cardiac perfusion in rats using a noninvasive MR spin-labeling method. *J Magn Reson Imaging* 1998;**8**:1240–5.

60. McCommis KS, Zhang H, Herrero P, Grapler RJ, Zheng J. Feasibility study of myocardial perfusion and oxygenation by noncontrast MRI: comparison with PET study in a canine model. *Magn Reson Imaging* 2008;**26**:11–19.

61. Golman K, Ardenkjaer-Larsen JH, Petersson JS, Mansson S, Leunbach I. Molecular imaging with endogenous substances. *Proc Natl Acad Sci U S A* 2003;**100**(18):10435–9.

62. Schwitter J. Myocardial perfusion imaging by cardiac magnetic resonance. *J Nucl Cardiol* 2006;**13**(6):841–54.

63. Schwitter J. Extending the frontiers of cardiac magnetic resonance. *Circulation* 2008;**118**:109–12.

64. Wahl A, Paetsch I, Gollesch A, *et al.* Safety and feasibility of high-dose dobutamine-atropine stress cardiovascular magnetic resonance for diagnosis of myocardial ischaemia: experience in 1000 consecutive cases. *Eur Heart J* 2004;**25**(14):1230–6.

65. Hundley WG, Hamilton CA, Thomas MS, *et al.* Utility of fast cine magnetic resonance imaging and display for the detection of myocardial ischemia in patients not well suited for second harmonic stress echocardiography. *Circulation* 1999;**100**(16):1697–702.

66. Wilkoff BL, Bello D, Taborsky M, *et al.* Magnetic resonance imaging in patients with a pacemaker system designed for the magnetic resonance environment. *Heart Rhythm* 2011;**8**(1):65–73.

67. Syed MA, Carlson K, Murphy M. Long-term safety of cardiac magnetic resonance imaging performed in the first few days after bare-metal stent implantation. *J Magn Reson Imaging* 2006;**24**(5):1056–61.

68. Kellman P, Derbyshire J, Agyeman K, McVeigh E, Arai A. Extended coverage first-pass perfusion imaging using slice-interleaved TSENSE. *Magn Reson Med* 2004;**51**:200–4.

69. Zaret BL, Rigo P, Wackers FJ, *et al.* Myocardial perfusion imaging with 99mTc tetrofosmin. Comparison to 201Tl imaging and coronary angiography in a phase III multicenter trial. Tetrofosmin International Trial Study Group. *Circulation* 1995;**91**:313–19.

70. Van Train KF, Garcia EV, Maddahi J, *et al.* Multicenter trial validation for quantitative analysis of same-day, rest-stress technetium-99m-sestamibi myocardial tomograms. *J Nucl Med* 1994;**35**:609–18.

71. Hendel RC, Berman DS, Cullon SJ, *et al.* Multicenter clinical trial to evaluate the efficacy of correction for photon attenuation and scatter in SPECT myocardial perfusion imaging. *Circulation* 1999;**99**:2742–9.

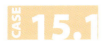

Cardiac stress perfusion MRI in a patient with exertional angina

History

A 63-year-old patient presented with a stable exertional angina (CCS grade II) and coronary artery bypass grafting (CABG) performed 16 years ago. There were no resting ECG changes, and stress ECG was clinically and electrocardiographically normal at maximal stress. Coronary angiography (Figures 15.7a and b) was performed and demonstrated a patent left internal mammary artery (LIMA) with both vein grafts occluded. The left anterior descending artery (LAD) was proximally occluded. The left circumflex artery (LCX) showed a severe proximal and mid-vessel stenosis (a, open arrows). The right coronal artery (RCA) had a distal 70% stenosis and 70% stenosis of a postero-lateral branch (b, open arrows). The RCA gave collaterals to the LCX and intermediate branch of the left coronary system. A patent vein graft segment that connects the LCX territory with the anterior wall of the LV was visualized. Global LV function was normal with an ejection fraction of 73% and a minimal anterior hypokinesia. Surgical revascularization was recommended due the complexity and multiplicity of the coronary artery stenoses.

Technique

A second opinion was obtained and a stress perfusion MRI study was performed to evaluate the extent of ischemic territories in this patient.

Image findings

The perfusion MRI (Figure 15.7c) study demonstrated a large ischemic region in the lateral wall of the LV extending into the anterior wall (open arrow heads), but no inferior ischemia was noted. A small basal-mid anterior subendocardial scar was observed on late gadolinium enhancement (arrows, bottom row).

Discussion

It was decided to revascularize the lateral wall with the assumption that the remaining graft between the first obtuse marginal branch and the intermediate should improve anterior wall perfusion. A percutaneous intervention (PCI) was judged to be suitable since no revascularization of the RCA and LAD was necessary.

Revascularization of the LCX was achieved by stenting of the mid-vessel stenosis and dilatation of the left main with a rotablator, and consequent stenting of the

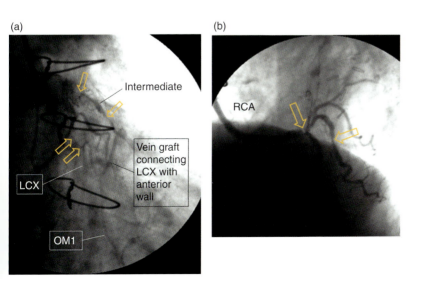

Figure 15.7 (a, b) Coronary angiogram, (c) stress-perfusion MRI at presentation, and (d) at follow-up.

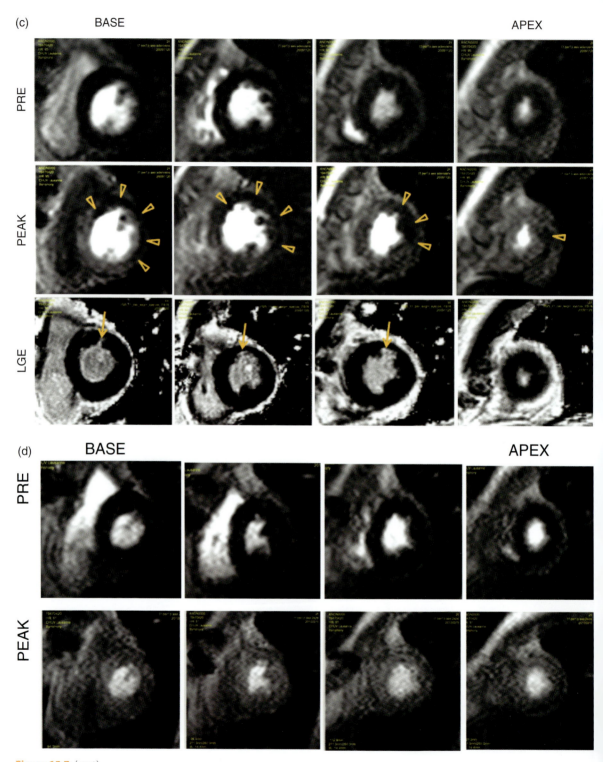

Figure 15.7 *(cont.)*

ostial LCX. A control stress perfusion MRI study performed 3 months later demonstrated intact perfusion in both the lateral and anterior LV wall (Figure 15.7d). The small subendocardial scar in the mid-anterior wall remained unchanged, and the patient was asymptomatic.

Key points

- ECG stress test is probably insufficient for ischemia assessment after CABG: stress imaging is recommended.

- Accurate assessment of myocardial viability and the distribution of inducible perfusion defects with MRI is of great value, especially in case of complex coronary lesions.
- MRI adds a functional assessment to the morphological picture provided by angiography, allowing better targeting of PCI, and avoiding unnecessary, potentially dangerous re-operations.

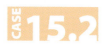

Cardiac stress perfusion MRI in a patient with stenoses of the left main coronary and anterior descending arteries

History

A 70-year-old woman presented to the emergency room with increasing recurrent pain in the lower left abdominal quadrant, of 6 weeks duration, with nausea and vomiting, loss of appetite, and a 20-kg weight loss over 3 months. Cardiovascular risk factors included arterial hypertension and heavy smoking. Resting ECG was normal and troponins were slightly elevated (0.21 mcg/l; normal <0.04). A diagnostic coronary angiogram (Figures 15.8a–c) revealed borderline significant stenoses of the left main (LM) and proximal LAD (filled red arrows in (a) and (b)), a sub-occlusion of the LCX (large open red arrow, (a)) with collaterals from the RCA. The RCA had only minor plaques without stenosis (c).

Technique

In order to assess the extent of ischemia a stress perfusion MRI study was performed.

Imaging findings

LV ejection fraction was supra-normal (73%) and without regional wall motion abnormalities. A septal hypertrophy of 14 mm was noted. No necrosis or scar tissue was detected on late gadolinium enhancement images. Perfusion MRI (Figure 15.8d) demonstrated a large ischemic territory in the lateral wall and anterior wall of the LV (open arrowheads).

Discussion

Due to the extensive ischemia in the anterior and lateral wall of the LV, the patient was sent for CABG. Further investigations for weight loss revealed a carcinoma of the oral mucosa with local metastasis to the inferior maxilla, without lung or liver metastasis. A duodenal ulcer was also diagnosed (*Helicobacter pylori* positive) without bleeding. The patient was referred for oncological surgery.

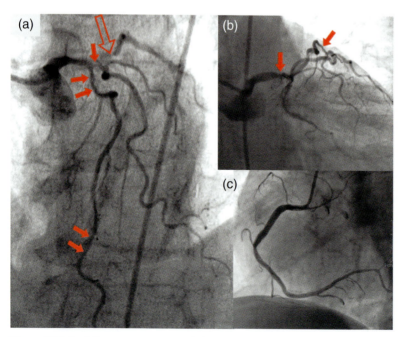

Figure 15.8 (a–c) Coronary angiogram and (d) stress-perfusion MRI.

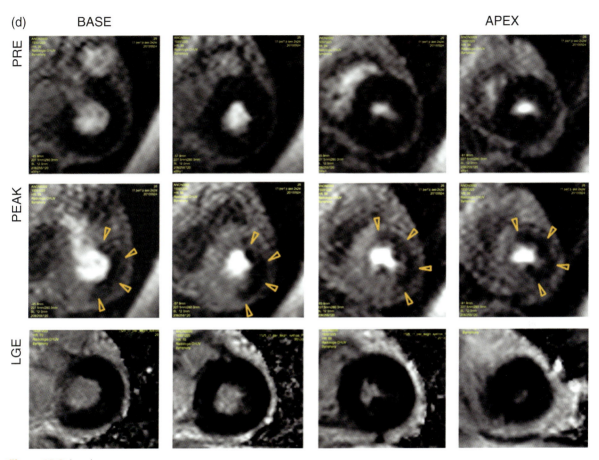

Figure 15.8 *(cont.)*

- Atypical acute coronary syndrome presentation with lower abdominal pain may be possible, especially in women.

- Angiographically borderline significant stenoses in series (LM and LAD, both <50%) may be hemodynamically significant and are well detected with perfusion MRI.

323

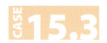
Cardiac stress perfusion MRI detects subtle ischemia in a patient with a stenosis of a branch of the left anterior descending artery

History

A 66-year-old female patient presented with atypical chest pain and dyspnea (NYHA class II) during physical exercise. Resting ECG showed a slight ST-segment depression in leads V3–V5. Troponins were negative. Cardiovascular risk factors included hypercholesterolemia, as well as smoking.

Technique

A stress perfusion MRI study was performed.

Imaging findings

Perfusion MRI demonstrated a distinct ischemic territory in the antero-lateral wall of the LV (Figure 15.9a), not involving the inter-ventricular septum

(a)

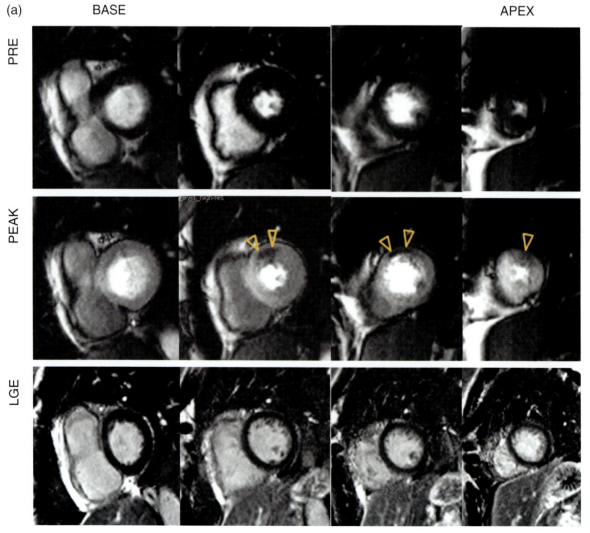

Figure 15.9 (a) Stress-perfusion MRI and (b–d) coronary angiogram.

Post-PCI Pre-PCI Pre-PCI

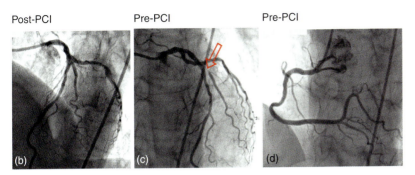

Figure 15.9 *(cont.)*

(open arrowheads). This finding was suggestive of a severe stenosis in an LAD branch.

Discussion

Coronary angiography (Figures 15.9b–d) then confirmed CAD with a severe stenosis of the first diagonal branch (b, open red arrow), which was successfully treated by PCI in the same session (d). The RCA was normal (c).

- Perfusion MRI is a sensitive test that can detect subtle ischemia corresponding to lesions in small coronary arteries.
- In patients with cardiovascular risk factors, even with atypical symptoms, a search for myocardial ischemia should be initiated to detect CAD in early stages.

MR perfusion imaging in pediatrics

Neel Madan and P. Ellen Grant

Key points

- Pediatric brains show perfusion changes with normal and abnormal development.
- Hyperperfusion is common in acute pediatric brain injury.
- Perfusion imaging has the potential to detect physiological changes not detected by other sequences and may therefore aid in early diagnosis and management of many disorders.
- ASL and DSC have unique challenges in pediatric patients and different pathologies than adults that must be taken into account for accurate quantification and interpretation.

Introduction

The MR perfusion techniques of dynamic susceptibility contrast (DSC; see Chapter 2) imaging and arterial spin labeling (ASL; see Chapter 3) imaging as applied to children will be discussed. While DSC perfusion is well established in the evaluation of adult neurological conditions, the use of both DSC and ASL perfusion imaging in pediatric neurological conditions remains in its infancy. While acute stroke imaging drove the adoption of DSC approaches in adults, the lack of demonstrated utility in children, the need for intravenous (IV) line placement, and the need for bolus injection has limited its adoption in children. While some groups extrapolate both DSC and ASL approaches and analysis from the adult literature in applying MR perfusion to pediatric disorders, there is still much unknown about pediatric cerebral perfusion and the changes that occur in pediatric diseases. For example, there are normal developmental changes in cerebral vasculature and cerebral perfusion as well as marked changes in body size, heart rate, vascular flow velocities, and capillary development which may impact optimization, quantification, and interpretation of both DSC and ASL. In addition, little is known about how these measures are affected by sedation, anesthesia, and hematocrit changes.

The normal changes of cerebral perfusion with age, current and potential uses of MR perfusion imaging in children, and limitations will be discussed in this chapter. For a more detailed discussion on the challenges of ASL quantification in general, we refer the reader to Chapter 3. And while bolus injection of contrast is required for DSC imaging to obtain relative cerebral blood flow (rCBF) and relative cerebral blood volume (CBV), ASL uses water as endogenous label and cerebral perfusion values in ml/100 g/min may be obtained.

Perfusion imaging of pediatric brain diseases

Perfusion imaging of normal development

While there is no longitudinal information on the normal evolution of DSC and ASL perfusion in pediatric patients, an understanding of the expected findings can be extrapolated from the literature, as the evolution of cerebral perfusion with age has been studied since the 1950s utilizing a number of different tools, including various nuclear medicine studies as well as computed tomography (CT) perfusion methods [1–5].

Using CT perfusion, it was demonstrated that increased perfusion in the gray matter compared with white matter occurred as early as 7 days of life [6]. Additionally, there is an age-related change in global cerebral perfusion such that cerebral perfusion at

Clinical Perfusion MRI: Techniques and Applications, ed. Peter B. Barker, Xavier Golay, and Greg Zaharchuk. Published by Cambridge University Press. © Peter B. Barker, Xavier Golay, and Greg Zaharchuk 2013.

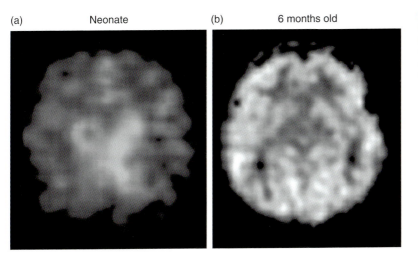

(a) Neonate (b) 6 months old

Figure 16.1 Normal development. (a) Neonatal pseudo-continuous ASL (pCASL) image shows marked regional variability with low cortical perfusion, compared with (b) a 6-month-old child where there is more uniform perfusion.

birth and in the early months of life is low, approximately 40 ml/100 g/min, increasing to a global peak of 130 ml/100 g/min at 2–4 years of life, and then declining to approximately 50 ml/100 g/min by 7–8 years of life, with regional variations (Figure 16.1). There may also be a second smaller global peak around puberty (12 years of age). Regional changes in cerebral glucose metabolism with age measured with ^{18}F-fluorodeoxyglucose (FDG)-positron emission tomography (PET) have also been previously described [7]. A recent ASL study [8] demonstrated similar perfusion patterns, with a peak around puberty in most brain areas, demonstrating a strong correlation with adjusted gray matter density.

Given that regional perfusion changes longitudinally in time in a similar order as the maturation of white matter, with areas of primary cortex maturing prior to association cortex, perfusion may reflect ongoing neuronal development, possibly related to known phenomena such as postnatal angiogenesis, polyneuronal innervations, and/or elective synaptic stabilization [4, 6]. As such, perfusion imaging, in particular ASL, provides a potential window into early brain development, which has been difficult to study fully due to radiation exposure that accompanies CT and PET studies. And indeed, the ASL study of Taki *et al.* [8] provided evidence for an ordered maturation of cortical areas, with low order association cortices maturing first, prior to higher association ones, assessed in over 200 young subjects.

One of the greatest difficulties in interpreting MR perfusion in pediatric patients is that there are few data as to how sedation or general anesthesia may alter perfusion parameters, either directly through vascular effects or indirectly through effects on neuronal metabolism [9, 10]. This, of course, is especially important given that many pediatric patients require sedation or anesthesia in order to be imaged. In nonsedated cases the impact of sleep state or video watching has also not been established. Further study into the influence of these factors is needed to provide reliable quantitative information on cerebral perfusion. Also with ASL, there are many additional issues that affect perfusion quantification, such as age-related changes in blood and parenchymal T_1 and arterial transit time (see Chapter 3). Finally, DSC also provides its own set of challenges for quantification of cortical rCBV and rCBF, given the prominence of cortical veins in infancy.

Perfusion imaging of pediatric brain injury

Ideally, ASL should be applied in the evaluation of acute pediatric brain injury as part of the routine protocol, given the non-invasive nature of the technique [11]. In neonatal brain injury, ASL has been used in the assessment of patients with global arterial ischemic injury or hypoxic ischemic injury (HII). Prior to therapeutic hypothermia becoming standard of care, HII, either profound (Figure 16.2) or partial (Figure 16.3), demonstrated increased perfusion in regions of decreased diffusion, with a larger territory of hyperperfusion compared with the area demonstrating slow diffusion [12]. This suggests that hyperperfusion accompanies the excitotoxic cascade that leads to secondary energy failure and

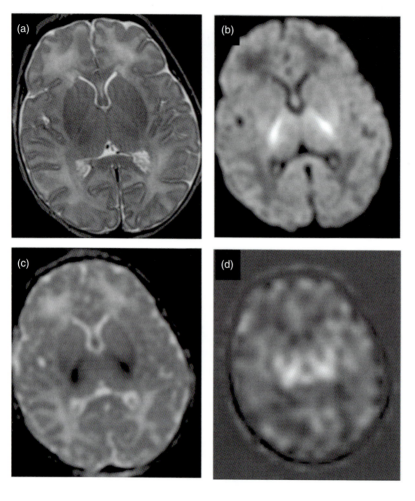

Figure 16.2 Profound hypoxic ischemic injury. Neonate born via Cesarean section after concerns of bradycardia on fetal cardiac monitoring, with Apgars of 2 at 1 min and 3 at 5 and 10 min. (a) Axial T_2-weighted MRI is normal in appearance, without evidence of edema. (b) Diffusion-weighted imaging (DWI) and corresponding (c) apparent diffusion coefficient (ADC) map demonstrate marked decreased diffusion in the ventrolateral portion of the thalamus and posterior limb of the internal capsule and to a lesser degree in the lateral putamen, consistent with profound hypoxic ischemic injury. (d) ASL image demonstrates corresponding hyperperfusion in similar regions.

results in increasing brain injury in these patients. Hypothermia treatment for HII patients is likely successful in part because it decreases metabolic demand and perhaps secondarily decreases cerebral perfusion; thereby decreasing delayed cell death and improving outcomes.

ASL imaging prior to treatment may serve as a biomarker of the severity and mechanisms of cell death by determining the presence and severity of hyperperfusion. In turn, hyperperfusion indicates reperfusion and restoration of oxygen and glucose supply, providing conditions which may delay cell death. More marked hyperperfusion that does not respond to hypothermia may portend a worse prognosis or metabolic etiology that does not respond to hypothermia. Thus ASL could potentially serve as a mechanism to evaluate the success of treatment, although it will be years before full outcome studies are available.

Neonatal focal arterial ischemic strokes are more variable in their presentation, with many areas of decreased diffusion having corresponding hyperperfusion or normal perfusion on ASL while fewer in our experience have hypoperfusion (Figures 16.4 and 16.5). ASL findings may help predict outcome, with hypoperfusion more likely to evolve to pan-necrosis. Few studies on DSC in neonates are available but in our experience, with DSC, the venous subarachnoid vessels dominate the reconstructed perfusion images, making it difficult to assess cortical perfusion (Figure 16.6).

Similar hyperperfusion may be seen in the early stages after cardiorespiratory arrest in older children as in neonatal profound HII (Figure 16.7). In such cases, hyperperfusion often portends delayed cell death and progression of the injury over the first week [13].

ASL may be equally useful in focal arterial ischemic stroke in older children as in neonates. In one series, the larger the lesion, the more likely hypoperfusion

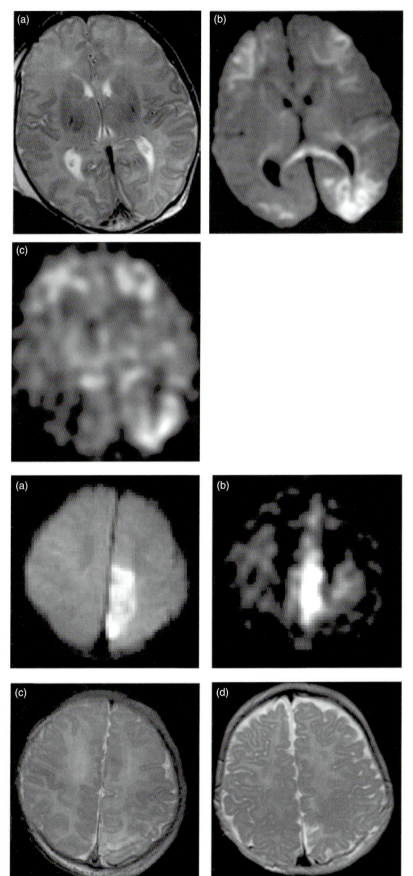

Figure 16.3 Partial hypoxic ischemic injury. A 41-week gestational age 3860-g neonate imaged at 22 hrs due to seizure activity at 8 hrs of life. Delivered by Cesarean section for failure to progress after scheduled induction. Apgars 9 at 5 and 10 min. (a) Axial T$_2$-weighted MRI shows patchy areas of loss of gray–white differentiation. On (b) axial DWI these areas and additional regions are bright due to decreased diffusion (ADC map not shown). (c) Hyperperfusion is associated with most regions of decreased diffusion on axial pCASL.

Figure 16.4 Neonatal stroke with hyperperfusion. (a) Axial DWI, (b) pCASL, and (c) T$_2$-weighted MRI in a neonate presenting with focal seizures. Note hyperperfusion associated with the anterior cerebral artery territory infarct. (d) Follow-up T$_2$ turbo spin echo (TSE) shows mild volume loss and gliosis with less injury than expected based on the DWI, possibly due to reperfusion.

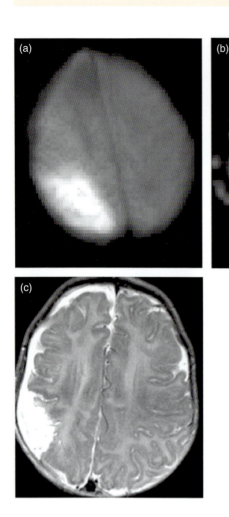

Figure 16.5 Neonatal stroke with hypoperfusion. In a neonate presenting with focal seizures, (a) motion-degraded DWI shows decreased diffusion in the posterior right middle cerebral artery distribution. (b) Corresponding slice on the axial pCASL shows hypoperfusion. (c) Cystic encephalomalacia is present on follow-up studies, likely due to the lack of reperfusion.

is seen, with corresponding larger volumes of infarcted tissue on follow-up [14]. On occasion, hypoperfusion may be observed centrally with hyperperfusion at the margin. This appearance is different than that typically observed in adult populations, where there tends to be predominantly hypoperfusion observed on ASL with increased transit time on DSC imaging [15, 16]. This suggests that the cascade of injury and/or the ability to develop collateral vessels may be different in pediatric than in adult patients, and that the diffusion-perfusion mismatch (core-penumbra) model often used in adults (see Chapter 8) may not be applicable in the pediatric population. Thus, ASL may help predict clinical outcome, identify treatment options for different patients, and possibly serve as a biomarker for following these injuries. This may be particularly true given that ASL seems to be more sensitive to hyperperfusion than DSC [17].

Other disease processes that can lead to infarction, including vasculopathies (Moyamoya, congenital absence or stenosis of the intracranial circulation, as well as vasculitis or HIV) and sickle cell disease, may also benefit from perfusion imaging in conjunction with diffusion-weighted imaging (DWI). Before an infarct occurs, perfusion imaging might be able to predict which patients are at risk for progression to clinical or subclinical infarcts and may help in treatment decisions [18, 19]. In the setting of an acute infarct, ASL perfusion imaging may help dichotomize patients into treatment categories based on cortical perfusion instead of more proximal vascular occlusion. However, in disorders that result in delayed arrival, caution should be used, since apparent decreases in rCBF maps may in fact be due to delays in arrival alone. In these situations, multiphase ASL or velocity-selective ASL (VS-ASL) may help in determining the true CBF (see Chapter 3).

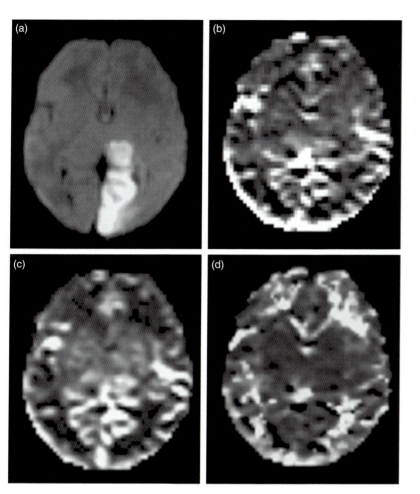

Figure 16.6. Neonatal stroke DSC. In a neonate presenting with focal seizures (a) axial DWI readily detects acute arterial ischemic stroke but (b) rCBV, (c) rCBF, and (d) mean transit time (MTT) maps are difficult to interpret as venous contrast appears to dominate.

Perfusion imaging is likely to provide additional complementary information in both accidental [20] and abusive head trauma. We have observed decreased ASL perfusion in association with high lactate and decreased diffusion in a child that did not survive abusive head trauma (Figure 16.8). In contrast, in a child with a skull fracture and multiple rib fractures, diffuse cerebral hyperperfusion was noted in the absence of any abnormality on routine imaging, including diffusion tensor imaging (DTI) (Figure 16.9). This suggests that ASL perfusion has the potential to detect physiological changes that may be of clinical relevance in the absence of other imaging abnormalities. Although there are no data that we could find in the literature on cerebral perfusion in accidental pediatric brain trauma, decreases in cerebral perfusion are thought to occur with concussion in the context of increased glucose consumption resulting in a state of energy deprivation [21]. ASL combined with magnetic resonance spectroscopy (MRS) may be well suited to evaluate this situation. In particular, if there is a "second impact syndrome" [22] in either abusive or accidental trauma, ASL perfusion imaging with MRS may be useful in detecting persistent physiological derangements that place the individual at higher risk for severe injury if another impact occurs.

Perfusion imaging in pediatric epilepsy

The evaluation of intractable epilepsy for possible surgical resection requires a multi-modality approach, incorporating high-resolution anatomical MRI, PET, ictal and inter-ictal single-photon emission computed tomography (SPECT), and, in some

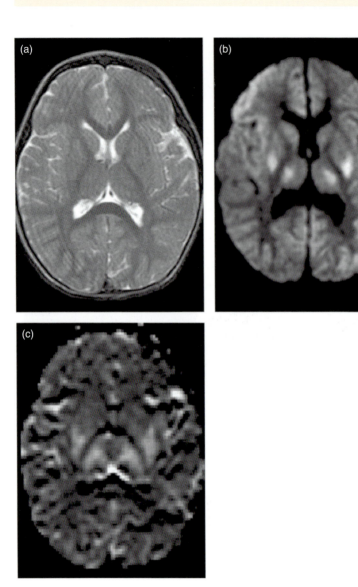

Figure 16.7 A 2-year-old child who choked on a candy. EMS arrived 30 min later and found the child in cardiorespiratory arrest. An MRI was obtained 18 hrs after the incident. (a) T_2-weighted images show no signal abnormality. (b) DWI shows decreased diffusion in the posterior putamen and in the ventrolateral thalamus. DSC was performed and (c) the rCBF maps showed increased rCBF in a slightly larger region than the regions of decreased diffusion. The injury evolved to diffuse cerebral necrosis and cerebral swelling, resulting in the child's demise.

centers, magnetoencephalography (MEG). SPECT imaging in epilepsy evaluation is based on assessment of the perfusion of the underlying epileptogenic substrate, which often has a decreased metabolic rate and CBF in the inter-ictal phase, and increased metabolic activity and blood flow in the ictal phase (Figure 16.10).

ASL provides a non-invasive method to assess the regional perfusion of the brain, which is easily co-registrable with anatomical MRI. As such, it is an easy addition to a standard seizure protocol that may provide additional benefit in the pre-surgical evaluation of patients. The main disadvantage of the technique is that patients rarely have concurrent electroencephalography (EEG) monitoring, thereby preventing assessment of ictal versus inter-ictal timing of imaging. Despite this, ASL is showing potential to aid in the localization of epileptogenic foci (Figure 16.10) [23, 24]. Anecdotally, we have also observed that ASL may be useful in the assessment of response to antiepileptic therapy, detecting transient perfusion changes that were associated with transient hemispheric EEG abnormalities and cognitive impairment (Figure 16.11).

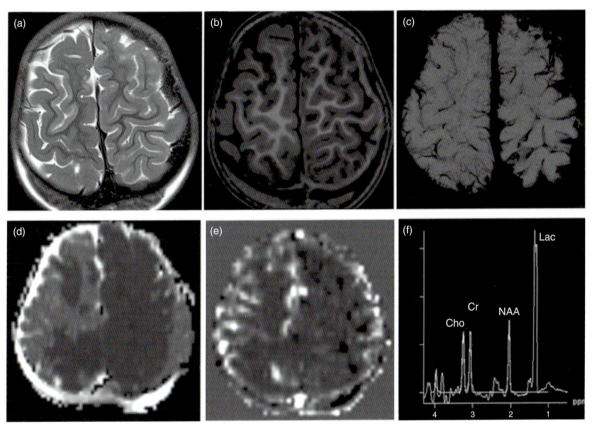

Figure 16.8 Abusive head trauma. Cortical edema is seen as increased cortical (a) T_2 and decreased cortical (b) T_1 signal. (c) Susceptibility-weighted image (SWI) shows subarachnoid venous prominence. (d) Low ADC is present throughout much of the brain with corresponding decreased (e) perfusion on ASL and increased (f) lactate (Lac) on MR spectroscopy. Lack of perfusion in regions of low ADC and a high lactate peak suggests irreversible pan-necrosis. The child did not survive.

Perfusion imaging in metabolic disorders

Although there are few reports of perfusion imaging in metabolic disorders, the ability to assess cerebral perfusion using ASL and in conjunction with information regarding metabolites in the brain obtained with MRS may be extremely helpful in better understanding these disorders. For example in mitochondrial disorders, identifying metabolic failure (high lactate) in the presence of perfusion could help to detect mitochondrial failure, as opposed to failure of oxygen delivery to the tissue (Figure 16.12).

Perfusion imaging in congenital heart disease

There has been great interest in assessing brain abnormalities in patients with congenital heart disease (CHD), as impaired neurodevelopment represents a major morbidity for patients successfully treated for cardiac disease. Periventricular leukomalacia (PVL) may occur in as many as 50% of all patients with CHD [25]. Inherent with the underlying pathology of the different forms of CHD, pulmonary-systemic shunts result in diminished CBF and perfusion.

ASL provides a non-invasive measurement of cerebral perfusion in patients, with measurements able to be made several times in response to a physiological challenge such as increased inspired carbon dioxide (CO_2, a potent cerebral arteriolar vasodilator and pulmonary arteriolar vasoconstrictor) in order to assess the physiological perfusion reserve [18, 26]. One study demonstrated that the mean cerebral perfusion in patients with CHD was below normal, and that patients who subsequently developed PVL were more likely to have a decreased baseline cerebral perfusion and CO_2 reactivity [27]. Thus, ASL may prove an important adjunct tool in the evaluation of

333

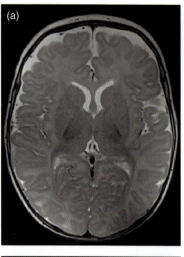

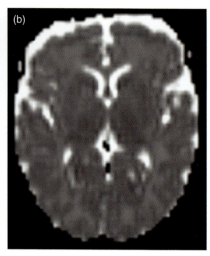

Figure 16.9 Abusive head trauma. Apart from small extra-axial fluid collections, the (a) T_2 TSE and (b) ADC map were normal. (c) Color-coded pCASL showed a marked increase in cerebral perfusion compared with an age-matched control (71 vs. 27 ml/100 g/min) in this child with an acute skull fracture and multiple rib fractures. The presence of perfusion abnormalities in the absence of any abnormality on conventional imaging suggests a central role for ASL in the evaluation of suspected or known acute brain injury.

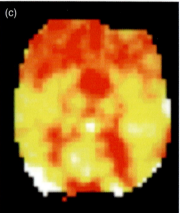

patients with CHD. One potential confounding factor is the role of changes in hematocrit and blood oxygenation that may accompany CHD and affect the ASL experiment by altering the blood T_1 values.

Perfusion imaging in developmental brain disorders

Although there are no data currently available, the fact that cerebral perfusion on ASL is correlated with FDG-PET glucose metabolism suggests that developmental brain disorders associated with altered regional cerebral metabolism may also show quantitative differences on ASL studies. However to detect such differences, high-quality studies will be required as well as extensive data in normal subjects, as the magnitude of the regional differences in perfusion in developmental disorders are likely to be less than those seen in major cerebral injury.

Perfusion imaging of pediatric brain tumors

Most research in perfusion imaging in pediatric neoplasms has been performed utilizing DSC, although ASL has a potential role in the future, as recent literature on adult brain tumors have begun to show the utility of this technique [28, 29]. ASL may play a complementary role to DSC, given that microvasculature characteristics of brain tumors are likely to have different characteristics on ASL compared to DSC, with ASL being insensitive to permeability effects and capillary blood volume, but providing information on capillary perfusion.

In adults, perfusion imaging has three main uses: (1) preoperative tumor grading, (2) guiding brain biopsies, and (3) differentiating between residual/recurrent neoplasm and post-treatment/radiation effects. Additionally, it remains to be seen whether perfusion imaging either by itself or in conjunction with other

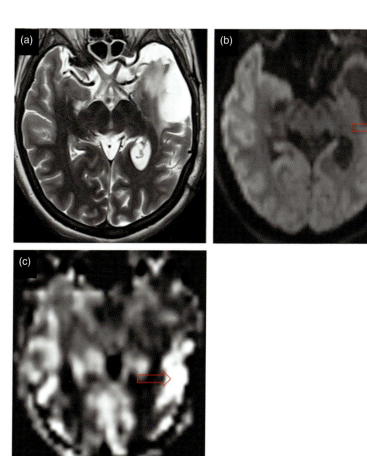

Figure 16.10 Status epilepticus. (a) Axial T_2 TSE, (b) axial DWI, and (c) axial pCASL in a 16-year-old girl with status epilepticus after prior left anterior temporal lobe resection show a focal area of decreased diffusion posterior to the resection cavity, as well as a much larger region of hyperperfusion in the temporal lobe (red arrows) in a region that correlated with regions of seizure activity on intraoperative grid placement.

MR techniques such as spectroscopy and DWI may serve as an effective biomarker to predict tumor response [30, 31]. Due to the different tumor biology in pediatric brain tumors, enhancement does not correlate with tumor grade. In fact grade I tumors such as pilocytic astrocytomas, dysembryoplasic neuroepithelial tumor, gangliogliomas, hemangioblastomas, and choroid plexus papillomas all enhance, whereas highgrade tumors such as atypical teratoid rhabdoid tumors (ATRT) and primitive neuroectodermal tumors (PNET) have heterogeneous enhancement, and highgrade diffuse infiltrating brainstem gliomas typically do not enhance. Therefore, caution should be used in pediatric tumor perfusion imaging as high rCBV, high rCBF, and increased leakage does not always correlate with high grade and vice versa (see Case Study 16.1 for an example of a PNET enhancing lesion).

Increased rCBV, rCBF, and ASL perfusion reflect increased vascular blood volume due to angiogenesis, whereas increased K^{trans} indicates breakdown in the blood–brain barrier (see Chapters 1, 4, and 11). Recently rCBV and K^{trans} have been correlated with tumor grade when studying adult glial tumors [32] but such correlations may not hold for all types of pediatric brain tumors due to different underlying biology. Further studies are needed in all types of pediatric brain tumors to develop general guidelines.

Juvenile pilocytic astrocytomas (JPAs) are a common neoplasm in pediatric patients. CBV can be relatively low with minimal leakage in the presence of enhancement (Figure 16.13). A recent study suggests that those with higher baseline rCBV values have a higher risk for early local recurrence or malignant transformation [33].

Resection and/or biopsy is the gold standard by which treatment decisions are made; but in those patients who are unable to have a resection, perfusion imaging may be able to help guide biopsy placement

335

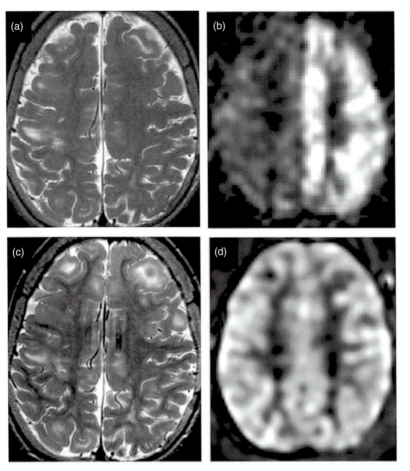

Figure 16.11 Reversible ASL changes. Child with tuberous sclerosis complex presenting with right hemispheric slowing on EEG and cognitive impairment. Initial (a) T_2 TSE and (b) pCASL show multiple tubers and hemispheric hypoperfusion (44 ml/100 g/min) with contralateral hyperperfusion (101 ml/100 g/min). (C) Follow-up imaging 5 years later after change in antiepileptic medication and improvement in cognitive status shows (d) symmetric cerebral perfusion (65 ml/100 g/min).

to potentially decrease the chance of a sampling error downgrading the tumor grade. Perfusion imaging can also serve as an additional parameter to monitor for tumor progression (Figure 16.14).

As in adults, once surgery, radiation, and/or chemotherapy have occurred, post-contrast enhancement surrounding the resection margin may be related either to treatment effects or tumor recurrence. Distinguishing between these two possibilities is vital in treatment decisions. Recurrent tumor will continue to have angiogenesis with breakdown in the blood–brain barrier, resulting in increased perfusion, while radiation necrosis results in vascular injury and ischemia, and thus is usually associated with hypoperfusion [34, 35]. Thus, perfusion imaging can be helpful in distinguishing between tumor recurrence and radiation-induced changes. However, if anti-angiogenesis agents (such as bevacizumab) are used

in the treatment of pediatric neoplasms, this can potentially confound the assessment of residual/recurrent tumor, given that the medication itself can decrease tumor vascularity. In the absence of an anti-angiogenic agent, perfusion imaging may be helpful in assessing treatment response (Figure 16.14).

As described above, JPAs are the most common pediatric neoplasm, and given angiogenesis, may have increased perfusion and signal recovery of greater than 70% [36]. Other tumors that also demonstrate increased perfusion include ependymomas and low-grade oligodendrogliomas. Medulloblastomas and PNETs demonstrate increased perfusion and variable capillary leakage (Figure 16.14, Case Study 16.1).

In order to accurately estimate CBV, a correction must be made to account for the capillary leakage (cCBV). However, care must be taken to not use cCBV measurements when there is no capillary

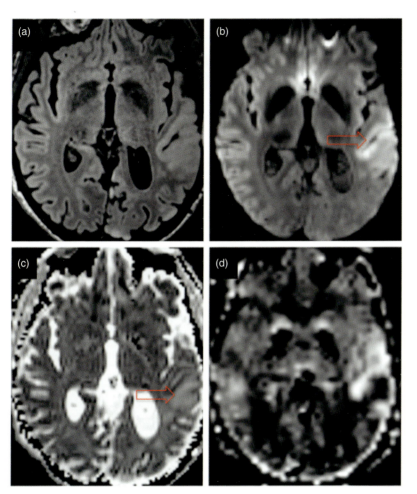

Figure 16.12 ASL in mitochondrial encephalopathy with lactic acidosis and stroke-like episodes (MELAS). (a) Cortical edema and swelling is present on the FLAIR images in the left temporal and parietal lobes. (b) On DWI the cortex is bright (red arrow) but (c) on the ADC map the cortex is isointense with normal brain, and subcortical white matter shows vasogenic edema (red arrow). (d) Pulsed ASL (PASL) CBF map shows increased cortical perfusion. Single voxel MRS (not shown) detected a large lactate peak.

leakage, since some of the correction algorithms may produce erroneous results in these cases. This may be relevant for some pediatric tumors (as in Case Study 16.1).

Brainstem gliomas represent another category of neoplasms where the lack of increased perfusion does not correlate with prognosis; most brainstem gliomas do not demonstrate enhancement or increased perfusion, and while the biological behavior of these tumors is heterogeneous, they generally are associated with greater morbidity/mortality. However, in a study on diffuse intrinsic pontine gliomas (DIPG), those with increased rCBV and rCBF on DSC at presentation had shorter survival times [37].

Finally, perfusion imaging may also be helpful in differentiating extra-axial neoplasms [38] as well as detecting recurrence after resection. While

meningiomas and choroid plexus papillomas demonstrate markedly increased perfusion, other extra-axial masses such as dural-based metastases and schwannomas do not. Thus, there may be a role for perfusion imaging in the evaluation of all intracranial masses.

Protocols and techniques in pediatric perfusion imaging

Both DSC and ASL imaging can be used in the evaluation of pediatric patients [39]. As with adult patients, both have advantages and disadvantages, which are discussed below. In addition, each modality presents particular challenges in the pediatric population, due both to the unique properties of the pediatric brain, and the different pathologies that are encountered.

337

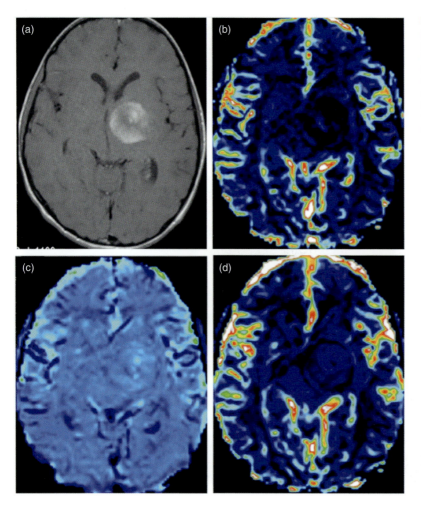

Figure 16.13 DSC in supratentorial pilocytic astrocytoma. A partially enhancing lesion on (a) T_1-weighted MRI is centered in the left thalamus. (b) The rCBV map is decreased in the lesion and (c) only minimal leakage is seen on the K2 map. (d) The leakage-corrected rCBV shows only mildly elevated rCBV. No vascular proliferation was noted on histology.

Dynamic susceptibility-weighted contrast-enhanced MRI

DSC uses the paramagnetic properties of a contrast agent as it transits through the cerebrovasculature to develop relative assessments of the CBV and mean transit time (MTT), and from which rCBF can be calculated (see Chapters 1 and 4). These measurements remain, however, relative due to multiple difficulties associated with the paramagnetic contrast agent, such as its lack of a linear relationship between MRI signal and concentration, or the uncertainties related to the choice and positioning of arterial input functions (for CBF).

For a well-defined contrast agent bolus, DSC-MRI is best performed using a power injector. However, this provides particular challenges in the pediatric

population. Gadolinium-based agents are typically administered at 0.1 mmol/kg of body weight (except for gadobutrol, which is administered at 0.05 mmol/kg). Because of the smaller caliber of the veins in children, IV catheters are typically smaller (although catheters should not be less than 24 gauge) than those used in adults, and thus, the rate of injection must be adjusted to a rate appropriate for the catheter size (not to exceed catheter manufacturer recommendations), typically 3–4 ml/s. However, in children under 2 years of age, power injection is often not feasible. In these cases, a hand injection can be done, but image quality and reproducibility may be significantly degraded. Additionally, it is important to ensure that baseline imaging prior to contrast administration is obtained as part of the perfusion acquisition. Finally, in younger pediatric patients who are imaged while

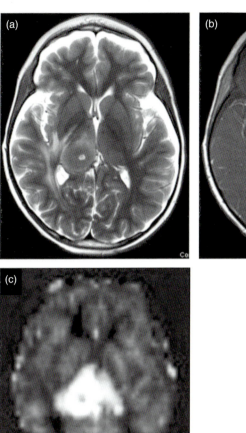

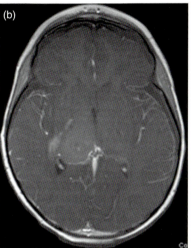

Figure 16.14 ASL in progressive PNET. A 3-year-old male diagnosed with right thalamic PNET, who developed worsening ataxia after radiation and chemotherapy. (a) Axial T_2-weighted and (b) post-contrast T_1-weighted imaging detect the right thalamic lesion with involvement of the adjacent white matter, but (c) PASL imaging better detects progression to the contralateral thalamus.

sedated/anesthetized, patients cannot respond when extravasation occurs. Thus, it is even more important to verify good flow through the IV catheter prior to contrast administration, as well as to monitor the patient's vital signs and the images to insure proper IV administration. Finally, contrast agents are not US Food and Drug Administration (FDA)-approved in children less than 2 years old and therefore if contrast is not strongly clinically indicated it is difficult to justify its use for perfusion purposes alone, even in the context of off-label utilization.

Because of the smaller size of the child, image optimization for pediatric patients is needed to maximize image quality. Compared to the adult brain, the smaller size of the pediatric head would benefit from a reduction in slice thickness from 5 mm typically used in adults to 3–4 mm with no gap, while maintaining the same number of slices (although older children could be scanned with parameters similar to those used in adults). However, signal-to-noise ratio (SNR) considerations often prevent decreasing the slice thickness in pediatric patients.

While both gradient-echo (GRE)- and spin-echo (SE)-based sequences can be utilized for DSC imaging, given the higher SNR of GRE and the need for double contrast dosage for better SNR with SE, most institutions have adopted GRE-based sequences for perfusion imaging. However, as this sequence is sensitive to magnetic susceptibility effects, lesions that have short T_2^* relaxation times are difficult to evaluate. Thus hemorrhage, calcium, metal, air, and bone can significantly degrade image quality in adjacent

339

tissue. This is especially relevant for lesions in the posterior fossa (particularly relevant in pediatric tumor imaging), but is also important for lesions at the skull base and near the paranasal sinuses or mastoid air cells. Susceptibility artifact can be partially reduced by using parallel imaging techniques (see Chapter 2) and decreasing slice thickness, although this may decrease SNR and also lead to incomplete coverage of the brain, depending on the number of slices used. DSC measures relative (rather than absolute) CBV, which prevents quantitative assessment. Finally, when a lesion results in a breakdown of the blood–brain barrier, this results in leakage of contrast material into the lesion from the capillary bed, and thus susceptibility related to the degree of leakage of contrast material rather than strictly related to perfusion. This can be overcome either by correcting for the amount of leakage by calculating K^{trans} and providing a cCBV or by pre-saturating the signal in the tissue by giving a portion of the contrast dose (0.05 mmol/kg) approximately 5 min prior to the power injection and subsequent perfusion imaging.

Arterial spin labeling

ASL is a non-invasive method for measuring CBF which uses magnetically labeled arterial blood water as an endogenous tracer, rather than gadolinium. The technical challenges of ASL in pediatric patients result from fundamental differences between pediatric and adult populations relative to the imaging parameters: differences in tissue T_1 relaxivity affecting both the label and control image, differences in transit time and capillary structure, differences in blood T_1, and finally differences in coverage of tissue included in the labeling band for pulsed ASL (PASL) techniques. As such, pseudo-continuous ASL (pCASL) techniques, as used in the images of this chapter, are better suited for pediatric populations in general.

Because ASL is based on a label that decays with the T_1 relaxation times of blood and tissue, it is important to consider the consequences of differences in T_1 relaxation times in the pediatric population compared with adults. The T_1 relaxation in gray matter (GM) and white matter (WM) is much higher in neonates (GM: 1140–1500 ms; WM: 1700–2300 ms) versus children (GM: 850–1150 ms; WM 650–650 ms) and adults (GM: 800–1100 ms; WM: 600–800 ms) [40, 41]. This is due to the high water and low lipid content of the pediatric brain, with T_1

decreasing as myelination progresses. This results in higher signal intensity in children relative to adults, and thus increased SNR, and offers a distinct advantage of using ASL in the pediatric population [42]. Additionally, the T_1 relaxation time of blood in children compared with adults is also higher, likely related to a lower hematocrit [42]. Also, at certain ages, children have increased cerebral perfusion compared with adults, and in ASL, this results in greater SNR. Additionally, because peak flow velocity is increased in children compared with adults, there is a decrease in transit time. For ASL, this results in less decay of signal between the labeling plane and the imaging plane, and thus further increases SNR [18].

Because of these differences between pediatric and adult brains, ASL calculations using an adult perfusion model may often overestimate the cerebral perfusion in pediatric populations. While the increased T_1 relaxation times in children may result in an overestimation of cerebral perfusion if an adult T_1 is assumed, an increase in the blood–brain partition coefficient may result in underestimation of cerebral perfusion[43]; these two assumptions may therefore balance each other out, and might result by chance in a close approximation of quantified cerebral perfusion, likely within 5–10% of its true value [42]. However, the quantified cerebral perfusion obtained via ASL is probably most inaccurate when the value is either very low or high.

This inaccuracy may be exacerbated in pathological states, including acute brain injury when perfusion may be very high and CHD when perfusion may be very low. Wang *et al.* [26] demonstrated that adjusting the traditional PASL sequence using a more restricted labeling volume produced more accurate CBF measurements in neonates with CHD, where systemic-pulmonary circulation hemodynamic shunts combined with a larger labeling volume resulted in increased spurious (negative) values.

Many of the parameters that help improve signal in adults (discussed in other sections) will have equivalent benefits in pediatric populations, including the use of pCASL versus PASL labeling as well as the use of higher magnetic field strengths (3 T versus 1.5 T). While both pCASL and increased magnetic field strength result in increased specific absorption rates (SAR) secondary to radiofrequency power deposition, which in children is further exacerbated by the smaller body size, optimization of imaging parameters allows safe imaging in children [18].

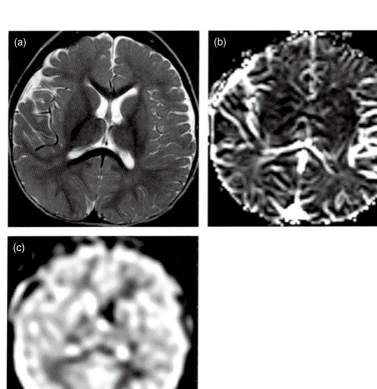

Figure 16.15 (a) Axial T$_2$-weighted MRI, (b) DSC, and (c) pCASL perfusion images in an 18-month-old infant with normal cerebral perfusion. DSC and ASL perfusion images have very different appearances, suggesting that DSC CBF is more sensitive to venous blood volume in the sulci, and ASL perfusion is more arterial/cortical in nature.

DSC versus ASL

While DSC is faster (typically less than 2 min versus about 5 min for ASL) and provides a larger SNR between the base and labeled images (20–50% change in signal in DSC versus 1–5% in ASL), it is invasive, requiring a catheter-based power injection and gadolinium administration. Therefore, particularly in infants, this technique can be difficult to perform. In contrast, non-invasive ASL is very appealing, especially in infants. Additionally, while DSC produces rCBF, rCBV, MTT, and time-to-peak (TTP) maps, it is a non-quantitative technique, whereas ASL provides absolute values and measures cerebral perfusion (although see above for discussion regarding limitations in quantifying measurements).

DSC and ASL also likely measure different aspects of perfusion imaging. Because DSC is based on assessing changes in susceptibility related to contrast infusion, GRE-based DSC is dependent on vascular diameter, and therefore will be weighted towards the venous component of perfusion imaging [44], whereas ASL depends on vascular inflow and therefore is weighted towards the arterial and capillary phase of perfusion [45–47]. In pediatric patients, this difference is particularly prominent (Figure 16.15). In our experience, this has led to hyperperfusion abnormalities detected in pediatric patients with ASL when comparison DSC perfusion images did not demonstrate any abnormality. Also given the large venous blood volume in infants, we suspect that ASL provides more accurate cortical perfusion measures, whereas DSC values may be more related to the subarachnoid venous compartment.

Assessment of permeability

Dynamic contrast-enhanced (DCE) T$_1$-weighted imaging represents another perfusion imaging technique, which is beginning to be used in pediatric patients for the evaluation of brain tumors. DCE allows for a better estimation of permeability, using the T$_1$ properties of the contrast agent (see Chapter 4). DCE-based permeability imaging evaluates capillary leakiness in brain tissue by calculating changes in concentration of the contrast agent to estimate the endothelial permeability surface area product or transfer coefficient, K^{trans}. As the estimation of capillary leakiness depends on models of vascular surface area and flow, permeability imaging represents an estimation of vascular density and angiogenic activity. This may be helpful in the evaluation of primary and recurrent neoplasms, especially those in the posterior fossa [48, 49]. An additional benefit in children is that this technique does not require a power injector since bolus injection of contrast does not need to be as rapid as in DSC-MRI.

Conclusion

MR perfusion imaging is a useful adjunct tool in the evaluation of pediatric neurological disease as it provides important physiological information not garnered by routine anatomical imaging. DSC and DCE have a potential role in the management of pediatric brain tumors. However, it is likely that ASL will begin to play a larger role in pediatric neuroimaging in general, as it provides a more quantitative measure of cerebral perfusion without the need for IV contrast administration.

References

1. Baird HW, Garfunkel JM. A method for the measurement of cerebral blood flow in infants and children. *J Pediatr* 1953;**42**(5): 570–5.

2. Kennedy C, Sokoloff L. An adaptation of the nitrous oxide method to the study of the cerebral circulation in children; normal values for cerebral blood flow and cerebral metabolic rate in childhood. *J Clin Invest* 1957; **36**(7):1130–7.

3. Chiron C, Raynaud C, Mazière B, *et al.* Changes in regional cerebral blood flow during brain maturation in children and adolescents. *J Nucl Med* 1992; **33**(5):696–703.

4. Takahashi T, Shirane R, Sato S, Yoshimoto T. Developmental changes of cerebral blood flow and oxygen metabolism in children. *AJNR Am J Neuroradiol* 1999;**20**(5):917–22.

5. Tokumaru AM, Barkovich AJ, O'uchi T, Matsuo T, Kusano S. The evolution of cerebral blood flow in the developing brain: evaluation with iodine-123 iodoamphetamine SPECT and correlation with MR imaging. *AJNR Am J Neuroradiol* 1999;**20** (5):845–52. Erratum in: *AJNR Am J Neuroradiol* 2000;**21**(5):990.

6. Wintermark M, Lepori D, Cotting J, *et al.* Brain perfusion in children: evolution with age assessed by quantitative perfusion computed tomography. *Pediatrics* 2004;**113**(6):1642–52.

7. Chugani HT, Phelps ME. Maturational changes in cerebral function in infants determined by 18FDG positron emission tomography. *Science* 1986; **231**(4740):840–3.

8. Taki Y, Hashizume H, Sassa Y, Takeuchi H, Wu K, Asano M, Asano K, Fukuda H, Kawashima R. Correlation between gray matter density-adjusted brain perfusion and age using brain MR images of 202 healthy children. *Hum Brain Mapp.* 2011 Nov; **32**(11):1973–85.

9. Harreld J, Kaddoum R, Sansgiri R, *et al.* Impact of sedation on pediatric MR brain perfusion imaging. Presented at the Radiological Society of North America 2011 meeting, Chicago, IL.

10. Todd MM, Weeks J. Comparative effects of propofol, pentobarbital, and isoflurane on cerebral blood flow and blood volume. *J Neurosurg Anesthesiol* 1996; **8**(4):296–303.

11. Pollock JM, Tan H, Kraft RA, *et al.* Arterial spin-labeled MR perfusion imaging: clinical applications. *Magn Reson Imaging Clin N Am* 2009;**17**(2):315–38.

12. Madan N, Pienaar R, Paladino M, Grant PE. Reperfusion in neonates with hypoxic ischemic injury. Presented at the 2011 meeting of the American Society of Neuroradiology, 2011.

13. Grant PE, Yu D. Acute injury to the immature brain with hypoxia with or without hypoperfusion. *Magn Reson Imaging Clin N Am* 2006;**14**(2):271–85.

14. Chen J, Licht DJ, Smith SE, *et al.* Arterial spin labeling perfusion MRI in pediatric arterial ischemic stroke: initial experiences. *J Magn Reson Imaging* 2009;**29**(2):282–90.

15. Chalela JA, Alsop DC, Gonzalez-Atavales JB, *et al.* Magnetic resonance perfusion imaging in acute ischemic stroke using continuous arterial spin labeling. *Stroke* 2000;**31**(3):680–7.

16. Wolf RL, Alsop DC, McGarvey ML, *et al.* Susceptibility contrast and arterial spin labeled perfusion MRI in cerebrovascular disease. *J Neuroimaging* 2003;**13**(1):17–27.

17. Wang DJJ, Alger JR, Qiao JX, *et al.* The value of arterial spin-labeled perfusion imaging in acute ischemic stroke: comparison with dynamic susceptibility contrast-enhanced MRI. *Stroke* 2012;**43**(4): 1018–24. Epub 2012/02/09.

18. Oguz KK, Golay X, Pizzini FB, *et al.* Sickle cell disease: continuous arterial spin-labeling perfusion MR imaging in children. *Radiology* 2003;**227**(2): 567–74.

19. Wang J, Licht DJ. Pediatric perfusion MR imaging using arterial spin labeling. *Neuroimaging Clin N Am* 2006; **16**(1):149–67.

20. Ashwal S, Schneider S, Tomasi L, Thompson J. Prognostic implications of hyperglycemia and reduced cerebral blood flow in childhood near-drowning. *Neurology* 1990;**40**(5):820–3.

21. Giza CC, Hovda DA. The neurometabolic cascade of concussion. *J Athl Train* 2001; **36**(3):228–35.

22. Cantu RC, Gean AD. Second-impact syndrome and a small subdural hematoma: an uncommon catastrophic result of repetitive head injury with a characteristic imaging appearance. *J Neurotrauma* 2010;**27**(9):1557–64.

23. Madan N, Grant PE. New directions in clinical imaging of cortical dysplasias. *Epilepsia* 2009;**50** Suppl 9:9–18.

24. Wolf RL, Alsop DC, Levy-Reis I, *et al.* Detection of mesial temporal lobe hypoperfusion in patients with temporal lobe epilepsy by use of arterial spin labeled perfusion MR imaging. *AJNR Am J Neuroradiol* 2001;**22**(7):1334–41.

25. Galli KK, Zimmerman RA, Jarvik GP, *et al.* Periventricular leukomalacia is common after neonatal cardiac surgery. *J Thorac Cardiovasc Surg* 2004;**127**(3): 692–704. Erratum in: *J Thorac Cardiovasc Surg* 2004;**128**(3):498.

26. Wang J, Licht DJ, Silvestre DW, Detre JA. Why perfusion in neonates with congenital heart defects is negative–technical issues related to pulsed arterial spin labeling. *Magn Reson Imaging* 2006;**24**(3):249–54.

27. Licht DJ, Wang J, Silvestre DW, *et al.* Preoperative cerebral blood flow is diminished in neonates with severe congenital heart defects. *J Thorac Cardiovasc Surg* 2004;**128**(6):841–9.

28. Warmuth C, Gunther M, Zimmer C. Quantification of blood flow in brain tumors: comparison of arterial spin labeling and dynamic susceptibility-weighted contrast-enhanced MR imaging. *Radiology* 2003;**228**(2):523–32.

29. Wolf RL, Wang J, Wang S, *et al.* Grading of CNS neoplasms using continuous arterial spin labeled perfusion MR imaging at 3 Tesla. *J Magn Reson Imaging* 2005; **22**(4):475–82.

30. Tzika AA, Astrakas LG, Zarifi MK, *et al.* Multiparametric MR assessment of pediatric brain tumors. *Neuroradiology* 2003; **45**(1):1–10.

31. Tzika AA, Astrakas LG, Zarifi MK, *et al.* Spectroscopic and perfusion magnetic resonance imaging predictors of progression in pediatric brain tumors. *Cancer* 2004;**100**(6):1246–56.

32. Server A, Graff BA, Orheim TED, *et al.* Measurements of diagnostic examination performance and correlation analysis using microvascular leakage, cerebral blood volume, and blood flow derived from 3T dynamic susceptibility-weighted contrast-enhanced perfusion MR imaging in glial tumor grading. *Neuroradiology* 2011;**53**(6):435–47.

33. Fuss M, Wenz F, Essig M, *et al.* Tumor angiogenesis of low-grade astrocytomas measured by dynamic susceptibility contrast-enhanced MRI (DSC-MRI) is predictive of local tumor control after radiation therapy. *Int J Radiat Oncol Biol Phys* 2001; **51**(2):478–82.

34. Ball WS, Jr., Holland SK. Perfusion imaging in the pediatric patient. *Magn Reson Imaging Clin N Am* 2001;**9**(1):207–30.

35. Poussaint TY, Rodriguez D. Advanced neuroimaging of pediatric brain tumors: MR diffusion, MR perfusion, and MR spectroscopy. *Neuroimaging Clin N Am* 2006;**16**(1):169–92.

36. Cha S. Dynamic susceptibility-weighted contrast-enhanced perfusion MR imaging in pediatric patients. *Neuroimaging Clin N Am* 2006;**16**(1):137–47.

37. Hipp SJ, Steffen-Smith E, Hammoud D, *et al.* Predicting outcome of children with diffuse intrinsic pontine gliomas using multiparametric imaging. *Neuro Oncol* 2011;**13**(8):904–9.

38. Zimny A, Sasiadek M. Contribution of perfusion-weighted magnetic resonance imaging in the differentiation of meningiomas and other extra-axial tumors: case reports and literature review. *J Neurooncol* 2011;**103**(3):777–83.

39. Huisman TA, Sorensen AG. Perfusion-weighted magnetic resonance imaging of the brain: techniques and application in children. *Eur Radiol* 2004; **14**(1):59–72.

40. Jones RA, Palasis S, Grattan-Smith JD. MRI of the neonatal brain: optimization of spin-echo parameters. *AJR Am J Roentgenol* 2004;**182**:367–72.

41. Steen RG, Hunte M, Traipe E, *et al.* Brain T1 in young children with sickle cell disease: evidence of early abnormalities in brain development. *Magn Reson Imaging* 2004;**22**:299–306.

42. Wang J, Licht DJ, Jahng GH, *et al.* Pediatric perfusion imaging using pulsed arterial spin labeling. *J Magn Reson Imaging* 2003; **18**(4):404–13.

43. Herscovitch P, Raichle ME. What is the correct value for the brain–blood partition coefficient for water? *J Cereb Blood Flow Metab* 1985;**5**(1):65–9.

44. Boxerman JL, Hamberg LM, Rosen BR, Weisskoff RM. MR contrast due to intravascular magnetic susceptibility

perturbations. *Magn Reson Med* 1995;**34**(4):555–66.

45. Li K, Zhu X, Hylton N, *et al.* Four-phase single-capillary stepwise model for kinetics in arterial spin labeling MRI. *Magn Reson Med* 2005;**53**(3):511–18.

46. Parkes LM, Tofts PS. Improved accuracy of human cerebral blood perfusion measurements using arterial spin labeling: accounting for capillary water permeability. *Magn Reson Med* 2002;**48**(1):27–41.

47. Ewing JR, Cao Y, Fenstermacher J. Single-coil arterial spin-tagging for estimating cerebral blood flow as viewed from the capillary: relative contributions of intra- and extravascular signal. *Magn Reson Med* 2001;**46**(3):465–75.

48. Gururangan S, Chi SN, Young Poussaint T, *et al.* Lack of efficacy of bevacizumab plus irinotecan in children with recurrent malignant glioma and diffuse brainstem glioma: a Pediatric Brain Tumor Consortium study. *J Clin Oncol* 2010;**28**(18):3069–75.

49. Meyzer C, Dhermain F, Ducreux D, *et al.* A case report of pseudoprogression followed by complete remission after proton-beam irradiation for a low-grade glioma in a teenager: the value of dynamic contrast-enhanced MRI. *Radiat Oncol* 2010;**5**:9.

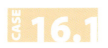
Pediatric primitive neuroectodermal tumor (PNET)

History

Child with new onset seizure.

Technique

Axial post-contrast T_1, DWI, and CBV and K2 maps estimated from DSC-MRI are shown.

Imaging findings

See Figure 16.16.

Discussion

Analysis of pediatric DSC-MRI experiments using parameters more appropriate for adults may result in artifacts in the reconstructed perfusion images, in this case the estimate of leakage "K2." Many pediatric brain tumors do not show enhancement. At pathology, this PNET showed vascular proliferation and a few erythrocytes among the small round blue cell tumor cells.

Key points

- DSC perfusion can be used to assess pediatric brain tumors and provide information on CBV, but care should be taken to use processing parameters appropriate for pediatric studies.
- Apparently negative contrast agent leakage (K2 values) can be generated by post-processing leakage correction schemes when a persistent low signal on T_2^*-weighted images occurs, with no corresponding T_1 effect to increase signal.

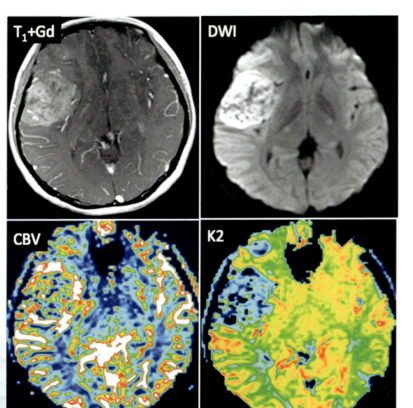

Figure 16.16 An enhancing lesion with decreased diffusion is noted in the right frontal lobe. DSC perfusion shows only slightly increased CBV and apparently negative K2 due to the lack of contrast agent leakage in the tumor.

Bibliography

Setty B, Snuderl M, Ferriera RM, Sagar P, Grant PE. *MR perfusion in pediatric brain tumors.* Presented at the Radiological Society of North America 2007, Chicago, IL, 2007.

Hipp SJ, Steffen-Smith E, Hammoud D, *et al.* Predicting outcome of children with diffuse intrinsic pontine gliomas using multiparametric imaging. *Neuro Oncol* 2011;**13**(8):904–9. Epub 2011/07/13. PMID: 21757444

Multifocal neonatal stroke

History

Neonate with seizure on day 2 after birth.

Technique

Axial T_2, DWI, ADC map, and pCASL CBF images are shown.

Imaging findings

See Figure 16.17.

Discussion

Arterial ischemic infarcts at different stages or with different severity of injury have different imaging appearances. Pan-necrosis is associated with cerebral edema on T_2 and markedly decreased perfusion and markedly decreased ADC. Less severe or earlier-stage injuries may present with no T_2 abnormality, but patchy decreased ADC and increased perfusion. Even milder injuries or earlier injuries present with no T_2 and no ADC abnormality but increased perfusion.

Key points

- Arterial ischemic infarcts have a variable appearance depending on age, severity, and degree of reperfusion.
- ASL perfusion imaging may detect abnormalities when other imaging sequences, including DWI and ADC, are normal.

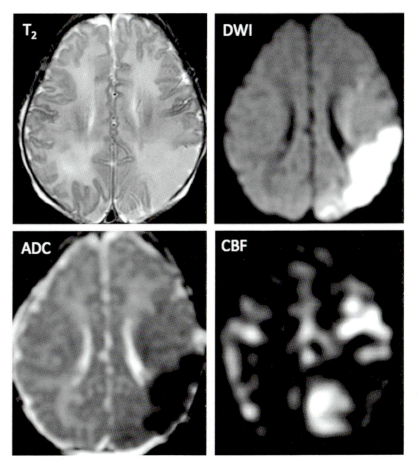

Figure 16.17 T_2-weighted image demonstrates loss of gray–white matter differentiation in the left parietal lobe, with corresponding wedge-shaped area of DWI hyperintensity and decreased diffusion on ADC map, and markedly decreased perfusion on ASL. The adjacent left frontoparietal region anterior to the DWI lesion shows no T_2 abnormality but has patchy decreased ADC and increased perfusion. The right frontoparietal region has no T_2, DWI, or ADC abnormality, but has increased perfusion on pCASL.

Bibliography

Grant PE, Yu D. Acute injury to the immature brain with hypoxia with or without hypoperfusion. *Magn Reson Imaging Clin N Am* 2006; **14**(2):271–85.

Wang DJ, Alger JR, Qiao JX, *et al.*; for the UCLA Stroke Investigators. The value of arterial spin-labeled perfusion imaging in acute ischemic stroke: comparison with dynamic susceptibility contrast-enhanced mRI. *Stroke* 2012:**43**(4):1018–24.

Index